ROBBINS
ESSENTIAL
PATHOLOGY

ROBBINS
ESSENTIAL
PATHOLOGY

Vinay Kumar, MBBS, MD, FRCPath
Alice Hogge and Arthur A. Baer Distinguished Service Professor
Department of Pathology
Biologic Science Division
The Pritzker School of Medicine
The University of Chicago
Chicago, Illinois

Abul K. Abbas, MBBS
Professor and Chairman Emeritus
Department of Pathology
University of California San Francisco
San Francisco, California

Jon C. Aster, MD, PhD
Professor of Pathology
Brigham and Women's Hospital
Harvard Medical School
Boston, Massachusetts

Andrea T. Deyrup, MD, PhD
Associate Professor
Department of Pathology
Duke University Medical Center
Durham, North Carolina

ELSEVIER

1600 John F. Kennedy Blvd.
Ste 1600
Philadelphia, PA 19103-2899

Notice

Practitioners and researchers must always rely on their own experience and knowledge in evaluating and using any information, methods, compounds or experiments described herein. Because of rapid advances in the medical sciences, in particular, independent verification of diagnoses and drug dosages should be made. To the fullest extent of the law, no responsibility is assumed by Elsevier, authors, editors or contributors for any injury and/or damage to persons or property as a matter of products liability, negligence or otherwise, or from any use or operation of any methods, products, instructions, or ideas contained in the material herein.

ISBN: 978-0-323-64025-1

Executive Content Strategist: Jim Merritt
Director, Content Development: Rebecca Gruliow
Publishing Services Manager: Catherine Jackson
Senior Project Manager: Kate Mannix
Design Direction: Brian Salisbury

Printed in India

Last digit is the print number: 9   8   7   6   5   4   3   2

Working together
to grow libraries in
developing countries

www.elsevier.com • www.bookaid.org

We are pleased to present a new member of the Robbins family connected to the roots.

In the preface of the first edition of *Textbook of Pathology–With Clinical Applications* (published in 1957), Stanley Robbins laid down the guiding principles of his new book: *"the subject matter is to be presented in a logical, concise, readable fashion, devoid of distracting detail and with considerable emphasis on relating pathology to clinical medicine."* While these time-honored fundamentals have remained embedded in medical education, two major changes have had an impact on how the discipline is taught now and how students learn it. First, in most medical schools, the basic and clinical sciences are taught in an integrated, organ system-based curriculum that blends basic principles with clinical relevance. Second, because of early clinical exposure, the time devoted to pathology (and other basic sciences) has progressively decreased. *Robbins Essential Pathology* is intended to satisfy the needs of today's medical students by distilling basic concepts of pathogenesis and morphology and providing clinical vignettes to highlight the relevance of pathology to the understanding of disease. To meet these goals, this new addition to the Robbins family consists of three integrated components:

- Nineteen text chapters in which the subject matter is presented in *"logical, concise, readable fashion, devoid of distracting details."* Core material is distilled to the information essential for every medical student, with an emphasis on mechanisms of disease.
- Each chapter is associated with five to six clinical cases that relate *"pathology to clinical medicine."* Cases highlight the scientific foundation of the practice of medicine and underscore the clinical relevance of pathogenic mechanisms. Clinical-pathologic correlations have always been the strength of the Robbins' family of books, and this core philosophy is woven into the fabric of *Robbins Essential Pathology*.

- More than 600 USMLE-style, multiple-choice questions are available to reinforce important concepts in the chapters and cases and to aid in board preparation. We hope that the organ system-based cases, linked to both the text and the questions, will facilitate an organic assimilation of critical information necessary for integrated curricula.

An all-electronic format enables interactive integration of text, cases and questions to promote active learning. The cases challenge the student to apply what has been learned from text and classwork. In effect, these are tutorials that allow students to learn at their own pace at a time and place of their choosing. Hot-spotting of gross and histologic features brings an expert pathologist to the student's side. Such interactivity is possible only in an electronic format. In addition, an extensive library of images (Supplemental eFigures) from the Robbins photo collection facilitates visual learning styles and augments the key images in the text.

Although the text is available in print form, the cases, questions, and expanded image collection are offered only in the interactive electronic form. We strongly encourage the readers to take advantage of the three components of *Essential Pathology*.

We hope that we have succeeded in providing a book that has adapted to the modern teaching of pathology. We welcome, and indeed appreciate, comments and feedback from students and their instructors. Partnership between authors and the readers is essential for excellence in education.

Vinay Kumar
Abul K. Abbas
Jon C. Aster
Andrea T. Deyrup

ACKNOWLEDGMENTS

Writing a new book is a significant effort. We have undertaken this task in response to numerous colleagues who asked for a short, clinically oriented textbook for integrated curricula in which pathology is not a standalone course

Several individuals provided us the impetus to develop this book. They are too numerous to mention individually but principal among them are Dr. Raga Ramachandran, UCSF, and Dr. Scott Lovitch, BWH. Jim Merritt, our editor at Elsevier, championed this book so that it could see the light of the day.

We are grateful to those who advised us on the content of individual chapters. They include Dr. Tony Chang, University of Chicago (kidney), Dr. Ryan Gill, UCSF (liver), and Dr. Marta Margeta, UCSF (nervous system). Several individuals at Duke University School of Medicine advised in the development of the clinical cases. They include Dr. Anna Lisa Crowley (cardiac), Dr. E. Wayne Massey (neurology), and Dr. John K. Roberts (kidney). Many of our colleagues provided us with images from their collections. These gems have been acknowledged where the images have been used in the book.

Some of the multiple-choice questions were originally published in *Robbins Review of Pathology* by Vinay Kumar and Ed Klatt, whom we wish to acknowledge.

The book developed as we wrote it from content to design. Several people at Elsevier worked tirelessly and patiently with us on the production of this text. Special mention should be made of Executive Content Strategist Jim Merritt; Director, Content Development Rebecca Gruliow; Senior Project Manager Kate Mannix; Designer Brian Salisbury; and Senior Manager Ebooks and Clinical Key Paul Dever.

Last but not least, we owe a deep debt of gratitude to our families: Raminder Kumar, Ann Abbas, Erin Malone, and Tony Williamson. Without their unwavering support, we could not have added one more book to the several with which we are already involved. Andrea T. Deyrup wishes to acknowledge the enduring mentorship and support of the late Dr Tony Montag (1954–2018). Finally, we wish to acknowledge each other for complementing and indeed enhancing our individual contributions.

Vinay Kumar
Abul K. Abbas
Jon C. Aster
Andrea T. Deyrup

To our students, who continually inspire and challenge us.

CONTENTS

1 Cell Injury and Cell Death, 1

2 Inflammation and Repair, 14

3 Hemodynamic Disorders, Thromboembolism, and Shock, 30

4 Diseases of the Immune System, 41

5 Neoplasia, 63

6 Genetic Diseases, 88

7 Diseases of Blood Vessels, 105

8 Heart, 118

9 Hematopoietic and Lymphoid Systems, 137

10 Lung and Upper Respiratory Tract, 163

11 Kidney, 186

12 Gastrointestinal System, 205

13 Liver, Biliary System, and Pancreas, 222

14 Male Genital Tract, Prostate, and Bladder, 240

15 Female Genital Tract and Breast, 250

16 Endocrine System, 264

17 Disorders of the Nervous System, 280

18 Musculoskeletal System and Skin, 296

19 Environmental Disease, 314

Index, 327

Cell Injury and Cell Death

OUTLINE

Overview of Cell Injury, 1
    Causes of Cell Injury, 1
Reversible Cell Injury, 1
Cell Death, 2
    Necrosis, 3
    Apoptosis, 3
    Other Pathways of Cell Death, 6
Mechanisms of Cell Injury and Death, 7

Oxidative Stress, 7
Hypoxia and Ischemia, 8
Toxin-Mediated Cell Injury, 9
Endoplasmic Reticulum (ER) Stress, 9
DNA Damage, 9
Cellular Aging, 9
Cellular Adaptations to Stress, 11
Pathologic Accumulations in Cells, 12

In medieval times, diseases were attributed to "evil humors," "miasma," and other equally nebulous and unprovable causes. One of the most fundamental advances in human biology and medicine was the realization that the cell is the structural and functional unit of living organisms and abnormalities in cells underlie all diseases: Individuals are sick because their cells are sick. All diseases share the common feature that they alter cellular function and structure. Therefore, the foundation of pathology and medicine is an understanding of how cells are injured, the theme of this first chapter.

OVERVIEW OF CELL INJURY

In response to stress, cells may adapt, may be injured reversibly and recover, or may be irreversibly damaged and die.

Cells normally maintain a steady state, called *homeostasis,* despite being constantly exposed to countless potentially damaging agents. Cells deal with external or internal stresses by undergoing changes that are grouped into three broad categories.

- *Adaptations* are alterations that enable cells to cope with stresses without damage, such as increased muscle mass in response to increased workload. The major cellular adaptations and their physiologic and pathologic significance are summarized at the end of the chapter.
- *Reversible injury* refers to structural and functional abnormalities that can be corrected if the injurious agent is removed. If the injury is persistent or severe, it can become irreversible and lead to cell death. In many cases, cells die without traversing a detectable reversible phase.
- *Cell death* is the end result of injury. As we discuss later, there are two major pathways of cell death, necrosis and apoptosis, and they occur upon exposure to a variety of injurious agents.

Causes of Cell Injury

Diverse insults cause cell injury or death and result in disease.
These injurious insults include:

- *Infectious pathogens,* which injure cells by producing toxins, interfering with critical cellular functions, or by stimulating immune responses that damage infected cells in the course of trying to eradicate the infection
- *Hypoxia* (reduced oxygen supply) and *ischemia* (reduced blood supply), which are caused by blockage of arteries or loss of blood; both deprive tissues of oxygen and, in the case of ischemia, cells are also denied essential nutrients and toxic metabolites are allowed to build up

- *Toxins,* which abound in the environment, as well as some *therapeutic drugs*
- *Environmental insults,* such as physical trauma, radiation exposure, and nutritional imbalances
- *Genetic abnormalities,* including mutations that impair the function of various essential proteins and other mutations that lead to the accumulation of damaged DNA or abnormal, misfolded proteins, both of which cause cell death if they cannot be repaired or corrected
- *Immunologic reactions* against self antigens (as in autoimmune diseases) or environmental antigens (as in allergies), which cause cell injury, often by triggering inflammation
- *Aging,* a form of slow, progressive cell injury

REVERSIBLE CELL INJURY

Reversible injury is characterized by functional and structural changes in cells that are not permanent.

The earliest changes associated with cell injury mostly affect cytoplasmic structures but do not damage nuclei (nuclear damage is usually irreversible) and include the following:

- *Swelling of cells* as a result of influx of water. This is usually caused by failure of the adenosine triphosphate (ATP)-dependent Na^+-K^+ plasma membrane pump due to decreased generation of ATP or plasma membrane damage. The loss of intracellular K^+ and compensatory influx of Na^+ brings water with it to maintain osmotic balance, resulting in plasma membrane alterations, including blebbing, loss of microvilli and swelling of mitochondria and the endoplasmic reticulum (ER) (Fig. 1.1). The histologic changes are subtle, but organs may appear grossly swollen and pale (due to compression of capillaries).
- *Fatty change.* In organs that are actively involved in metabolism (e.g., liver, heart), toxic injury disrupts metabolic pathways and leads to rapid accumulation of triglyceride-filled lipid vacuoles.
- *Eosinophilia.* The cytoplasm of injured cells appears eosinophilic (red in hematoxylin-and-eosin [H&E] stains) because of loss of

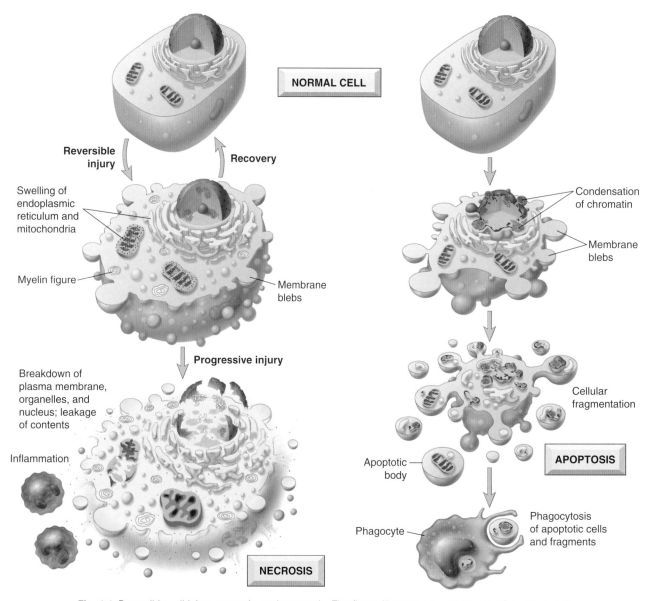

Fig. 1.1 Reversible cell injury, necrosis, and apoptosis. The figure illustrates the sequence of events in cell injury that culminate in necrosis or apoptosis. Myelin figures are collections of phospholipids in concentric layers released from damaged plasma membranes. In cells undergoing necrosis, mitochondria often contain amorphous densities visible by electron microscopy, of unknown significance.

RNA, which binds the blue hematoxylin stain. The eosinophilia becomes more pronounced with progression toward necrosis.

- *"Myelin figures"* composed of phospholipids derived from damaged cellular *membranes* appear in the cytosol.
- The *mitochondria* may swell.
- The *ER* may become dilated, with detachment of ribosomes and dissociation of polysomes, halting protein synthesis.
- *Nuclear chromatin* may clump.
- These alterations become more severe if the injury progresses to the irreversible phase of necrosis, culminating in loss of plasma membrane integrity and breakdown of the nucleus.

With persistent or excessive noxious exposures, injured cells pass a nebulous "point of no return" and undergo cell death. Although there are no definitive morphologic or biochemical correlates of irreversibility, it is consistently characterized by three phenomena: the *inability to restore mitochondrial function* (oxidative phosphorylation and ATP generation) even after resolution of the original injury; *altered structure and function of the plasma membrane and intracellular membranes*; and *DNA damage and loss of chromatin structural integrity*.

CELL DEATH

Necrosis and apoptosis, the two main forms of cell death, differ in causes, mechanisms, and functional consequences.

Necrosis and apoptosis are usually distinct forms of cell death, with different morphologic changes and other distinguishing features (Table 1.1). Necrosis may be thought of as "accidental" cell death, reflecting severe injury that irreparably damages so many cellular components that the cells simply "fall apart". When cells die by necrosis, there is a local inflammatory response that clears the scene of the "accident." By contrast, apoptosis is "regulated" cell death, because it is mediated by defined molecular

Table 1.1 Features of Necrosis and Apoptosis

Feature	Necrosis	Apoptosis
Cell size	Enlarged (swelling)	Reduced (shrinkage)
Nucleus	Pyknosis → karyorrhexis → karyolysis	Fragmentation into nucleosome-sized fragments
Plasma membrane	Disrupted	Intact; altered structure, especially orientation of lipids
Cellular contents	Enzymatic digestion; may leak out of cell	Intact; may be released in apoptotic bodies
Adjacent inflammation	Frequent	No
Physiologic or pathologic role	Invariably pathologic (culmination of irreversible cell injury)	Often physiologic means of eliminating unwanted cells; may be pathologic after some forms of cell injury, especially DNA and protein damage

pathways that are activated under specific circumstances and kill cells with surgical precision, without inflammation or the associated collateral damage. In some situations, cell death may show features of both necrosis and apoptosis, or may start with apoptosis and progress to necrosis, so the distinctions may not be as absolute as once thought. Nevertheless, it is useful to consider the two forms as largely nonoverlapping pathways of cell death because their principal mechanisms and functional consequences are usually different.

Necrosis

Necrosis is the result of severe injury and is a pathologic process in which cells spill their contents into the extracellular milieu, causing local inflammation.

The hallmarks of necrosis are:
- *Dissolution of cellular membranes,* including the plasma membrane and lysosomal membranes, because of damage to membrane lipids and activity of phospholipases
- *Leakage of lysosomal enzymes* that digest the cell
- *Local inflammation* in response to the released contents of dead cells. Some specific components of these contents have been called damage-associated molecular patterns (DAMPs). These released factors include ATP (from damaged mitochondria), uric acid (a breakdown product of DNA), and numerous other molecules that are normally contained within healthy cells and whose release indicates severe cell injury. These molecules are recognized by receptors expressed by macrophages and most other cell types, and trigger phagocytosis of the debris, as well as the production of cytokines that induce inflammation (see Chapter 2). Inflammatory cells produce more proteolytic enzymes that exacerbate the damage and the subsequent reaction, until the necrotic tissue has been cleared.

The main causes of necrosis include ischemia, exposure to microbial toxins, burns and other forms of chemical and physical injury, and unusual situations in which enzymes leak out of cells and injure adjacent tissues (as in pancreatitis). All these initiating triggers lead to irreparable damage to numerous cellular components, which culminate in membrane damage, the basis for the subsequent steps in necrosis.

Morphology. Necrotic cells show more diffuse cytoplasmic eosinophilia compared with that seen in reversible injury (Fig. 1.2). Nuclei undergo sequential changes, from condensation of chromatin (*pyknosis*) to fragmentation of nuclei *(karyorrhexis)* to their complete dissolution *(karyolysis).*

Necrosis from different causes is manifested by different morphologies, and recognition of these patterns is helpful for determining the underlying etiology:
- In *coagulative necrosis,* the underlying tissue architecture is preserved, at least for some time, even though the constituent

cells are dead (Fig. 1.3). This form of necrosis is characteristic of hypoxia-induced cell death, caused most commonly by a loss of blood supply (ischemia). The resultant necrosis, called *infarction,* is seen in most solid organs, such as the heart and kidneys.
- In *liquefactive necrosis,* the dead cells are digested by released enzymes (Fig. 1.4). This is seen in necrosis resulting from bacterial and fungal infections and in ischemic infarcts of the brain (even if sterile).
- *Gangrenous necrosis* is a clinical term used for the death of soft tissue and is often applied to a limb that has lost its blood supply and has undergone coagulative necrosis involving multiple tissue layers. It results from ischemia (e.g., from diabetic vascular disease, affecting the lower limbs) and is called *dry gangrene* if the dead tissue remains intact or *wet gangrene* if the tissue liquefies, as is common following superimposed bacterial infection.
- *Caseous necrosis* is characteristic of tuberculosis and some fungal infections such as histoplasmosis. The dead tissue breaks down, creating a cheesy consistency on gross examination (Fig. 1.5). Microscopically, the necrotic focus is a collection of fragmented or lysed cells with an amorphous granular pink (eosinophilic) appearance. Cellular outlines cannot be discerned, and there is often a peripheral collection of macrophages forming a *granuloma.*
- *Fat necrosis* refers to focal areas of fat destruction, typically resulting from the release of activated pancreatic lipases into the substance of the pancreas and the peritoneal cavity. This occurs in acute pancreatitis (Chapter 13). Fatty acids are released and combine with calcium to produce grossly visible chalky white areas (fat saponification), which enable the surgeon and the pathologist to identify the lesions (Supplemental eFig. 1.1). On histologic examination, the foci of necrosis contain shadowy outlines of necrotic fat cells surrounded by basophilic calcium deposits and an inflammatory reaction.
- *Fibrinoid necrosis* is a characteristic microscopic finding seen most commonly in immune reactions in which complexes of antigens and antibodies and extravasated plasma proteins are deposited in the walls of blood vessels, where they have a bright pink, amorphous appearance reminiscent of fibrin (Fig. 1.6).

The laboratory diagnosis of necrosis may be made by detecting an increase in serum levels of intracellular proteins, which leak out of the necrotic cells because of membrane damage. This is the basis of measuring serum troponin for diagnosis of myocardial infarction, transaminases for liver disease, and pancreatic enzymes such as amylase for pancreatitis.

Apoptosis

Apoptosis is a form of cellular suicide that eliminates cells that are no longer needed or are damaged beyond repair, without eliciting a potentially harmful inflammatory response.

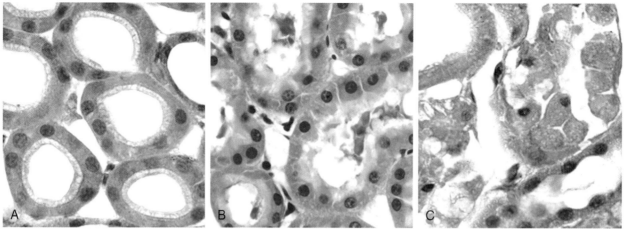

Fig. 1.2 Morphologic changes in reversible and irreversible cell injury (necrosis). (A) Normal kidney tubules with viable epithelial cells. (B) Early (reversible) ischemic injury showing surface blebs, increased eosinophilia of cytoplasm, and swelling of occasional cells. (C) Necrotic (irreversible) injury of epithelial cells, with loss of nuclei and fragmentation of cells and leakage of contents. (Courtesy of Drs. Neal Pinckard and M.A. Venkatachalam, University of Texas Health Sciences Center, San Antonio.)

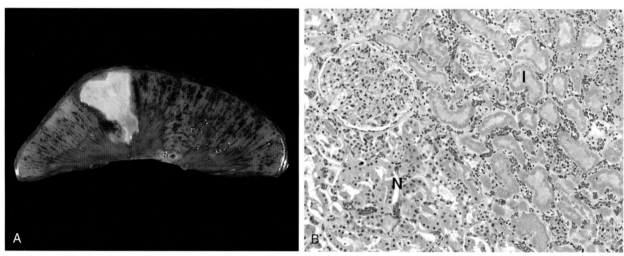

Fig. 1.3 Coagulative necrosis. (A) A wedge-shaped kidney infarct *(yellow)*. (B) Microscopic view of the edge of the infarct, with normal kidney *(N)* and necrotic cells in the infarct *(I)*. The necrotic cells show preserved outlines with loss of nuclei, and an inflammatory infiltrate (dark nuclei interspersed between necrotic tubules) is present.

In this pathway of cell death, enzymes activated by specific signals dismantle the nucleus and cytoplasm, generating fragments that are recognized and rapidly cleared by phagocytes.

Causes of Apoptosis

Apoptosis occurs in many physiologic situations and serves to eliminate potentially harmful cells and cells that have outlived their usefulness (Table 1.2). It also occurs as a pathologic event when cells are damaged, especially when the damage affects the cell's DNA or proteins; thus, the irreparably damaged cell is eliminated.

- *Physiologic apoptosis*
  - Death of cells during the development of organisms, such as cells of primordial tissues that are replaced by mature tissues
  - Death of leukocytes (neutrophils and lymphocytes) after inflammatory and immune responses have eliminated offending agents
  - Elimination of dysfunctional or autoreactive lymphocytes or lymphocyte precursors, particularly in the bone marrow and the thymus

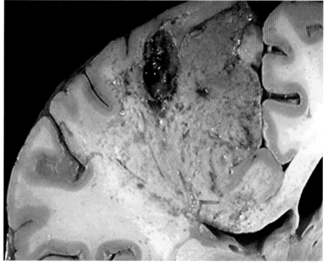

Fig. 1.4 Liquefactive necrosis. An infarct in the brain showing dissolution of the tissue.

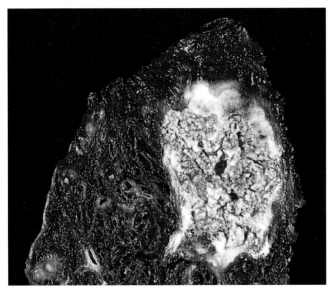

Fig. 1.5 Caseous necrosis. Tuberculosis of the lung, with a large area of caseous necrosis containing yellow-white (cheesy) debris.

Table 1.2 Physiologic and Pathologic Conditions Associated With Apoptosis

Condition	Mechanism of apoptosis
Physiologic	
During embryogenesis	Loss of growth factor signaling (presumed mechanism)
Turnover of proliferative tissues (e.g., lymphocytes in bone marrow and thymus)	Absence of survival signals or activation of death-inducing signals
Involution of hormone-dependent tissues (e.g., endometrium)	Decreased hormone levels lead to reduced survival signals
Decline of leukocyte numbers at the end of immune and inflammatory responses	Loss of survival signals as stimulus for leukocyte activation is eliminated
Elimination of potentially harmful self-reactive lymphocytes	Strong recognition of self antigens induces apoptosis by both the mitochondrial and death receptor pathways
Pathologic	
DNA damage	Activation of proapoptotic proteins
Accumulation of misfolded proteins	Activation of proapoptotic proteins, possibly direct activation of caspases
Infections, especially certain viral infections	Activation of the mitochondrial pathway by viral proteins Killing of infected cells by cytotoxic T lymphocytes, which activate caspases

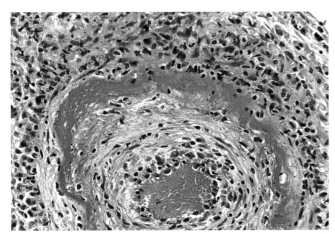

Fig. 1.6 Fibrinoid necrosis in an artery in a patient with polyarteritis nodosa. The wall of the artery shows a circumferential bright pink area of necrosis with protein deposition and inflammation.

- Cell loss that alternates with cell proliferation in hormone-responsive tissues such as the endometrium
- Elimination of lymphocytes that recognize self antigens
- *Pathologic apoptosis*
    - Severe DNA damage, after exposure to radiation or cytotoxic drugs
    - Accumulation of misfolded proteins, giving rise to ER stress
    - Certain infectious agents, particularly some viruses such as hepatitis B and C, which trigger immune responses that destroy infected cells.

Mechanisms of Apoptosis

There are two pathways of apoptosis, the mitochondrial (or intrinsic) pathway and the death receptor (or extrinsic) pathway, which differ in their initiation and molecular signals (Fig. 1.7).

The biochemical pathways of apoptosis control the balance of death- and survival-inducing signals and ultimately the activation of enzymes called *caspases*. Caspases are cysteine proteases that cleave

proteins after aspartic acid residues. The end result of apoptotic cell death is the clearance of apoptotic bodies by phagocytes.

- *The mitochondrial (intrinsic) pathway* seems to be responsible for apoptosis in most physiologic and pathologic situations. Molecular sensors in the cytoplasm detect the lack of survival signals, DNA damage, or the accumulation of misfolded proteins. These activated sensors induce the dimerization of two proteins (called BAX and BAK) that insert into the mitochondrial membrane and form channels, leading to increased mitochondrial permeability. The channels allow proapoptotic factors (i.e., cytochrome c and other proteins) to leak into the cytosol, where they activate the enzyme caspase-9. A cascade of additional caspases is activated, culminating in the enzymatic breakdown of nuclei and cytoplasmic structures. Fragments of nuclei and other organelles such as mitochondria are extruded into fragments (called apoptotic bodies) that are subsequently phagocytosed. Because cellular membranes remain intact, enzymes and other cell contents do not leak out (as they do in necrosis), and there is no inflammation. The dimerization of the effector molecules BAX and BAK is normally prevented by antiapoptotic molecules of the BCL family, notably BCL-2 and BCL-x. These are activated by growth factors, which is one way that growth factors promote cell survival and subsequent proliferation. Constitutive activation of BCL-2 by genetic aberrations is seen in tumors; in fact, BCL-2 stands for B cell lymphoma-2, so named for the tumor in which it was discovered as an oncogene (see Chapter 5).
- *The death receptor (extrinsic) pathway of apoptosis.* Death receptors are plasma membrane receptors of the tumor necrosis factor (TNF)

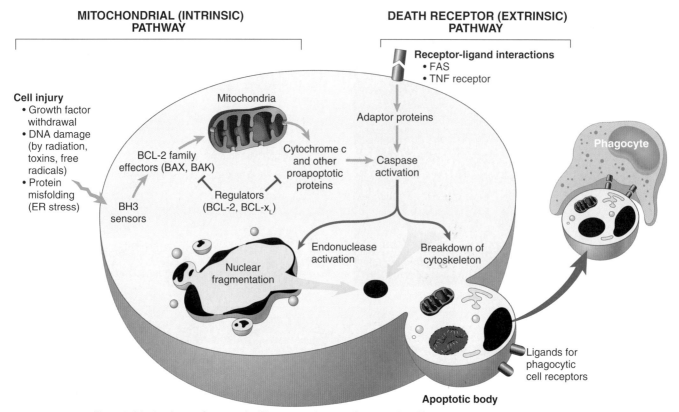

Fig. 1.7 Mechanisms of apoptosis. The two pathways of apoptosis differ in their induction and regulation, and both culminate in the activation of caspases. In the mitochondrial pathway, BH3-only proteins, which are related to members of the BCL-2 family, sense a lack of survival signals or DNA or protein damage. These BH3-only proteins activate effector molecules that increase mitochondrial permeability. In concert with a deficiency of BCL-2 and other proteins that maintain mitochondrial permeability, the mitochondria become leaky and various substances, such as cytochrome c, enter the cytosol and activate caspases. Activated caspases induce the changes that culminate in cell death and fragmentation. In the death receptor pathway, signals from plasma membrane receptors lead to the assembly of adaptor proteins into a "death-inducing signaling complex," which activates caspases, and the end result is the same. *ER,* Endoplasmic reticulum; *TNF,* tumor necrosis factor.

receptor family found on many cells. These receptors have a conserved cytoplasmic "death domain" that mediates interaction with other proteins involved in cell death. The prototypic death receptors are the type I TNF receptor and FAS (CD95). FAS ligand (FASL) is a membrane protein expressed mainly on activated T lymphocytes. When these T cells recognize FAS-expressing targets, FAS molecules are cross-linked by FASL and bind adaptor proteins via the death domain. These then recruit and activate caspase-8, which, in turn, activates downstream caspases. The death receptor pathway is involved in the elimination of self-reactive lymphocytes and in the killing of target cells by some cytotoxic T lymphocytes that express FASL

- *Clearance of apoptotic fragments.* When cells undergo apoptosis, they begin to express a number of molecules that are recognized by receptors on phagocytes. Phagocytes ingest and destroy the fragments of apoptotic cells, often within minutes, before the cells undergo membrane damage and release their contents. The phagocytosis of apoptotic cells is so efficient that dead cells disappear without leaving a trace, and inflammation is virtually absent.

The morphologic appearance of apoptotic cells is distinctive and different from necrosis. In H&E-stained sections, the nuclei appear pyknotic, because of the condensation of chromatin, and the cells are shrunken, appearing to lie in vacuoles (Fig. 1.8). However, apoptotic

cells are removed so quickly and efficiently that they are often not identified in histologic specimens, even in tissues in which many cells are dying by apoptosis.

Other Pathways of Cell Death

Although necrosis and apoptosis are the best-defined pathways of cell death, several other mechanisms have also been described recently. Their importance in human diseases remains a topic of investigation, but students should be aware of their names and unique features.

- *Necroptosis* is induced by activation of specific kinases in response to the cytokine tumor necrosis factor (TNF), which is produced as part of the host response to microbes and other irritants. Signals from these kinases lead to plasma membrane injury, as in necrosis, but the process is regulated by specific molecules, like apoptosis, so it is considered to have features of both.
- *Pyroptosis* is a form of cell death induced by bacterial toxins in which the dying cell releases cytokines, such as interleukin-1, that induce local inflammation and fever (hence *pyro* in the name).
- *Autophagy* is a form of "self-eating" (Greek, *phagia* = to eat) in which cells starved of nutrients digest their own organelles and recycle the material to provide energy for survival. In this process, organelles and portions of the cytosol are enclosed within vacuoles, which fuse with lysosomes, and the contents are destroyed by lysosomal

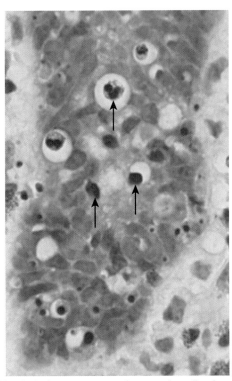

Fig. 1.8 Morphologic appearance of apoptotic cells. Apoptotic cells (some indicated by *arrows*) in a crypt in the colonic epithelium are shown. (The preparative regimen for colonoscopy frequently induces apoptosis in epithelial cells, which explains the abundance of dead cells in this normal tissue.) Note the fragmented nuclei with condensed chromatin and the shrunken cell bodies, some with pieces falling off of them. (Courtesy of Dr. Sanjay Kakar, Department of Pathology, University of California San Francisco.)

enzymes. If the process continues because the nutrient deficiency is not corrected, it can trigger apoptosis by the mitochondrial pathway.

MECHANISMS OF CELL INJURY AND DEATH

The degree of injury from any injurious stimulus varies depending on the type of the offending agent, its severity, and its duration, as well as the adaptive ability and genetic makeup of the target cell.

Small amounts of a toxin or brief periods of ischemia may cause reversible injury but larger doses of the toxin or more prolonged ischemia may cause necrosis. Striated muscle in the leg survives ischemia for 2 to 3 hours, whereas cardiac muscle, with its higher metabolic needs, dies after 20 to 30 minutes of ischemia. The genetic makeup of the individual may also determine the reaction to injurious agents. Polymorphisms in genes encoding members of the cytochrome P450 family affect the rate of metabolism of many chemicals and hence the effects of toxins. One of the goals of precision medicine is to use genetics to predict how individuals will react to different types of injurious stimuli.

Cell injury results from abnormalities in one or more essential cellular components, mainly mitochondria, membranes, and the nucleus (Fig. 1.9).

The consequences of impairment of each of these cellular organelles are distinct but overlapping.

- *Mitochondria* are the sites where ATP, the primary carrier of energy in cells, is produced by oxidative phosphorylation. Injury due to hypoxia, ischemia, radiation, or other insults impairs oxidative phosphorylation, leading to the formation of reactive oxygen species (ROS) (see

later) and decreased ATP production. Mitochondria also sequester molecules, such as cytochrome c, whose release into the cytosol is an indicator of damage and, as described earlier, a trigger for apoptosis.
- *Cellular membranes* are composed of lipids and contain protein and carbohydrate molecules. They maintain the structure of cells and organelles and serve numerous critical transport functions such as fluid and ion homeostasis. Damage to lysosomal membranes, by ROS or other agents, leads to release of enzymes that digest the injured cell, the hallmark of necrosis. Damage to the plasma membrane results in loss of cellular constituents, the end result of necrosis.
- *Nuclei* store most of the cell's genetic material. Nuclear damage disrupts transcription-dependent cellular functions (i.e., protein synthesis), as well as cell proliferation. Irreparable damage to DNA triggers apoptosis.
- *Other cellular components* that suffer damage upon exposure to various injurious agents include the ER (one site of protein synthesis and post-translation processing) and the cytoskeleton (the structural scaffold and "motor" of cells).
- In addition to cell injury resulting from impairment of these intrinsic structures, cells may be damaged from the outside, for example, by the products of leukocytes during inflammatory reactions.

Oxidative Stress

Oxidative stress refers to cellular abnormalities that are induced by ROS, which belong to a group of molecules called free radicals.

Free radicals are highly reactive molecules with an unpaired electron in an outer orbit. They react with all inorganic and organic molecules (e.g., proteins, lipids, and nucleic acids) and remove electrons from other molecules, converting them into free radicals. Biologically important free radicals include ROS and nitric oxide (Fig. 1.10).

- *ROS are produced normally in small amounts in all cells during the reduction–oxidation (redox) reactions* that occur during mitochondrial respiration and energy generation. In this process, molecular oxygen is reduced in mitochondria to generate water by the sequential addition of four electrons. This reaction is imperfect, however, and small amounts of highly reactive but short-lived toxic intermediates are generated when oxygen is only partially reduced. These intermediates include superoxide $O_2^{\cdot-}$, which is converted to hydrogen peroxide (H_2O_2) spontaneously and by the action of the enzyme superoxide dismutase. H_2O_2 is more stable than $O_2^{\cdot-}$ and can cross biologic membranes. In the presence of metals, such as Fe^{2+}, H_2O_2 is converted to the highly reactive hydroxyl radical by the Fenton reaction. The generation of free radicals is increased by exposure to UV light, radiation and toxins, and during normal cellular aging, all of which may impair mitochondrial functions. Oxygen deprivation also leads to ROS production because of incomplete reduction of oxygen.
- *ROS are produced in phagocytic leukocytes, mainly neutrophils and macrophages,* to destroy ingested microbes and other substances during inflammation. In the "respiratory" or "oxidative" burst, following ingestion of a microbe, a phagosome membrane enzyme catalyzes the generation of $O_2^{\cdot-}$, which is converted to H_2O_2. H_2O_2 is in turn converted to a highly reactive compound, hypochlorite (the major component of household bleach), by the enzyme myeloperoxidase, which is present in leukocyte granules. This is one reason why inflammation intended to kill infectious pathogens is often associated with injury to normal tissues.
- *Nitric oxide* is another reactive free radical produced in macrophages and other leukocytes during inflammatory reactions. It can combine with $O_2^{\cdot-}$ to form a highly reactive compound, peroxynitrite, which also participates in cell injury.

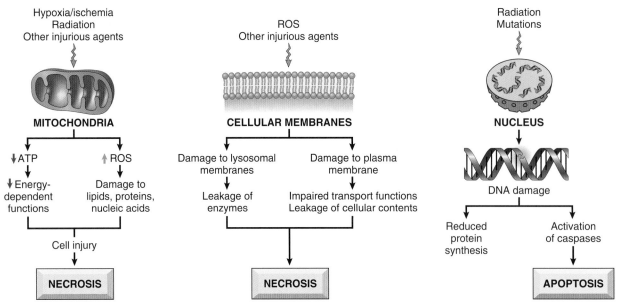

Fig. 1.9 Principal cellular targets of injurious stimuli. Most injurious stimuli affect mitochondria, cellular membranes, or nuclear DNA. Injury to these structures may progress to necrosis or apoptosis. *ATP,* Adenosine triphosphate; *ROS,* reactive oxygen species.

ROS can damage lipids (by peroxidation), proteins (mainly by cross-linking), and DNA (by creating breaks at deoxythymidine residues), and thus affect all cellular components. Their accumulation is controlled by enzymes such as glutathione peroxidase and catalase, which break down hydrogen peroxide. Increased generation of free radicals during pathologic injury overwhelms these scavenging mechanisms.

Hypoxia and Ischemia

Oxygen deficiency leads to reduced generation of ATP and failure of energy-dependent cellular systems (Fig. 1.11).

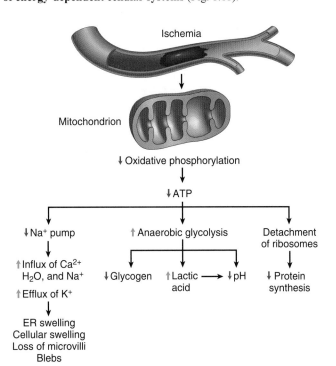

Fig. 1.10 The functional and morphologic consequences of hypoxia and ischemia. *ATP,* Adenosine triphosphate. *ER,* endoplasmic reticulum.

Hypoxia (reduced availability of oxygen) is seen in situations of blood loss, anemia, and carbon monoxide poisoning (which interferes with the oxygen-carrying capacity of hemoglobin). Ischemia, or reduced blood flow, may be a consequence of arterial obstruction (as in coronary artery disease, the major cause of myocardial infarction, or cerebral artery disease, the major cause of stroke) or a severe drop in blood pressure (shock). These are some of the most frequent and serious problems in clinical medicine.

ATP is produced in mitochondria in an electrochemical reaction that depends on the reduction of oxygen (oxidative phosphorylation) and its high-energy phosphate is required for membrane transport, synthesis of proteins and lipids, and turnover of phospholipids. It is estimated that the cells of a healthy individual burn 50 to 75 kg of ATP every day. Therefore, oxygen deprivation and the resulting depletion of ATP damages many cellular components, as follows:

- Reduced activity of the plasma membrane ATP-dependent Na^+-K^+ *pump* results in the influx of Na^+ and water, as discussed earlier, leading to cell swelling and dilation of the ER, which are some of the earliest manifestations of cell injury (see Fig. 1.1).
- *Anaerobic glycolysis* increases in an attempt to generate ATP in the absence of oxygen, resulting in increased production of lactic acid, decreased intracellular pH, and, consequently, reduced activity of many intracellular enzymes.
- *Ribosomes* detach from the ER, leading to reduced protein synthesis.
- Hypoxia may increase the generation of *ROS,* which have many damaging effects.
- Ultimately, lysosomal and mitochondrial membranes are damaged, lysosomal acid hydrolases are activated by low pH, and the cell begins to digest itself, culminating in *necrosis.*

Ischemia–Reperfusion Injury

Restoration of blood flow to an ischemic tissue sometimes paradoxically exacerbates tissue injury.

The cell injury that may follow reperfusion is likely due to increased production of ROS by injured cells with damaged mitochondria and by leukocytes, which are recruited to get rid of the necrotic cells. These inflammatory cells may release enzymes that cause yet more tissue damage (see Chapter 2). Complement proteins, which enter the

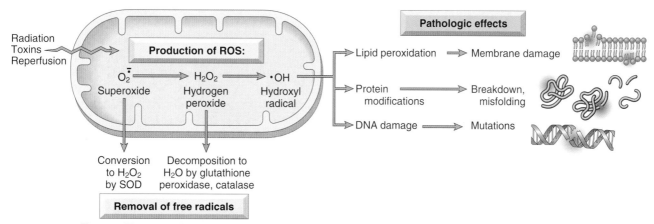

Fig. 1.11 The generation, removal, and role of reactive oxygen species (ROS) in cell injury. The production of ROS is increased by many injurious stimuli. These free radicals are removed by spontaneous decay and by specialized enzymatic systems. Excessive production or inadequate removal leads to accumulation of free radicals in cells, which may damage lipids (by peroxidation), proteins, and DNA, resulting in cell injury. *SOD,* superoxide dismutase.

reperfused tissue, may also contribute to the injury, as in other inflammatory reactions.

Toxin-Mediated Cell Injury

Many environmental and microbial toxins damage cellular components directly or after conversion to reactive metabolites, often by cytochrome P450 in liver cells.

A classic, now mainly historical, example of toxin-mediated cell injury is liver damage following inhalation of carbon tetrachloride, a chemical once used in the dry cleaning industry but now banned. This molecule is converted in the liver into a free radical that is the cause of cell injury, mainly by membrane phospholipid peroxidation. Damage to the ER membrane causes a decline in the synthesis of enzymes and plasma proteins, as well as apoproteins, which are transport proteins that form complexes with triglycerides, facilitating triglyceride secretion; this defect results in the accumulation of lipids in hepatocytes and other cells (steatosis; see later). The analgesic acetaminophen has a similar mechanism of action. It is metabolized to a free radical by cytochrome P450 enzymes, and acute overdose of this drug is the most frequent cause of serious liver damage in the United States and other developed countries.

Endoplasmic Reticulum (ER) Stress

The accumulation of misfolded proteins in the ER can stress adaptive mechanisms and trigger apoptosis.

When improperly folded proteins accumulate in the ER, they first activate a protective reaction called the *unfolded protein response*, in which protein translation is reduced and the production of chaperones (molecules that maintain newly synthesized proteins in their proper shape) is increased (Fig. 1.12). If the load of misfolded proteins is too great, the cell dies by the mitochondrial pathway of apoptosis; in this way, cells that can no longer function are eliminated.

Intracellular accumulation of misfolded proteins may be caused by abnormalities that increase the production of misfolded proteins or reduce the ability to eliminate them. These may result from gene mutations, such as those responsible for cystic fibrosis, that lead to the production of proteins that cannot fold properly: aging, which is associated with a decreased capacity to correct misfolding; infections, especially viral infections, when large amounts of microbial proteins are synthesized within cells, exceeding the cell's protein-folding capacity; increased demand for secretory proteins such as insulin in insulin-resistant states; changes in the intracellular pH and redox

state; and certain neoplasms of protein-secreting cells, particularly plasma cell neoplasms such as multiple myeloma. Protein misfolding is thought to be the fundamental cellular abnormality in several neurodegenerative diseases (see Chapter 17). Deprivation of glucose and oxygen, as in ischemia and hypoxia, also may increase the burden of misfolded proteins. Diseases caused by misfolded proteins are listed in Table 1.3.

DNA Damage

DNA damage that is too great to be corrected by DNA repair mechanisms leads to apoptosis.

Damage to nuclear DNA occurs upon exposure to radiation, chemotherapeutic (anticancer) drugs, and ROS and as a result of mutations. Damaged DNA activates p53, which arrests cells in the G1 phase of the cell cycle to allow the damage to be repaired and also activates DNA repair mechanisms. If these mechanisms fail to correct the DNA damage, p53 triggers apoptosis by the mitochondrial pathway. Thus, the cell "chooses" to die rather than survive with abnormal DNA that has the potential to induce malignant transformation of the cell. Predictably, mutations in p53 that interfere with its ability to arrest cell cycling or to induce apoptosis are associated with numerous cancers (see Chapter 5).

Cellular Aging

Cells age because of accumulation of mutations, progressively decreased replication, and defective protein homeostasis.

People age because their cells age. Although much of the public's attention on aging is focused on its cosmetic and physical consequences, the greatest danger of cellular aging is that it promotes the development of many degenerative, metabolic, and neoplastic disorders. Numerous intrinsic molecular abnormalities are believed to cause the aging of cells (Fig. 1.13).

- Accumulation of *mutations* in DNA, which occurs naturally and may be enhanced by ROS and environmental mutagens.
- *Decreased replication of cells* because of progressive loss of the enzyme telomerase, which maintains the normal length of the enzyme telomeres. These short DNA sequences at the ends of chromosomes protect the ends from fusion and degradation. Telomeres shorten with every replication but can be maintained by the activity of the enzyme telomerase. Because most cells (except germ cells) contain little or no telomerase, telomere shortening is inevitable in dividing cells. With complete loss of telomeres during cellular

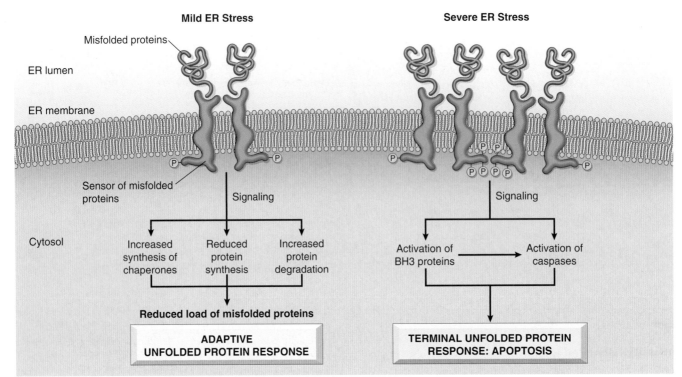

Fig. 1.12 The unfolded protein response and endoplasmic reticulum (er) stress. The presence of misfolded proteins in the ER is detected by sensors in the ER membrane (BH3-only proteins, mentioned earlier) that trigger an adaptive unfolded protein response, which can protect the cell from the harmful consequences of the misfolded proteins. When the amount of misfolded proteins is too great to be corrected, the mitochondrial pathway of apoptosis is induced and the irreparably damaged cell dies; this is also called the terminal unfolded protein response.

Table 1.3 Diseases Caused by Misfolded Proteins

Disease	Affected protein	Pathogenesis
Diseases Caused by Mutant Proteins That are Degraded, Leading to Their Deficiency		
Cystic fibrosis	CFTR	Loss of CFTR leads to defects in chloride transport
Familial hypercholesterolemia	LDL receptor	Loss of LDL receptor leads to hypercholesterolemia
Tay-Sachs disease	Hexosaminidase α subunit	Lack of the lysosomal enzyme leads to storage of GM_2 gangliosides in neurons
Diseases Caused by Misfolded Proteins That Result in ER Stress–Induced Cell Loss		
Retinitis pigmentosa	Rhodopsin	Abnormal folding of rhodopsin causes photoreceptor loss and cell death, resulting in blindness
Creutzfeldt-Jakob disease	Prions	Abnormal folding and aggregation of PrP^{sc} causes neuronal cell death
Alzheimer disease	Aβ peptide	Abnormal folding of Aβ peptide causes aggregation within neurons and apoptosis
Diseases Caused by Misfolded Proteins That Result From Both ER Stress–Induced Cell Loss and Functional Deficiency of the Protein		
Alpha-1-antitrypsin deficiency	α-1 antitrypsin	Storage of nonfunctional protein in hepatocytes causes apoptosis; absence of enzymatic activity in lungs causes destruction of elastic tissue, giving rise to emphysema

Selected illustrative examples of diseases are shown in which protein misfolding is thought to be the major mechanism of functional derangement or cell or tissue injury.
CFTR, Cystic fibrosis transmembrane conductance regulator; *LDL*, low-density lipoprotein.

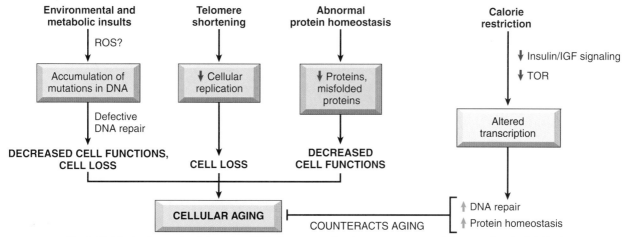

Fig. 1.13 Mechanisms of cellular aging. DNA damage, replicative senescence, and decreased and misfolded proteins are among the best-described mechanisms of cellular aging. Some environmental stresses, such as calorie restriction, counteract aging by activating various signaling pathways and transcription factors. *IGF,* Insulin-like growth factor; *ROS,* reactive oxygen species; *TOR,* target of rapamycin.

aging, the "naked" chromosome ends activate the DNA damage response, causing the cells to enter a state of replicative senescence.

- *Defective protein homeostasis,* due to increased turnover and decreased synthesis of intracellular proteins, together with accumulation of misfolded proteins.
- *Altered signaling pathways* that may affect responses to growth factors. There has been great interest in defining these pathways, in part because of the intriguing observation that calorie restriction prolongs life. One possibility is that calorie restriction reduces signaling by insulin-like growth factor, so cells cycle less and suffer fewer DNA replication–related errors.
- In addition to these intrinsic abnormalities, damaged and dying cells induce low-level *inflammation,* and chronic inflammation predisposes to many diseases, such as atherosclerosis, type 2 diabetes, and some types of cancer.

CELLULAR ADAPTATIONS TO STRESS

Adaptations are reversible changes in the number, size, phenotype, metabolic activity, or functions of cells in response to changes in their environment.

Cellular adaptations may be part of physiologic cellular responses or may be pathologic. *Physiologic adaptations* usually represent responses of cells to normal stimulation by hormones or endogenous chemical mediators (e.g., the hormone-induced enlargement of the breast and uterus during pregnancy), or to the demands of mechanical stress (in the case of bones and muscles). *Pathologic adaptations* are responses to stress that allow cells to modulate their structure and function and thus escape injury, but at the expense of normal function. Physiologic and pathophysiologic adaptations can take several distinct forms.

- *Hypertrophy* is an increase in the size of cells resulting in enlargement of the organ (Fig. 1.14). It can be physiologic or pathologic and is caused either by an increased functional demand or by hormonal stimulation. For example, physiologic enlargement of the uterus during pregnancy is caused by increased estrogen levels. Muscle hypertrophy following weight lifting is an adaptation to increased mechanical stress. Cardiac hypertrophy in hypertension or aortic valve disease is an example of pathologic hypertrophy resulting from increased work load. In all forms, hormones and mechanical sensors activate signaling pathways that lead to increased protein synthesis and assembly of more organelles, and thus enlargement of the cell. Although an adaptation to stress, hypertrophy can progress to functionally significant cell or organ injury if the stress is not relieved. For example, cardiac hypertrophy can

cause myocardial ischemia due to relative lack of oxygen delivery, and eventually give rise to cardiac failure.

- *Hyperplasia* is an increase in the number of cells in an organ that stems from increased proliferation, either of less-differentiated progenitor cells or, in some instances, differentiated cells. Hyperplasia occurs if the tissue contains cell populations capable of replication and may occur concurrently with hypertrophy and often in response to the same stimuli. Hyperplasia can be physiologic or pathologic and, in both situations, cellular proliferation is stimulated by hormones and growth factors that are produced by a variety of cell types. Postpartum enlargement of the breast due to increased proliferation of ductular epithelium is an example of physiologic hyperplasia induced by hormones. Growth factors are responsible for stimulating proliferation of surviving cells after death or removal of some of the cells in an organ (e.g., growth of residual liver following partial hepatectomy, called *compensatory hyperplasia*). Pathologic hyperplasia is typically the result of inappropriate and excessive stimulation by hormones and growth factors, as in endometrial hyperplasia resulting from a disturbed estrogen–progesterone balance. Benign prostatic hyperplasia is induced by androgens and can cause obstruction to the flow of urine and predispose to urinary tract infections. It is important to distinguish hyperplasia from neoplasia: Unlike neoplastic growths, hyperplasia is reversible when the growth signals abate. In some cases, persistent pathologic hyperplasia, such as that affecting the endometrium, sets the stage for the development of cancer because proliferating cells are susceptible to mutations and oncogenic transformation.
- *Atrophy* is a decrease in the size and number of cells that may cause an organ to shrink. It is caused by decreased protein synthesis (due to reduced metabolic activity) and increased protein breakdown mediated by the ubiquitin–proteasome pathway. Causes include a diminished workload (as in immobilization or denervation of muscle, leading to disuse atrophy), progressive ischemia, reduced nutrition, and loss of hormone stimulation (as in menopause). Faced with malnutrition, cells undergo atrophy rather than death as an adaptation to reduced energy supply, but may die with persistent stress. It is often associated with increased autophagy.
- *Metaplasia* is a change of one adult cell type to another. It is a response to stress in which a cell that is sensitive to that stress is replaced by another cell type that is better able to survive the adverse environment. The mechanism is thought to be reprogramming of tissue stem cells to differentiate along a new pathway. Examples include squamous metaplasia of the bronchial columnar epithelium

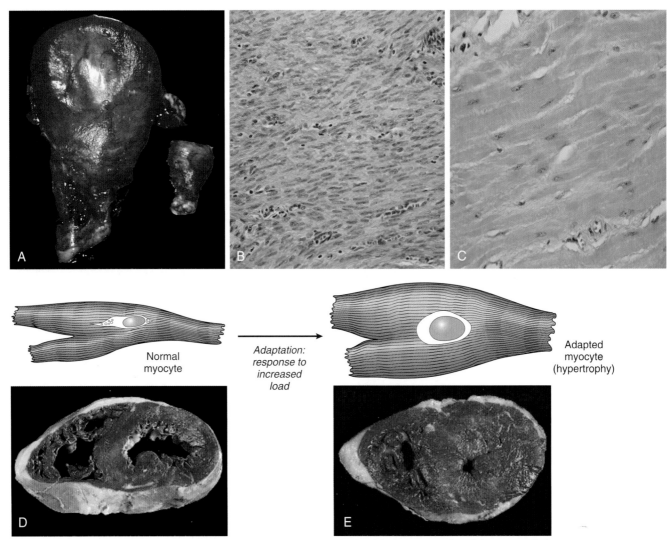

Fig. 1.14 Physiologic and pathologic hypertrophy. (A-C) Physiologic hypertrophy of the uterus during pregnancy. (A) Gross appearance of a normal uterus (right) and a gravid uterus (left) that was removed for postpartum bleeding. (B) Small spindle-shaped uterine smooth muscle cells from a non-gravid uterus. (C) Large, plump, hypertrophied smooth muscle cells from a gravid uterus; compare with (B). (B and C, same magnification.) (D, E) Myocardial hypertrophy in a patient with severe hypertension. (D) Normal myocardium (thickness 1 to 1.5 cm). (E) Myocardial hypertrophy. The left ventricular wall is thicker than 2 cm.

in chronic smokers and columnar metaplasia of the esophageal squamous epithelium in patients with chronic gastric reflux (Fig. 1.15). Although metaplasia allows cells to survive, it often compromises their function; for instance, squamous epithelium in the bronchus cannot produce mucus and provide ciliary action, two important functions of normal bronchial epithelium that protect the airways from infection. Also, with the persistence of triggering stimuli, metaplastic epithelium can be the site of neoplastic transformation, as in the bronchi (squamous cell carcinoma of the lung) and upper gastrointestinal tract (esophageal adenocarcinoma arising in the setting of Barrett esophagus).

PATHOLOGIC ACCUMULATIONS IN CELLS

Cells may accumulate abnormal amounts of various substances, which may be harmless (e.g., carbon particles in the lungs and mediastinal lymph nodes of city dwellers) or may cause varying degrees of injury.

The substance may be located in the cytoplasm, within organelles (typically lysosomes), or in the nucleus, and it may be synthesized by the affected cells or it may be produced elsewhere.

The main pathways of abnormal intracellular accumulations are inadequate removal and degradation or excessive production of an endogenous substance, or deposition of an abnormal exogenous material. Some examples are described in the following.

- *Fatty change (steatosis).* Steatosis is the accumulation of lipids (Supplemental eFig. 1.2), most often in the liver following prolonged alcohol consumption or in obese individuals as a component of nonalcoholic fatty liver disease (see Chapter 13).
- *Cholesterol* and cholesteryl esters. Phagocytic cells may become overloaded with lipid (triglycerides, cholesterol, and cholesteryl esters) in several different pathologic processes (Supplemental eFig. 1.3), mostly characterized by increased intake or decreased catabolism of lipids. Of these, atherosclerosis is the most important (see Chapter 8).

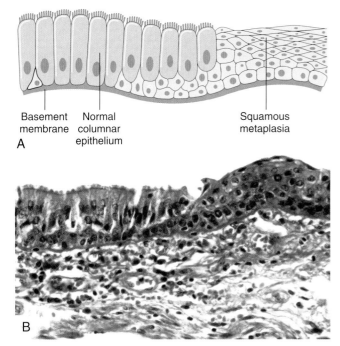

Fig. 1.15 Metaplasia of normal columnar (left) to squamous epithelium (right) in a bronchus, shown schematically (A) and histologically (B).

- *Proteins.* Morphologically visible protein accumulations are less common than lipid accumulations; they may occur when cells take up or synthesize excessive amounts. For example, *protein droplets* are visible in renal tubular epithelial cells when the tubules resorb excessive amounts of proteins from the urine, which occurs with glomerular damage leading to the nephrotic syndrome (see Chapter 11) (Supplemental eFig. 1.4). Other examples include Russell bodies, eosinophilic inclusions comprised of newly synthesized immunoglobulins that misfold and accumulate in the rough ER of some plasma cells; neurofibrillary tangles in neurons; and "alcoholic hyaline" (see Chapter 13).

- *Pigments.* Pigments of several types may accumulate in cells. *Lipofuscin* is a brownish, granular material composed of lipids and proteins that is produced by free radical–mediated lipid peroxidation (Supplemental eFig. 1.5). Its accumulation in cells is a sign of free radical–mediated injury, so it is often seen in older individuals and in atrophic tissues. *Hemosiderin* is a hemoglobin-derived brown pigment (Supplemental eFig. 1.6) that accumulates in phagocytes and other cells in conditions of increased red cell breakdown or iron overload (see Chapter 9).

- *Glycogen.* Excessive intracellular deposits of glycogen are associated with abnormalities in the metabolism of either glucose or glycogen. Glycogen may accumulate in poorly controlled diabetes or in glycogen storage diseases (see Chapter 13).

- *Calcium.* Calcium salt deposits are seen in a variety of disease states. *Dystrophic calcification* occurs in the setting of normal serum calcium and is the deposition of calcium salts in injured tissue (e.g., in areas of caseous necrosis and in advanced atherosclerosis). Dystrophic calcification can have functional consequences, as in calcific stenosis of the aortic valve causing left ventricular hypertrophy due to pressure overload (Supplemental eFig. 1.7). *Metastatic calcification* occurs in the setting of hypercalcemia, which is seen in states of hyperparathyroidism (see Chapter 16), or increased bone destruction, as in cancers involving the bone. Metastatic calcification occurs widely throughout the body but principally affects the interstitial tissues of the vasculature, kidneys, lungs, and gastric mucosa. It usually does not cause clinical dysfunction.

- *Amyloid.* Amyloid consists of one of many different proteins that assume a fibrillar conformation and are deposited in extracellular tissues, where they may interfere with the normal functions of organs (Supplemental eFig. 1.8). Amyloid deposition is often related to immune processes and is discussed in Chapter 4.

2

Inflammation and Repair

OUTLINE

Overview of Inflammation, 14
    Causes of Inflammation, 14
    Sequence of Events in Inflammation, 14
    Features of Acute and Chronic Inflammation, 15
    Cells of Inflammation, 15
Acute Inflammation, 16
    Vascular Reactions, 16
    Cellular Reactions, 17
    Resolution of Acute Inflammation, 20

Mediators of Inflammation, 20
    Clinicopathologic Features of Acute Inflammation, 23
    Outcomes of Acute Inflammation, 25
Chronic Inflammation, 26
    Cellular Reactions of Chronic Inflammation, 26
    Clinicopathologic Features of Chronic Inflammation, 27
Tissue Repair, 27
    Angiogenesis, 28
    Clinicopathologic Features of Tissue Repair, 28

OVERVIEW OF INFLAMMATION

Inflammation is a host response to infections and tissue damage that brings cells and molecules to the sites where they are needed to eliminate the cause of injury (e.g., microbes or toxins) and the consequences of such injury (e.g., necrotic cells and tissues).

The mediators of defense include leukocytes (white blood cells), antibodies, and complement proteins. Most of these normally circulate in the blood, where they are sequestered to prevent damage to normal tissues, but they can be rapidly recruited to any site in the body. Some of the cells involved in inflammatory responses also reside in tissues, where they function as sentinels on the lookout for threats.

In clinical medicine, much of the emphasis on this useful response has been on its harmful consequences (e.g., pain, fever, and functional impairments), but it is important to note that an appropriately regulated inflammatory response is a critical part of normal health and tissue maintenance. The suffix *itis* after an organ denotes inflammation in that site (e.g., appendicitis, conjunctivitis, meningitis). Inflammation can be damaging if:

- It is *inadequately controlled*
- It is *misdirected* (e.g., against normally harmless environmental substances [as in allergies] or commensal microbes, or against self tissues [as in autoimmune diseases])
- The stimulus is *persistent* and cannot readily be eliminated (e.g., the mycobacterium that causes tuberculosis)

Too little inflammation, which is typically manifested by increased susceptibility to infections, is also problematic and is most often caused by quantitative or qualitative defects in leukocytes, which may result from replacement of the marrow by cancers, destruction of normal leukocytes by cancer therapies, or use of immunosuppressive drugs.

After the noxious stimuli and the damage they cause are eliminated, the inflammatory reaction sets in motion the process of repair, which restores tissue integrity.

Causes of Inflammation

The major causes of inflammation are infections, immunologic reactions, tissue necrosis, and environmental substances.

Infections (bacterial, viral, fungal, parasitic) and microbial toxins are among the most common and medically important causes of inflammation. Different infectious pathogens elicit a range of inflammatory responses, from mild acute inflammation that causes little or no lasting damage, to severe systemic reactions that can be fatal, to prolonged chronic reactions that cause extensive tissue injury.

Immune reactions occur when the normally protective immune system damages the individual's own tissues either by attacking self antigens (autoimmune diseases) or reacting to environmental substances (allergies*)*. Inflammation is a major cause of tissue injury in these diseases (see Chapter 4). Because the stimuli for the inflammatory responses in autoimmune and allergic diseases cannot be eliminated, these reactions tend to be persistent and difficult to cure and are often associated with chronic inflammation.

Necrosis from any cause, even sterile injury as in infarction caused by loss of blood supply, elicits inflammation due to molecules released from necrotic cells.

Foreign bodies (e.g., splinters, dirt, sutures) may elicit inflammation, and even some *endogenous substances* stimulate potentially harmful inflammation if large amounts are deposited in tissues (e.g., urate crystals in gout and cholesterol crystals in atherosclerosis).

Sequence of Events in Inflammation

The inflammatory response consists of sequential events involving vascular reactions and recruitment of leukocytes.

The major steps in the response are recognition, recruitment, removal, regulation, and repair (the 5 Rs), described next (Fig. 2.1). These steps are mediated by the coordinated actions of chemical mediators that will be described later.

1. *Recognition* of the noxious agent that is the initiating stimulus for inflammation. The cells that trigger inflammation (tissue-resident sentinel cells, phagocytes, and others, described later) are equipped with receptors that recognize microbial products and substances released from damaged cells. Cellular receptors for microbes can be located in plasma membranes (for extracellular

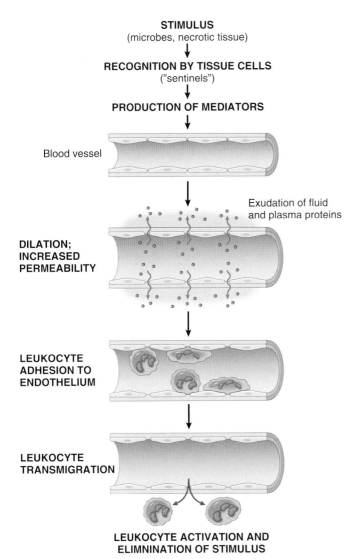

STIMULUS
(microbes, necrotic tissue)
↓
RECOGNITION BY TISSUE CELLS
("sentinels")
↓
PRODUCTION OF MEDIATORS
↓

Blood vessel

DILATION;
INCREASED
PERMEABILITY

Exudation of fluid
and plasma proteins

LEUKOCYTE
ADHESION TO
ENDOTHELIUM

LEUKOCYTE
TRANSMIGRATION

LEUKOCYTE ACTIVATION AND
ELIMNINATION OF STIMULUS

Fig. 2.1 Sequence of events in inflammation. In most inflammatory reactions, recognition of an offending agent (the stimulus for inflammation) leads to the production of chemical mediators, which elicit the vascular and cellular reactions that serve to eliminate the offenders.

and for complement proteins, which recognize microbes coated (opsonized) with antibodies and complement.

2. *Recruitment* of leukocytes and plasma proteins into the tissues. Because blood perfuses every tissue, leukocytes and proteins such as complement can be delivered to any vascularized site of microbial invasion. When pathogenic microbes invade the tissues, or tissue cells die, leukocytes (first, mainly neutrophils; later, monocytes and lymphocytes) and plasma proteins are rapidly recruited from the circulation to the extravascular site where the offending agent is located. The exodus of cells and plasma proteins from blood requires coordinated changes in blood vessels and the secretion of mediators, described in more detail later.

3. *Removal* of the stimulus for inflammation is accomplished mainly by phagocytic cells, which ingest and destroy microbes and dead cells. Phagocytosis, described later, involves three sequential steps: (1) recognition and attachment of the particle to be ingested by the leukocyte; (2) engulfment, with subsequent formation of a phagocytic vacuole; and (3) destruction of the ingested material.

4. *Regulation* of the response is important for terminating the reaction when it has accomplished its purpose. In large part, termination is because of the decay of mediators and death of leukocytes after the stimulus is eliminated. It is likely that, in concert with the inflammatory response, active regulatory mechanisms also are triggered that serve to turn off the response.

5. *Repair* heals the damage, and is discussed at the end of the chapter.

Features of Acute and Chronic Inflammation

The two principal patterns of inflammation, acute and chronic, differ in kinetics and many other features.

Acute inflammation is a rapid, often self-limited, response to infections and tissue damage. It typically develops within minutes or hours and is of short duration (several hours to a few days). It is characterized by the exudation of fluid and plasma proteins (edema) and the emigration of leukocytes, predominantly neutrophils. If the offending stimulus is eliminated, the reaction subsides and residual injury is repaired. But if the initial response fails to clear the stimulus, the reaction progresses to a protracted type of inflammation that is called chronic inflammation.

Chronic inflammation may follow acute inflammation or arise de novo (and acute inflammation may be superimposed on a background of chronic inflammation). Chronic inflammation is of longer duration and is associated with more tissue destruction, the presence of lymphocytes and macrophages, the proliferation of blood vessels, and fibrosis.

Although the distinction between acute and chronic inflammation was originally based on the duration of the reaction, we now know that they differ in several ways (Table 2.1). Acute inflammation is the response to offending agents that are readily eliminated, such as many bacterial and viral infections and dead cells, and chronic infection is a response to agents that are difficult to eradicate, such as some bacteria and other pathogens, as well as self and environmental antigens.

Cells of Inflammation

The principal cells of inflammation are leukocytes (white blood cells) in the circulation and tissues.

The major cells of inflammation are (1) tissue-resident sentinels that detect pathogenic microbes, toxins, and products of cell damage,

pathogens), endosomes (for ingested microbes), or the cytosol (for intracellular agents). Sensors of cell damage are present in the cytosol of all cells: They recognize molecules that result from cell injury (e.g., uric acid, a product of DNA breakdown). These receptors belong to several molecular families, including Toll-like receptors, NOD-like receptors, and others. They are called pattern recognition receptors because they recognize and are activated by microbial and dead cell products called pathogen-associated and damage-associated molecular patterns (PAMPs and DAMPs, respectively). Engagement of the receptors leads to the production of mediators of inflammation, including cytokines, whose functions are described later. A subset of cytosolic NOD-like receptors activates a multiprotein complex called the *inflammasome,* which stimulates the production of the proinflammatory and fever-inducing cytokine interleukin-1 (IL-1). Leukocytes also express receptors for the Fc portion of antibodies

Table 2.1 Acute and Chronic Inflammation

	Acute Inflammation	Chronic Inflammation
Onset	Rapid: minutes to hours	Slower: days
Duration	Typically brief (days)	Prolonged
Cellular infiltrate	Mainly neutrophils	Macrophages (derived from blood monocytes), lymphocytes
Tissue injury	Usually self-limited	May be extensive
Scarring	Uncommon	Prominent
Major mediators	Histamine, prostaglandins and leukotrienes, cytokines, complement proteins	Cytokines, other mediators involved in acute inflammation
Local and systemic signs	Prominent	Usually milder
Common causes:		
Infections	Pyogenic bacteria (e.g., staphylococci), fungi, some viruses (e.g., influenza).	Intracellular bacteria (e.g., *Mycobacterium tuberculosis*), viruses (e.g., hepatitis), fungi
Cell death	Ischemic necrosis of tissues	Not a frequent underlying cause
Immune reactions	Antibody deposition in tissues (in autoimmune diseases), IgE-mediated immediate hypersensitivity	T cell–mediated inflammatory diseases
Trauma	Physical injury, burns, radiation	Sometimes, repeated low-dose radiation exposure
Environmental toxins		Inhaled particles (e.g., silica, beryllium)
Others	Crystal deposition in tissues (e.g., gout)	
Examples of human diseases	Infections, acute respiratory distress syndrome	Rheumatoid arthritis, atherosclerosis, asthma, pulmonary fibrosis

and also produce many of the mediators of inflammation, and (2) phagocytic cells that eliminate the noxious substances.
- The major *sentinel cells* are:
  - *Dendritic cells*, so named because of their dendrite-like projections, recognize microbes and dead cells and also capture and display protein antigens to T cells, to initiate immune responses.
  - *Mast cells* are located adjacent to blood vessels.
  - *Tissue-resident macrophages* are present in all connective tissues and most organs. They are given special names in different organs (e.g., *Kupffer cells* in the liver, *microglia* in the central nervous system, *alveolar macrophages* in the lung). During inflammation, most macrophages are derived from blood monocytes, which originate from hematopoietic stem cells in the bone marrow. Many of the tissue-resident macrophages are derived from hematopoietic progenitors in the yolk sac and fetal liver early during development and are long-lived.
- *Phagocytes* are cells specialized for eating and killing offending agents. The two major classes of circulating phagocytes, *neutrophils* (polymorphonuclear leukocytes, or PMNs) and *monocytes,* are recruited from the blood into the site of inflammation. Following their entry into tissues, monocytes mature into macrophages. Neutrophils are more abundant early in the reaction because they are more numerous in the blood and respond more rapidly to chemotactic mediators, but with time macrophages become progressively dominant because they are longer lived. Although both cell types share the common function of phagocytosis, they differ in life span and specialized activities (Table 2.2).
- Other cells play diverse roles in various inflammatory reactions:
  - *Lymphocytes*, especially *T lymphocytes*, are prominent when the offending agent elicits an adaptive immune response. This is often the case with viral infections and autoimmune and allergic reactions. Antibody-producing *B lymphocytes* and *plasma cells* may also be prominent in reactions to particular stimuli.

- *Eosinophils* are often seen in allergic reactions and infections with helminthic parasites.

ACUTE INFLAMMATION

Acute inflammation is a rapid tissue response to microbes, toxins, necrotic cells, and antibody deposition.

Acute inflammation consists of vascular and cellular reactions that deliver leukocytes and plasma proteins from the blood into the tissues, where these cells and proteins get rid of the noxious substances that elicited the response.

Vascular Reactions

The major changes in blood vessels during acute inflammation are dilation and increased permeability.

The exit of cells and plasma proteins from the blood into tissues requires alterations in blood vessels. The initial changes are dilation and increased permeability of the vessels, followed by changes that promote the exit of leukocytes.
- *Vasodilation* is induced by the action of several mediators, notably histamine, on vascular smooth muscle. It first involves the arterioles and then leads to the opening of new capillary beds in the area. The result is increased blood flow, which is the cause of heat and redness (erythema) at the site of inflammation.
- *Increase in vascular permeability* can occur by two mechanisms: contraction of endothelial cells and direct endothelial injury. Contraction of endothelial cells with opening of interendothelial spaces is the most common mechanism of vascular leakage. This response is elicited by histamine, bradykinin, leukotrienes, and other chemical mediators that also cause vasodilation, and occurs rapidly after exposure to the mediator (within 15 to 30 minutes). The blood flow slows, allowing plasma proteins that mediate host defense to pass through the vessels into the tissue. Direct endothelial injury is the

Table 2.2 Phagocytes

	Neutrophils	Macrophages
Origin	HSCs in bone marrow	HSCs in bone marrow (in inflammatory reactions) Many tissue-resident macrophages: stem cells in yolk sac or fetal liver (early in development)
Life span in tissues	1–2 days	Inflammatory macrophages: days or weeks Tissue-resident macrophages: years
Responses to activating stimuli	Rapid, short-lived, mostly degranulation and enzymatic activity	More prolonged, slower, often dependent on new gene transcription
Reactive oxygen species	Rapidly induced by assembly of phagocyte oxidase (respiratory burst)	Less prominent
Nitric oxide	Low levels or none	Induced following transcriptional activation of iNOS
Degranulation	Major response; induced by cytoskeletal rearrangement	Not prominent
Cytokine production	Low levels or none	Major functional activity, requires transcriptional activation of cytokine genes
NET formation	Rapidly induced, by extrusion of nuclear contents	Less
Secretion of lysosomal enzymes	Prominent	Less

This table lists the major differences between neutrophils and macrophages. The reactions summarized above are described in the text. Note that the two cell types share many features, such as phagocytosis, the ability to migrate through blood vessels into tissues, and chemotaxis. The images show a typical blood neutrophil and monocyte (the precursor of tissue macrophages in inflammatory reactions).
HSC, Hematopoietic stem cells; *iNOS,* inducible nitric oxide synthase; *NET,* neutrophil extracellular trap.

mechanism by which cells and proteins escape venules, capillaries, and arterioles in cases of severe necrotizing injury (e.g., burns) and exposure to some microbial toxins.

The protein-rich fluid that escapes into the tissue *(exudate)* results in edema at the site of inflammation. The loss of fluid and increased vessel diameter lead to slower blood flow, increased concentration of red cells in small vessels, and increased viscosity of the blood. These changes result in the engorgement of small vessels with slowly moving red cells, a condition termed *stasis,* which is seen histologically as *vascular congestion* and externally as localized redness *(erythema)* of the involved tissue. As stasis develops, blood leukocytes, principally neutrophils, begin to adhere to the vascular endothelium, the first step in their migration out of the vessels.

Lymphatic vessels also participate in inflammatory reactions and help to remove the exudate. Vessels draining sites of acute inflammation are often engorged and congested (lymphangitis), and the draining lymph nodes are swollen and tender (lymphadenitis).

Cellular Reactions

Cytokines and other mediators activate endothelial cells at the site of inflammation and stimulate the binding of leukocytes to endothelium and the subsequent migration of cells through the endothelium into the tissue.

The type of leukocyte that emigrates into a site of infection or injury depends on the nature of the original stimulus and the duration of the response. Bacterial infections tend to initially recruit neutrophils, whereas viral infections recruit lymphocytes, allergic reactions have increased eosinophils, and in some cases a mixed infiltrate. In acute inflammation, neutrophils predominate during the first 6 to 24 hours, and then undergo apoptosis (in 24 to 48 hours), to be replaced by monocytes.

The process of leukocyte emigration can be divided into phases, consisting first of adhesion of leukocytes to endothelium at the site of inflammation, then transmigration of the leukocytes through the vessel wall, and finally movement of the cells toward the offending agent. Each step involves soluble mediators and adhesion molecules, the latter expressed on leukocytes and endothelial cells, allowing leukocytes to latch on to endothelial cells and leave the vasculature. The principal adhesion molecules belong to two families of proteins, selectins and integrins, and their ligands (Fig. 2.2 and Table 2.3). The steps in leukocyte recruitment are the following:

- *Leukocyte margination.* As the blood flow slows, leukocytes, being larger than red cells, slow down the most and accumulate near the vessel wall, allowing the leukocytes to bind to the endothelium.

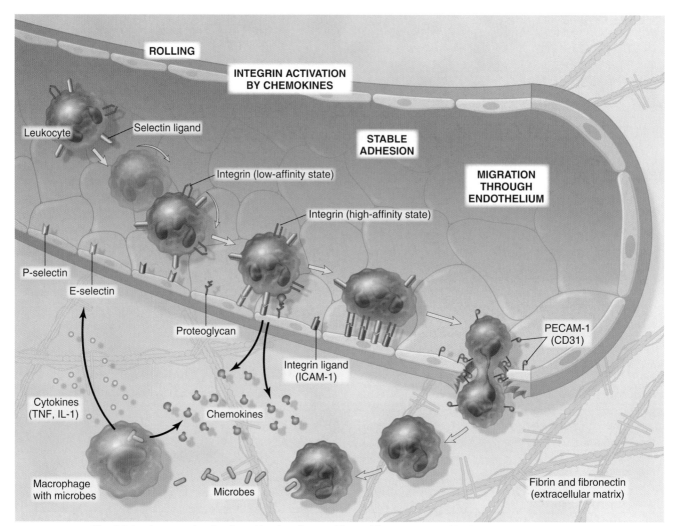

Fig. 2.2 Leukocyte migration from blood to tissues. The multistep process of leukocyte migration through blood vessels is shown here for neutrophils. The leukocytes first roll; then become activated and adhere to the endothelium; and then transmigrate across the endothelium, pierce the basement membrane, and migrate toward chemoattractants emanating from the source of injury. Different molecules play predominant roles in different steps of this process: selectins in rolling; chemokines (usually displayed bound to proteoglycans on endothelium) in activating the neutrophils to increase the avidity of integrins; integrins in firm adhesion; and CD31 (PECAM-1) in transmigration. *ICAM-1*, Intercellular adhesion molecule 1; *IL-1*, interleukin 1; *PECAM-1 (CD31)*, platelet endothelial cell adhesion molecule-1; *TNF*, tumor necrosis factor.

Table 2.3   Selected Adhesion Molecules in Leukocyte Migration

Family	Adhesion Molecule	Major Cell Type	Principal Ligands
Selectin	L-selectin	Lymphocytes	Sialyl-Lewis X on various glycoproteins expressed on endothelium
	E-selectin	Activated endothelium	Sialyl-Lewis X on glycoproteins expressed on neutrophils, monocytes, T lymphocytes
	P-selectin	Activated endothelium	Sialyl-Lewis X on glycoproteins expressed on neutrophils, monocytes, T lymphocytes
Integrin	LFA-1	T lymphocytes, neutrophils	ICAM-1 expressed on activated endothelium
	MAC-1	Monocytes, dendritic cells	ICAM-1 expressed on activated endothelium
	VLA-4	T lymphocytes	VCAM-1 expressed on activated endothelium
	α4β7	T lymphocytes, monocytes	MAdCAM-1; expressed on endothelium in gut and gut-associated lymphoid tissues

Most of the integrins are expressed on many leukocytes; only the cell types that are most dependent on a particular integrin for adhesion are listed. All the selectins, integrins, and their ligands are also named according to the CD nomenclature, but their CD numbers are not shown for simplicity.
ICAM, intercellular adhesion molecule; *Ig*, immunoglobulin; *IL-1*, interleukin-1; *TNF*, tumor necrosis factor; *VCAM*, vascular cell adhesion molecule.

- *Endothelial activation.* Two of the cytokines secreted in response to microbes and other stimuli, tumor necrosis factor (TNF) and IL-1, act on nearby endothelial cells to increase the expression of selectins and ligands for integrins. Cytokines also convert the endothelial surface from its normal antithrombotic state to a prothrombotic state. Local thrombosis may prevent dissemination of microbes and toxins.
- *Leukocyte rolling.* Selectin ligands on the tips of neutrophil microvilli bind to selectins on the endothelium. This is a low-affinity interaction that is easily disrupted by the flowing blood. Therefore, the leukocytes bind, detach, and bind again, and thus slowly roll along the endothelium.
- *Integrin activation.* Chemokines secreted by sentinel cells in the tissue and also by activated endothelial cells bind to and are displayed on the surface of the endothelium. These chemokines are recognized by receptors on the rolling leukocytes, which deliver signals that change the conformation of integrins on the leukocytes from a low-affinity to a high-affinity state.

- *Stable adhesion* of leukocytes. The activated integrins on the leukocytes bind tightly to their ligands, which are induced on endothelial cells by cytokines, leading to the arrest and firm attachment of leukocytes to the endothelium.
- *Leukocyte transmigration.* Chemokines and other mediators, such as leukotrienes, complement products, and some microbial products, stimulate leukocyte chemotaxis (directed movement along a chemical gradient). The leukocytes migrate between endothelial spaces, through the vessel wall, to the site of inflammation. This process of leukocyte extravasation has been called *diapedesis.*

The noxious substances that triggered inflammation are cleared by phagocytosis followed by intracellular destruction, which proceeds through the following steps (Fig. 2.3).

- *Recognition, attachment, and engulfment.* Activated neutrophils and macrophages bind microbes and other particles (such as fragments of dead cells, crystals, and foreign material), wrap their plasma membranes around the particles, and internalize the particles into

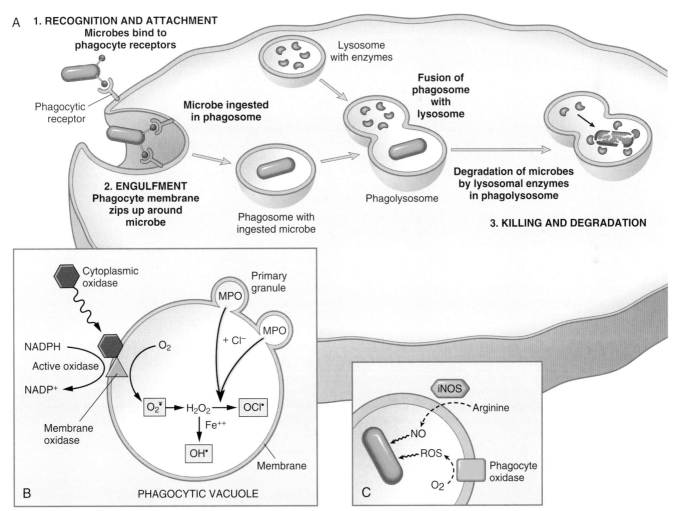

Fig. 2.3 Phagocytosis and intracellular destruction of microbes. (A) Phagocytosis of a particle (e.g., a bacterium) involves binding to receptors on the leukocyte membrane, engulfment, and fusion of the phagocytic vacuoles with lysosomes. This is followed by destruction of ingested particles within the phagolysosomes by lysosomal enzymes and by reactive oxygen and nitrogen species. (B) In activated phagocytes, cytoplasmic components of the phagocyte oxidase enzyme assemble in the membrane of the phagosome to form the active enzyme, which catalyzes the conversion of oxygen into superoxide (O_2^-) and H_2O_2. Myeloperoxidase, present in the granules of neutrophils, converts H_2O_2 to hypochlorite (OCl'). In the presence of metals such as Fe^{++}, H_2O_2 can also be converted to highly reactive hydroxyl radicals (OH'). (C) Microbicidal reactive oxygen species *(ROS)* and nitric oxide *(NO)* kill ingested microbes. During phagocytosis, granule contents may be released into extracellular tissues (not shown). *iNOS,* Inducible NO synthase; *MPO,* myeloperoxidase; *NADPH,* nicotinamide adenine dinucleotide phosphate; *ROS,* reactive oxygen species.

vesicles called endosomes or phagosomes. Phagocytes use a variety of receptors to bind to microbes, such as mannose receptors that bind to terminal mannose on microbial cell wall glycoproteins. The efficiency of this process is greatly increased if the particles are opsonized with tags for which the phagocytes have receptors, such as IgG antibodies (which bind to IgG-specific Fc receptors on the phagocytes) and complement products C3b and C4b (which bind to complement receptors).

- *Killing and destruction.* Phagosomes fuse with lysosomes, and several enzymes are activated in the confines of these vesicles (where they destroy the ingested substances without damaging the phagocyte itself). Neutrophils have two types of granules, called azurophil (or primary) and specific (or secondary) granules. These granules contain enzymes that destroy ingested substances (e.g., elastase, a serine protease that cleaves the matrix protein elastin, and many other proteases) and other enzymes that activate killing mechanisms (e.g., myeloperoxidase, which converts reactive oxygen species to more destructive free radicals, described next).
- *Leukocyte activation.* Circulating leukocytes are in a quiescent state so that they do not cause injury to tissues. After activation by microbial products such as lipopolysaccharides, cytokines such as inteferon-γ (IFN-γ) and chemokines, and phagocytic receptors such as mannose receptors or receptors for opsonins, the leukocytes acquire the ability to destroy ingested microbes and dead cells.
- The major killing mechanisms of neutrophils and macrophages include reactive oxygen species (ROS) (see Chapter 1), nitric oxide, and lysosomal enzymes.
  - *ROS* are produced mainly in neutrophils by the respiratory burst, a process initiated by rapid assembly of the phagocyte oxidase enzyme in the membrane of the phagolysosome. This enzyme catalyzes the generation of the ROS superoxide, which can be converted to hydrogen peroxide or, under the action of neutrophil myeloperoxidase, to highly reactive halides. All of these substances damage proteins, DNA, and lipid membranes and thus destroy microbes and aid in the cleanup of debris from necrotic cells. Healthy tissues are normally protected from ROS-mediated damage by the action of antioxidant enzymes that degrade ROS, such as superoxide dismutase, which degrades superoxide, and catalase, which detoxifies hydrogen peroxide, as well as serum proteins that scavenge the free radicals.
  - *Nitric oxide (NO)* is made mostly in macrophages following transcriptional activation of the enzyme inducible nitric oxide synthase (iNOS). NO is converted to free radicals that act much like ROS.
  - *Lysosomal enzymes,* including elastase and other proteases, gain access to the ingested particles and digest them.
- *Extracellular destruction.* Some of these molecules, especially lysosomal enzymes, are released into the extracellular space, where they destroy microbes and clear dead tissues. Neutrophils also extrude their nuclear contents, forming a mesh of histones and DNA called neutrophil extracellular traps (NETs). Microbes are trapped in this mesh and destroyed by antimicrobial substances that are also released into the NETs.

Some collateral damage is an inevitable consequence of protective host responses, but this is usually self-limited. Pathologic lesions develop when the inflammation is targeted abnormally (e.g., against self antigens or against usually harmless environmental substances such as pollen and other allergens).

Resolution of Acute Inflammation

Normally, following clearance of the offending agent, the acute inflammatory response spontaneously subsides, because the activating stimulus is gone and because mediators (see the following) and neutrophils are short lived. In addition, as inflammation develops, the process itself triggers a variety of stop signals that actively terminate the reaction, including a switch in the type of arachidonic acid metabolite produced, from proinflammatory leukotrienes to antiinflammatory lipoxins (described later), and the liberation of antiinflammatory cytokines, including transforming growth factor-β (TGF-β) and IL-10, from macrophages and other cells.

Mediators of Inflammation

The reactions of inflammation described previously are induced by chemicals, called the mediators of inflammation, that are produced or activated at the site of the reaction (Table 2.4).

These mediators may be produced by cells residing at the site of the inflammatory reaction or that are recruited from the blood and activated at the site of inflammation. They are produced only in response to molecules that stimulate inflammation, including microbial products and substances released from necrotic cells. One mediator can stimulate the release of other mediators. For instance, products of complement activation stimulate the release of histamine, and the cytokine TNF acts on endothelial cells to stimulate the production of another cytokine, IL-1, and many chemokines. They quickly decay, are inactivated by enzymes, or are otherwise scavenged or inhibited. There is thus a system of checks and balances that regulates mediator actions.

Cell-Derived Mediators

These are produced locally by the sentinel cells that recognize pathogens and dead cells, and by recruited leukocytes. The major classes of these mediators are the following.

Histamine is a small molecule that dilates arterioles by acting on smooth muscle cells and increases the permeability of capillaries and venules by causing retraction of endothelial cells. It is stored in mast cell granules and released rapidly upon mast cell activation by pathogens and other signals, such as binding of allergens to IgE on mast cell Fc receptors, exposure to the complement products C5a and C3a, and physical trauma and heat.

Prostaglandins and leukotrienes are derived from arachidonic acid. In many cell types, inflammatory stimuli induce the enzyme phospholipase A2, which liberates arachidonic acid from membrane phospholipids. Arachidonic acid is then converted by the enzyme cyclooxygenase into prostaglandins and by lipoxygenase into leukotrienes. These chemicals have diverse actions on blood vessels and leukocytes, as summarized in Table 2.4. The therapeutic action of many clinically useful antiinflammatory drugs depends on their ability to inhibit the production or activity of these mediators.

- *Prostaglandins* are named based on structural features coded by a letter (e.g., PGD, PGE, PGF, PGG, and PGH) and a subscript numeral (e.g., 1, 2), which indicates the number of double bonds in the compound. The most important prostaglandins in inflammation are PGE_2, PGD_2, PGF_{2a}, PGI_2 (prostacyclin), and TXA_2 (thromboxane A_2).
- *Leukotrienes* are involved in vascular and smooth muscle reactions and leukocyte recruitment. The synthesis of leukotrienes involves multiple steps, the first of which generates leukotriene A_4 (LTA_4), which in turn gives rise to LTB_4 or LTC_4. LTB_4 is produced by neutrophils and some macrophages, and is a potent chemotactic agent and activator of neutrophils, causing aggregation and adhesion of the cells to the venular endothelium, the generation of ROS, and the release of lysosomal enzymes. LTC_4 and its metabolites, LTD_4 and LTE_4, are produced mainly in mast cells and cause intense vasoconstriction, bronchospasm (important in asthma), and increased permeability of venules. In general, leukotrienes are far more potent than histamine.

Table 2.4   Mediators of Inflammation

Mediator	Production	Role in Inflammation	Pharmacologic Antagonists
Cell-Derived Mediators			
Histamine	Stored as a preformed molecule in granules of mast cells and basophils; released rapidly upon degranulation in response to IgE cross-linking (allergy), trauma, complement products	Dilation of blood vessels, increased vascular permeability	Antihistamines for allergy; bind to histamine receptors and competitively inhibit histamine binding
Arachidonic acid derived	PLA_2 production is induced in many cell types by complement products, cytokines, other stimuli → releases arachidonic acid from membrane phospholipids → converted to active mediators		
Prostaglandins	Produced in mast cells, leukocytes, endothelial cells, and other cells by cyclooxygenase; activated by trauma, complement products, cytokines, microbial products	Vasodilation and increased vascular permeability (PGD_2, PGE_2); inhibit (PGI_2) or stimulate (TXA_2) platelet aggregation; pain, fever (PGD_2, PGE_2)	Many nonsteroidal antiinflammatory drugs (NSAIDs) inhibit cyclooxygenase
Leukotrienes	Produced in mast cells, leukocytes, endothelial cells, and other cells by lipoxygenase; activated by trauma, complement products, cytokines, microbial products	Neutrophil chemotaxis (LTB_4); smooth muscle (e.g., bronchial) contraction (LTC_4, LTD_4), involved in asthma	Leukotriene receptor antagonists for asthma
Cytokines: see Table 2.5			
Platelet-activating factor (PAF)	Produced in mast cells, leukocytes, endothelial cells, and platelets by action of PLA_2 on membrane phospholipids	Vasodilation, increased vascular permeability, constriction of bronchi, platelet aggregation (promotes thrombosis)	
Plasma Protein–Derived Mediators			
Complement proteins (see Chapter 4)	Produced at site of complement activation by sequential enzymatic (protease) activity	C5a, C3a are chemotactic for leukocytes (especially neutrophils), dilate vessels C3b coats microbes and promotes their phagocytosis	Anti-C5 for diseases caused by excessive complement activation (in trials)
Pentraxins	Synthesized in the liver in response to cytokines C-reactive protein (CRP) Serum amyloid protein (SAP)	Markers of inflammation (acute-phase proteins) CRP: opsonizes microbes for phagocytosis SAP: unknown	
Kinins	Bradykinin: peptide produced in activated endothelial cells by the kinin–kallikrein system	Vasodilation, increased vascular permeability, bronchial constriction, pain	

- *Lipoxins* are also generated from arachidonic acid by the lipoxygenase pathway, but unlike prostaglandins and leukotrienes, the lipoxins suppress inflammation by inhibiting the recruitment of leukocytes, neutrophil chemotaxis, and adhesion to the endothelium.

Cytokines are proteins that direct communication among leukocytes and other cells, and are therefore considered the messenger molecules that regulate immunity and inflammation (Table 2.5). One subset of cytokines consists of the chemoattractant cytokines, known as *chemokines*, whose function is to direct the movement of leukocytes to the site of inflammation (chemotaxis). Recognition of microbes and products of dead cells by the pattern recognition receptors of sentinels, macrophages, and other cells, mentioned earlier, leads to the activation of signaling pathways that induce the synthesis and secretion of cytokines. Various cytokines have distinct or overlapping roles in acute and chronic inflammation, as described later. Chemokines are classified into four major groups according to the arrangement of the conserved cysteine (C) residues. Each group acts preferentially on neutrophils, monocytes, eosinophils, or lymphocytes.

Plasma Protein–Derived Mediators

These mediators are products of plasma proteins that are synthesized in the liver and other tissues and activated at the site of inflammation. The most important of these mediators are described in the following (see Table 2.4).

The *complement system* consists of several circulating proteins that are activated by microbes and by antibodies or plasma lectins bound to microbes and other antigenic substances. Complement activation leads to sequential enzymatic modification of the proteins, culminating in the deposition of products that variously coat (opsonize) microbes and other cells for phagocytosis; recruit leukocytes; and lyse thin-walled microbes. Complement activation is described in more detail in Chapter 4, in the context of hypersensitivity reactions.

Table 2.5   Major Cytokines of Acute and Chronic Inflammation

Cytokine	Principal Cell Sources	Principal Functions and Role in Inflammation	Use of Therapeutic Antagonists[a]
Cytokines in Acute Inflammation			
Tumor necrosis factor (TNF)	Macrophages, dendritic cells, T cells	Endothelial cells: activation → expression of adhesion molecules, secretion of chemokines, reduced anticoagulant properties (inflammation, coagulation) Neutrophils: activation Hypothalamus: fever Muscle, fat: catabolism (cachexia)	Rheumatoid arthritis, inflammatory bowel disease, psoriasis
Interleukin-1 (IL-1)	Macrophages, dendritic cells, fibroblasts, endothelial cells, keratinocytes	Endothelial cells: activation (inflammation, coagulation), similar to TNF Hypothalamus: fever Liver: synthesis of acute-phase proteins T cells: Th17 differentiation	Rheumatoid arthritis, autoinflammatory syndromes (rare genetic diseases)
Interleukin-6 (IL-6)	Macrophages, dendritic cells, T cells	Liver: synthesis of acute-phase protein B cells: proliferation of antibody-producing cells T cells: Th17 differentiation	Rheumatoid arthritis (juvenile and adult)
Chemokines (many)	Virtually all cell types	Recruitment of leukocytes from the circulation into tissues Maintenance of lymphoid tissue architecture (segregation of T and B cells in secondary lymphoid organs)	Inflammatory bowel disease (in clinical trials)
Cytokines in Chronic Inflammation			
Interleukin-2 (IL-2)	T cells (mainly CD4+ helper T cells)	T cells: proliferation and differentiation into effector and memory cells; promotes regulatory T-cell development, survival, and function	Anti-IL-2 receptor used to prevent acute organ transplant rejection
Interleukin-4 (IL-4)	CD4+ T cells (Th2), mast cells	B cells: isotype switching to IgE T cells: Th2 differentiation, proliferation Macrophages: alternative activation Role in allergic inflammation	Asthma, atopic dermatitis
Interleukin-5 (IL-5)	CD4+ T cells (Th2)	Eosinophils: activation, increased generation Role in allergic inflammation	Asthma
Interleukin-12 (IL-12)	Macrophages, dendritic cells	T cells: Th1 differentiation NK cells and T cells: IFN-γ synthesis	
Interleukin-17	CD4+ T cells (Th17)	Epithelial cells, macrophages, and other cell types: increased chemokine and cytokine production; GM-CSF and G-CSF production → recruitment and activation of neutrophils	Psoriasis; some effect in multiple sclerosis
Interferon-γ (IFN-γ)	T cells (Th1, CD8+ T cells), NK cells	Macrophages: classical activation (increased microbicidal functions) T cells: Th1 differentiation	Hemophagocytic syndromes
Interleukin-10 (IL-10)	Macrophages, T cells (mainly regulatory T cells)	Macrophages, dendritic cells: inhibition Role in termination of inflammation	
Transforming growth factor-β (TGF-β)	T cells, macrophages, other cell types	T cells: inhibition of proliferation and effector functions; differentiation of Th17 and Treg Macrophages: inhibition of activation; stimulation of angiogenic factors Fibroblasts: increased collagen synthesis	

[a]Specific for the cytokine or its receptor.

Pentraxins are plasma proteins that include C-reactive protein (CRP) and serum amyloid protein (see below). They recognize phospholipids expressed on bacterial membranes (and apoptotic cells) and promote phagocytosis or activate the complement system, thus causing the elimination of these microbes and dead cells. The plasma levels of these proteins increase during the acute-phase response that accompanies inflammatory reactions, discussed later. *Kinins* are produced from circulating precursor proteins and contribute to vascular dilation and pain at the site of inflammation.

The four major features of inflammation (initially described in the 1st century AD by the Roman encyclopedist Celsus), *rubor* (redness), *calor* (warmth), *tumor* (swelling), and *dolor* (pain), can be explained by the actions of particular mediators (Table 2.6). A fifth sign, loss of function, was added later.

Because of their essential role in the inflammatory process, drugs that inhibit mediators are part of the physician's armamentarium (see Tables 2.4 and 2.5). Most of these drugs block the production or function of individual mediators. An exception is corticosteroids that are widely used to suppress inflammation, which are thought to inhibit the synthesis of arachidonic acid–derived mediators (by inhibiting phospholipase A$_2$), as well as the production of multiple cytokines. Lymphocytes are also sensitive to corticosteroid-induced apoptosis, an effect that is useful in treating various autoimmune disorders as well as lymphocytic malignancies.

Clinicopathologic Features of Acute Inflammation

Acute inflammatory reactions show distinct morphologic patterns that are typically associated with different inciting conditions and clinical manifestations (Table 2.7).

Morphology. Special morphologic patterns are often superimposed on the general features of acute inflammation (vasodilation, leukocyte recruitment, and edema), depending on the severity of the reaction, its specific cause, and the particular tissue and site involved. The importance of recognizing the gross and microscopic patterns is that they often provide valuable clues about the underlying cause.

- In *serous inflammation* (Fig. 2.4), exuded fluid is cell poor and it accumulates in body cavities such as the pleura or pericardium (forming an effusion) or under epithelia such as the skin (forming blisters or vesicles). This reaction is typical of mild injury (e.g., thermal burns of skin), infections that damage the adjacent tissue (such as pleuritis accompanying pneumonia) or relatively nondestructive infections (such as viral pericarditis). The fluid is resorbed when the inflammation subsides.
- *Fibrinous inflammation,* like serous inflammation, occurs on the surface of organs such as the lung or heart, but in this case the vascular leaks are large and hence, the exudate contains large-molecular-weight plasma proteins such as fibrinogen and coagulation pathway factors, which become activated and convert fibrinogen to insoluble fibrin clot. Fibrin is deposited on the surface of the organ (Fig. 2.5), and may either be removed by enzymatic lysis (called *resolution)* or, if extensive, be replaced by scar tissue that can cause significant functional impairment. Replacement of fibrinous exudate by scar tissue is called *organization.*
- *Purulent (suppurative) inflammation* is characterized by destructive inflammation leading to the formation of *pus,* a liquefied collection of dead tissues and neutrophils. It is most often caused by infections by pyogenic (pus-producing) bacteria that elicit a neutrophil exudate.
- An *abscess* is a localized collection of purulent inflammation (Fig. 2.6) with central necrosis and acute inflammation often surrounded by inflammatory cells and scar tissue (if it is chronic). Abscesses may form in any organ as a result of seeding by bacteria or lodging of septic emboli. Because they are poorly vascularized, they may have to be drained surgically for healing to occur.
- An *ulcer* (Fig. 2.7) is a localized defect in the surface of a tissue, usually as a result of necrosis and loss of the epithelium, as in the stomach or duodenum (often caused by *Helicobacter pylori* infection and exacerbated by gastric acid), or in the extremities (often seen in diabetics because of reduced blood supply, or as bed sores in elderly individuals because of prolonged immobility and pressure). Most ulcers show features of acute and chronic inflammation. Healing of ulcers requires treatment of the underlying condition.

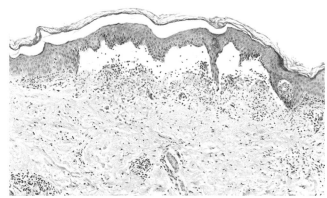

Fig. 2.4 Serous inflammation. Low-power view of a cross section of a skin blister showing the epidermis separated from the dermis by a focal collection of pale pink-staining or clear serous effusion.

Table 2.6 Role of Mediators in Cardinal Features of Acute Inflammation

Feature	Mechanism
Redness *(rubor)*	Vasodilation (caused by histamine, prostaglandins) and stasis of blood (erythema in the skin, congestion in parenchymal organs)
Warmth *(calor)*	Increased blood flow in the affected organ
Swelling *(tumor)*	Exudation of fluid due to increased vascular permeability (caused by histamine, prostaglandins); leakage of fibrinogen and formation of fibrin deposits in extravascular tissue (responsible for induration in chronic inflammatory reactions)
Pain *(dolor)*	Action of prostaglandins and kinins on sensory nerve endings

Table 2.7 Patterns of Acute Inflammation

Type of Inflammation	Morphology	Examples of Diseases
Serous	Accumulation of cell-poor fluid exudate	Pleuritis, pericarditis, mild burns, skin diseases (pemphigus)
Fibrinous	Deposition of fibrin	Pericarditis, meningitis, pleuritis
Suppurative (purulent)	Necrosis with accumulation of leukocytes and formation of pus (containing dead leukocytes and tissue cells)	Bacterial pneumonias, appendicitis, abscesses
Ulcer	Epithelial defect with underlying acute and chronic inflammation	Gastric ulcer, diabetic ulcer, venous and arterial ulcers (typically in lower extremities)

Systemic Manifestations

Acute inflammation is usually accompanied by systemic manifestations that may cause clinical problems and provide valuable diagnostic clues (Table 2.8).

Inflammation, even if it is localized, may be associated with cytokine-induced systemic reactions that are collectively called the

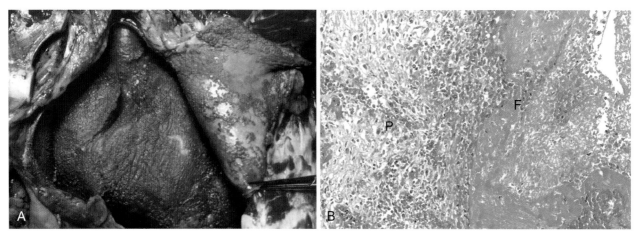

Fig. 2.5 Fibrinous pericarditis. (A) Deposits of fibrin on the pericardium. (B) A pink meshwork of fibrin *(F)* overlies the pericardial surface *(P)*.

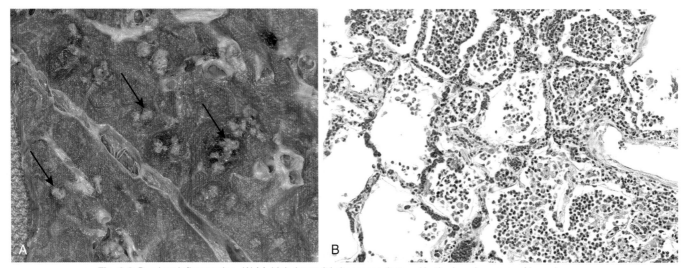

Fig. 2.6 Purulent inflammation. (A) Multiple bacterial abscesses *(arrows)* in the lung in a case of bronchopneumonia. (B) The abscess contains neutrophils and cellular debris resulting from destruction of alveoli, and is surrounded by congested blood vessels. Alveolar destruction is seen in the lower right corner. Above left shows intensely congested alveolar walls and intra-alveolar exudate.

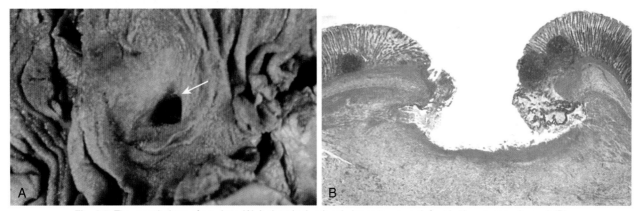

Fig. 2.7 The morphology of an ulcer. (A) A chronic duodenal ulcer seen as a defect in the mucosa *(arrow)*. (B) Low-power cross-sectional view of a duodenal ulcer crater with an acute and chronic inflammatory exudate in the base.

Table 2.8 Systemic Manifestations of Inflammation

	Mechanism	Clinical Features
Fever	Cytokines (IL-1, TNF) stimulate prostaglandin production in the hypothalamus, act on body temperature control center	In severe cases, increased body temperature can cause mental disturbances and coma Treated with NSAIDs
Leukocytosis	Initially, TNF stimulates release of leukocytes from the bone marrow. Later, colony-stimulating factors (GM-CSF, G-CSF) produced by activated macrophages and T cells act on hemopoietic stem cells in bone marrow and stimulate production of neutrophils and monocytes	Marker for inflammation; not by itself a cause of clinical problems
Increased plasma levels of acute-phase proteins	Increased liver synthesis in response to cytokines (IL-6, IL-1, TNF)	C-reactive protein: marker of inflammation Fibrinogen: increases erythrocyte sedimentation rate Serum amyloid protein: may lead to amyloidosis in prolonged, chronic inflammation
Hypotension, disseminated intravascular coagulation, generalized edema, organ failure	High levels of TNF and other cytokines → vasodilation, increased procoagulant activity of endothelium	Life-threatening complication of disseminated infections and other causes of severe acute inflammation (burns, acute pancreatitis)

G-CSF, Granulocyte colony-stimulating factor; *GM-CSF,* granulocyte-macrophage colony-stimulating factor; *IL-1,* interleukin 1; *NSAID,* nonsteroidal antiinflammatory drug; *TNF,* tumor necrosis factor.

acute-phase response and are manifested by fever, leukocytosis, and increased plasma levels of acute-phase proteins.

Fever is a cytokine response that alters the body temperature set point. The physiologic function of fever remains unclear, but it is a valuable clinical sign in assessing whether an underlying inflammatory process is present. Bacterial products, such as lipopolysaccharide (called exogenous pyrogens), stimulate leukocytes to release cytokines such as IL-1 and TNF (called endogenous pyrogens) that increase the enzymes (cyclooxygenases) that convert arachidonic acid into prostaglandins. In the hypothalamus, the prostaglandins, especially PGE$_2$, stimulate the production of neurotransmitters that reset the temperature set point at a higher level. Nonsteroidal anti-inflammatory drugs (NSAIDs), including aspirin, reduce fever by inhibiting prostaglandin synthesis. Excessive production of IL-1 is associated with periodic fever syndromes, also called autoinflammatory syndromes, some of which are the result of gain-of-function mutations in the Nod-like receptor family of proteins that sense microbes and necrotic cells.

Leukocytosis is an increase in circulating white blood cells that is most often induced by cytokines produced by activated leukocytes. Cytokines stimulate the rapid appearance of leukocytosis (in minutes to hours) by enhancing the release of preformed leukocytes from the marginal pool of the bone marrow, and may also produce a more sustained leukocytosis (over days to weeks) by acting on progenitor cells in the bone marrow to increase leukocyte production. These activities serve to replace cells that die during the inflammatory reaction and to increase the numbers of cells that are available to eliminate the offending agent. White blood cell counts are widely used in the clinic to diagnose inflammation, which is presumed to be of infectious origin until proved otherwise. In acute inflammation, the most prominent increase is in blood neutrophils, which, in severe cases, can reach numbers approximating those in leukemias (the so-called leukemoid reaction).

Plasma levels of *acute-phase proteins* rise when the liver is stimulated by cytokines (mainly IL-6) to increase their synthesis. The three main proteins are C-reactive protein (CRP), serum amyloid A (SAA) protein, and fibrinogen. CRP and SAA bind to microbial cell walls and may act as opsonins and fix complement. Fibrinogen binds to red cells and causes them to form stacks (rouleaux) that sediment more rapidly than individual red cells. This is the basis for measuring the erythrocyte sedimentation rate (ESR) as an indicator of inflammation. Another peptide whose production is increased in the acute-phase response is the iron-regulating peptide hepcidin. Chronically elevated plasma concentrations of hepcidin reduce the availability of iron and are responsible for the anemia associated with chronic inflammation (see Chapter 9). Acute-phase proteins have beneficial effects during acute inflammation, but prolonged production of these proteins (especially SAA) in states of chronic inflammation can, in some cases, cause secondary amyloidosis (see Chapter 4).

Severe systemic acute inflammation is seen in *sepsis,* caused by disseminated infections (see Chapter 3), and in the *systemic inflammatory response syndrome,* caused by noninfectious conditions such as severe burns, trauma, and inflammatory reactions such as pancreatitis. The classic clinical triad in these conditions is hypotension, disseminated intravascular coagulation, generalized edema, and metabolic disturbances leading to organ dysfunction, all caused by the massive production of cytokines, principally TNF.

Outcomes of Acute Inflammation

Most acute inflammatory responses have one of three outcomes.

- *Resolution.* The response ends because the stimuli that initiated it (microbes, necrotic cells) are eliminated. Because most of the cells and molecules in inflammation are short lived and need stimulation to be active, once the offending agents are no longer present the reaction subsides. Typically, there is minimal tissue destruction, hence the normal tissue structure is retained.
- *Organization.* Some types of acute inflammation are replaced by fibrosis (scarring), described in more detail later.
- *Progression to chronic inflammation* may occur if the stimulus is persistent and cannot be eliminated. In most instances, however,

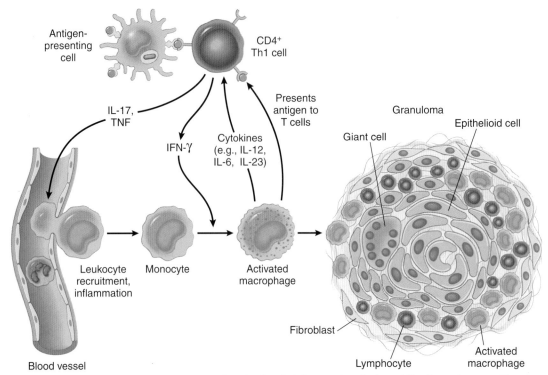

Fig. 2.8 Macrophage–lymphocyte interactions in chronic inflammation. Activated T cells produce cytokines that recruit macrophages (tumor necrosis factor *[TNF]*, interleukin 17 *[IL-17]*, chemokines) and others that activate macrophages (interferon gamma *[IFN-γ]*). Activated macrophages in turn stimulate T cells by presenting antigens and via cytokines such as IL-12. Prolonged activation of macrophages may lead to the formation of granulomas.

chronic inflammation is a distinct reaction that does not necessarily follow an acute phase.

CHRONIC INFLAMMATION

Chronic inflammation is a prolonged reaction to persistent stimuli in which inflammation, tissue injury, and scarring usually coexist.

Chronic inflammation develops in the setting of persistent infections (e.g., tuberculosis), autoimmune diseases (e.g., rheumatoid arthritis, multiple sclerosis), and prolonged exposure to toxic agents that may be exogenous (e.g., silica particles) or endogenous (e.g., cholesterol crystals). In many cases, there is a strong component of adaptive immunity, especially activation of cytokine-producing T cells, which contribute to the persistent and prominent activation of other leukocytes, especially macrophages. The most frequent causes of chronic inflammation are summarized in Table 2.1.

Cellular Reactions of Chronic Inflammation
Chronic inflammatory reactions are dominated by infiltration of mononuclear cells.

Chronic inflammatory reactions develop as a consequence of prolonged bidirectional interactions between macrophages, T lymphocytes, and other immune cells (Fig. 2.8).

Macrophages are the central cells of chronic inflammation. They are activated by cytokines produced by T cells, mostly IFN-γ, and other signals provided by T cells. Persistent innate immune stimulation by Toll-like receptors and other receptors may also contribute. These macrophages have been called classically activated (M1) macrophages (in contrast to alternatively activated [M2] macrophages, which are involved in tissue repair, discussed later).

The macrophages try to destroy or wall off the offending agent by producing NO, lysosomal enzymes, and cytokines that recruit more leukocytes.

T lymphocytes are activated by microbial protein antigens, environmental chemicals (which sometimes bind to and modify self proteins), and self antigens (in autoimmune diseases). Macrophages and dendritic cells display these antigens to T cells and respond to signals from the T cells. Subsets of activated T cells produce many cytokines that contribute to inflammation:

- *IFN-γ* activates macrophages.
- *IL-5* activates eosinophils.
- *IL-17* stimulates the production of chemokines that recruit neutrophils.
- *TNF* activates endothelial cells and promotes recruitment of leukocytes (as in acute inflammation).

Other cells in chronic inflammatory reactions include plasma cells. If there are superimposed episodes of acute inflammation, neutrophils also may be prominent.

Chronic inflammation is accompanied by tissue injury and repair occurring at the same time.

Tissue injury is caused by the numerous mediators that macrophages produce in the attempt to eliminate the offending agent. When the response is strong and prolonged, there is often considerable damage to otherwise healthy tissues at the site of inflammation.

Repair of injured tissues often accompanies chronic inflammation. Proliferation of blood vessels (angiogenesis) and fibrosis are induced by growth factors and cytokines, notably vascular endothelial growth factor (VEGF) and TGF-β, produced by the activated macrophages. This process is discussed later in the context of tissue repair.

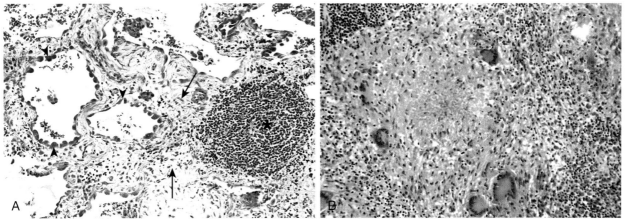

Fig. 2.9 Chronic inflammation. (A) Chronic inflammation in the lung, showing all three characteristic histologic features: (1) collection of chronic inflammatory cells (*), (2) destruction of parenchyma (normal alveoli are replaced by spaces lined by cuboidal epithelium, *arrowheads*), and (3) replacement by connective tissue (fibrosis, *arrows*). (B) Typical tuberculous granuloma showing an area of central necrosis surrounded by multiple Langhans-type giant cells, epithelioid cells, and lymphocytes.

Clinicopathologic Features of Chronic Inflammation

Chronic inflammation underlies many important diseases.

Some of the most vexing diseases of humans, such as pulmonary fibrosis, atherosclerotic coronary artery disease, liver cirrhosis, end-stage renal disease, and various autoimmune and allergic diseases, are caused at least in part by chronic inflammation. Despite impressive advances in immunotherapy for some of these diseases, they remain important clinical challenges and major causes of morbidity and mortality. These disorders are discussed in chapters on the different organ systems.

Morphology. Most chronic inflammatory diseases show mononuclear cell (lymphocyte and macrophage) infiltration with fibrosis and tissue injury (Fig. 2.9A). Under some circumstances, such as infection with tubercle bacilli, the reaction may develop a particular morphology referred to as granulomatous inflammation. Granulomas are circumscribed collections of activated macrophages with abundant cytoplasm, called *epithelioid cells* because they have a flattened, epithelium-like shape. Activated macrophages also may fuse to form multinucleate *giant cells* (Fig. 2.9B). Granuloma formation is a classic example of a special type of chronic inflammation in which macrophages are strongly activated either by T cells or by recognition of persistent foreign bodies. Granulomas are seen in only a few conditions, and recognizing their presence has important therapeutic implications. Where tuberculosis is endemic, it may be the most frequent cause of granulomatous inflammation. In the western world, granulomas are more often seen in Crohn disease, a type of inflammatory bowel disease, in sarcoidosis, a rare but protean disease of unknown etiology, and in some fungal diseases such as histoplasmosis.

Systemic Manifestations

The systemic reactions of chronic inflammation are similar to but typically less severe than those of acute inflammation. Fever is common; in fact, recurrent fever and night sweats are a classic manifestation of tuberculosis. In severe and prolonged cases, high levels of TNF may interfere with appetite and increase the catabolism of lipids, resulting in weight loss (called *cachexia* when severe). Infrequently, chronic inflammation is also associated with deposition of amyloid protein in tissues, because the precursor serum amyloid protein is an acute-phase protein whose production increases during inflammation. In some cases of chronic inflammation, such as chronic viral hepatitis, obvious physical signs are absent, and the diagnosis requires laboratory assessment and tissue biopsy.

TISSUE REPAIR

After the offending agent is eliminated and inflammation subsides, damaged tissue is repaired by two processes, regeneration and scarring.

The terms *repair, healing,* and *resolution* are often used interchangeably, although healing generally refers to skin wounds and resolution refers to restoration of normal tissue architecture without scarring. Under different conditions of tissue injury, the repair is mainly by regeneration or scarring (described below and shown in Fig. 2.10). Both processes are triggered by cytokines and growth factors that are produced mainly by macrophages. In some situations, the macrophages that initiate repair belong to the alternatively activated (M2) subset, which produces various antiinflammatory cytokines (to terminate inflammation) and growth factors (to promote repair). One secreted cytokine that can both suppress inflammation and stimulate fibrosis (scarring) is TGF-β.

Regeneration is the proliferation of residual cells to restore the damaged tissue. It occurs when the injured tissue is capable of proliferation or contains stem cells that can differentiate into functional cells, and when the connective tissue stroma is sufficiently intact to provide a scaffold for the architectural restoration. Regeneration is most often seen in epithelia of the skin, intestines, and liver, which have a high proliferative capacity and contain abundant tissue stem cells. Their proliferation is stimulated by growth factors secreted by macrophages and other cells. By contrast, cardiac muscle and neurons are incapable of proliferation and regeneration.

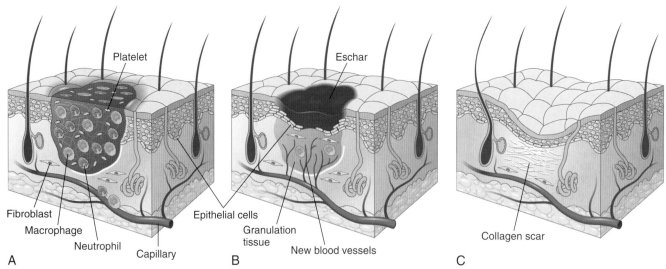

Fig. 2.10 Tissue repair. Following mild injury, which damages the epithelium but not the underlying tissue, resolution occurs by regeneration, but after more severe injury with damage to the connective tissue, repair is by scar formation. Steps in repair by scar formation are shown, specifically during wound healing in the skin. (A) Inflammation and clot formation. (B) Formation of granulation tissue by vessel growth and proliferating fibroblasts. (C) Remodeling to produce the fibrous scar.

Fibrous scar is formed if the tissue is unable to regenerate or if the structural framework is irreversibly damaged. Although a scar lacks the functions of the healthy tissue, it provides adequate structural integrity to maintain some tissue function. Growth factors such as TGF-β and fibroblast growth factor (FGF) are produced by activated macrophages and other cells, and act on fibroblasts in the connective tissue to stimulate their proliferation and collagen synthesis. Concomitantly, VEGF, also produced by macrophages, leads to the formation of new blood vessels that provide nutrition to the proliferating fibroblasts (see below). During the initial 3 to 5 days of repair, the area of injury is filled with newly formed capillaries, macrophages, and fibroblasts embedded in loose extracellular matrix, called *granulation tissue*. The amount of granulation tissue depends on the size of the tissue defect and intensity of inflammation. Gradually, collagen is laid down by the fibroblasts to form the scar, which over time is modified by enzymes in the extracellular matrix through a process called remodeling. This process involves the cross-linking of collagen fibers to strengthen the tissue and subsequent reshaping and partial resorption by matrix metalloproteases. Remodeling leads to structurally strong and well-compacted collagen. Collagen deposited in a peripheral site (limb, skin) is usually called a *scar*, but when it occurs in a parenchymal organ in abnormally large amounts (liver, lung), it is referred to as *fibrosis*. The fundamental underlying processes in all these reactions are essentially the same.

Angiogenesis

Angiogenesis is the process of new blood vessel development from existing vessels. It is not only critical in healing at sites of injury but also in the development of collateral circulations at sites of ischemia and in allowing tumors to increase in size beyond the constraints of their original blood supply. Angiogenesis involves sprouting of new vessels from existing ones and consists of the following steps (Fig. 2.11):

- *Vasodilation* in response to nitric oxide (NO) and increased permeability induced by vascular endothelial growth factor (VEGF)
- *Separation of pericytes* from the abluminal surface and breakdown of the basement membrane to allow formation of a vessel sprout
- *Migration of endothelial cells* toward the area of tissue injury
- *Proliferation of endothelial cells* just behind the leading front (tip) of migrating cells
- *Remodeling* into capillary tubes
- *Recruitment of periendothelial cells* (pericytes for small capillaries and smooth muscle cells for larger vessels) to form the mature vessel
- *Suppression of endothelial proliferation* and deposition of the basement membrane

Clinicopathologic Features of Tissue Repair

The appearance of repaired tissue varies according to the nature and extent of injury.

When the injury is mild, acute, and in a tissue capable of proliferation, it is repaired by cell regeneration, so the edges are closed. Examples include regeneration of the liver and the epithelium of the skin and gut. No scar tissue is formed.

Healing by first intention occurs in a clean, uninfected surgical incision of the skin that is closed with surgical sutures. The wound is initially sealed by a blood clot, followed by the arrival of neutrophils and macrophages and the formation of a small amount of granulation tissue that is replaced by a thin scar. Concomitantly, the surface epithelial cells regenerate and bridge the incisional gap.

Healing by second intention occurs in more severe and deep injuries of the skin, when the edges cannot be closed. The sequence of events is identical to the one described previously, with the exception that the amount of granulation tissue is much larger and persists for a longer period, and, hence, more collagen is laid down and the fibrous scar is thicker. By about 4 to 6 weeks, the skin wound

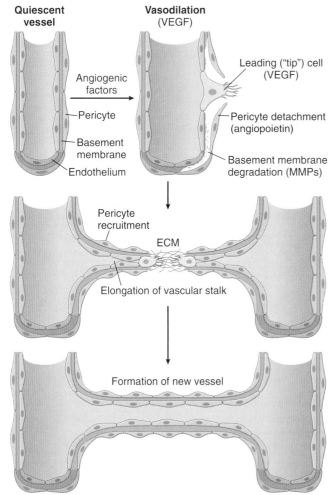

Quiescent vessel

Vasodilation (VEGF)

Angiogenic factors

Leading ("tip") cell (VEGF)

Pericyte

Pericyte detachment (angiopoietin)

Basement membrane

Endothelium

Basement membrane degradation (MMPs)

Pericyte recruitment

ECM

Elongation of vascular stalk

Formation of new vessel

Fig. 2.11 Angiogenesis. In tissue repair, angiogenesis occurs mainly by the sprouting of new vessels. The steps in the process, and the major signals involved, are illustrated. The newly formed vessel joins up with other vessels (not shown) to form the new vascular bed. *ECM*, extracellular matrix; *MMP*, matrix metalloproteinases; *VEGF*, vascular endothelial growth factor.

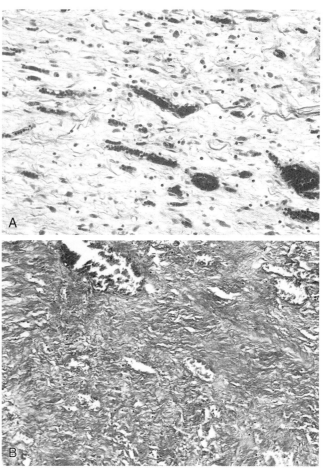

Fig. 2.12 Tissue repair. (A) Granulation tissue showing numerous blood vessels, edema, and a loose extracellular matrix containing occasional inflammatory cells. Collagen is stained blue by the trichrome stain; minimal mature collagen can be seen at this point. (B) Trichrome stain of mature scar, showing dense collagen, with only scattered vascular channels.

contracts because of the action of myofibroblasts in the connective tissue, shrinking the area of injury (Fig. 2.12).

Repair can be impaired by numerous factors.

These include:

• *Mechanical factors* such as excessive movement or pressure
• *Infection,* which prolongs the inflammation and causes progressive tissue injury
• *Diabetes,* a disease in which healing is retarded because of the underlying metabolic abnormality and vascular narrowing, leading to a reduced blood supply. Furthermore, diabetics are susceptible to infections because of decreased neutrophil function and impaired

cytokine production by macrophages. Diabetic skin ulcers do not heal normally and contain extensive granulation tissue.

• *Compromised blood supply,* which can cause ulcers in the lower extremities.

In contrast to these situations of defective repair, there are conditions in which the repair process becomes excessive. This can give rise to hypertrophic scars following injury, which usually regress slowly, and scar tissue that grows beyond the margins of the injury and fails to regress, called keloid (Supplemental eFig. 2.1). Excessive scarring in organs results in functional compromise and is the basis of serious disorders such as pulmonary fibrosis (Chapter 10) and cirrhosis of the liver (Chapter 13).

3

Hemodynamic Disorders, Thromboembolism, and Shock

OUTLINE

Hyperemia, Congestion, and Edema, 30
   Edema, 30
Hemostasis and Hemorrhage, 31
   Platelets, 32
   Coagulation Cascade, 33
   Coagulation Control, 34
Thrombosis, 35

Embolism, 36
   Pulmonary Thromboembolism, 37
   Systemic Thromboembolism, 37
   Nonthrombotic Emboli, 37
Infarction, 37
Shock, 38
   Septic Shock, 39

The health of tissues depends on adequate blood circulation, which delivers oxygen and nutrients and removes carbon dioxide and metabolic waste products. Blood has two major constituents: cellular elements made in the marrow (white cells, red cells, and platelets) and a fluid phase (plasma), consisting of water, inorganic salts, organic metabolites, and numerous proteins, most of which are made by the liver. Important plasma proteins include albumin, the most abundant protein in plasma; immunoglobulins and components of the complement system (discussed in Chapter 4); and coagulation factors, which upon activation catalyze a series of reactions that cause the blood to clot.

Disorders that disturb normal fluid balances between the blood and tissues or that compromise the integrity or patency of blood vessels are very common, and may cause dysfunction or necrosis of affected tissues. In this chapter, we will first discuss disorders of fluid balance, including the accumulation of excessive fluid within tissues or body cavities and the loss of blood, and then turn to disorders of inadequate or excessive clotting, including pathologic intravascular clotting (thrombosis) and the shedding of clots into the circulation (embolism), and their downstream consequences. We will finish by discussing shock, a disorder with several different causes that have in common a systemic failure of tissue perfusion.

HYPEREMIA, CONGESTION, AND EDEMA

Swelling of tissues may stem from increased blood volume due to hyeperemia or congestion, or from increased fluid within the interstitium, a condition called edema.

Hyperemia is defined by increased flow of arterial blood into a tissue, generally due to arteriolar dilation. It is a normal adaptation to certain environmental challenges (e.g., increased workload in exercising skeletal muscle, or cold in exposed skin). By contrast, congestion is an abnormal process caused by decreased venous outflow from a tissue. Congested tissues have poor blood delivery and are prone to dysfunction and even necrosis. Edema refers to an abnormal accumulation of fluid in tissues. Through similar mechanisms as those that cause edema (described in the following), abnormal fluid accumulations called effusions may also gather in body cavities such as the pleural, pericardial, and peritoneal spaces.

Edema

In normal tissues, endothelial junctions in capillaries are permeable to water and salts and other small molecules, but not to proteins. High intravascular hydrostatic pressure tends to push water and salts into the tissues, but this is nearly balanced by osmotic pressure, which is generated by plasma proteins and pulls water back into the vessels (Fig. 3.1). The small amount of fluid that does accumulate in normal tissues is taken up by lymphatic vessels and returned to the circulation through the thoracic duct.

Edema and effusions may occur with increased hydrostatic pressure, decreased osmotic pressure, or lymphatic obstruction. Common causes are listed in Table 3.1. Note that some factors cause fluid accumulations through several direct or indirect effects.

- *Inflammation* (discussed in Chapter 2) promotes edema by increasing both blood flow and vascular permeability to proteins. The protein-rich fluid of inflammation is referred to as an *exudate,* whereas protein-poor noninflammatory edema fluid is referred to as a *transudate.*
- *Cardiac failure,* which takes two forms:
  - *Right-sided cardiac failure* causes passive venous congestion in the systemic circulation, raising the hydrostatic pressure in the microcirculation, which in turn causes egress of protein-poor fluid in the interstitium, resulting in subcutaneous edema.
  - *Left-sided cardiac failure* is a common cause of pulmonary edema and pleural effusion and also diminishes the blood supply to the kidney, which responds by increasing renin production. Renin activates angiotensin, thereby increasing arteriolar smooth muscle tone and stimulating the production of aldosterone by the adrenal cortex, which promotes reabsorption of sodium and water by the kidney. The retention of sodium and water increases the hydrostatic pressure, often worsening edema throughout the body.

Morphology. Edema is easily recognized. Tissues (particularly the subcutaneous tissue, lungs, and brain) are swollen and heavy. Subcutaneous edema is accentuated in dependent parts of the body (e.g., the sacrum in recumbent patients and the feet following prolonged sitting or standing). Pulmonary edema is marked by heavy lungs, which release frothy, blood-tinged fluid when cut. Brain edema, if generalized, leads to the narrowing of sulci because of compression of the swollen gyri against the skull. **Anasarca** (generalized edema) is seen in chronic heart failure. By contrast, the edema that accompanies renal failure sometimes preferentially affects loose tissues (e.g., the eyelids). Various forms of heart failure are associated with congestion as well as edema. In patients with severe right-sided heart failure, congestion produces necrosis of the hepatic lobules (**centrilobular necrosis**). The gross appearance is known as nutmeg liver (Fig. 3.2). In left-sided heart failure, pulmonary congestion produces blood-engorged capillaries, interstitial edema, and the presence of hemosiderin-laden intraalveolar macrophages (**heart failure cells**), the latter stemming from small bleeds.

Clinical Features. The clinical effects of fluid accumulations vary widely depending on their size and location. Subcutaneous edema may signal an important underlying disorder (e.g., heart or kidney failure) and if severe may interfere with wound healing and clearance of infections. Pulmonary edema impairs gas exchange (potentially exacerbating underlying conditions such as heart failure) and also increases the risk of infections. Brain edema may be fatal since the brain cannot expand within the enclosed skull. Increases in CNS pressure may compromise the blood supply to the brain or cause herniation through the foramen magnum, injuring medullary centers that control respiration (see Chapter 17).

HEMOSTASIS AND HEMORRHAGE

Hemorrhage is caused by injuries that disrupt blood vessels, allowing blood to extravasate into tissues or outside of the body. It represents failure of hemostasis.

The integrity of blood vessels may be disrupted by trauma or disorders that destroy vessel walls (e.g., vasculitis, erosion by cancers). Disorders that impair blood clotting exacerbate bleeding tendencies, even in the absence of obvious trauma.

The terms listed describe bleeds according to their size and appearance:

- *Hematoma* describes a bleed into tissues and may range from skin bruises to fatal intracerebral hemorrhages (Fig. 3.3).
- *Petechiae* are pinpoint, 1- to 2-mm bleeds into the skin, mucous membranes, or serosal surfaces (see Fig. 3.3), usually seen in patients with inadequate platelet function.

Table 3.1 Causes of Edema and Effusions

Increased Hydrostatic Pressure
Impaired Venous Return
Congestive heart failure
Constrictive pericarditis
Liver cirrhosis (ascites)
Venous obstruction or compression (e.g., by a mass)
Venous thrombosis
Lower extremity inactivity with prolonged dependency
Sodium retention (e.g., renal failure, left-sided heart failure)
Sodium Retention
Renal failure
Left-sided heart failure
Arteriolar Dilation
Inflammation
Reduced Osmotic Pressure
Protein-losing glomerulopathies (nephrotic syndrome)
Liver failure
Malnutrition
Protein-losing gastroenteropathy
Lymphatic Obstruction
Inflammatory
Neoplastic
Postsurgical
Postirradiation

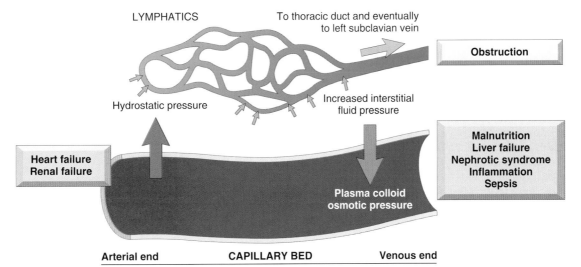

Fig. 3.1 Factors influencing fluid movement across capillary walls. Capillary hydrostatic and osmotic forces are normally balanced, so there is little net movement of fluid into the interstitium. What little fluid accumulates is cleared by lymphatic drainage. Edema may result when hydrostatic pressures rise (as in renal failure or heart failure), osmotic pressures fall (as in malnutrition, liver failure, or nephrotic syndrome), vascular permeability increases (as with inflammation or sepsis), or lymphatic vessels are obstructed.

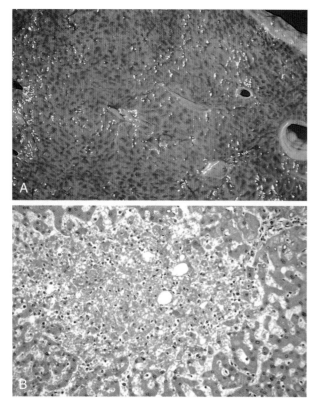

Fig. 3.2 Liver with chronic passive congestion and hemorrhagic necrosis. (A) In this autopsy specimen, central areas are red and slightly depressed compared with the surrounding tan viable parenchyma, creating "nutmeg liver" (so called because it resembles the cut surface of a nutmeg). (B) Microscopic preparation shows centrilobular hepatic necrosis with hemorrhage and scattered inflammatory cells. (Courtesy of Dr. James Crawford, Hofstra/Northwell School of Medicine, Hempstead, NY.)

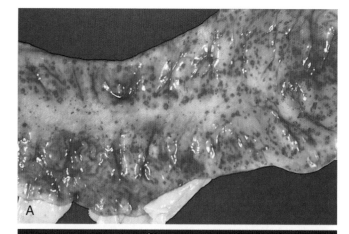

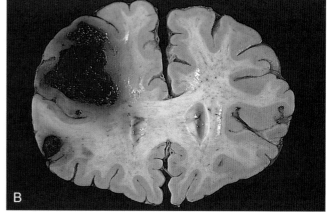

Fig. 3.3 (A) Punctate petechial hemorrhages of the colonic mucosa, a consequence of thrombocytopenia. (B) Fatal intracerebral hemorrhage.

- *Purpura* are 3- to 5-mm bleeds that may stem from defects in platelet function, trauma, vascular inflammation, or vascular fragility.
- *Ecchymoses* are 1-2 cm in size and correspond to "bruises"; they are usually caused by trauma.

Hemostasis, the clotting of blood following blood vessel trauma, is essential for life.

Under normal circumstances, blood clotting occurs at sites where the walls of blood vessels have been physically disrupted. The initial steps in clot formation are two mutually reinforcing processes (Fig. 3.4):

- *Primary hemostasis* is initiated by the exposure of subendothelial collagen and von Willebrand factor (vWF) within injured vessel walls. These factors lead to the adhesion and activation of platelets, which form a platelet-rich plug.
- *Secondary hemostasis* is triggered by the exposure of tissue factor within the subendothelium and tissues. Tissue factor acts in conjunction with factor VII (described later) to initiate the coagulation cascade, which uses cofactors that are present on the surfaces of activated platelets and leads to the deposition of fibrin. Fibrin reinforces and stabilizes the platelet plug, sealing the area of vascular damage and preventing further bleeding.

Once a clot has formed, its extent must be limited to the area of damage. This is mediated by counterregulatory mechanisms, which we will discuss later in this chapter.

Platelets

Platelets are anucleate fragments derived from megakaryocytes that form the primary hemostatic plug and provide a procoagulant surface that promotes secondary hemostasis.

Platelet function depends on surface glycoprotein receptors, a contractile cytoskeleton, and cytoplasmic granules that contain a number of procoagulant substances. In the setting of vascular injury, platelets undergo a series of stereotypic events:

- *Adhesion.* Platelet adhesion is mediated largely by interactions with vWF, which acts as a bridge between exposed subendothelail collagen and platelet surface receptor glycoprotein 1b (Gp1b).
- *Activation.* Platelets change shape from smooth discs to spiky spheres and release the contents of their granules, which include coagulation cofactors (calcium, factor V) and platelet activators such as adenosine diphosphate (ADP), which recruit other platelets to the growing platelet plug.
- *Aggregation.* The shape change associated with activation exposes negatively charged phospholipids, which are required by certain coagulation factors (described later), and also alters the conformation of surface glycoprotein IIb/IIIa (GpIIb/IIIa), converting IIb/IIIa to a high-affinity receptor for fibrinogen. Bivalent bridging interactions involving IIb/IIIa receptors and fibrinogen then cause platelets to clump into aggregates.

Deficiencies of GpIb, IIb/IIIa, or vWF are associated with abnormal bleeding (Fig. 3.5).

A. VASOCONSTRICTION

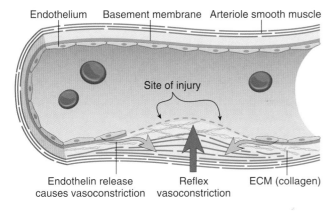

B. PLATELET ACTIVATION AND AGGREGATION

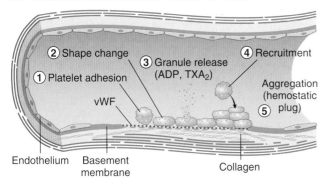

C. ACTIVATION OF CLOTTING FACTORS AND FORMATION OF FIBRIN

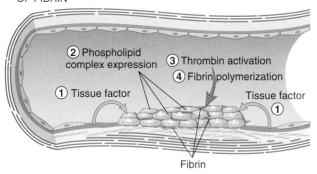

Fig. 3.4 Normal hemostasis. (A) After vascular injury, local neurohumoral factors induce a transient vasoconstriction. (B) Platelets bind via glycoprotein Ib (GpIb) receptors to von Willebrand factor (vWF) on exposed extracellular matrix and are activated, undergoing a shape change and a granule release. Released adenosine diphosphate (ADP) and thromboxane A₂ *(TxA₂)* induce additional platelet aggregation through platelet GpIIb-IIIa receptor binding to fibrinogen, and form the primary hemostatic plug. (C) Local activation of the coagulation cascade (involving tissue factor and platelet phospholipids) results in fibrin polymerization, "cementing" the platelets into a definitive *secondary* hemostatic plug. *ECM,* extracellular matrix.

Platelet aggregation occurs in parallel with coagulation factor activation, and the two systems work together. Most notably, thrombin, the protease that cleaves fibrinogen to create fibrin, also cleaves a protease-activated receptor on the surface of platelets, triggering signals that augment platelet activation and aggregation. Another factor

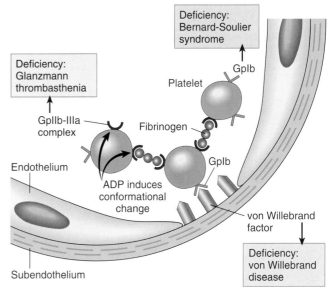

Fig. 3.5 Platelet adhesion and aggregation. vWF functions as an adhesive bridge between subendothelial collagen and the glycoprotein Ib (GpIb) platelet receptor. Platelet aggregation is accomplished by fibrinogen binding to platelet GpIIb-IIIa receptors on different platelets. Congenital deficiencies in the various receptors or bridging molecules lead to the diseases indicated in the colored boxes. *ADP,* Adenosine diphosphate.

released by activated platelets is thromboxane A₂, a potent agonist of platelet aggregation. Aspirin's antiplatelet effects are due to its irreversible inhibition of *cyclooxygenase,* an enzyme required for thromboxane A₂ synthesis.

Coagulation Cascade

The coagulation cascade is a series of enzymatic reactions that culminate in the deposition of fibrin. In the laboratory, the cascade has two initiation points, one involving factor XII (contact factor) and the second one involving factor VII (Fig. 3.6).

- *The intrinsic pathway* starts with factor XII and is initiated in the laboratory by the addition of negatively charged material such as glass beads, along with calcium and phospholipids, to plasma. The time until the formation of a fibrin clot is recorded as the partial thromboplastin time (PTT).
- *The extrinsic pathway* starts with factor VII and is initiated by the addition of tissue factor, calcium, and phospholipids to plasma. Calcium is a cofactor for prothrombin and factors VII, IX, and X, all of which contain specially modified glutamate residues that bind calcium, whereas phospholipids (provided by platelets in the body) are required by factor IX and factor X complexes. The time until the formation of a fibrin clot is recorded as the prothrombin time (PT). The key steps in the coagulation cascade, common to both pathways are:
  - conversion of factor X to activated factor X (Xa), which is mediated by a complex of factor IXa and factor VIIIa
  - conversion of prothrombin to thrombin by a complex of factor Xa and Va
  - conversion of fibrinogen to fibrin mediated by thrombin
- The elements shared by the extrinsic and intrinsic pathways (factor X, cofactor factor V, prothrombin, and fibrinogen) comprise the common pathway.

The PT and the PTT are useful for evaluating the coagulation factor function but do not recapitulate the events that lead to clotting in vivo.

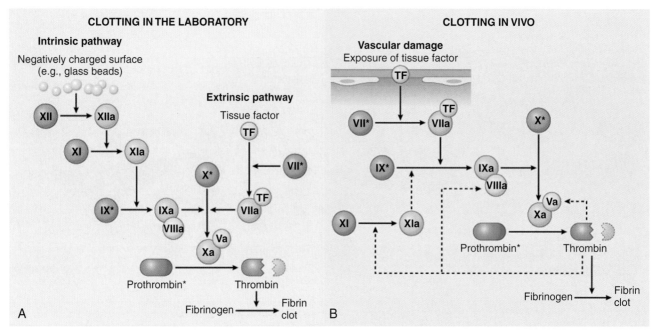

Fig. 3.6 The coagulation cascade in the laboratory and in vivo. (A) Clotting is initiated in the laboratory by adding phospholipids, calcium, and either a negative charged substance such as glass beads (intrinsic pathway) or a source of tissue factor (extrinsic pathway). (B) In vivo, tissue factor is the major initiator of coagulation, which is amplified by feedback loops involving thrombin *(dotted lines)*. The *red* polypeptides are inactive factors, the *dark green* polypeptides are active factors, and the *light green* polypeptides correspond to cofactors. Factors marked with an asterisk (*) are vitamin K dependent, as are proteins C and S (not depicted). Warfarin acts as an anticoagulant by inhibiting the γ-carboxylation of the vitamin K–dependent coagulation factors. Vitamin K is an essential cofactor for the synthesis of all of these vitamin K–dependent clotting factors.

For example, rare patients with factor XII deficiency do not bleed, whereas patients with factor XI deficiency have a mild bleeding disorder. In contrast, deficiencies of other factors are associated with severe bleeding disorders (the hemophilias [see Chapter 9]) or are incompatible with life. This suggests that the major initiator of coagulation in vivo is tissue factor, and that tissue factor/factor VII complexes act in vivo by activating factor IX rather than factor X (Fig. 3.6).

Coagulation Control

Once the activation of coagulation factors and platelets commences, it must be confined to the immediate site of injury to prevent serious consequences. This involves a number of negative regulators, the most important of which are constitutively produced by intact normal endothelium cells near the site of injury. These endothelium-derived anticoagulants include surface molecules that inhibit or inactivate various clotting factors, as well as platelet inhibitors and soluble factors that promote the dissolution of clot (Fig. 3.7).

Remarkably, several of the most important counter-regulatory mechanisms involving normal endothelium are activated by thrombin, which becomes an anticoagulant as it is washed away from areas of vascular damage. One way that this occurs is through binding of thrombin to a surface protein on endothelium called

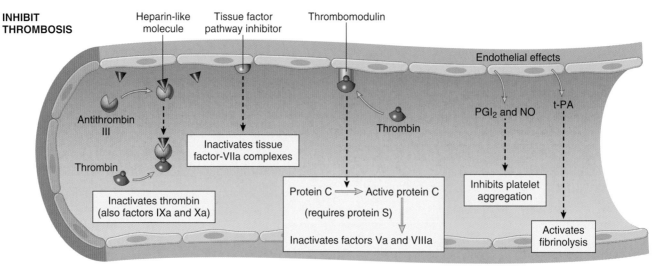

Fig. 3.7 Anticoagulant properties of normal endothelium. Highlighted are multiple inhibitors of the coagulation cascade that are expressed on (heparin-like molecules, thrombomodulin) or secreted from (tissue factor pathway inhibitor) endothelium, as well as secreted inhibitors of platelets (PGI$_2$ and NO) and t-PA (tissue plasminogen activator), which stimulates the breakdown of fibrin clot.

thrombomodulin. Bound thrombin no longer is able to cleave fibrinogen and instead acquires the ability to cleave protein C. Protein C and its cofactor, protein S, in turn inactivate factor V, a critical cofactor for factor X. The importance of this reaction is made evident by the increased risk of deep venous thrombosis (DVT) that is seen in patients with a variant of factor V called factor V Leiden, which is resistant to inactivation by protein C. We will return to risk factors for DVT later. Thrombin also cleaves and activates the thrombin receptor on endothelium, stimulating the release of tissue plasminogen activation (t-PA), an important activator of the breakdown of fibrin clots (fibrinolysis).

THROMBOSIS

Thrombosis, the abnormal clotting of blood within intact vessels, is associated with a serious risk of mortality.

Pathogenesis. Thrombosis reflects some abnormality involving the vessel wall, the flow of blood (specifically, stasis or turbulent flow), or blood coagulability, an alteration referred to as hypercoagulability. These three factors make up the *Virchow triad* (Fig. 3.8), named for the famous 18th century pathologist Rudolf Virchow.

- *Abnormalities of the vessel wall (endothelial injury).* In vessels carrying blood at high pressures and under high shear forces, such as the aorta and its major branches, the coronary arteries, and the arteries supplying the CNS, clot formation is most commonly due to atherosclerotic lesions (see Chapter 7). Rupture of atherosclerotic plaques exposes collagen and tissue factor and leads to activation of platelets and coagulation factors. The endothelial abnormalities associated with atherosclerosis lead to the increased expression of procoagulant factors and the decreased expression of anticoagulant factors by endothelial cells, which may contribute to the prothrombotic state seen in atherosclerosis. Trauma or inflammatory processes such as vasculitis that damage vessels also may lead to thrombus formation.
- *Abnormal blood flow.* Turbulence and stasis contribute to thrombosis in the heart and the arterial side of the circulation, whereas stasis is the major factor in the development of venous thrombi. Stasis and turbulent blood flow cause changes in endothelial cell gene expression that favor thrombosis. *Stasis* allows platelets extended contact with the vessel wall, where they may encounter dysfunctional endothelium or areas denuded of endothelium; stasis also slows the

washout of activated coagulation factors and impedes the inflow of clotting factor inhibitors.

Numerous abnormalities affecting the heart and the vessels can lead to stasis or turbulent blood flow: aneurysmal dilations of the heart following myocardial infarction, or of atherosclerotic arteries; left atrial dilation due to mitral stenosis; and atrial fibrillation.

- *Hypercoagulability.* Hypercoagulability is any alteration that renders the blood more prone to thrombosis than normal. The causes may be inherited or acquired (Table 3.2). The most common inherited risk factors include *factor V Leiden* (already mentioned), which is found in 2% to 15% of people of Northern European descent, and a genetic variant that increases plasma levels of prothrombin. Inherited risk factors are associated with thrombosis at a young age; in general, the occurrence of a thrombotic event in an individual less than 50 years of age is an indication for a genetic workup. Even more common are acquired risk factors: age over 50 years, male sex, immobilization, hyperestrogenic states (e.g., pregnancy and use of oral contraceptives), and smoking. Estrogens increase synthesis of procoagulant proteins and reduce formation of anticoagulant proteins in the liver.

Among other causes of hypercoagulable states, two deserve brief mention because of their unique pathogenesis and clinical importance:

- *Heparin-induced thrombocytopenia (HIT) syndrome* occurs in up to 5% of patients treated with unfractionated heparin and a lower fraction of patients treated with low-molecular-weight heparin. HIT is caused by antibodies that bind to complexes composed of heparin and platelet factor 4. Through unclear mechanisms, this leads to platelet activation, platelet consumption, and deposition of platelet-rich clots in the arterial and venous circulation. These

Table 3.2 Hypercoagulable States

Primary (Genetic)
Common (>1% of the Population)
Factor V mutation (factor V Leiden)
Prothrombin mutation
Rare
Antithrombin III deficiency
Protein C deficiency
Protein S deficiency
Secondary (Acquired)
Higher Risk for Thrombosis
Prolonged bed rest or immobilization
Cardiac dysmotility (myocardial infarction, atrial fibrillation)
Tissue injury (surgery, fracture, burn)
Disseminated cancer
Prosthetic cardiac valves
Disseminated intravascular coagulation
Heparin-induced thrombocytopenia
Antiphospholipid antibody syndrome
Lower Risk for Thrombosis
Nephrotic syndrome (due to loss of antithrombin III)
Hyperestrogenic states (during pregnancy and following delivery)
Oral contraceptive use
Sickle cell anemia
Smoking

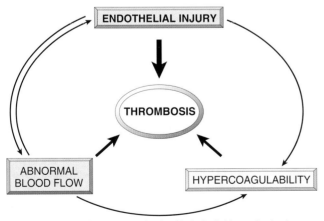

Fig. 3.8 Virchow triad in thrombosis. Endothelial integrity is the most important factor. Abnormalities of procoagulants or anticoagulants can tip the balance in favor of thrombosis. Abnormal blood flow (stasis or turbulence) can lead to hypercoagulability directly and also indirectly through endothelial dysfunction.

clots may lead to loss of limbs or life, and recognition of the HIT syndrome and cessation of heparin therapy are therefore critical.

• *Antiphospholipid antibody syndrome,* associated with recurrent thrombosis, repeated miscarriages, and cardiac valve vegetations, may be an isolated anomaly or secondary to an autoimmune disorder (e.g., systemic lupus erythematosus). The name of this disorder came from the detection of circulating antibodies that bind to phospholipids in the lab. It is believed that the most important pathologic effects in patients are mediated through binding of these antibodies to epitopes on proteins that are somehow induced or "unveiled" by phospholipids. In vivo, it is suspected that these antibodies bind to various proteins and induce a hypercoagulable state through uncertain mechanisms. However, in vitro, the antibodies interfere with phospholipids and thus inhibit coagulation (hence the name *lupus anticoagulant* is a misnomer). The antibodies often cross-react with cardiolipin, a component of the test for syphilis, producing a false-positive result.

Morphology. Arterial thrombi typically overlie atherosclerotic lesions, whereas venous and cardiac thrombi characteristically occur at sites of stasis. At sites of initiation, thrombi are attached to the underlying vessel or cardiac wall. When located in partially obstructed vessels and exposed to flowing blood, thrombi tend to propagate toward the heart (even arterial thrombi, which grow in a retrograde direction). Venous thrombi are particularly likely to propagate some distance, forming long casts within the vessel lumen. The propagating portions are not attached to vessel walls and are prone to fragmentation and embolization.

Microscopically, thrombi have laminations called *lines of Zahn,* which represent alternating pale layers rich in platelets and fibrin, and darker layers rich in red cells. Layered thrombi only form in flowing blood, and the presence of these layers, as well as the firm attachment of the clot to the vessel wall, distinguish antemortem thrombi from postmortem clots. Venous thrombi contain a higher fraction of red cells entrapped in fibrin (red clots) than arterial thrombi. In the days and weeks following an initial thrombotic or embolic event, vascular thrombi may undergo dissolution; continue to shed emboli; or undergo organization (Supplemental eFig. 3.1). In organizing thrombi, the ingrowth of stromal cells and the deposition of extracellular matrix are accompanied by varying degrees of recanalization.

Nonobstructive thrombi occurring in the heart or aorta bear special designations. Thrombi occurring in the heart and the aortic lumen (Fig. 3.9) are referred to as **mural thrombi,** whereas thrombi on heart valves are called **vegetations.** Some vegetations occur in hypercoagulable states and are sterile, but others are caused by bacterial or fungal infections (infective endocarditis; see Chapter 8) and may lead to the development of large thrombotic masses.

Clinical Features. Clinical symptoms caused by thrombi are due to the obstruction of vessels and clot embolization and vary according to the vessels and organs that are affected. The most feared complication of thrombi is embolization (discussed later), whereas thrombi in smaller arteries are occlusive and hence more likely to cause a local infarction due to obstruction of the blood supply to organs such as the heart and the brain. The relationship between arterial thrombosis, atherosclerosis, and cardiac disease is discussed in detail in Chapter 8.

More than 90% of venous thromboses occur in the lower extremities. Thrombi in superficial veins rarely embolize, but they may be painful and cause congestion and edema, predisposing the overlying

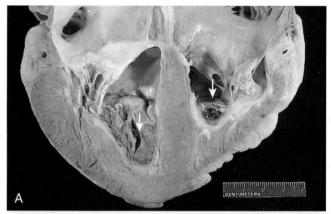

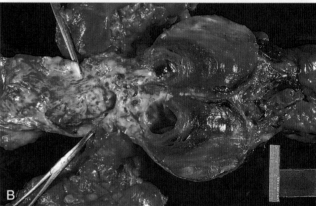

Fig. 3.9 Mural thrombi. (A) Thrombus in the left and right ventricular apices, overlying white fibrous scar. (B) Laminated thrombus in a dilated abdominal aortic aneurysm. Numerous friable mural thrombi are also superimposed on advanced atherosclerotic lesions of the more proximal aorta *(left side of photograph).*

skin to infection and varicose ulcers. By contrast, deep venous thromboses (DVTs) in large leg veins at or above the level of the knee often embolize. DVTs also may cause pain and edema, but collateral venous channels frequently circumvent the obstruction. Consequently, approximately 50% of DVTs are asymptomatic and are recognized only after they have embolized to the lungs.

The clinical importance of thromboembolic disease cannot be overstated. The greatest toll is taken by coronary artery thrombosis secondary to atherosclerosis, which is the major cause of myocardial infarction (heart attack) in the Western world. Emboli shed from the heart and thromboembolic disease due to atherosclerosis of the carotid arteries and other great vessels supplying the central nervous system (CNS) are an important cause of stroke. Pulmonary embolization of DVTs is fatal in approximately 3% of affected patients.

EMBOLISM

An embolus is a detached intravascular solid, liquid, or gaseous mass that is carried by the blood from its point of origin to a distant site, where it may cause vascular obstruction and organ dysfunction or infarction.

The vast majority of emboli are derived from dislodged thrombi; hence, the term *thromboembolism.* Less common types of emboli include fat droplets, bubbles of air or nitrogen, atherosclerotic debris (i.e., cholesterol emboli), tumor fragments, bits of bone marrow, and amniotic fluid. Emboli are transported through the blood from their site of origin until they lodge in the first vessel that is too narrow to permit further passage, where they result in partial or complete occlusion. The major consequence of embolization in most vascular beds is ischemic necrosis *(infarction)* of affected tissues; one exception is the lung, which has a dual blood supply that protects against infarction. Nevertheless, circulatory changes associated with pulmonary thromboembolism often cause significant clinical disease.

Pulmonary Thromboembolism

Pulmonary emboli originate from DVTs and are frequent causes of morbidity and mortality.

Pulmonary emboli cause about 100,000 deaths per year in the United States. In more than 95% of cases, the emboli originate from thrombi within deep leg veins proximal to the knee. Fragmented thrombi from DVTs usually pass through the right side of the heart and become arrested in the pulmonary vasculature. A more complete discussion of pulmonary embolism is found in Chapter 10. The clinical and pathologic features associated with pulmonary emboli vary according to the size and number, as follows:

- *Most pulmonary emboli (60% to 80%) are small and clinically silent.* With time, they undergo organization and either become incorporated into the vascular wall or undergo recanalization, sometimes leaving behind bridging fibrous webs (Supplemental eFig. 3.1).
- *A large embolus* may occlude the main pulmonary artery or lodge at the bifurcation of the right and left pulmonary arteries *(saddle embolus),* sometimes causing virtually instantaneous death.
- *Smaller emboli* may obstruct smaller, branching arteries (Fig. 3.10). The subsequent rupture of capillaries may cause pulmonary hemorrhage, but infarction is uncommon because the area also receives blood through an intact bronchial circulation (dual circulation).
- *Lodging of emboli in the small end-arteriolar pulmonary branches often results in infarction*, particularly in individuals in whom oxygenation of the lung is compromised by congestive heart failure.
- *Multiple small emboli* occurring over time may obstruct a sufficient portion of the pulmonary vascular bed to cause pulmonary hypertension and right ventricular heart failure *(cor pulmonale).*

Rarely, an embolus passes through an atrial or ventricular defect and enters the systemic circulation, where it may cause infarcts by lodging in end-arterial vascular beds in the brain (stroke) or elsewhere (paradoxical embolism).

Systemic Thromboembolism

The most common source of systemic thromboemboli is the heart (80%), followed by atherosclerotic aortic lesions, aortic aneurysms, valvular vegetations, and DVTs (by paradoxical embolization). Most emboli lodge in the lower extremities (75%) or brain (10%), but no organ is spared.

The consequences of embolization depend on the caliber of the occluded vessel, the collateral supply, and the affected tissue's vulnerability to anoxia. Because arterial emboli often lodge in end arteries, infarction is a common outcome.

Nonthrombotic Emboli

In addition to thrombus, emboli may be composed of other substances. These other forms of embolic disease tend to occur in distinct clinical settings:

- *Fat embolism.* Soft tissue crush injuries or fracture of long bones (which have abundant fat in their marrow) can release microscopic fat globules into the circulation, causing fat embolism syndrome in a minority of patients (Supplemental eFig. 3.2). This syndrome is fatal in 10% of cases and is characterized by pulmonary insufficiency, neurologic symptoms, anemia, thrombocytopenia, and petechial bleeding. Both the mechanical obstruction of small vessels and toxic effects of fatty acids released from the lipid globules on nearby endothelial cells cause injury.
- *Amniotic fluid embolism.* Amniotic fluid embolism is a rare but serious complication of labor and delivery (1 in 40,000 births) that has a mortality rate of approximately 80%. It is responsible for 10% of maternal deaths in the United States, and 85% of survivors have permanent neurologic deficits. Amniotic fluid and its contents enter the maternal circulation through tears in the placental membranes or the uterine vein (Supplemental eFig. 3.3). The onset is sudden and is characterized by severe dyspnea, cyanosis, and shock, followed by seizures and coma. The pathogenesis involves activation of components of the innate immune system and coagulation, rather than mechanical obstruction. If the patient survives the initial crisis, disseminated intravascular coagulation (Chapter 9) often develops secondary to the release of thrombogenic substances in amniotic fluid.
- *Air embolism.* Gas bubbles within the circulation can coalesce and obstruct vascular flow, causing distal ischemic injury. Gas may be introduced into the vasculature accidentally during surgical, obstetric, or laparoscopic procedures; following a severe chest wall injury; or as a consequence of sudden decreases in the atmospheric pressure (e.g., when divers surface too rapidly, dissolved nitrogen comes out of solution, forming gas bubbles in the blood and the tissues, a condition known as the bends).

INFARCTION

An infarct is an area of ischemic necrosis caused by occlusion of the vascular supply to the affected tissue; infarction is a common and important cause of clinical disease.

Arterial thromboembolism underlies the vast majority of infarctions. Venous thrombosis can cause infarction, but more commonly, there is simply congestion, as collateral channels open rapidly and restore the arterial inflow. Infarcts caused by venous thrombosis occur in organs with a single efferent vein (e.g., testis or ovary) and typically stem from a mechanical problem (e.g., twisting of a testicle, leading to venous obstruction).

Not all vascular occlusions lead to infarction. Determinants of whether infarction occurs include the following:

- *Anatomy of the vascular supply.* The presence or absence of an alternative blood supply is the most important factor in determining whether occlusion of an individual vessel causes damage. Tissues with dual blood supplies (lung, liver, and hand and forearm) are resistant to infarction, whereas those with end-arterial circulations (heart, kidney, and spleen) are likely to infarct.

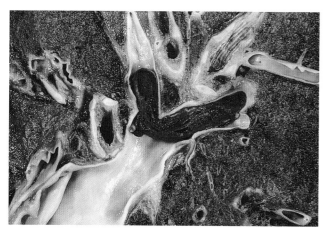

Fig. 3.10 Embolus derived from a lower-extremity deep venous thrombus lodged in a pulmonary artery branch.

- *Rate of occlusion.* Slowly developing occlusions are less likely to cause infarction due to the development of collateral circulations.
- *Cellular vulnerability to hypoxia.* Cells range in their susceptibility to damage from vascular occlusion: Neurons die after only 3 to 4 minutes, myocardial cells can last for 20 to 30 minutes, and fibroblasts remain viable after many hours of ischemia.

Morphology. Infarcts may be either red (hemorrhagic) or white (anemic) and may be either septic or bland. **Red infarcts** (Fig. 3.11A) occur with venous occlusions (as in ovarian torsion); in tissues with collateral blood supplies (e.g., the lung); and following reestablishment of flow after infarction has occurred (e.g., after angioplasty of an arterial obstruction). **White infarcts** occur with arterial occlusions in organs with end-arterial circulations (e.g., heart, spleen, and kidney) (Fig. 3.11B). Infarcts tend to be wedge shaped, with the occluded vessel at the apex and the organ periphery forming the base (Fig. 3.11A); when the base is a serosal surface, there is often an overlying fibrinous exudate.

In most tissues, infarcts display coagulative necrosis (see Chapter 1). Within a few hours, an inflammatory response develops along the margins of infarcts; the lesion is usually well defined within 1 to 2 days. Inflammation is followed by repair, beginning in the preserved margins (see Chapter 2). Most infarcts are ultimately replaced by scar tissue (Fig. 3.12). The brain is an exception to these generalizations, as ischemic tissue injury in the CNS results in liquefactive necrosis followed by gliosis (see Chapter 17).

Septic infarcts occur when infected cardiac valve vegetations embolize or when microbes seed necrotic tissue. In these cases, the infarct is converted into an abscess, with a greater inflammatory response and healing by organization and fibrosis (see Chapter 2).

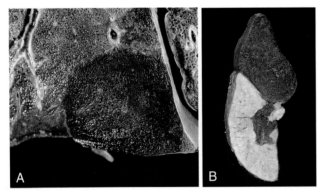

Fig. 3.11 Red and white infarcts. (A) Hemorrhagic, roughly wedge-shaped pulmonary infarct *(red infarct)*. (B) Sharply demarcated pale infarct in the spleen *(white infarct)*.

SHOCK

Shock is a state in which diminished cardiac output or effective circulating volume causes a fall in blood pressure, resulting in diminished tissue perfusion and consequent cellular hypoxia.

Prolonged shock eventually leads to irreversible tissue injury and is often fatal. Its causes fall into several categories (Table 3.3):

- *Cardiogenic shock* results from cardiac pump failure. It may be caused by myocardial damage (infarction), ventricular arrhythmias,

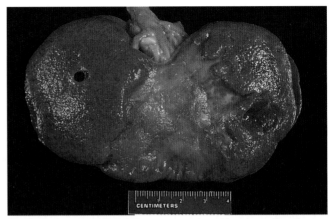

Fig. 3.12 Remote kidney infarct, now replaced by a large fibrotic scar.

extrinsic compression (cardiac tamponade) (see Chapter 8), or outflow obstruction (e.g., pulmonary embolism).
- *Hypovolemic shock* results from loss of blood or plasma volume (e.g., due to hemorrhage or fluid loss from severe burns).
- *Septic shock* is triggered by microbial infections and is associated with the systemic inflammatory response syndrome (SIRS). In addition to microbes, SIRS may be triggered by severe burns, trauma, and pancreatitis. The pathogenesis of septic shock is discussed later.
- *Neurogenic shock* results from the loss of vascular tone, as may occur following spinal cord injury.
- *Anaphylactic shock* results from systemic vasodilation and increased vascular permeability that is triggered by immunoglobulin E–mediated immediate hypersensitivity reactions (see Chapter 4).

Pathogenesis. Shock, regardless of its cause, has certain common features. It is a progressive disorder that leads to death if the underlying problem is not corrected. Shock tends to evolve through stages, except in the setting of massive injury (e.g., exsanguination from a ruptured aortic aneurysm). These stages are best documented in hypovolemic shock but are seen in other types, as well:

- Initial *nonprogressive stage:* reflex compensatory mechanisms are activated and vital organ perfusion is maintained
- *Progressive stage:* tissue hypoperfusion occurs, with worsening circulatory and metabolic derangements
- *Irreversible stage,* in which cellular and tissue injury is so severe that even if the hemodynamic defects are corrected, survival is not possible

In the early nonprogressive phase, neural and hormonal feedback loops maintain the cardiac output and blood pressure by increasing the heart rate, constricting the arterioles (in hypovolemic and cardiogenic shock), and decreasing the urine output. Coronary and cerebral vessels are less sensitive to sympathetic signals and maintain a relatively normal caliber, blood flow, and oxygen delivery. Thus, blood is shunted away from the skin to the vital organs such as the heart and the brain.

Without correction of the underlying cause, shock proceeds to the progressive phase, characterized by widespread tissue hypoxia. Due to a persistent oxygen deficit, cells are forced to rely on anaerobic glycolysis instead of aerobic respiration, causing lactic acidosis. The lowered tissue pH blunts the vasomotor response; as a result, arterioles dilate and blood pools in the microcirculation, worsening the cardiac output, lowering blood pressure, and putting endothelial cells at risk for anoxic injury. Endothelial dysfunction then sets the stage for the development of widespread tissue edema and disseminated intravascular

Table 3.3 Major Types of Shock

Type of Shock	Clinical Examples	Principal Pathogenic Mechanisms
Cardiogenic	Myocardial infarction Ventricular rupture Arrhythmia Cardiac tamponade Pulmonary embolism	Failure of myocardial pump resulting from intrinsic myocardial damage, extrinsic pressure, or obstruction to outflow
Hypovolemic	Hemorrhage Fluid loss (e.g., vomiting, diarrhea, burns)	Inadequate blood or plasma volume
Septic	Overwhelming microbial infections	Activation of cytokine cascades; endothelial activation/injury; peripheral vasodilation and pooling of blood; leukocyte-induced damage; disseminated intravascular coagulation

coagulation, both of which may further compromise the tissue perfusion. With widespread tissue hypoxia, vital organs are affected and begin to fail.

In the absence of appropriate intervention or in severe cases, the myocardial contractile function worsens, partly owing to increased nitric oxide synthesis. Progression to renal failure occurs because of renal ischemia (see Chapter 11). The downward spiral often culminates in death.

Morphology. The effects of shock on cells and tissues resemble those of hypoxic injury (see Chapter 1) and are caused by a combination of hypoperfusion and microvascular thrombosis. Any organ may be affected; the brain, heart, kidneys, adrenals, and gastrointestinal tract are most commonly involved. Fibrin thrombi are readily visualized in kidney glomeruli but may be found throughout the body. The lungs are resistant to hypoxic injury in hypovolemic shock occurring after hemorrhage, but sepsis and trauma often precipitate **diffuse alveolar damage** and acute respiratory distress syndrome (see Chapter 10). Except for irreversible neuronal and cardiomyocyte loss, affected tissues can recover completely if the patient survives.

Clinical Features. The manifestations of shock depend on the precipitating insult. In hypovolemic and cardiogenic shock, patients exhibit hypotension, a weak rapid pulse, tachypnea, and cool, clammy, cyanotic skin. By contrast, in septic shock, the skin may be warm and flushed due to peripheral vasodilation. The primary initial threat to life is the triggering event (e.g., myocardial infarction, severe hemorrhage, bacterial infection). However, secondary cardiac, cerebral, renal, and pulmonary changes rapidly aggravate the situation.

The prognosis varies with the origin of shock and its duration. More than 90% of young, otherwise healthy patients with hypovolemic shock survive with appropriate management; by comparison, septic or cardiogenic shock is associated with substantially worse outcomes, even with state-of-the-art care.

Septic Shock

In the United States, there are more than 750,000 cases per year of septic shock, which is responsible for approximately 2% of all hospital admissions. Despite improvements in care, 20% to 30% of affected patients die.

Pathogenesis. Septic shock is triggered by constituents of microbes (most commonly, gram-positive bacteria, followed by gram-negative bacteria and fungi) that activate the innate immune system (i.e., macrophages, neutrophils, dendritic cells, endothelial cells, and soluble components such as complement). These cells and factors recognize and are activated by microbial pathogen–associated molecular patterns (PAMPs). Following activation, a number of inflammatory responses ensue that, when massive or widespread, interact in a complex, incompletely understood fashion to produce septic shock and multiorgan dysfunction (Fig. 3.13). Factors believed to play major roles in the pathophysiology of septic shock include the following:

- *Inflammatory responses.* PAMPs activate inflammatory responses by engaging receptors on innate immune cells, such as *Toll-like receptors* (see Chapter 2), which recognize a host of microbe-derived PAMPs. Activated innate immune cells produce cytokines such as tumor necrosis factor (TNF) and other proinflammatory mediators that induce endothelial cells (and other cell types) to upregulate adhesion molecule expression and further stimulate cytokine and chemokine production. The complement cascade is also activated by microbial components, both directly and through the proteolytic activity of plasmin, resulting in the production of anaphylatoxins (C3a, C5a), chemotactic fragments (C5a), and opsonins (C3b), all of which contribute to the proinflammatory state.

- *Endothelial activation and injury.* Inflammatory cytokines loosen endothelial cell tight junctions, resulting in the accumulation of protein-rich edema that limits nutrient delivery and waste removal throughout the body. Activated endothelium also produces nitric oxide and other vasoactive inflammatory mediators, which may contribute to vascular smooth muscle relaxation and systemic hypotension.

- *Induction of a procoagulant state.* Microbial components can activate coagulation directly through factor XII and indirectly through altered endothelial function. Moreover, sepsis alters the expression of many factors so as to favor coagulation. Proinflammatory cytokines increase tissue factor production by monocytes (and possibly endothelial cells) and decrease the production of endothelial anticoagulant factors (e.g., thrombomodulin and protein C). Blood flow in small vessels decreases, producing stasis and diminishing the washout of activated coagulation factors. These derangements cause disseminated intravascular coagulation (see Chapter 9) in up to half of septic patients. Tissue perfusion is further compromised by the systemic activation of thrombin and the deposition of fibrin-rich thrombi in small vessels. In full-blown disseminated

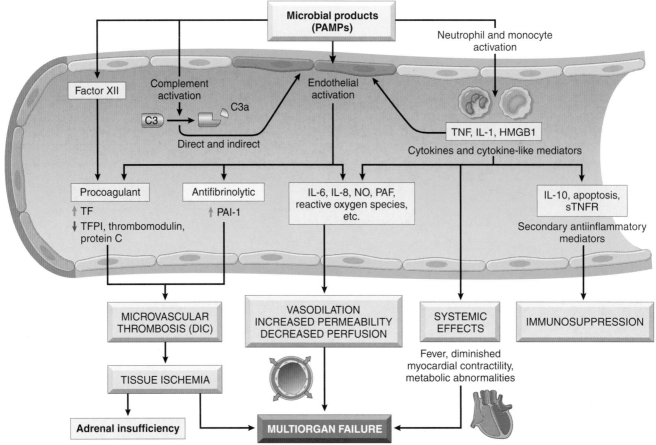

Fig. 3.13 Major pathogenic pathways in septic shock. Microbial products activate endothelial cells and cellular and humoral elements of the innate immune system, initiating a cascade of events that lead to end-stage multiorgan failure. Additional details are provided in the text. *DIC,* Disseminated intravascular coagulation; *NO,* nitric oxide; *PAI-1,* plasminogen activator inhibitor-1; *sTNFR,* soluble TNF receptor; *TF,* tissue factor; *TFPI,* tissue factor pathway inhibitor; *TNF,* tumor necrosis factor.

intravascular coagulation, the consumption of coagulation factors and platelets causes deficiencies of these factors, resulting in a superimposed bleeding disorder that may be life threatening.

- *Metabolic abnormalities.* Septic patients exhibit insulin resistance and hyperglycemia. Cytokines such as tumor necrosis factor and IL-1, stress-induced hormones such as glucagon, growth hormone, and glucocorticoids, and catecholamines all drive gluconeogenesis. At the same time, the proinflammatory cytokines suppress insulin release and promote insulin resistance in the liver and other tissues. If severe, cellular hypoxia and diminished oxidative phosphorylation lead to increased lactate production and lactic acidosis.
- *Organ dysfunction.* Systemic hypotension, interstitial edema, and small-vessel thrombosis decrease the delivery of oxygen and

nutrients to tissues. High cytokine levels and secondary mediators diminish myocardial contractility and cardiac output, further compromising tissue perfusion. Increased vascular permeability and endothelial injury may lead to the acute respiratory distress syndrome (see Chapter 10). Ultimately, these factors may conspire to cause the failure of multiple organs, particularly the kidneys, liver, lungs, and heart, culminating in death.

The multiplicity of factors and the complexity of the interactions that underlie sepsis preclude therapeutic intervention with antagonists to specific mediators, such as tumor necrosis factor. The standard of care remains antibiotics to treat the underlying infection and intravenous fluids, pressors, and supplemental oxygen to maintain the blood pressure and limit tissue hypoxia. Even in the best centers, septic shock remains a daunting clinical challenge.

4

Diseases of the Immune System

OUTLINE

Hypersensitivity Disorders, 41
  Immediate (Type I) Hypersensitivity, 42
  Antibody-Mediated (Type II) Hypersensitivity, 44
  Immune Complex–Mediated (Type III) Hypersensitivity, 47
  T Cell-Mediated (Type IV) Hypersensitivity, 47
Autoimmune Diseases, 49
  Mechanisms of Autoimmunity, 49
  Systemic Lupus Erythematosus (SLE), 50
  Systemic Sclerosis (Scleroderma), 51
  Sjögren Syndrome, 51

Rejection of Transplants, 52
  Immune Responses to Organ Allografts, 53
  Mechanisms of Rejection of Solid-Organ Allografts, 53
  Hematopoietic Stem Cell Transplantation, 54
Immunodeficiency Disorders, 56
  Primary (Congenital) Immunodeficiencies, 56
Acquired Immunodeficiency Syndrome, 58
  Human Immunodeficiency Virus: Structure and
    Life Cycle, 58
Amyloidosis, 59

The immune system protects us against infections and cancers by two types of mechanisms: innate immunity and adaptive immunity.

Innate immunity is the rapid response to infections mediated by cells and plasma proteins that are always present and ready to attack (hence, *innate*). The principal cells of innate immunity are myeloid cells, including macrophages, neutrophils, and dendritic cells, but lymphocytes, epithelial cells, and other cell types also possess intrinsic defense mechanisms. These cells express receptors such as Toll-like receptors that recognize microbial products and products of necrotic cells. These receptors, unlike the antigen receptors of T and B lymphocytes, are not pathogen specific and have limited diversity. They are triggered by molecules shared by many pathogens (pathogen-associated molecular patterns [PAMPs]) and substances released from damaged cells (damage-associated molecular patterns [DAMPs]). The major reaction of innate immunity is acute inflammation (see Chapter 2).

Adaptive immunity is the more powerful and specialized set of responses mediated by T and B lymphocytes. These cells express specific and highly diverse receptors for antigens. Each T and B lymphocyte and its clonal progeny express a unique receptor and, hence, have a unique specificity. The diversity of the receptors is created by rearrangements of antigen-receptor genes that occur during the maturation of the lymphocytes. Thus, the presence of rearranged antigen-receptor genes is a reliable marker of T and B lymphocytes and of tumors derived from these cells. Lymphocytes are normally silent and are activated by (adapt to) antigens (hence, the term adaptive immunity). Following activation, the lymphocytes produce effector cells that possess mechanisms that function to eliminate microbes and tumor cells. These mechanisms include:

- *Humoral immunity* mediated by antibodies, which are produced by B cells and their differentiated progeny, plasma cells. Antibodies neutralize microbes, opsonize them for phagocytosis, and activate the complement system.

- *Cell-mediated immunity* mediated by T cells. T cells are activated by protein antigens displayed by antigen-presenting cells (APCs), and require repeat antigen stimulation to perform their functions. Two major types of T cells, CD4+ and CD8+, function differently in host defense and pathologic reactions. CD4+ helper T cells secrete cytokines that activate macrophages to destroy phagocytosed microbes, help B cells to make potent antibodies, and stimulate inflammation. Helper T cells consist of several subsets that produce different cytokines and induce different types of inflammatory reactions: Th1 cells activate macrophages, Th2 cells activate eosinophils, and Th17 cells stimulate neutrophil-rich inflammation. CD8+ cytotoxic T lymphocytes (CTLs) kill infected and transformed cells.

Although the immune system evolved as a protective force, at times it can go awry and cause tissue injury and clinical disease. In this chapter, we discuss the most important pathologic reactions and diseases that are caused by immune responses, mainly adaptive immune responses, as well as deficiencies of the immune system and their consequences.

HYPERSENSITIVITY DISORDERS

Persistent, misdirected, or inadequately regulated immune reactions against a variety of antigens may cause tissue injury.

An individual who has been exposed to and reacts against an antigen is said to be sensitized, so injurious immune reactions are called *hypersensitivity reactions*. Hypersensitivity diseases tend to be chronic and difficult to control, and are therefore important clinical problems. These diseases may be caused by reactions to three main types of antigens.

- *Reactions against self antigens* are called autoimmunity, and the diseases they cause are *autoimmune diseases*. As we shall discuss later, individuals are normally tolerant to their own (self) antigens, and autoimmunity results when self-tolerance breaks down.

Table 4.1 Hypersensitivity Reactions

Type	Immune Mechanisms	Histopathologic Lesions	Prototypical Disorders
Immediate (type I) hypersensitivity	Production of IgE antibody → immediate release of histamine and other mediators from mast cells; later recruitment of inflammatory cells	Vascular dilation, edema, smooth muscle contraction, mucus production, tissue injury, inflammation	Anaphylaxis; allergies; bronchial asthma (atopic forms)
Antibody-mediated (type II) hypersensitivity	Production of IgG, IgM → binds to antigen on target cell or tissue → phagocytosis or lysis of target cell by activated complement or Fc receptors; recruitment of leukocytes	Phagocytosis and lysis of cells; inflammation; in some diseases, functional derangements without cell or tissue injury	Autoimmune hemolytic anemia; Goodpasture syndrome
Immune complex–mediated (type III) hypersensitivity	Deposition of antigen–antibody complexes → complement activation → recruitment of leukocytes by complement products and Fc receptors → release of enzymes and other toxic molecules	Inflammation, necrotizing vasculitis (fibrinoid necrosis)	Systemic lupus erythematosus; some forms of glomerulonephritis; serum sickness; Arthus reaction
Cell-mediated (type IV) hypersensitivity	Activated T lymphocytes → (1) release of cytokines, inflammation and macrophage activation; (2) T cell–mediated cytotoxicity	Perivascular cellular infiltrates; edema; granuloma formation; cell destruction	Contact dermatitis; multiple sclerosis; type 1 diabetes; tuberculosis

Ig, Immunoglobulin.

- *Reactions against environmental antigens* include allergy, which is an abnormal reaction against common and normally harmless environmental substances, and contact sensitivity, which is a cutaneous immune reaction against chemicals and drugs.
- *Excessive reactions against microbes* also cause hypersensitivity reactions. Although defense against microbes is the normal function of the immune system, in some cases, such as tuberculosis, the microbe is unusually persistent and the immune response itself becomes the cause of tissue injury. Inflammatory bowel diseases are thought to be caused by reactions against commensal bacteria, which may activate immune cells when normal protective mechanisms are defective.

The terms *hypersensitivity* and *autoimmunity* are often used interchangeably, but they are not synonymous. Hypersensitivity refers to an immunologically mediated tissue reaction that is dominated by inflammation. It is frequently associated with autoimmunity, but it also may be caused by microbes and other environmental agents. Conversely, some autoimmune reactions do not have a component of hypersensitivity, such as depletion of red cells and platelets by autoantibodies without accompanying inflammation.

Hypersensitivity reactions are classified into four major types based on the nature of the adaptive immune reaction.

This classification is useful because each type has distinct mechanisms and pathologic and clinical features (Table 4.1).

- *Immediate (type I) hypersensitivity* is caused by Th2 cells and immunoglobulin E (IgE) antibodies. Inflammation is triggered mainly by mediators released by mast cells.
- *Antibody-mediated (type II) hypersensitivity* is caused by antibodies that bind to target antigens on cells or in tissues and destroy cells, trigger inflammation, or induce functional abnormalities.
- *Immune complex–mediated (type III) hypersensitivity* is caused by complexes of antibodies and antigens that become deposited in vessels and tissues and elicit inflammation.
- *T cell–mediated (type IV) hypersensitivity* is caused by CD4+ T cells, which induce chronic inflammation, or CD8+ T cells, which destroy host cells.

Immediate (Type I) Hypersensitivity

This inflammatory reaction, also called *allergy*, is caused by IgE antibodies that recognize environmental antigens and sensitize mast cells, leading to the release of mediators.

Allergies, the most common immunologic diseases, are reactions to antigens in the environment, foods, and insect venoms, and are most frequent in urban areas in industrialized societies (where such antigens are abundant). In most individuals, the immune system does not react against environmental antigens, but in some individuals, these normally harmless antigens elicit strong reactions that can lead to significant morbidity and even death. The propensity to develop these reactions is called *atopy*. The typical allergic reaction consists of an early (within minutes) vascular and smooth muscle response, which may be followed by a slower (late-phase) inflammatory response over the next few hours (Fig. 4.1).

Pathogenesis. Most immediate hypersensitivity reactions follow a stereotypic sequence of cellular responses (Fig. 4.2).

- *Activation of Th2 cells and production of IgE antibody.* Atopic individuals make strong Th2 responses to some antigens. Th2 cells secrete the cytokines IL-4, IL-5, and IL-13, which act on several cell types with integral roles in immediate hypersensitivity. IL-4 stimulates B cells specific for the allergen to produce the IgE immunoglobulin isotype. IL-5 activates eosinophils that are recruited to the reaction, and IL-13 acts on epithelial cells and stimulates mucus secretion.
- *Sensitization of mast cells by IgE antibody.* Mast cells express a high-affinity receptor for the Fc portion of the ε heavy chain of IgE. The receptor is also expressed on blood basophils, but because allergic reactions occur in tissues and not in the circulation, it is likely that mast cells are the major cell type involved in these reactions. Mast cells bind IgE and retain it on their surfaces.
- *Activation of mast cells and release of mediators.* When the antigen is reintroduced, it binds to the IgE, thus cross-linking the associated Fc receptors, which in turn transmit intracellular signals that lead to the secretion of mediators from the mast cells.

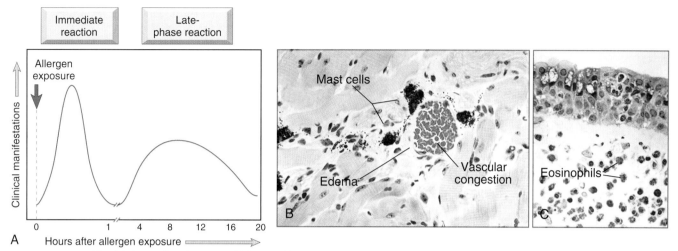

Fig. 4.1 Immediate hypersensitivity. (A) Kinetics of the immediate and late-phase reactions. The immediate vascular and smooth muscle reaction to an allergen develops within minutes after challenge (allergen exposure in a previously sensitized individual), and the late-phase reaction develops 2 to 24 hours later. (B) Morphology of the immediate reaction is characterized by vasodilation, congestion, and edema. (C) The late-phase reaction is characterized by an inflammatory infiltrate rich in eosinophils, neutrophils, and T cells. (Micrographs courtesy Dr. Daniel Friend, Department of Pathology, Brigham and Women's Hospital, Boston.)

Three groups of mediators are important in immediate hypersensitivity reactions:

- *Vasoactive amines, mainly histamine,* are stored in mast cell granules and rapidly released upon mast cell degranulation. Histamine causes rapid vasodilation and increased vascular permeability and causes smooth muscles to contract. Chemotactic factors and proteases are also released. The latter may damage tissues and also generate kinins and cleave complement components to produce additional chemotactic and inflammatory factors.
- *Lipid mediators, including prostaglandins and leukotrienes,* are synthesized from membrane arachidonic acid and have multiple actions in inflammation, described in Chapter 2. Prostaglandin D_2 (PGD_2) is the most abundant mediator generated by the cyclooxygenase pathway in mast cells. It causes intense bronchospasm, as well as increased mucous secretion. The leukotrienes LTC_4 and LTD_4 are the most potent vasoactive and spasmogenic agents known.
- *Cytokines* are synthesized and secreted following mast cell activation. These include tumor necrosis factor (TNF) and chemokines, which recruit and activate leukocytes in the late-phase reaction, and IL-4 and IL-5, which amplify the Th2-initiated immune reaction.

The combined actions of these mediators account for the manifestations of immediate hypersensitivity. It is not clear why some individuals develop injurious reactions to antigens that are ignored in most people. The many factors accounting for atopy include genetic susceptibility and exposure to antigens during childhood. Twenty percent to 30% of immediate hypersensitivity reactions, especially asthma, are triggered by nonantigenic stimuli, such as temperature extremes and exercise, and do not involve Th2 cells or IgE. It is believed that in these cases (called *nonatopic allergy*), mast cells are abnormally sensitive to activation by various nonimmune stimuli.

Morphology. The histologic appearance of type I hypersensitivity is typically unimpressive. Congestion and excessive secretion of mucus triggered by histamine may be the only manifestations. In asthma, there may be significant bronchial gland hypertrophy, eosinophil-rich inflammatory infiltrates in bronchial walls, and mucous plugs that obstruct the lumens (see Chapter 10).

Clinical Features. Immediate hypersensitivity reactions range in severity from the mild nuisance of hives (urticaria) and hay fever (allergic rhinitis), to serious, sometimes fatal, acute anaphylaxis and chronic diseases such as bronchial asthma (Table 4.2). The reaction is localized when the antigen is confined to a particular site, such as the skin (following contact) or the gastrointestinal tract (following ingestion). Systemic exposure to protein antigens (e.g., in bee venom) or drugs (e.g., penicillin) may result in systemic anaphylaxis. In anaphylaxis, within minutes of the exposure in a sensitized host, itching, urticaria, and skin erythema appear, followed by profound respiratory difficulty caused by pulmonary bronchoconstriction and accentuated by the hypersecretion of mucus. Laryngeal edema may exacerbate difficulty in breathing by causing upper airway obstruction. The musculature of the entire gastrointestinal tract may be affected, with resultant vomiting, abdominal cramps, and diarrhea. Without immediate intervention, there may be systemic vasodilation with a fall in blood pressure (anaphylactic shock), and the patient may progress to circulatory collapse and death within minutes.

Treatment for these conditions relies on blocking or counteracting the actions of various mediators. Commonly used drugs are antihistamines, corticosteroids (to treat inflammation), epinephrine (to correct the precipitous drop in blood pressure in

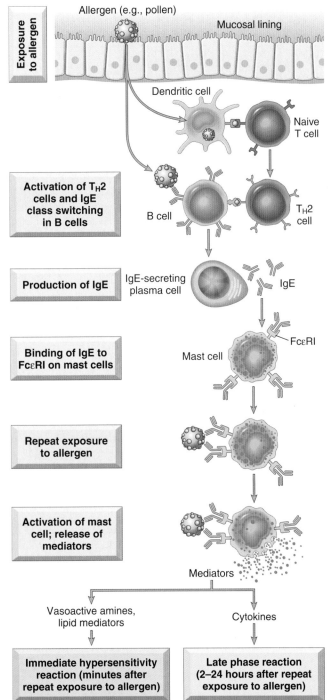

Fig. 4.2 The sequence of events in immediate hypersensitivity. Immediate hypersensitivity reactions are initiated by the introduction of an allergen, which stimulates Th2 cells and immunoglobulin E (IgE) production. IgE binds to Fc receptors (FcεRI) on mast cells, and subsequent exposure to the allergen activates the mast cells to secrete the mediators that are responsible for the pathologic reactions of immediate hypersensitivity.

anaphylaxis, and to relieve bronchospasm), and, more recently, anti-IgE antibody to inhibit the primary initiator of the allergic reaction. Antibodies that block the cytokines IL-4, IL-5, and IL-13 or their receptors are used to treat asthma and atopic dermatitis. Early childhood exposure to an allergen (e.g., peanut extract) reduces the incidence of allergy to that agent later in life, although the mechanism is not understood.

Table 4.2 Immediate Hypersensitivity (Allergic) Disorders

Clinical Syndrome	Clinical and Pathologic Manifestations
Anaphylaxis (may be caused by drugs, bee sting, food)	Fall in blood pressure (shock) caused by vascular dilation; airway obstruction due to laryngeal edema
Bronchial asthma	Airway obstruction caused by bronchial smooth muscle hyperactivity; inflammation and tissue injury caused by late-phase reaction
Allergic rhinitis, sinusitis (hay fever)	Increased mucus secretion; inflammation of upper airways and sinuses
Food allergies	Increased peristalsis due to contraction of intestinal muscles, resulting in vomiting and diarrhea

Antibody-Mediated (Type II) Hypersensitivity

Antibody-mediated (type II) hypersensitivity disorders are caused by antibodies, usually IgG or IgM autoantibodies, directed against target antigens on the surface of cells or other tissue components.

Pathogenesis. The antigens may be normal molecules intrinsic to cell membranes or in the extracellular matrix, or they may be adsorbed exogenous antigens (e.g., a drug metabolite). Rarely, antibodies to microbial or other antigens that cross-react with host antigens may be responsible. The mechanisms of cell injury in this form of hypersensitivity are the following:

- *Phagocytosis:* Antibodies may coat (opsonize) circulating cells (such as red cells or platelets) and target them for phagocytosis or complement-mediated destruction. Opsonized blood elements are mostly eliminated in the spleen, explaining why splenectomy is of clinical benefit in antibody-mediated diseases marked by low blood counts.
- *Inflammation:* Antibodies that are deposited in extracellular tissues bind leukocyte Fc receptors or activate complement (described later), both resulting in the recruitment and activation of leukocytes (neutrophils and macrophages) and acute inflammation.
- *Cellular dysfunction:* Antibodies can also cause cellular dysfunction when they bind to and activate or inhibit receptors on the surface of cells, or bind to and deplete essential molecules, producing functional deficiencies without cell or tissue injury.

Because complement proteins play an essential role in type II and III forms of hypersensitivity, a brief discussion of complement activation and function follows.

Activation and Functions of Complement

The complement system consists of several circulating and membrane proteins that play important roles in host defense, as well as in inflammation and tissue injury in immunologic diseases.

There are three pathways of complement activation, only one of which involves antibodies (Fig. 4.4). The phylogenetically older *alternative pathway* is activated by microbial molecules that stably bind complement proteins. The *classical pathway* is activated by binding of complement proteins to antibodies that are deposited on surfaces and form complexes with antigens. This is important in adaptive immunity and is the only pathway that participates in the antibody-mediated (type II) and immune complex–mediated (type III) forms of hypersensitivity. The *lectin pathway* is activated by a plasma lectin that binds to microbial

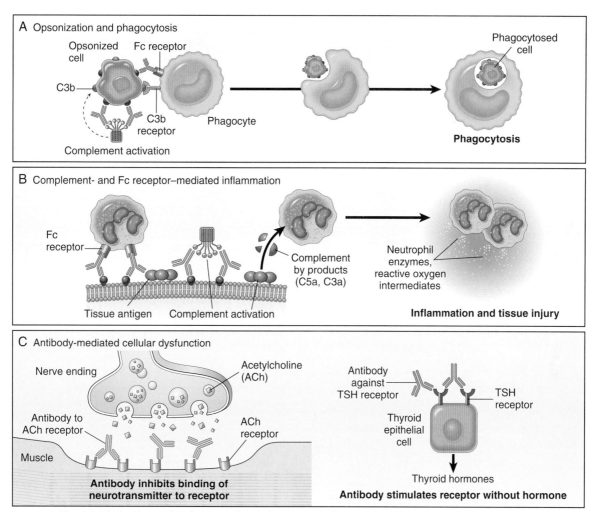

Fig. 4.3 Mechanisms of antibody-mediated diseases. (A) Opsonization of cells by antibodies and complement components and ingestion by phagocytes. (B) Inflammation induced by antibody binding to Fc receptors of leukocytes and by complement breakdown products. (C) Antireceptor antibodies disturb the normal function of receptors. In these examples, antibodies to the acetylcholine (ACh) receptor impair neuromuscular transmission in myasthenia gravis, and antibodies against the thyroid-stimulating hormone (TSH) receptor activate thyroid cells in Graves disease.

carbohydrates. The functions of complement are mediated by various proteolytic cleavage products. All three pathways lead to the cleavage of the most abundant complement protein, C3, to generate a fragment, C3b, that is deposited on nearby surfaces (microbes or sites of antibody binding). C3b opsonizes cells for phagocytosis by binding to C3b receptors that are expressed on phagocytes. C3b also is a component of a protease that cleaves later complement components. Among the other proteolytic products are C5a and C3a, which stimulate the release of histamine from mast cells, as well as other proinflammatory activities. The terminal steps in complement activation lead to the formation of a large protein channel, the membrane attack complex, which creates holes in lipid membranes and leads to osmotic lysis of cells.

Complement activation is controlled by several cell-associated and secreted proteins that prevent collateral damage to normal cells and unrestrained complement activation during normal defense. Predictably, deficiencies of these complement regulators lead to cell injury and inflammation. *Paroxysmal nocturnal hemoglobinuria (PNH)* is caused by an acquired deficiency of an enzyme involved in synthesis of a

regulator called *decay accelerating factor,* which normally limits the formation of the enzyme that cleaves C3. In the absence of this regulator, there is excessive C3 breakdown and formation of the membrane attack complex. Red blood cells are especially sensitive to complement-mediated lysis because of their thin cell walls, accounting for urinary excretion of hemoglobin released from lysed red cells. The susceptibility of red cells to complement-mediated lysis increases when the pH of the blood decreases during sleep, hence the nocturnal nature of the red cell breakdown. *Hereditary angioedema* results from inherited deficiency of C1 inhibitor, a plasma serine protease inhibitor that limits the proteolytic activity of early complement proteins, mainly C1. Deficiency of this inhibitor leads to excessive production of numerous vasoactive proteins, which increase vascular permeability and cause episodes of fluid accumulation in the skin, gastrointestinal tract, and larynx (the most serious feature because it could lead to airway obstruction).

Clinical Features. In many autoimmune diseases, the clinical problems are caused by autoantibodies (Table 4.3). The pathology may be dominated by inflammation (as in antibody-mediated

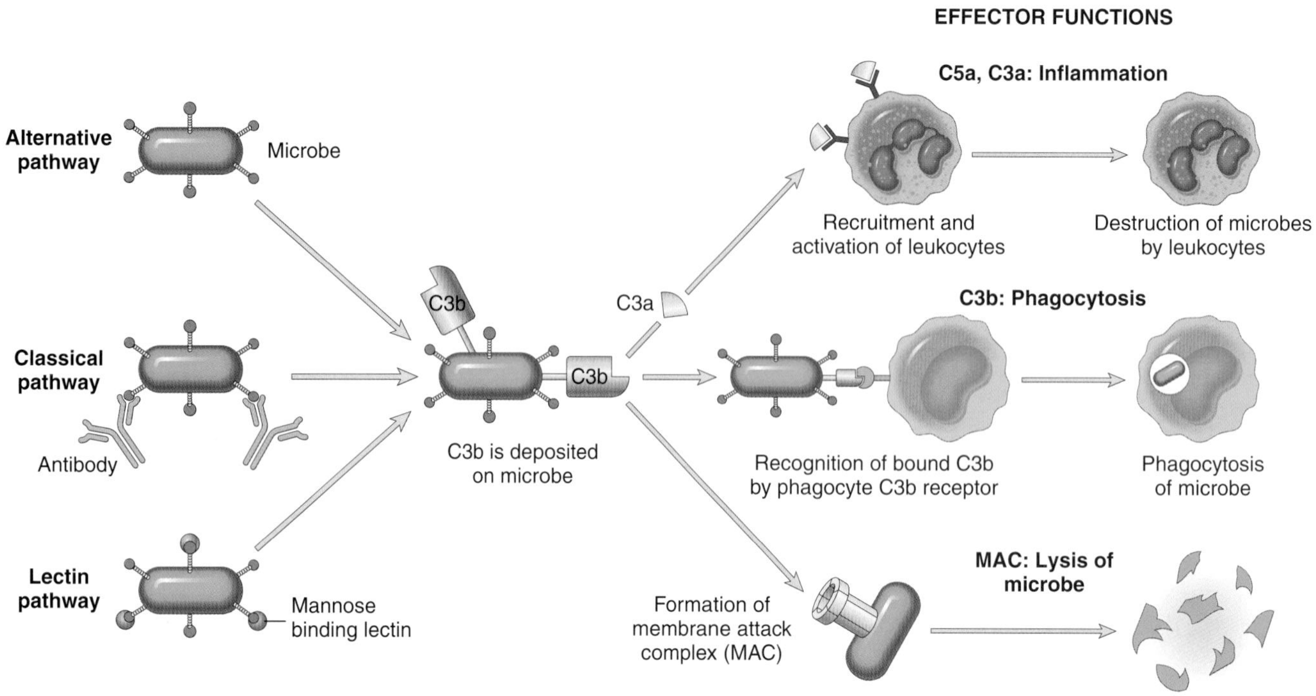

EFFECTOR FUNCTIONS

Fig. 4.4 Pathways of complement activation and functions of complement. The activation of the complement system (the early steps) may be initiated by three distinct pathways, all of which lead to the production of C3b. C3b initiates the late steps of complement activation, culminating in the formation of a multiprotein complex called the membrane attack complex (MAC), which is a transmembrane channel composed of polymerized C9 molecules that causes lysis of thin-walled microbes. Peptide by-products released during complement activation are the inflammation-inducing C3a and C5a. The principal functions of proteins produced at different steps are shown.

Table 4.3 Antibody-Mediated Diseases

Disease	Target Antigen	Mechanisms of Disease	Clinicopathologic Manifestations
Autoimmune hemolytic anemia	Red cell membrane proteins	Opsonization and phagocytosis of red blood cells	Hemolysis, anemia
Autoimmune thrombocytopenic purpura	Platelet membrane proteins (GpIIb: IIIa integrin)	Opsonization and phagocytosis of platelets	Bleeding
Pemphigus vulgaris	Proteins in intercellular junctions of epidermal cells (desmogleins)	Antibody-mediated activation of proteases, disruption of intercellular adhesions	Skin vesicles (bullae)
Vasculitis caused by ANCA	Neutrophil granule proteins, presumably released from activated neutrophils	Neutrophil degranulation and inflammation	Vasculitis
Goodpasture syndrome	Protein in basement membranes of kidney glomeruli and lung alveoli	Complement- and Fc receptor–mediated inflammation	Nephritis, lung hemorrhage
Acute rheumatic fever	Streptococcal cell wall antigen; antibody cross-reacts with myocardial antigen	Inflammation, macrophage activation	Myocarditis, arthritis
Myasthenia gravis	Acetylcholine receptor	Antibody inhibits acetylcholine binding, down-modulates receptors	Muscle weakness, paralysis
Graves disease (hyperthyroidism)	TSH receptor	Antibody-mediated stimulation of TSH receptors	Hyperthyroidism
Pernicious anemia	Intrinsic factor of gastric parietal cells	Neutralization of intrinsic factor, decreased absorption of vitamin B_{12}	Abnormal erythropoiesis, anemia

ANCA, Antineutrophil cytoplasmic antibodies; *TSH,* thyroid-stimulating hormone.

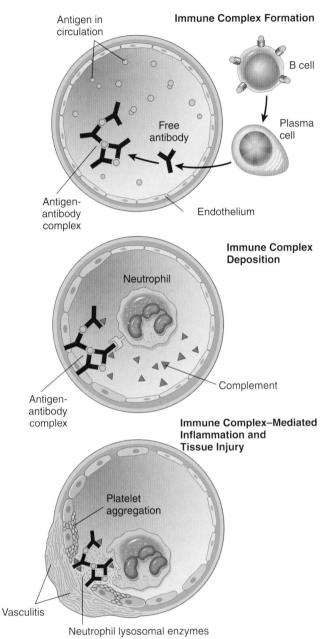

Fig. 4.5 Immune complex disease. The sequential phases in the induction of systemic immune complex–mediated diseases (type III hypersensitivity).

glomerulonephritis), the secondary effects of cell depletion (autoimmune hemolytic anemia and thrombocytopenia), or functional derangements (myasthenia gravis and Graves disease). In myasthenia gravis, antibodies against acetylcholine (ACh) receptors in the motor end plates of skeletal muscles inhibit neuromuscular transmission, with resultant muscle weakness. Antibodies can also stimulate excessive cellular responses: In Graves disease, antibodies against the thyroid-stimulating hormone (TSH) receptor stimulate thyroid epithelial cells to secrete thyroid hormones, resulting in hyperthyroidism.

Immune Complex–Mediated (Type III) Hypersensitivity

Antigen–antibody (immune) complexes that are formed in the circulation may become deposited in blood vessels and induce inflammation.

Table 4.4 Immune Complex Diseases

Disease	Antigen Involved	Clinicopathologic Manifestations
Systemic lupus erythematosus	Nuclear antigens (circulating or "planted" in kidney)	Nephritis, skin lesions, arthritis, others
Poststreptococcal glomerulonephritis	Streptococcal cell wall antigen(s); may be "planted" in glomerular basement membrane	Nephritis
Polyarteritis nodosa	Hepatitis B virus antigens in some cases	Systemic vasculitis
Reactive arthritis	Bacterial antigens (e.g., *Yersinia*)	Acute arthritis
Serum sickness	Various proteins (e.g., foreign serum protein, such as horse antithymocyte globulin)	Arthritis, vasculitis, nephritis
Arthus reaction (experimental)	Various foreign proteins	Cutaneous vasculitis

Pathogenesis. Typically, pathogenic immune complexes are produced in antibody excess and are of a size such that they avoid elimination by phagocytes but are capable of depositing in vessels. Tissue deposition leads to complement activation and acute inflammation (Fig. 4.5). Consumption of complement during the active phase of the disease leads to decreased serum levels of C3, which can be used as a marker of disease activity. *Serum sickness* is a systemic immune complex disease in which a single large dose of a foreign antigen, such as an antibody produced in other species, is injected into an individual. Immune complexes form in the blood, become deposited in tissues, activate complement, and induce inflammation. The *Arthus reaction* is an experimental model of cutaneous vasculitis that resembles human vasculitides (Chapter 7).

Morphology. The principal morphologic manifestation of immune complex injury is acute vasculitis, which may be associated with fibrinoid necrosis of the vessel wall and neutrophilic infiltration. When deposited in the kidney, the complexes can be seen on immunofluorescence microscopy as granular deposits of immunoglobulin and complement and on electron microscopy as electron-dense deposits along the glomerular basement membrane.

Clinical Features. Many systemic immunologic diseases are associated with the formation and tissue deposition of immune complexes (Table 4.4). The pathologic picture is of acute inflammation in the sites of deposition of complexes, typically the capillaries of the kidneys (causing glomerulonephritis), synovium of joints (arthritis), and blood vessels in any tissue (vasculitis). The prototypic human immune complex disease is systemic lupus erythematosus (SLE), associated with persistent antibody responses to autoantigens.

T Cell-Mediated (Type IV) Hypersensitivity

Two types of T-cell reactions are capable of causing tissue injury and disease: (1) cytokine-mediated inflammation (also called delayed-type hypersensitivity), in which the cytokines are produced mainly by CD4+ T cells, and (2) cytotoxicity, mediated by CD8+ T cells (Fig. 4.6).

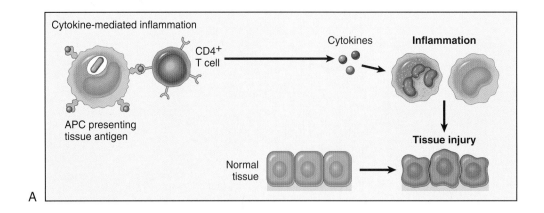

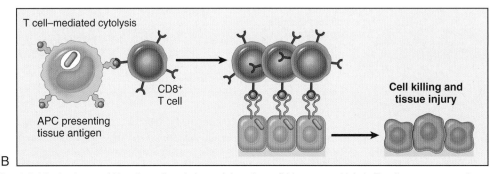

Fig. 4.6 Mechanisms of T cell–mediated tissue injury (type IV hypersensitivity). T cells may cause tissue injury and disease by two mechanisms. (A) Inflammation may be triggered by cytokines produced mainly by CD4⁺ T cells in which tissue injury is caused by activated macrophages and inflammatory cells. (B) Direct killing of target cells is mediated by CD8⁺ cytotoxic T lymphocytes (CTLs). *APC,* Antigen-presenting cell.

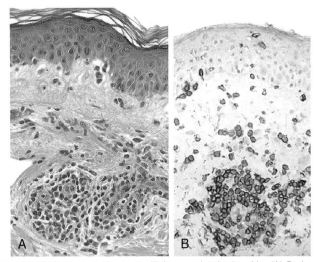

Fig. 4.7 Delayed-type hypersensitivity reaction in the skin. (A) Perivascular accumulation (cuffing) of mononuclear inflammatory cells (lymphocytes and macrophages), with associated dermal edema and fibrin deposition. (B) Immunoperoxidase staining reveals a predominantly perivascular cellular infiltrate that marks positively with anti-CD4 antibodies. (B, Courtesy Dr. Louis Picker, Department of Pathology, Oregon Health Sciences University, Portland.)

Pathogenesis. Cytokine-mediated hypersensitivity is a reaction of Th1 effector cells, but Th17 cells also may contribute to the reaction, especially in cases where neutrophils are prominent in the inflammatory infiltrate. Th1 cells secrete cytokines, mainly interferon-γ (IFN-γ), which are responsible for many of the manifestations of delayed-type hypersensitivity. IFN-γ–activated (classically activated) macrophages produce substances that destroy microbes and damage tissues, and mediators that promote inflammation. Activated Th17 cells secrete cytokines that recruit neutrophils and monocytes. In cell-mediated cytotoxicity, CD8+ T cells kill antigen-expressing target cells. CD8+ T cells also produce cytokines, notably IFN-γ, and are involved in inflammatory reactions resembling delayed-type hypersensitivity, especially following virus infections and exposure to some contact-sensitizing agents.

Clinical Features. The typical manifestation of this form of hypersensitivity is chronic inflammation (Fig. 4.7). It is called delayed-type hypersensitivity because it develops over 1 to 2 days after an antigen challenge in a previously sensitized individual (in contrast with immediate hypersensitivity). This time lag is due to the multiple steps involved in the reaction, including the capture, processing, and presentation of the antigen, activation of T cells, migration of effector T cells to the site of antigen challenge, and production of cytokines. This type of reaction is seen in many immunologic diseases (Table 4.5). The advent of cytokine antagonists as therapeutic agents has revolutionized the treatment and prognosis for patients with these disorders. For example, neutralization of TNF is highly effective in the treatment of rheumatoid arthritis.

Table 4.5   T Cell–Mediated Hypersensitivity Diseases

Disease	Specificity of Pathogenic T Cells	Principal Mechanisms of Tissue Injury	Clinicopathologic Manifestations
Rheumatoid arthritis	Collagen (postulated) Citrullinated self proteins	Inflammation mediated by Th17 (and Th1?) cytokines; role of antibodies and immune complexes	Chronic arthritis with synovial inflammation, destruction of articular cartilage
Multiple sclerosis	Protein antigens in myelin (e.g., myelin basic protein)	Inflammation mediated by Th1 and Th17 cytokines, myelin destruction by activated macrophages	Demyelination in central nervous system with perivascular inflammation; paralysis
Type 1 diabetes mellitus	Antigens of pancreatic islet β cells	T cell–mediated inflammation, destruction of islet cells by cytotoxic lymphocytes	Insulitis (chronic inflammation in islets), destruction of β cells; diabetes
Inflammatory bowel disease	Enteric bacteria; self antigens (unknown)	Inflammation mediated by Th1 and Th17 cytokines	Chronic intestinal inflammation, obstruction
Psoriasis	Self antigen (unknown)	Inflammation mediated mainly by Th17 cytokines	Cutaneous plaques
Contact sensitivity	Various environmental chemicals (e.g., urushiol from poison ivy, therapeutic drugs)	Inflammation mediated by Th1 (and Th17?) cytokines	Epidermal necrosis, dermal inflammation, causing skin rash and blisters

Examples of human T cell–mediated diseases are listed.

AUTOIMMUNE DISEASES

Autoimmune diseases are caused by adaptive immune responses against self antigens.

It is estimated that these diseases affect 1% to 5% of Western populations, and their incidence seems to be increasing, for unknown reasons. Based on the involved tissues and clinical manifestations, autoimmune diseases are broadly divided into organ-specific and systemic diseases (summarized in Table 4.6). In systemic diseases that are caused by immune complexes and autoantibodies, the lesions principally affect the connective tissues and blood vessels of involved organs. Therefore, these diseases are often referred to as collagen vascular diseases or connective tissue diseases, even though the immunologic reactions are not specifically directed against constituents of connective tissue or blood vessels.

Mechanisms of Autoimmunity

Self-tolerance in T and B lymphocytes prevents harmful reactions against self tissues.

The normal immune system can react to an enormous diversity of foreign antigens but does not recognize or respond to self antigens. The lack of reactivity is called *tolerance* (implying that the cells "tolerate" the presence of the antigen); the absence of immune responsiveness against one's own tissues is called *self-tolerance*. Because autoimmunity results from a breakdown of self-tolerance, we first discuss the major mechanisms of tolerance.

- *Central tolerance.* Self-reactive lymphocytes are eliminated (deleted) before they complete their maturation in the thymus (for T cells) and bone marrow (for B cells). Numerous self antigens are present in these organs, and when immature lymphocytes with high-affinity receptors for these antigens encounter them, the cells die. Central tolerance eliminates many potentially dangerous self-reactive lymphocytes but is imperfect, and some of these cells mature and enter peripheral tissues.
- *Regulatory T cells.* The response of self-reactive lymphocytes that escape deletion is prevented by the actions of regulatory T cells (Tregs) in peripheral tissues. The best-defined Tregs are CD4+ cells that express the transcription factor Foxp3. A severe autoimmune disease affecting many organs occurs in boys who inherit deleterious mutations in the X-linked *FOXP3* gene.

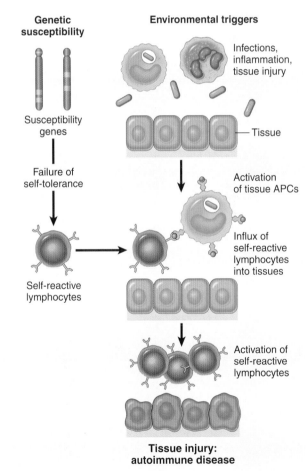

Genetic susceptibility

Susceptibility genes

Failure of self-tolerance

Self-reactive lymphocytes

Environmental triggers

Infections, inflammation, tissue injury

Tissue

Activation of tissue APCs

Influx of self-reactive lymphocytes into tissues

Activation of self-reactive lymphocytes

Tissue injury: autoimmune disease

Fig. 4.8 Postulated mechanisms of autoimmunity. In this proposed model of organ-specific T cell–mediated autoimmunity, various genetic loci may confer susceptibility to autoimmunity, probably by influencing the maintenance of self-tolerance. Environmental triggers, such as infections and other inflammatory stimuli, promote the influx of lymphocytes into tissues and the activation of antigen-presenting cells (APCs) and subsequently of self-reactive T cells, resulting in tissue injury.

Table 4.6 Organ-Specific and Systemic Autoimmune Diseases

Organ-Specific Diseases	Systemic Diseases
Diseases Mediated by Antibodies	
Autoimmune hemolytic anemia	Systemic lupus erythematosus
Autoimmune thrombocytopenia	
Autoimmune atrophic gastritis of pernicious anemia	
Myasthenia gravis	
Graves disease	
Goodpasture syndrome	
Diseases Mediated by T Cells[a]	
Type 1 diabetes	Rheumatoid arthritis
Multiple sclerosis	Systemic sclerosis (scleroderma)[b]
	Sjögren syndrome[b]
Diseases Postulated to Be Autoimmune	
Inflammatory bowel diseases (Crohn disease, ulcerative colitis)[c]	
Primary biliary cholangitis[b]	Polyarteritis nodosa[b]
Autoimmune (chronic active) hepatitis	Inflammatory myopathies[b]

[a]A role for T cells has been demonstrated in these disorders, but antibodies may also be involved in tissue injury.
[b]An autoimmune basis of these disorders is suspected but not established.
[c]These disorders may result from excessive immune responses to commensal enteric microbes, autoimmunity, or a combination of the two.
The features of many of these diseases have been summarized in Tables 4.3, 4.4, and 4.5.

- *Inhibitory receptors.* Self-reactive lymphocytes that have matured can also be inactivated upon recognition of self antigens in peripheral tissues. One of the mechanisms of inactivation is that T lymphocytes that respond to self antigens express inhibitory receptors (also called *coinhibitors*), notably two named CTLA-4 and PD-1, that shut off further lymphocyte activation, thus establishing "checkpoints" in immune responses. As we will discuss in Chapter 5, tumors also induce the expression of these receptors, and blocking them is a strategy for stimulating immune responses against cancer cells. Predictably, patients treated with checkpoint blockade for cancer immunotherapy also develop autoimmunity.

Numerous factors contribute to the breakdown of self-tolerance and the development of autoimmunity, including susceptibility genes and environmental insults (Fig. 4.8).

The susceptibility genes may influence lymphocyte tolerance, and environmental factors, such as infections or tissue injury, may alter the display of and responses to self antigens. The complex interactions between these diverse genetic and environmental factors in autoimmune diseases are not completely understood.

Genetic Susceptibility

Autoimmune diseases are multigenic, meaning that polymorphisms in many different genes are associated with an increased or decreased risk of the disease.

Except for some rare mendelian causes of autoimmune disease, no autoimmune disease can be attributed to a single gene. Among the polymorphic genes linked to autoimmunity, by far the most

commonly incriminated is the *HLA* locus, with specific *HLA* alleles showing "odds ratios" (relative risk of developing a disease compared to individuals who do not inherit that allele) of less than 2 to more than 100 for different diseases. It is reasonable to postulate that a variation in HLA molecules affects the presentation of self antigens, but how a given *HLA* allele influences the risk of developing a particular disease remains unknown.

Environmental Factors

Environmental factors participate in causing autoimmunity in a genetically susceptible host.

A link between infections and autoimmunity has been postulated based on results from experimental models and because of the fact that infectious prodromes sometimes precede autoimmune diseases in patients. It may be that microbial pathogens activate immune cells and overcome the normal mechanisms of self-tolerance.

In addition to infections, the display of tissue antigens also may be altered by a variety of environmental insults. For instance, ultraviolet radiation causes cell death and may lead to the exposure of nuclear antigens that elicit pathologic immune responses (e.g., in SLE; see later). Smoking is a risk factor for rheumatoid arthritis, perhaps due to chemical modification of self antigens. Local tissue injury for any reason may lead to the release of self antigens, with subsequent autoimmune responses. Many autoimmune diseases are more common in women than in men, suggesting that hormones influence the development of autoimmunity, but the underlying mechanisms are obscure.

In the following sections, we discuss selected autoimmune diseases that affect multiple organs and illustrate important aspects of the pathogenesis and manifestations of this group of disorders. Other organ-specific diseases are discussed in relevant chapters.

Systemic Lupus Erythematosus (SLE)

SLE is characterized by the production of autoantibodies and immune complexes, which elicit inflammation and damage many cells and tissues.

It is more common in women than in men (~10:1 ratio) and tends to occur in women of reproductive age. The pathogenesis of the disease is best understood in terms of the antibodies that are produced.

Pathogenesis. **The hallmark of SLE is autoantibodies produced against nuclear antigens, including double-stranded DNA (present in about 50% of cases), nucleoproteins, and others.**

The antibodies form complexes with released antigens, and the complexes deposit in the kidneys and other organs (type III hypersensitivity). Antibodies also bind to and opsonize blood cells, leading to their destruction by phagocytes (type II hypersensitivity). These antibodies and immune complexes usually activate the complement system, which may lead to a fall in serum complement levels.

Although the etiology and mechanisms of SLE are not established, a plausible hypothesis is the following: Exposure to ultraviolet light (a known risk factor) leads to apoptosis of various cells; improper clearance of nuclear fragments combined with failure of B and T cell tolerance causes activation of lymphocytes specific for self nuclear antigens. High-affinity antibodies produced against these antigens form immune complexes, which are endocytosed by dendritic cells and B lymphocytes. The nuclear DNA and RNA stimulate production of type I interferons, which activate lymphocytes and APCs, setting up a cycle of persistent autoantibody production.

Morphology. SLE can affect virtually any organ. The most characteristic lesions result from immune complex deposition in blood vessels, kidneys, and skin:

- *Blood vessels.* An acute necrotizing vasculitis involving capillaries, small arteries, and arterioles may be present in any tissue. The arteritis leads to fibrinoid necrosis of the vessel walls. In chronic stages, vessels undergo fibrous thickening with luminal narrowing.
- *Kidney.* Up to 50% of SLE patients have clinically significant renal involvement, and the kidney virtually always shows evidence of abnormality if examined by electron microscopy and immunofluorescence (Supplemental eFig. 4.1). Renal involvement takes a number of forms, all of which are associated with the deposition of immune complexes within the glomeruli. Proliferative glomerulonephritis is the most common manifestation of renal pathology (see Chapter 11).
- *Skin.* Characteristic erythema affecting the face along the bridge of the nose and cheeks (the butterfly or malar rash) is seen in approximately 50% of patients, but a similar rash also may be seen on the extremities and trunk. Exposure to sunlight incites or accentuates the erythema. Histologically, the involved areas show vacuolar degeneration of the basal layer of the epidermis (Supplemental eFig. 4.2). In the dermis, there is variable edema and perivascular inflammation. Vasculitis with fibrinoid necrosis may be prominent. Immunofluorescence microscopy shows deposits of immunoglobulin and complement along the dermoepidermal junction (Supplemental eFig. 4.3).
- *Cardiovascular system.* There may be damage to any layer of the heart. Symptomatic or asymptomatic pericardial involvement is present in up to 50% of patients and may be acute, subacute, or chronic. During the acute phase, fibrinous exudate is seen on the pericardial surface and an effusion may be present. With time, organization of the exudate may lead to fibrosis and a restrictive pericarditis. Myocarditis is less common and may cause resting tachycardia and electrocardiographic abnormalities. Valvular (so-called Libman-Sacks) endocarditis (Supplemental eFig. 4.4) was more common prior to the widespread use of steroids. This sterile endocarditis takes the form of single or multiple, 1- to 3-mm verrucous deposits, which may form on either surface of any heart valve, distinctively on either surface of the leaflets.
- *Other serosal cavity involvement.* Inflammation similar to that seen in the pericardium may involve the pleura, leading to fibrinous exudates, effusions, and fibrosis.
- *Other organs.* The joints may be involved by a nonerosive synovitis. Noninflammatory occlusion of small vessels by intimal proliferation may be seen in the CNS.

Clinical Features. SLE is a highly variable multisystem disease, and its diagnosis relies on clinical, serologic, and morphologic findings. It may be acute or insidious in onset. Many patients present with vague and puzzling symptoms that require an astute physician to diagnose. So-called generic antinuclear antibodies (ANAs) that bind to a variety of nuclear antigens are found in virtually 100% of patients but are not specific, whereas antibodies to double-stranded DNA, detected in 40% to 60% of cases, are highly specific for SLE, and hence a useful diagnostic test. Renal involvement may produce a variety of findings, including hematuria, red cell casts, proteinuria, and nephrotic syndrome (see Chapter 11). Anemia or thrombocytopenia is a presenting manifestation in some patients and may be a dominant clinical problem. Thromboembolic phenomena are secondary to antibodies that bind to phospholipid–protein complexes involved in clotting, a form of the antiphospholipid antibody syndrome (see Chapter 3). Neuropsychiatric manifestations (including seizures, psychosis, and neuropathy) and systemic manifestations such as fever are common. Mild arthritis may occur secondary to immune complex deposition.

Systemic Sclerosis (Scleroderma)

Systemic sclerosis is characterized by fibrosis of the skin and walls of the gastrointestinal tract and vascular abnormalities.

Pathogenesis. The development of this puzzling disease involves a poorly defined interplay of the immune system, small blood vessels, and fibroblasts. The presence of circulating autoantibodies, especially antinuclear antibodies, and T-cell infiltrates in affected skin suggest an autoimmune etiology, but neither the relevant self antigen nor the reason for the failure of self-tolerance is known. The immune infiltrates often contain CD4+ Th2 cells and macrophages that produce profibrotic cytokines such as transforming growth factor-β. Microvascular disease with evidence of endothelial activation and platelet aggregation is a consistent feature, but its basis is also not known. One hypothesis states that the vascular disease is the initiating event, and that it causes the chronic ischemia that ultimately results in tissue injury and fibrosis. Alternatively, the primary defect may lie in fibroblasts that are spontaneously activated to produce excessive collagen.

Morphology. Systemic sclerosis is a multi-system disease. The most prominent changes occur in the skin, alimentary tract, musculoskeletal system, and kidney, but lesions also are often present in the blood vessels, heart, lungs, and peripheral nerves. Most patients have diffuse fibrosis of the skin and associated atrophy (Fig. 4.9), which usually begins in the fingers and distal regions of the upper extremities and extends proximally to involve the upper arms, shoulders, neck, and face. Fibrosis often is accompanied by thinning of the epidermis, loss of rete pegs, atrophy of the dermal appendages, and hyaline thickening of the walls of dermal arterioles and capillaries.

Clinical Features. Diffuse skin fibrosis causes immobilization of the fingers and stiff facial features. Involvement of the esophagus leads to dysphagia and obstruction. Vascular narrowing is responsible for ischemia of fingers and toes, especially in cold weather, called Raynaud phenomenon. Mild proteinuria is frequent, indicating renal involvement. For unclear reasons, patients sometimes develop pulmonary or systemic hypertension. Most patients have a slowly progressive course, but development of hypertension is an ominous sign. Two ANAs are strongly associated with systemic sclerosis. One, directed against DNA topoisomerase I, is highly specific and is associated with a greater likelihood of pulmonary fibrosis and peripheral vascular disease. The other, an anticentromere antibody, is associated with the CREST syndrome, in which there are limited skin disease, often confined to fingers, forearms, and face; subcutaneous calcifications; and late or no esophageal lesions and pulmonary hypertension.

Sjögren Syndrome

In this disease, chronic inflammation and destruction of lacrimal and salivary glands lead to reduced production of tears and saliva.

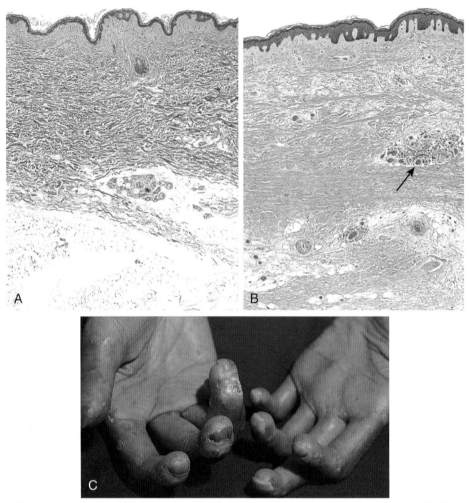

Fig. 4.9 Systemic sclerosis. (A) Normal skin. (B) Skin biopsy from a patient with systemic sclerosis. Note the extensive deposition of dense collagen in the dermis with virtual absence of appendages (e.g., hair follicles) and foci of inflammation *(arrow)*. (C) The extensive subcutaneous fibrosis has virtually immobilized the fingers, creating a clawlike flexion deformity. Loss of blood supply has led to cutaneous ulcerations. (C, Courtesy Dr. Richard Sontheimer, Department of Dermatology, University of Texas Southwestern Medical School, Dallas.)

Pathogenesis. The disease is often associated with other autoimmune disorders and the presence of serum autoantibodies, supporting an autoimmune etiology. Of the various autoantibodies, two directed towards ribonucleoprotein antigens SS-A and SS-B are specific for this disease. The triggers for antibody formation are not known, and it has even been suggested that the disease is initiated by viral infection of the salivary glands, with a persistent autoimmune T-cell reaction developing subsequently.

Morphology. The lacrimal and salivary glands are the major targets of the disease, but other exocrine glands, including those lining the respiratory and gastrointestinal tracts and the vagina, also may be involved. The lacrimal and salivary glands contain dense infiltrates of CD4+ T cells (Fig. 4.10); in the larger salivary glands, lymphoid follicles with germinal centers, indicative of a B cell reaction, may also be seen. Salivary glands may be visibly enlarged.

Clinical Features. Because of destruction of the lacrimal glands, there is dryness of the eyes and secondary inflammation and ulceration of the cornea (keratoconjunctivitis sicca). Lack of saliva causes dryness of the mouth (xerostomia). Nasal dryness may lead to ulceration and, in some cases, perforation of the septum. Lesions outside the glands, seen in about half of patients, include synovitis, peripheral neuropathy, and pulmonary fibrosis. More than half of the patients have another autoimmune disease, most frequently rheumatoid arthritis.

REJECTION OF TRANSPLANTS

The replacement of damaged or functionally impaired organs by transplantation of organs from other individuals has become standard medical practice. About 30,000 organ transplants are performed yearly in the United States, the most common being the kidney (accounting for almost half), followed by the heart, liver, lung, and pancreas. Transplantation of hematopoietic stem cells is widely used to treat both neoplastic and nonneoplastic disorders of blood cells. Except in rare cases of identical twins, the graft donor and recipient are genetically

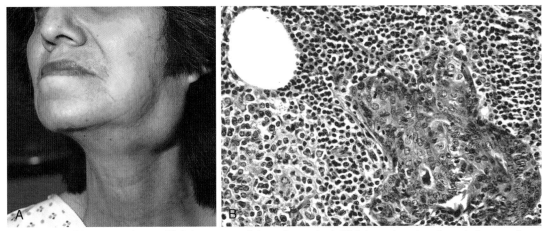

Fig. 4.10 Sjögren syndrome. (A) Enlargement of the salivary gland. (B) Intense lymphocytic and plasma cell infiltration with ductal epithelial hyperplasia in a salivary gland. (A, Courtesy Dr. Richard Sontheimer, Department of Dermatology, University of Texas Southwestern Medical School, Dallas. B, Courtesy Dr. Dennis Burns, Department of Pathology, University of Texas Southwestern Medical School, Dallas.)

different. Some of these differences are recognized by the immune system and are responsible for immune destruction of the graft, called *rejection*. Grafts exchanged between nonidentical individuals of the same species are called *allografts*.

Immune Responses to Organ Allografts

The principal graft antigens recognized by the recipient's immune system are histocompatibility molecules, which evoke both cellular and humoral immune responses.

As the name implies, histocompatibility molecules were discovered as the molecules that determine whether or not tissue grafts (*histo,* tissue) exchanged between individuals would be accepted (compatible). The major histocompatibility complex (MHC, or HLA in humans) is a collection of highly polymorphic genes that differ among individuals. The physiologic function of MHC proteins encoded by these genes is to display peptide antigens for recognition by T cells. If the graft donor expresses MHC molecules that differ from those in the recipient, the graft is recognized as foreign by the recipient's T cells. MHC molecules in the graft may be presented on graft cells (parenchymal cells and APCs) and be recognized by recipient T cells (direct recognition), or graft MHC molecules may be taken up by the recipient's APCs and presented to T cells (indirect recognition). In both cases, the recipient's CD4+ and CD8+ T cells specific for graft antigens are activated, migrate back into the transplant, and cause its rejection. Recipient B cells also recognize molecules in the graft as foreign, resulting in the production of antibodies specific for these molecules.

Mechanisms of Rejection of Solid-Organ Allografts

Rejection of allografts is mediated by T cells and antibodies.

CD4+ T cells specific for graft antigens secrete cytokines that induce inflammation in the graft; CD8+ CTLs kill graft cells; and antibodies bind to graft tissues (notably endothelium because it is the most accessible to circulating antibodies), activate complement, and cause injury to the tissues. All three mechanisms may be involved simultaneously, but as is discussed later, they play dominant roles in different types of rejection.

The major patterns of rejection reflect different mechanisms of graft injury and have different morphologic and clinical features.

These patterns were first described and are best established for kidney transplants, but the same principles apply to the rejection of all solid organ transplants. The utility of classifying rejection into

different types is that, although the patterns were defined on the basis of pathologic and clinical features, each is caused by specific immune mechanisms.

- *Hyperacute rejection.* This is mediated by antibodies specific for donor antigens that are present in the recipient prior to transplantation. It occurs very rapidly following connection of the graft vasculature to the host circulation, when preformed antibodies flood the graft. These antibodies bind to graft endothelium, activating the complement system and coagulation cascade, causing rapid thrombosis of the vessels and ischemic necrosis of the graft (Fig. 4.11). In the past, ABO blood group incompatibility was the greatest risk for hyperacute rejection, since individuals lacking a particular ABO antigen make antibodies against that antigen. Recipients who have been sensitized by blood transfusions or previous transplant are also at risk. Careful blood group matching of recipients and prospective donors and cross-match testing for serum antibodies in the recipient reactive with donor tissue have largely eliminated this problem.
- *Acute rejection.* This form of rejection develops days to weeks after transplantation and leads to graft failure. In *acute cellular rejection,* CD8+ CTLs kill graft parenchymal cells (Fig. 4.12). At the same time, CD4+ T cells stimulate inflammation in the graft, which exacerbates the damage. In *acute humoral* (or *vascular) rejection,* antibodies are produced against donor antigens, bind to graft endothelium, and cause damage mainly by complement-dependent mechanisms (Fig. 4.13). Often, the cellular and humoral reactions coexist. Immunosuppressive therapy has been more successful in treating acute rejection than any other form.
- *Chronic rejection.* With increasingly effective therapy of acute rejection, chronic rejection, which develops over months to years, has become the major cause of graft failure. Chronic rejection is characterized by vascular injury and intimal fibrosis, leading to narrowing of vessels and ischemia, and interstitial fibrosis due to prolonged inflammation and ischemic tissue injury (Fig. 4.14).

Treatment of Graft Rejection

In all except identical twins, immunosuppression is needed to prolong graft survival. Corticosteroids, anti–T-cell antibodies, and drugs that inhibit T-cell function are the mainstays of treatment. Immunosuppression carries the risk of opportunistic fungal and viral infections. Reactivation of latent viruses (e.g., polyomavirus and cytomegalovirus), as

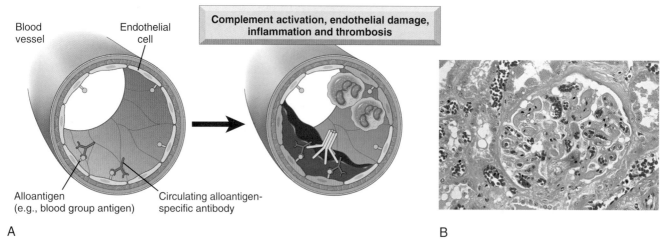

Blood vessel — Endothelial cell

Complement activation, endothelial damage, inflammation and thrombosis

Alloantigen (e.g., blood group antigen) — Circulating alloantigen-specific antibody

A

B

Fig. 4.11 Hyperacute rejection. (A) Deposition of antibody on endothelium and activation of complement causes thrombosis. (B) Hyperacute rejection of a kidney allograft showing platelet and fibrin thrombi, early neutrophil infiltration, and severe ischemic injury (necrosis) in a glomerulus.

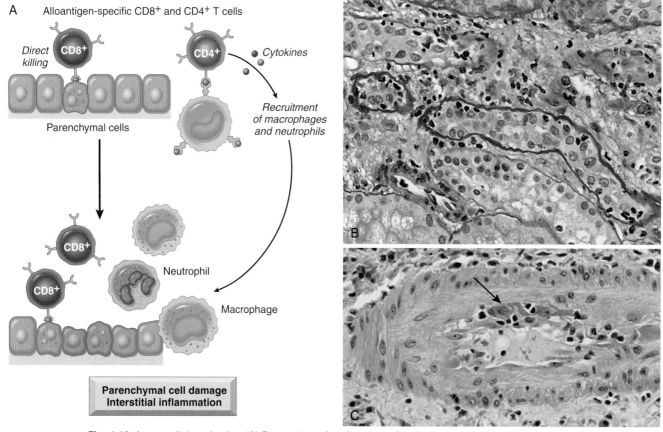

A Alloantigen-specific CD8+ and CD4+ T cells

Direct killing — CD8+ — CD4+ — Cytokines

Parenchymal cells

Recruitment of macrophages and neutrophils

CD8+

CD8+

Neutrophil

Macrophage

Parenchymal cell damage Interstitial inflammation

B

C

Fig. 4.12 Acute cellular rejection. (A) Destruction of graft cells by T cells. Acute T cell–mediated rejection involves direct killing of graft cells by CD8+ CTLs and inflammation caused by cytokines produced by CD4+ T cells. (B) Acute cellular rejection of a kidney graft, manifested by inflammatory cells in the interstitium and between epithelial cells of the tubules (tubulitis). (C) Acute cellular rejection involving an artery with inflammatory cells damaging the endothelium *(arrow)*.

well as an increased risk of cancers, are also seen in immunosuppressed patients.

Hematopoietic Stem Cell Transplantation

The transplantation of hematopoietic stem cells (HSCs) is used to treat leukemias and other hematologic malignancies, and to correct numerical or functional deficiencies of blood cells.

The process was historically called bone marrow transplantation because the HSCs were isolated from the donor's bone marrow, but now these stem cells are mobilized from the marrow of donors by treatment with growth factors or agents that inhibit binding of HSCs to their marrow "niche", allowing HSCs to be harvested in most instances from the peripheral blood.

Recipients of HSCs need "conditioning" to ablate their own immune system (to prevent graft rejection), create "space" for the transplanted

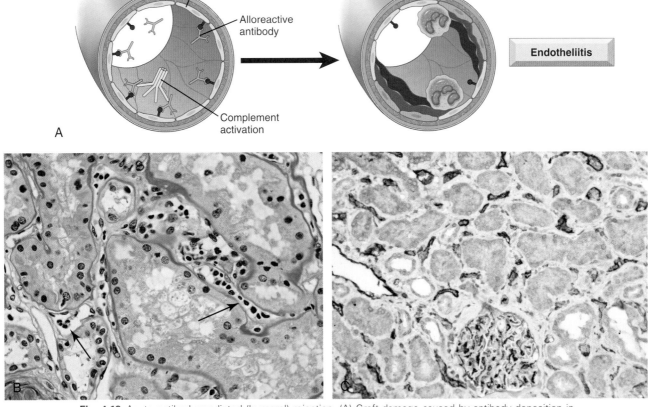

Fig. 4.13 Acute antibody-mediated (humoral) rejection. (A) Graft damage caused by antibody deposition in vessels. (B) Light micrograph showing inflammation (capillaritis) in peritubular capillaries *(arrows)* in a kidney graft. (C) Immunoperoxidase staining shows C4d deposition in peritubular capillaries and a glomerulus. (Courtesy Dr. Zoltan Laszik, Department of Pathology, University of California San Francisco.)

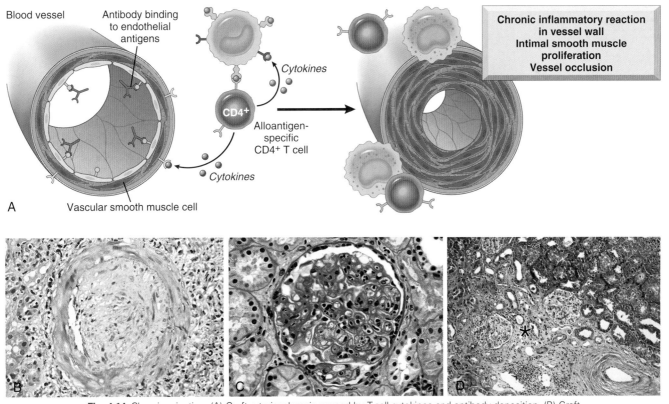

Fig. 4.14 Chronic rejection. (A) Graft arteriosclerosis caused by T-cell cytokines and antibody deposition. (B) Graft arteriosclerosis in a cardiac transplant. (C) Transplant glomerulopathy, the characteristic manifestation of chronic antibody-mediated rejection in the kidney. The glomerulus shows inflammatory cells within the capillary loops (glomerulitis), accumulation of mesangial matrix, and duplication of the capillary basement membrane. (D) Interstitial fibrosis and tubular atrophy, resulting from vascular narrowing and ischemia. In this trichrome stain, the blue area *(asterisk)* shows fibrosis, contrasted with the normal kidney on the top right. At the bottom right is an artery showing prominent arteriosclerosis. (B, Courtesy Dr. Richard Mitchell, Department of Pathology, Brigham and Women's Hospital, Boston; C, courtesy Dr. Zoltan Laszik, Department of Pathology, University of California San Francisco.)

stem cells, and (in the case of leukemia and other malignancies) kill tumor cells. The major problem with HSC transplantation is graft-versus-host disease (GVHD). Grafts contain not only HSCs but also mature T cells, and these cells can attack host tissues and cause serious and even fatal clinical problems. Even small, non-MHC differences between donor and recipient can elicit this response. The recipient, being immunodeficient, cannot reject the foreign, attacking cells. *Acute GVHD* is characterized by T cell–mediated killing of epithelial cells of the liver, gastrointestinal tract, and skin, producing liver failure with jaundice, bloody diarrhea, and rashes. *Chronic GVHD* is a more indolent condition in which fibrosis of the skin and other tissues is prominent (probably due to chronic inflammation) and there are various manifestations of autoimmunity (because of prolonged activation of lymphocytes). The clinical and histologic picture may resemble systemic sclerosis.

Recipients of HSC transplants also may have profound immunodeficiency before the transplanted cells produce adequate numbers of granulocytes and T lymphocytes. Recovery of immune competence may take several months.

IMMUNODEFICIENCY DISORDERS

Immunodeficiencies make individuals susceptible to infections and cancers.

Although mild deficiencies of the immune system seem to be quite common, clinically significant defects are relatively rare. The infectious diseases these patients get may be the result of new infections with opportunistic and pathogenic microbes or reactivation of latent infections. The cancers are most often virus induced but can be quite diverse. Paradoxically, some patients with defective immune systems develop autoimmunity, a reflection of a hyperactive immune system. The reason for this association is unclear; it may be because tolerance mechanisms are lost or because persistent infections induce excessive immune activation.

Immunodeficiency diseases may be primary (resulting from mutations) or secondary to other disorders.

Primary immunodeficiencies are caused by mutations that are usually inherited, so the term *congenital immunodeficiency* is often used, but sometimes the mutation is a new one in the affected patient. Patients typically present with recurrent infections in infancy or early childhood, but in some diseases the first symptoms appear later in life.

Secondary immunodeficiencies are much more common than primary ones. In higher-income countries, the most frequent cause of immunodeficiency is therapy that destroys the immune system (e.g., chemotherapy and radiation for cancer) or that is used to intentionally suppress the immune system (e.g., for graft rejection and autoimmune diseases). In lower-income countries, malnutrition is a major cause of immunodeficiency. The acquired immunodeficiency syndrome (AIDS) is an important cause of immunodeficiency worldwide, and is discussed later.

Primary (Congenital) Immunodeficiencies

Primary immunodeficiencies are caused by mutations that impact one or more components of innate or adaptive immunity.

Because of the increasing use of DNA sequencing technology in medicine, the genetic basis of many primary immunodeficiencies is now known. Table 4.7 and Supplemental eFig. 4.5 summarize the most common of these. Selected diseases that illustrate important principles are discussed below.

- *Severe combined immunodeficiency (SCID)* presents in infancy with defects in humoral and cell-mediated immunity and susceptibility to a diverse range of infections. It is most often caused by defects in T-cell maturation, and the absence of T-cell help leads to reduced antibody production. About half the cases are X-linked (X-SCID), caused by a mutation in the gene on the X chromosome that encodes the common γ chain (γc), one of the chains for the receptors for many cytokines, including interleukins IL-2 and IL-7. Because IL-7 is required for the proliferation of T-cell progenitors, the absence of IL-7 signaling leads to a profound deficiency of mature T cells. As with all X-linked diseases, boys are affected and girls are carriers.

  The remaining cases of SCID are autosomal recessive. The most frequent mutation in these cases is in the gene encoding the enzyme adenosine deaminase, which is expressed at high levels in developing T cells in the thymus. Adenosine deaminase deficiency leads to the accumulation of toxic purine metabolites, which are especially damaging to rapidly proliferating cells such as immature lymphocytes. Many other genes have been identified in rare cases of autosomal recessive SCID.

  Because both T-cell and B-cell responses are impaired, patients present with recurrent infections with a wide range of pathogens, including fungi *(Candida, Pneumocystis),* bacteria *(Pseudomonas),* and viruses (cytomegalovirus, varicella). HSC transplantation can repopulate the patients with normal immune cells and is the mainstay of treatment. X-SCID is the first disease that has been treated with gene therapy, in which a normal *γc* gene is introduced into HSCs of patients and the cells are transplanted into the patients.

- *X-linked agammaglobulinemia* is due to a defect in B-cell maturation and a resultant failure to produce antibodies (gamma globulins is an old name for circulating antibodies). The defect is caused by mutations in the gene encoding a signaling molecule, Bruton tyrosine kinase. This kinase is associated with the B-cell receptor in mature B cells and the pre-B cell receptor in B cell progenitors, and delivers signals that are required for B-cell proliferation and maturation. Without these signals, B cells die at the pre-B stage, resulting in the absence of antibody-producing B cells and plasma cells. Affected children are susceptible to many bacterial and viral infections.

- *X-linked hyper-IgM syndrome* was originally identified by the absence of class-switched IgG and IgA antibodies, and, hence, the dominance of IgM. It is usually associated with a profound deficiency of cell-mediated immunity. The disease is most frequently caused by mutations in the gene for CD40-ligand (CD40L), which is expressed on helper T cells and is a mechanism by which CD4+ T cells activate (help) B cells and macrophages. CD40L binds to CD40 on B cells and macrophages, and delivers signals that stimulate B-cell responses as well as macrophage activation (the central reaction of cell-mediated immunity). Affected children suffer from infections by pyogenic and intracellular bacteria, viruses, and fungi.

- *Common variable immunodeficiency* is more frequent than the other immunodeficiencies discussed, but its basis is obscure. Patients have deficiencies of plasma cells and antibodies, although the number of B cells is virtually normal, suggesting a block in the differentiation of mature B cells. The genetic basis is known in fewer than 10% of cases; mutations affecting receptors for growth factors and other lymphocyte signaling pathways have been reported. Patients are susceptible to bacterial infections.

Table 4.7   The Major Primary Immunodeficiency Diseases

Disease	Functional Deficiencies	Mechanism of Defect
A. Defects in lymphocyte maturation		
Severe combined immunodeficiency (SCID)		
X-linked SCID	Markedly decreased T cells; normal or increased B cells; reduced serum Ig	Cytokine receptor common γ-chain gene mutations, defective T-cell maturation due to lack of IL-7 signals
B cell immunodeficiencies		
X-linked agammaglobulinemia	Decrease in all serum Ig isotypes; reduced B-cell numbers	Failure of maturation beyond pre-B cells, because of mutation in Bruton tyrosine kinase
Ig heavy-chain deficiencies	Deficiency of IgG subclasses; sometimes associated with absent IgA or IgE	Chromosomal deletion involving Ig heavy-chain locus
Disorders of T-cell maturation		
DiGeorge syndrome	Decreased T cells; normal B cells; normal or decreased serum Ig	Anomalous development of 3rd and 4th branchial pouches, leading to thymic hypoplasia
B. Defects in lymphocyte activation		
X-linked hyper-IgM syndrome	Defects in helper T-cell–dependent B-cell and macrophage activation	Mutations in CD40 ligand
Common variable immunodeficiency	Reduced or no production of selective isotypes or subtypes of immunoglobulins; susceptibility to bacterial infections or no clinical problems	Mutations in receptors for B-cell growth factors, costimulators
Defective class II MHC expression: the bare lymphocyte syndrome	Lack of class II MHC expression and impaired CD4$^+$ T-cell activation; defective cell-mediated immunity and T cell–dependent humoral immunity	Mutations in genes encoding transcription factors required for class II MHC gene expressions
X-linked lymphoproliferative disease	Uncontrolled EBV-induced B-cell proliferation and cytotoxic lymphocyte (CTL) activation; defective NK-cell and CTL function and antibody responses	Mutations in gene encoding SAP (an adaptor protein involved in signaling in lymphocytes)
C. Defects in innate immunity		
Chronic granulomatous disease	Defective production of reactive oxygen intermediates by phagocytes	Mutations in genes encoding components of the phagocyte oxidase enzyme
Leukocyte adhesion deficiency-1	Absent or deficient expression of β2 integrins causing defective leukocyte adhesion-dependent functions	Mutations in gene encoding the β chain (CD 18) of β2 integrins
Leukocyte adhesion deficiency-2	Absent or deficient expression of leukocyte ligands for endothelial E- and P-selectins, causing failure of leukocyte migration into tissues	Mutations in gene encoding a protein required for synthesis of the sialyl-Lewis X component of E- and P-selectin ligands
Complement C3 deficiency	Defect in complement cascade activation	Mutations in *C3* gene
Complement C2, C4 deficiency	Deficient activation of classical pathway of complement, leading to failure to clear immune complexes and development of lupus-like disease	Mutations in *C2* or *C4* gene

EBV, Epstein-Barr disease; *Ig,* immunoglobulin; *IL,* interleukin; *MHC,* major histocompatibility complex. From Abbas AK, Lichtman AH, Pillai S: Basic Immunology: Function and Disorders of the Immune System, 5th ed., Philadelphia: Elsevier, 2016.

- *DiGeorge syndrome (thymic hypoplasia)* is caused by a congenital defect in the development of the thymus, resulting in deficient T-cell maturation. T cells are absent in the lymph nodes, spleen, and peripheral blood, and infants with this defect are vulnerable to viral, fungal, and protozoal infections. The disorder is a consequence of a developmental defect affecting the third and fourth pharyngeal pouches, structures that give rise to the thymus, parathyroid glands, and portions of the face and aortic arch. Thus, in addition to the thymic and T-cell defects, there may be parathyroid gland hypoplasia, resulting in hypocalcemic tetany, as well as additional midline developmental abnormalities. In 90% of cases of DiGeorge syndrome, there is a deletion affecting chromosomal region 22q11 (see Chapter 6). Most patients improve with age and do not require treatment (other than for infections). Unlike most other primary immunodeficiencies, DiGeorge syndrome is a developmental defect but is not heritable.

- *Defects in innate immunity.* Defective production of reactive oxygen species in neutrophils is caused by mutations affecting the phagocyte oxidase enzyme (Chapter 2). This disease is called *chronic granulomatous disease (CGD)* because strong macrophage activation, often resulting in granuloma formation, compensates for the inability of neutrophils to destroy phagocytosed microbes. The *leukocyte adhesion deficiencies* are caused by mutations affecting the functions of the adhesion molecules integrins and selectins (Chapter 2). Leukocyte recruitment into tissues, and hence acute inflammation, are impaired in these disorders. Deficient recruitment and functions of neutrophils result in increased susceptibility to bacterial infections.

ACQUIRED IMMUNODEFICIENCY SYNDROME

AIDS is caused by infection with human immunodeficiency virus (HIV), which destroys CD4+ T cells and leads to profound immunodeficiency.

This disease was first identified in the 1980s, and has become one of the great scourges of the modern world. Recent successes of antiviral drugs have provided hope to patients, but it remains a major medical and societal problem, especially in developing countries. It is estimated that there are more than 35 million HIV-infected individuals in the world, of whom 70% are in Africa and 20% in Asia, and almost 1 million die each year from the disease.

The disease is transmitted by direct transfer of infected fluids. The three main modes of transmission are:

- *Sexual transmission:* This is the dominant mode of infection, accounting for more than 75% of all cases. About 50% of the reported cases are in homosexual or bisexual men, but heterosexual transmission has rapidly increased, especially in Africa and Asia, where it accounts for half or more of new infections in adults. The virus is carried in the semen and enters the body through mucosal abrasions.
- *Parenteral transmission:* Another 20% of cases are in intravenous drug users. Transmission occurs by sharing of needles and syringes contaminated with HIV-infected blood. Transmission by blood or blood products can occur but is now very uncommon because of routine screening.
- *Mother-to-infant transmission* is the major cause of pediatric AIDS. It can occur by transplacental spread during delivery and through breast milk. About 2% of new cases are in babies born of infected mothers.

Human Immunodeficiency Virus: Structure and Life Cycle

HIV is a retrovirus that infects cells via CD4 and coreceptors, integrates into the host cell genome, and kills cells when it is activated to replicate.

Like other retroviruses, HIV is an enveloped virus whose core contains structural capsid proteins, enzymes involved in viral integration, and two strands of viral RNA, which encode all these proteins, as well as numerous regulators of viral gene expression and replication (Fig. 4.15). There are two genetically different but related forms of HIV, called HIV-1 (the most frequent cause of AIDS) and HIV-2. To enter cells, the outer capsid protein gp120 binds to CD4 and subsequently to the chemokine receptors CXCR4 or CCR5 (called coreceptors for the virus). The virus then fuses with the host cell membrane and is internalized. Therefore, the cells that are infected are those that express CD4 and the coreceptors, mainly T cells and some macrophages and dendritic cells. Polymorphisms in the gene encoding CCR5 alter the susceptibility to HIV infection, while certain rare mutations in *CCR5* confer resistance.

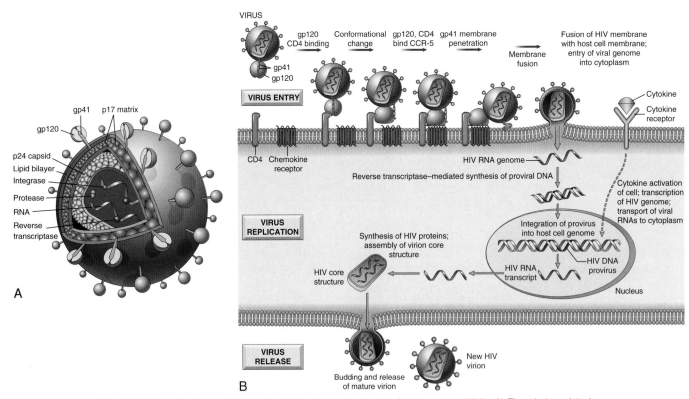

Fig. 4.15 The structure and life cycle of the human immunodeficiency virus (HIV). (A) The viral particle is covered by a lipid bilayer derived from the host cell and studded with viral glycoproteins gp41 and gp120. (B) The life cycle of HIV showing the steps from viral entry to the production of infectious virions. (Adapted with permission from Wain-Hobson S: HIV. One on one meets two. *Nature* 1996;384:117. Copyright 1996, Macmillan Magazines Limited.)

After entry of HIV into the cell, viral RNA is reverse transcribed to produce proviral DNA, which persists in episomal form in the cytoplasm or integrates into the genome of the infected cell. The virus may be silent in infected cells for years, establishing a latent infection. If the infected cell is activated (e.g., by an infection or inflammatory stimulus), the proviral DNA is transcribed, viral proteins are produced, and complete virions are released to continue the cycle of infection.

Pathogenesis. **HIV depletes CD4+ cells, mainly as a consequence of viral replication in infected cells.**

Exactly how the replicating virus mediates its cytopathic effect is still unclear; possibilities include an increase in membrane permeability caused by budding virions and competitive interference with host cell protein synthesis. The consequence is a progressive loss of T cells, primarily CD4+ cells. This decline is initially most prominent in mucosal tissues (the major site of virus entry), then is seen in draining lymph nodes, and only later is detected in blood T cells.

In addition to the direct loss of infected T cells, other mechanisms of immune deficiency have been postulated to account for the frequent observation that the severity of the immune deficits is much greater than the numbers of infected cells (measured mostly in the blood). These other mechanisms include the death of uninfected cells as a consequence of their chronic activation, defects in APCs, and the destruction of lymphoid tissue architecture.

Other cell types that are affected include B cells (which are not infected but show excessive activation), macrophages, and microglia in the CNS. Macrophages and microglia may be reservoirs of infection; in late stages of HIV infection, when CD4+ T-cell numbers decline greatly, macrophages may be an important site of continued viral replication.

Clinical Course. HIV disease may be divided into three sequential phases (Fig. 4.16).
- *Acute phase.* Virus enters through mucosa and infects and destroys CD4+ T cells at the site. Dendritic cells at mucosal sites carry the virus to regional lymph nodes, where the virus replicates and eventually spreads to other tissues. The individual mounts antiviral humoral and cell-mediated responses, resulting in seroconversion (usually within 3 to 7 weeks of exposure) and the development of virus-specific CD8+ CTLs. Around this time, patients develop a self-limited acute HIV syndrome, with systemic symptoms resembling those in many other acute infections. This typically resolves in 2 to 4 weeks.
- *Chronic phase.* The virus replicates mainly in secondary lymphoid organs and destroys T cells in these tissues, but infected cells are not numerous in the blood. Because infected patients do not have severe symptoms, this is often called the phase of clinical latency. Lymph nodes show lymphocyte depletion, and eventually, over a period of years, there is a decline in the number of CD4+ T cells in the blood.
- *AIDS.* The progressive loss of CD4+ T cells ultimately leads to profound immune deficiency. Patients with AIDS have a high incidence of opportunistic infections (e.g., *Pneumocystis jiroveci*, cytomegalovirus infections, cryptococcosis, candidiasis, and mycobacterial infections) and of certain tumors, many of which are caused by oncogenic DNA viruses, including Kaposi sarcoma (Kaposi sarcoma herpesvirus), B-cell lymphoma (Epstein-Barr virus), and cervical and anal carcinoma (human papillomavirus). Involvement of the CNS is a common and important manifestation of AIDS. Lesions include an initial self-limited presumed viral meningoencephalitis or aseptic meningitis, vacuolar myelopathy, peripheral neuropathies, and, most commonly, a progressive encephalopathy called HIV-associated neurocognitive disorder.

Because the loss of immune containment is associated with declining CD4+ T-cell counts, the Centers for Disease Control and Prevention (CDC) classification of HIV infection stratifies patients into three groups based on CD4+ cell counts: greater than or equal to 500 cells/μL, 200 to 499 cells/μL, and fewer than 200 cells/μL. The extent of viremia, measured as HIV-1 RNA levels in the blood, is a useful marker of HIV disease progression and is of value in the management of HIV-infected individuals.

The disease course described previously is typical of untreated patients. Currently, individuals treated with combinations of antiviral drugs (highly active antiretroviral therapy [HAART]) do not develop immune deficiency or AIDS with its attendant complications. However, the virus is not eradicated, so the treatment is not a cure, and there are significant side effects to these medications, including elevated lipids, insulin resistance, peripheral neuropathy, and premature cardiovascular, kidney, and liver disease. Furthermore, with long-term therapy, patients are at increased risk for diseases such as cancer and cardiovascular disease, for unknown reasons.

AMYLOIDOSIS

Amyloid is an extracellular deposit of fibrillar protein that can affect many organs and tissues.

These insoluble fibrils are produced by the aggregation of various proteins that are produced in excess amounts, are not cleared adequately, or fold improperly. The protein deposits bind carbohydrate-rich molecules, imparting staining properties that resemble starch (hence, the name). Amyloidosis, referring to amyloid deposits and their pathologic effects, is discussed here because some of the most common forms are composed of antibody molecules.

There are several forms of the disease, each associated with a morphologically identical but chemically distinct protein in the deposits (Fig. 4.17).
- *Primary amyloidosis.* The deposits are made of immunoglobulin light chains (called *AL [amyloid light chain]*), which are produced in excessive amounts by a neoplasm of plasma cells called myeloma, or by clonal proliferations of plasma cells without overt myeloma (see Chapter 9).
- *Reactive secondary amyloidosis.* The deposits are composed of the *amyloid A (AA)* protein, which is generated by proteolysis of its precursor serum amyloid A (SAA) protein. SAA is an acute-phase protein produced during inflammation. Prolonged production of large amounts of SAA is seen in chronic inflammation, so this form of amyloidosis is an infrequent complication of chronic inflammatory disorders (tuberculosis in the past; rheumatoid arthritis more frequently now, especially in developed countries).
- *Other forms of amyloidosis.* Deposits of Aβ amyloid are seen in the brains of patients with Alzheimer disease and some other forms of dementia. Several familial forms of amyloidosis are known, perhaps the most common of which is associated with familial Mediterranean fever, an inherited "autoinflammatory" disease in which patients spontaneously develop systemic inflammation, one consequence of which is increased production of the amyloid precursor SAA. In other familial forms, the amyloid is made up of mutant transthyretin, a transporter of thyroxine. It is deposited in autonomic and peripheral nerves, giving rise to polyneuropathies. In the past, patients undergoing hemodialysis developed amyloid deposits composed of the β2-microglobulin protein because it did

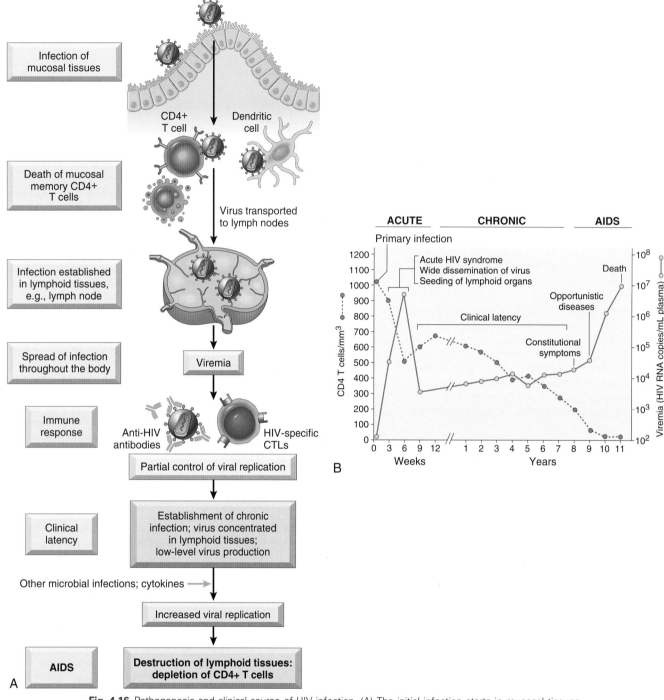

Fig. 4.16 Pathogenesis and clinical course of HIV infection. (A) The initial infection starts in mucosal tissues, involving mainly memory CD4+ T cells and dendritic cells, and spreads to lymph nodes. Viral replication leads to viremia and widespread seeding of lymphoid tissue. The viremia is controlled by the host immune response, and the patient then enters a phase of clinical latency. During this phase, viral replication in both T cells and macrophages continues unabated, but there is some immune containment of virus (not illustrated). There continues a gradual erosion of CD4+ cells, and ultimately, CD4+ T-cell numbers decline and the patient develops clinical symptoms of full-blown AIDS. (B) Clinical course of HIV infection. CTL, Cytotoxic T lymphocyte. (B, from Pantelo G, et al: *N Engl J Med* 328:327, 1993. Copyright 1993 Massachusetts Medical Society. All rights reserved.)

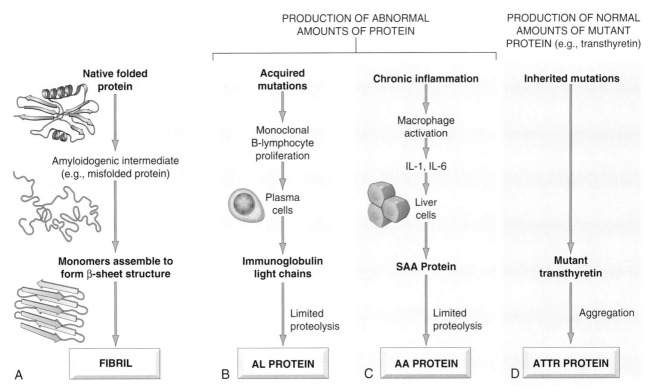

Fig. 4.17 Pathogenesis of amyloidosis. (A) General mechanism of formation of amyloid fibrils. (B) Primary amyloidosis, in which unknown mutations cause monoclonal B cell or plasma cell proliferations, resulting in excessive production of one immunoglobulin, and the light chains form the AL (amyloid light chain) form of amyloid. (C) Reactive systemic amyloidosis, in which chronic inflammation leads to production of serum amyloid A (SAA), which is converted to the amyloid A (AA) protein. (D) Mutations in transthyretin (TTR) lead to deposition as amyloid fibrils (ATTR, amyloid TTR) in amyloid of aging, especially affecting the heart.

not pass through older dialysis membranes, but newer filters have largely eliminated this problem.

- *Localized amyloidosis.* The primary and secondary amyloidoses described earlier are systemic in nature and affect many tissues and sites. By contrast, in some cases the amyloid deposits are limited to a single organ or site (e.g., skin, lung, tongue). At least in some localized forms, the amyloid consists of AL amyloid and may thus be a manifestation of primary amyloidosis.

- *Amyloid of aging.* Amyloid associated with aging affects elderly patients (in their seventies and eighties) and in many cases there is dominant involvement of the heart, presenting as a restrictive cardiomyopathy. Biochemically, the amyloid is comprised of transthyretin. Unlike in familial forms, transthyretin is wild type.

In all these types of amyloidosis, the responsible protein is produced in excess or has an unusual sequence. In the case of AL amyloid, experimental data suggest that particular light chains are amyloidogenic and others are not, implying that the primary amino acid sequence of the light chain determines whether amyloid fibrils form. But in any particular case, why amyloid forms (or not) is unknown.

Morphology. Extracellular deposits of amyloid may be present in virtually any parenchymal organ. In routine sections, they appear as pink, glassy, acellular material, often in vessel walls. Deposits can be distinguished from other substances by the Congo red stain, which imparts a characteristic color and yellow-green birefringence to the deposits (Fig. 4.18).

Clinical Features. Amyloid interferes with the normal function of the organ where it is deposited. The most frequent clinical complications result from deposition in the kidneys (nephrotic syndrome), heart (congestive heart failure), and gastrointestinal tract (malabsorption). The diagnosis of amyloidosis depends on demonstration of amyloid in tissues. The prognosis of individuals with systemic amyloidosis is poor, particularly those with systemic AL amyloidosis. The course of reactive systemic amyloidosis depends on the control of the underlying condition.

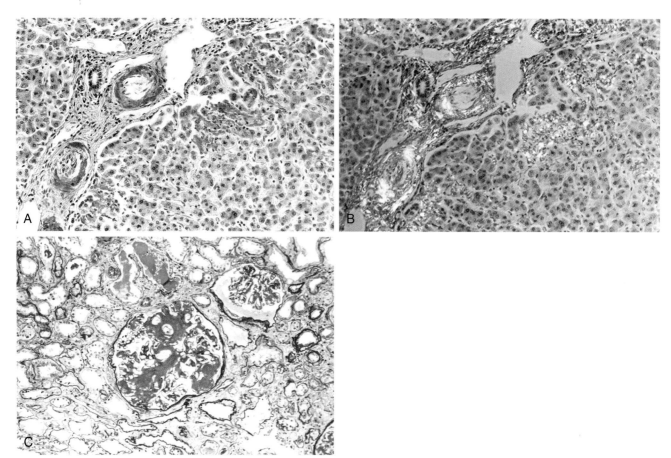

Fig. 4.18 Amyloidosis. (A) A section of liver stained with Congo red reveals pink-red deposits of amyloid in the walls of blood vessels and along sinusoids. (B) Note the yellow-green birefringence of the deposits when observed by a polarizing microscope. (C) In the kidney, the glomerular architecture is almost totally obliterated by the massive accumulation of amyloid. The stain, called a PAS stain, reveals glycogen-rich deposits. (B, Courtesy Dr. Trace Worrell and Sandy Hinton, Department of Pathology, University of Texas Southwestern Medical School, Dallas.)

5

Neoplasia

OUTLINE

Definition of Neoplasia, 63
Benign and Malignant Neoplasms, 63
Nomenclature, 64
    Nomenclature of Benign Tumors, 64
    Nomenclature of Malignant Tumors, 64
Characteristics of Benign and Malignant Neoplasms, 66
    Differentiation of Neoplasms, 66
    Local Invasion, 68
    Metastasis, 68
Molecular Basis of Neoplasia, 69
    Cancer Genes and "Driver" Mutations, 69
    Epigenetic Alterations in Cancer, 70
    Carcinogenesis: A Multistep Process Directed
      by Darwinian Evolution, 70
    Origin of Carcinogenic Mutations, 71
    Role of Infectious Agents in Cancer, 72
    Significance of Passenger Mutations, 73

Hallmarks of Cancer, 73
    Self-Sufficiency in Growth Signals, 74
    Insensitivity to Growth-Inhibitory Signals, 75
    Altered Cellular Metabolism, 77
    Evasion of Cell Death, 79
    Limitless Replicative Potential (Immortality), 79
    Sustained Angiogenesis, 80
    Invasion and Metastasis, 80
    Evasion of Immune Surveillance, 81
    Genomic Instability as an Enabler of Malignancy, 83
    Tumor-Promoting Inflammation as an Enabler
      of Malignancy, 83
Clinical Aspects of Neoplasia, 83
    Clinical Effects of Tumors, 84
    Grading and Staging of Cancer, 84
    Cancer Diagnosis, 85

Cancer, the most feared form of neoplasia, remains the second leading cause of death in both children and adults.

Despite considerable progress in understanding the biology of neoplasms and in their diagnosis and treatment, cancer trails only cardiovascular disease as a cause of morbidity and mortality in the United States. Approximately 1.69 million new cases of cancer and over 600,000 cancer deaths were recorded in 2017 in the country. Incidence data for the most common forms of cancer, with the major killers identified, are presented in Fig. 5.1.

Our study of neoplasia begins with the defining biologic and morphologic characteristics of benign and malignant neoplasms. This is followed by a discussion of the genetic and molecular basis of cancer and the common features that are shared by all malignant neoplasms, the so-called "hallmarks of cancer." Finally, we discuss the clinical manifestations and laboratory diagnosis of cancer.

DEFINITION OF NEOPLASIA

Neoplasia (literally, new growth) refers to a clonal proliferation of cells that have "escaped" from normal growth control mechanisms because of the acquisition of genetic aberrations.

In virtually all instances, every cell within a given neoplasm shares a set of pathogenic mutations, indicating that neoplasms are composed of genetically related "daughter" cells derived from a single aberrant founding cell. Because of their origin from a single progenitor cell, neoplastic cells are said to be clonal in origin. The mutations that cause neoplasia alter the function of genes that regulate cell growth and survival (described later), thereby conferring the most striking property of neoplasms, their ability to produce a localized mass referred to as a tumor (from the Latin *tumere,* to swell). The study of tumors is called *oncology* (from the Greek *oncos,* "tumor," and *logos,* "study of"). The mutations that cause neoplasms are usually acquired but also may be inherited. We will return to the issue of mutations and cancer later.

In contrast to neoplasia, hyperplasia occurs when many cells within affected tissues begin to proliferate simultaneously in response to physiologic or pathophysiologic growth signals; as a result, hyperplasias are polyclonal. Examples of hyperplasias include enlargements of lymphoid tissues caused by inflammatory mediators and of the uterus in response to gestational hormones during pregnancy. Unlike neoplasias, hyperplasias are reversible: Lymph node swelling abates as an infection is cleared, and the uterus reverts to its prior state after delivery of the fetus.

BENIGN AND MALIGNANT NEOPLASMS

Benign neoplasms generally are well circumscribed, are easily excised, and do not spread from their site of origin, whereas malignant neoplasms often infiltrate surrounding tissues and have the capacity to spread to distant sites (metastasize).

Neoplasms are defined as benign and malignant based on the gross and microscopic appearance of the proliferation (described later), which is predictive of a given tumor's probable clinical behavior.

- *Benign* implies that a tumor will remain localized and is amenable to complete surgical removal. Affected patients generally survive, but even "benign" tumors may occasionally cause serious morbidity

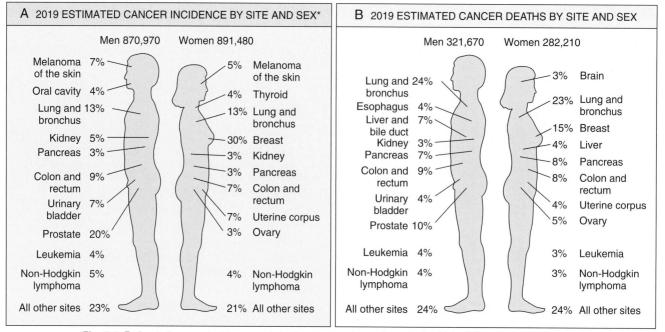

Fig. 5.1 Estimated cancer incidence and death rates by site and sex in the United States. Excludes basal cell and squamous cell skin cancers and in situ carcinomas, except those of urinary bladder. (Adapted from Cancer Facts and Figures 2019. American Cancer Society. www.cancer.org/research/cancer-facts-statistics/all-cancer-facts-figures/cancer-facts-figures-2019.html)

or even mortality, for example, by causing a local mass effect in a critical organ (e.g., the brain).

- *Malignant* is applied to lesions that can invade and destroy adjacent tissues and metastasize to distant sites, ultimately resulting in death. Malignant tumors are collectively referred to as *cancers* (derived from the Latin word for "crab") because their infiltrative growth causes them to "grab" onto normal tissues and adhere tightly, similar to a crab's behavior. Although not all cancers pursue a deadly course and some of the most aggressive are also among the most curable, the designation *malignant* is a red flag.

All tumors, benign and malignant, are composed of two components: (1) neoplastic cells and (2) a nonneoplastic stroma, made up of connective tissue, blood vessels, and inflammatory cells. As will be discussed in the Hallmarks of Cancer section, the behavior of a neoplasm depends not only on the intrinsic properties of the neoplastic cells but also on the nature of the stromal response, which tumor cells "manipulate" in order to favor their growth and survival.

NOMENCLATURE

The nomenclature of various neoplasms is important because each name carries with it certain associated characteristics that are related to the biology of the neoplasm and its likely clinical behavior.

Nomenclature of Benign Tumors

Most benign tumors are designated by attaching the suffix "-oma" to the cell type from which the tumor arises (Table 5.1). Others have names that reflect their growth patterns. A *papilloma* is a benign epithelial neoplasm growing on a surface that produces microscopic or macroscopic finger-like projections. A *polyp* is a mass that projects above a mucosal surface, as in the gut, to form a macroscopically visible structure (Fig.

5.2). Although this term commonly is used for benign tumors, some malignant tumors begin as polypoid growths, particularly in the gut.

Nomenclature of Malignant Tumors

The nomenclature of malignant tumors essentially follows that of benign tumors (see Table 5.1), with certain additions and exceptions:

- *Carcinomas* are malignant neoplasms of epithelial cells, and are further subdivided based on patterns of growth and differentiation.
- *Sarcomas* are malignant neoplasms composed of cells similar to those found in solid mesenchymal tissues. Sarcomas are designated based on the normal cell type or tissue they most closely resemble.
- *Leukemias* and *lymphomas* are malignant neoplasms derived from the hematopoietic progenitor cells that give rise to blood and immune cells. Leukemias preferentially involve marrow and blood, and lymphomas involve lymphoid tissues (lymph node and spleen) (see Chapter 9).

The transformed cells in a neoplasm, whether benign or malignant, usually resemble the cells of a single lineage. In some tumors, however, the neoplastic cells follow more than one line of differentiation. These include pleomorphic adenoma of the salivary gland, a classic *mixed tumor*, which (although clonal) is comprised of neoplastic epithelial and mesenchymal elements (Fig. 5.3). Uncommonly, malignant tumors consist of malignant elements from different lineages, such as *carcinosarcomas*, which are composed of both mesenchymal and epithelial components. *Teratoma* is another type of tumor that shows multiple lines of differentiation (Supplemental eFig. 5.1). Teratomas originate from totipotential germ cells that have the capacity to differentiate into any cell type and may contain haphazardly arranged elements resembling many different tissues.

Some glaring inconsistencies in the naming conventions laid out above may be noted in Table 5.1. For example, lymphoma, mesothelioma, melanoma, and seminoma "sound" benign but are all malignant neoplasms.

Table 5.1 Nomenclature of Tumors

Tissue of Origin	Benign	Malignant
Composed of One Parenchymal Cell Type		
Connective tissue and derivatives	Lipoma	Liposarcoma
	Chondroma	Chondrosarcoma
	Osteoma	Osteosarcoma
Blood vessels	Hemangioma	Angiosarcoma
Mesothelium		Mesothelioma
Brain coverings	Meningioma	Invasive meningioma
Hematolymphoid cells		Leukemias, lymphomas
Smooth muscle	Leiomyoma	Leiomyosarcoma
Stratified squamous	Squamous cell papilloma	Squamous cell carcinoma
Basal cells of skin or adnexa		Basal cell carcinoma
Epithelial lining of glands or ducts	Adenoma Papilloma Cystadenoma	Adenocarcinoma
Liver cells	Hepatic adenoma	Hepatocellular carcinoma
Urinary tract epithelium (transitional)	Urothelial papilloma	Urothelial carcinoma
Placental epithelium	Hydatidiform mole	Choriocarcinoma
Testicular epithelium (germ cells)		Seminoma Embryonal carcinoma
Tumors of melanocytes	Nevus	Malignant melanoma
Composed of More Than One Neoplastic Cell Type: Mixed Tumors, Usually Derived from One Germ Cell Layer		
Salivary gland	Pleomorphic adenoma (mixed tumor of salivary gland)	Malignant mixed tumor of salivary gland
Renal anlage		Wilms tumor
More Than One Neoplastic Cell Type Derived from More Than One Germ Cell Layer: Teratogenous		
Totipotential cells in gonads or in embryonic rests	Mature teratoma, dermoid cyst	Immature teratoma, teratocarcinoma

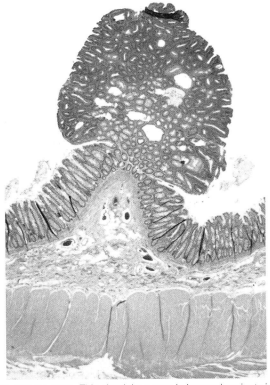

Fig. 5.2 Colonic polyp. This glandular tumor (adenoma) projects into the colonic lumen and is attached to the mucosa by a distinct stalk.

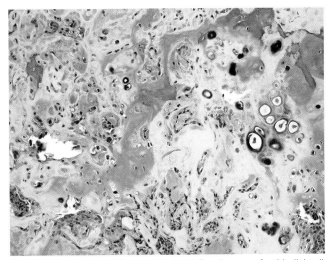

Fig. 5.3 Mixed tumor of the parotid gland. Small nests of epithelial cells and myxoid stroma forming cartilage and bone (an unusual feature) are present in this field. (Courtesy of Dr. Vicky Jo, Department of Pathology, Brigham and Women's Hospital, Boston.)

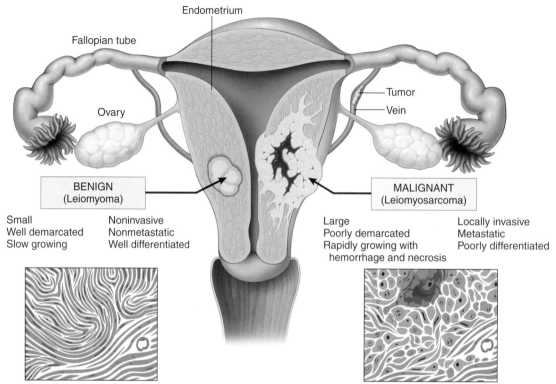

Fig. 5.4 Comparison between a benign tumor of the myometrium (leiomyoma) and a malignant tumor of similar origin (leiomyosarcoma).

CHARACTERISTICS OF BENIGN AND MALIGNANT NEOPLASMS

Most benign and malignant tumors can be distinguished based on the evaluation of three features: degree of differentiation, local invasion, and metastasis.

In most instances, the determination of benign versus malignant is made with remarkable accuracy using long-established clinical and anatomic criteria. The features that usually permit the differentiation of benign and malignant neoplasms, using tumors of the myometrium as an example, are summarized in Fig. 5.4 and described in detail next.

Differentiation of Neoplasms

Differentiation refers to the extent to which tumor cells resemble their parenchymal cells of origin, both morphologically and functionally.

In general, benign neoplasms are composed of well-differentiated cells that closely resemble their normal counterparts. By contrast, most malignant neoplasms exhibit morphologic alterations that betray their malignant nature. Tumors composed of undifferentiated cells are said to be anaplastic, a feature that is a reliable indicator of malignancy. *Anaplasia* literally means "backward formation," implying dedifferentiation, or loss of the structural and functional characteristics of normal differentiated cells. Anaplastic cells often display one or more of the following features:

- *Pleomorphism* (variation in cell size and shape; Fig. 5.5). Extreme examples include tumor giant cells that are considerably larger than their neighbors, with each possessing either one enormous nucleus or several nuclei.

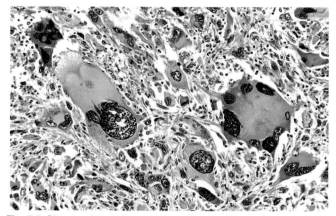

Fig. 5.5 Pleomorphic malignant tumor (poorly differentiated sarcoma). Note the marked variation in cell and nuclear sizes, the hyperchromatic nuclei, and the presence of tumor giant cells. (Courtesy Dr. Trace Worrell, Department of Pathology, University of Texas Southwestern Medical School, Dallas.)

- *Nuclear abnormalities*, including hyperchromatism (dark-staining), variation in nuclear size and shape, or unusually prominent single or multiple nucleoli. Enlargement of nuclei may result in an increased nuclear-to-cytoplasmic ratio, and nucleoli may attain astounding sizes that approach the diameter of normal lymphocytes.
- *Atypical mitoses*, which may be numerous. Abnormal separation of chromatids during cell division may produce tripolar or quadripolar mitotic figures (Fig. 5.6).
- *Loss of polarity,* such that groups of neoplastic cells lack normal patterns of orientation to one another. In the most anaplastic

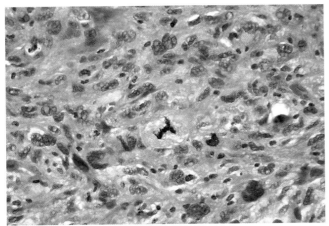

Fig. 5.6 High-power detail view of anaplastic tumor cells shows cellular and nuclear variation in size and shape. The prominent cell in the center field has an abnormal tripolar spindle.

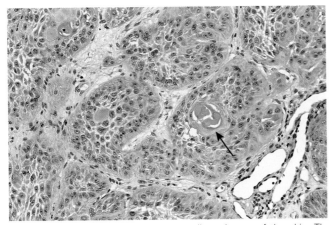

Fig. 5.7 Well-differentiated squamous cell carcinoma of the skin. The tumor cells are strikingly similar to normal squamous epithelial cells, with intercellular bridges and nests of keratin *(arrow)*.

tumors, cells grow in disorganized sheets, with total loss of organized structures such as glands or stratified squamous architecture.

Well-differentiated tumor cells are likely to retain the functional capabilities of their normal counterparts, whereas anaplastic tumor cells are much less likely to do so (discussed later, regarding tumor grading). For example, benign neoplasms and well-differentiated cancers of endocrine glands frequently elaborate the hormones characteristic of their cell of origin. Similarly, well-differentiated squamous cell carcinomas produce keratin (Fig. 5.7) and well-differentiated hepatocellular carcinomas secrete bile. In other instances, unanticipated functions emerge. Most notably, cancers of nonendocrine origin may cause signs and symptoms by secreting so-called ectopic hormones, such as adrenocorticotropic hormone (ACTH), parathyroid hormone-related protein (PTrP), insulin, glucagon, and others. More is said about these so-called paraneoplastic syndromes later.

Dysplasia is disordered growth of epithelial cells that are abnormal but not malignant.

Dysplasia is important to recognize because it is a well-documented precursor of carcinoma in many tissues, such as the cervix, endometrium, and gastrointestinal tract. Features that are used to assess dysplasia include the following:

- *Cellular and nuclear pleomorphism,* typically in the form of abnormally large, hyperchromatic nuclei
- *Abnormal mitotic activity,* including more numerous mitotic figures and mitoses in superficial layers of stratified squamous epithelium, where they are not normally seen
- *Architectural disarray.* Examples include the partial or complete loss of the usual progressive maturation of cells in stratified squamous epithelium or transitional epithelium in the bladder, resulting in a disordered hodgepodge of dark basal-appearing cells. When dysplastic changes are severe and involve the entire thickness of the epithelium, the lesion is referred to as carcinoma in situ, a preinvasive stage of cancer (Fig. 5.8).

The progression of dysplasia to cancer is not inevitable, and dysplasias may regress completely, particularly if inciting causes are removed. Nevertheless, as a general rule, the presence of dysplasia marks a tissue as being at increased risk for developing an invasive cancer.

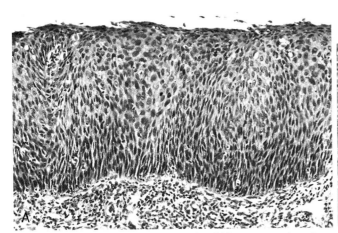
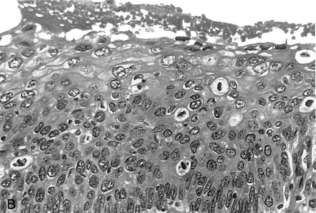

Fig. 5.8 Carcinoma in situ. (A) Low-power view shows that the entire thickness of the epithelium consists of dysplastic cells lacking orderly differentiation. The basement membrane is intact and there is no tumor in the subepithelial stroma. (B) High-power view of another region shows failure of normal differentiation, marked nuclear and cellular pleomorphism, and numerous mitotic figures extending toward the surface.

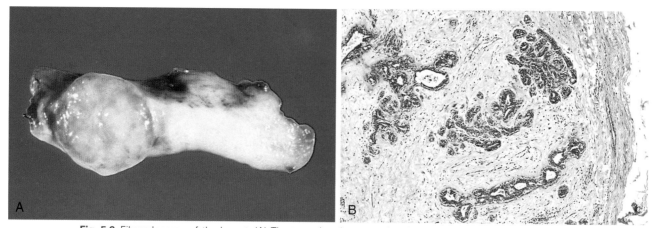

Fig. 5.9 Fibroadenoma of the breast. (A) The tan-colored, encapsulated small tumor is sharply demarcated from the whiter breast tissue. (B) Microscopic appearance. The fibrous capsule (*right*) sharply delimits the tumor from the surrounding tissue. (B, Courtesy Dr. Trace Worrell, Department of Pathology, University of Texas Southwestern Medical School, Dallas.)

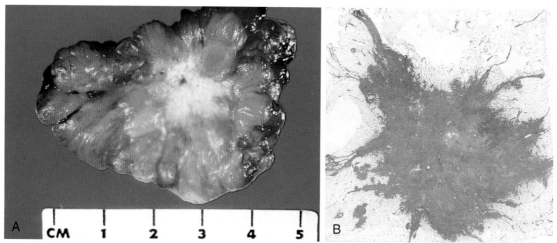

Fig. 5.10 Invasive ductal carcinoma of the breast. (A) The lesion infiltrates the surrounding breast substance, causing tissue retraction, and is stony-hard on palpation. (B) Microscopic view illustrates the invasion of breast stroma and fat by nests and cords of tumor cells. (B, Courtesy Dr. Trace Worrell, Department of Pathology, University of Texas Southwestern Medical School, Dallas.)

Local Invasion

Next to the development of metastases, invasiveness is the feature that most reliably distinguishes cancers from benign tumors.

As benign tumors slowly grow and expand, most develop a rim of fibrous tissue called a *capsule* (Fig. 5.9). The capsule is formed by deposition of collagen by stromal cells, such as fibroblasts. Benign encapsulated tumors are discrete, movable (nonfixed), and usually easy to excise. Invasive cancers can also induce a stromal response associated with fibrosis, and slowly growing malignant tumors on gross inspection may appear to be encapsulated. However, cancers, even those that appear to be circumscribed, lack true capsules and progressively invade, infiltrate, and destroy surrounding tissues (Fig. 5.10). This infiltrative growth necessitates removal of a wide margin of surrounding "normal" tissue when surgical excision of a malignant tumor is attempted. These distinguishing features are not absolute: Some benign tumors (e.g., hemangiomas) lack capsules and are not discretely defined.

Metastasis

Metastasis is defined by the spread of a tumor to sites that are physically discontinuous with the primary tumor and the ability to metastasize marks a tumor as malignant.

The invasiveness of cancer cells permits them to penetrate into blood vessels, lymphatic channels, and body cavities, providing opportunities for spread (Fig. 5.11). Approximately 30% of patients with newly diagnosed malignant solid tumors (excluding skin cancers other than melanomas) have clinically evident metastases, and an additional 20% have occult (hidden) metastases at the time of diagnosis. In general, large, anaplastic cancers are more likely to metastasize, but even small primary tumors may be associated with metastatic disease. Certain cancers, such as basal cell carcinoma of the skin and most primary tumors of the central nervous system, are locally aggressive but metastasize only rarely. Thus, the ability to invade is not always predictive of metastatic potential.

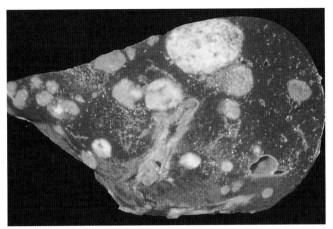

Fig. 5.11 A liver studded with metastatic cancer.

Malignancies of the blood (leukemias and lymphomas) are a special circumstance: These tumors are derived from blood-forming cells that circulate through the bloodstream and migrate to distant tissues. Therefore, with only rare exceptions, leukemias and lymphomas are disseminated diseases at diagnosis and are always considered to be malignant.

Malignant neoplasms spread by one of three pathways:

- *Seeding within body cavities.* This mode of dissemination is particularly characteristic of ovarian carcinomas, which often spread along peritoneal surfaces, and certain neoplasms of the central nervous system (e.g., medulloblastoma, ependymoma) that may enter the cerebral ventricles, travel through the cerebrospinal fluid, and implant on meningeal surfaces adjacent to the brain or the spinal cord.
- *Lymphatic spread.* Although this is most typical of carcinomas, all forms of cancer may disseminate through lymphatic channels. The pattern of lymph node involvement depends on the site of the primary neoplasm and the natural pathways of local lymphatic drainage. A *"sentinel" lymph node* is the first regional lymph node that receives lymph flow from a primary tumor. The results of sentinel lymph node biopsy are used to gauge tumor spread via lymphatics, which in turn guides treatment. Lymph node enlargement near a primary tumor may stem from the metastatic spread of cancer cells or from immunologic reactions to tumor antigens. Thus, the cause of lymph node enlargement can only be determined with certainty by biopsy and histopathologic examination of the affected nodes.
- *Hematogenous spread.* Spread through blood vessels is the favored pathway for sarcomas, but carcinomas follow this course, as well. Thin-walled veins are penetrated more easily than thick-walled arteries and are the usual avenue of spread. Blood-borne tumor cells are often arrested in the first capillary bed they encounter: Gastrointestinal cancers frequently spread through the portal system to the liver, whereas other cancers often metastasize first to the lungs. Cancers arising near the vertebral column often embolize through the paravertebral plexus; this pathway probably explains the high frequency of vertebral metastases in patients with carcinomas of the thyroid and prostate. However, the anatomic localization of a neoplasm and its venous drainage cannot wholly explain the systemic distribution of metastases. For example, lung carcinoma tends to spread to the adrenal glands and the brain, and neuroblastoma often spreads to the liver and bones. Conversely, skeletal muscles, although rich in capillaries, are rarely sites of tumor metastases.

MOLECULAR BASIS OF NEOPLASIA

Cancer Genes and "Driver" Mutations

All forms of neoplasia stem from mutations that alter the function of genes that regulate the behavior of normal cells.

Thus, in essence, cancer is a genetic disease. Genes that are recurrently mutated or dysregulated in cancer cells can be referred to as *cancer genes.* These number in the hundreds and are not only numerous but often have unpronounceable acronyms for names that are difficult to remember, even for the expert. One way to simplify this complexity is to consider that cancer genes fall into four major functional classes:

- *Oncogenes* are genes that when overexpressed or mutated promote increased cell growth. Their normal cellular counterparts are called *protooncogenes.* Most oncogenes encode transcription factors or signaling molecules that participate in progrowth pathways. They are considered dominant genes because a mutation involving a single allele is sufficient to produce a prooncogenic effect.
- *Tumor suppressor genes* are genes that normally prevent uncontrolled growth; the function of such genes is lost in neoplasms due to disruptive mutations or epigenetic silencing (gene repression). In most instances, the function of both alleles of a tumor suppressor gene must be lost to allow unregulated cell growth.
- *Genes that regulate apoptosis* primarily act by enhancing cell survival, rather than by stimulating proliferation per se. Genes that protect against apoptosis are often overexpressed in cancer cells, whereas those that promote apoptosis tend to be underexpressed.
- *Genes that regulate interactions between tumor cells and host cells* also are recurrently mutated or functionally altered in certain cancers. Particularly important are genes that enhance or inhibit the recognition of tumor cells by the host immune system.

Mutations that promote the development or progression of cancers are referred to as *driver mutations.* Most driver mutations affect genes that encode proteins, but genes that encode regulatory RNAs, such as microRNAs, also can be affected by driver mutations. Driver mutations are structurally diverse and include:

- *Single-nucleotide substitutions and small insertions and deletions.* Depending on their precise location and type, these may either activate an oncoprotein or inactivate a tumor suppressor protein.
- *Large deletions,* which frequently remove one or more genes with tumor suppressor function.
- *Chromosome rearrangements* (often in the form of chromosome translocations) produce gross changes in the chromosome structure (Fig. 5.12). In some instances involving oncogenes, the rearrangement places a strong regulatory element (either a promoter or an enhancer) near an oncogene, leading to overexpression of a normal protein. In other instances, a chimeric gene is created that encodes an oncogenic fusion protein composed of portions of two different proteins. These types of rearrangements are particularly common in blood cancers and sarcomas, but may be found in carcinomas, as well.
- *Gene amplifications* produce extra copies of one or more oncogenes and represent another way to increase the level of a protein with oncogenic activity (Fig. 5.13). The amplified genes may be carried in extrachromosomal DNA fragments known as double minute chromosomes, or may be present within a chromosome and appear as an abnormal homogeneous-staining region, detected by staining a metaphase chromosome with special dyes.

Another common genetic aberration that is found in cancer cells is *aneuploidy,* which is defined as gains or losses of whole chromosomes or large portions thereof (see Chapter 6). How this causes

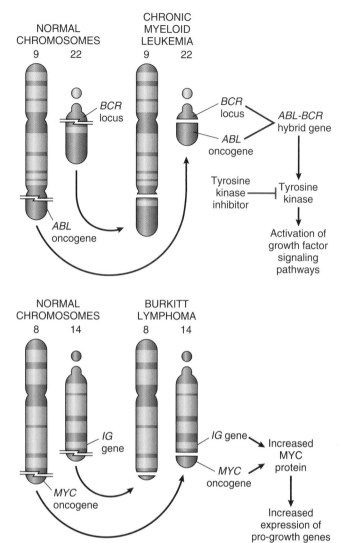

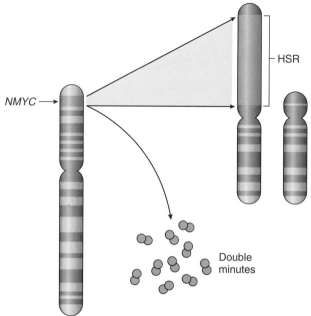

Fig. 5.13 Amplification of the *NMYC* gene in human neuroblastoma. The *NMYC* gene, present normally on chromosome 2p, becomes amplified and is seen either as extrachromosomal double minutes or as a chromosomally integrated homogeneous-staining region, usually on a chromosome other than chromosome 2. NMYC is closely related in structure to MYC and also is an oncogenic transcription factor. (Modified from Brodeur GM, Seeger RC, Sather H, et al: Clinical implications of oncogene activation in human neuroblastomas. *Cancer* 58:541, 1986. Reprinted by permission of Wiley-Liss, Inc., a subsidiary of John Wiley & Sons, Inc.)

Fig. 5.12 Chromosomal translocations and associated oncogenes. In chronic myeloid leukemia, a balanced translocation involving chromosomes 9 and 22 creates a chimeric gene containing pieces of the *BCR* and *ABL* genes that encode a chimeric BCR-ABL fusion protein with constitutively active tyrosine kinase activity. In Burkitt lymphoma, a balanced translocation involving chromosomes 8 and 14 places the coding sequence for the *MYC* gene adjacent to strong regulatory elements in the immunoglobulin heavy-chain gene, leading to overexpression of MYC, an oncogenic transcription factor.

cancer is incompletely understood, but it is believed to involve changes in the expression of cancer genes that reside in affected chromosomal regions.

Epigenetic Alterations in Cancer

Epigenetic changes are defined as heritable changes in the expression of a gene that occur without mutation of the gene.

Gene expression is regulated by posttranslational modifications of histones and by DNA methylation, both of which are frequently altered in cancer cells when compared with their normal cellular counterparts. How these alterations in the epigenome contribute to neoplasia is poorly understood, but are likely in most, if not all, instances to stem from the altered expression of cancer genes.

Carcinogenesis: A Multistep Process Directed by Darwinian Evolution

Cancers are initiated and subsequently progress by the stepwise acquisition of multiple genetic aberrations that disrupt sets of cancer genes with complementary prooncogenic functions.

Even though tumor formation is initiated from a single founding cell, cancers continue to evolve genetically (Fig. 5.14), a process that contributes to a phenomenon referred to as tumor progression. At the molecular level, tumor progression is believed to result from additional mutations that accumulate independently in different cancer cells. Some of these mutations may alter the function of cancer genes, thereby making the affected cells more adept at growth, survival, invasion, metastasis, or immune evasion, resulting in progression akin to Darwinian evolution (survival of the fittest). Due to this selective advantage, subclones may come to dominate a tumor, either at the primary site or at sites of metastasis. Because of continuing mutation and selection, malignant tumors that were monoclonal in origin are typically genetically heterogeneous at the time of clinical presentation.

Genetic heterogeneity has implications not only for cancer progression but also for the response to therapy.

When tumors recur after chemotherapy, the recurrent tumor is almost always resistant to the original drug regimen. This acquired resistance stems from the outgrowth of subclones that have mutations (or epigenetic alterations) that impart drug resistance. Thus, genetic evolution forged by darwinian selection can explain the two most

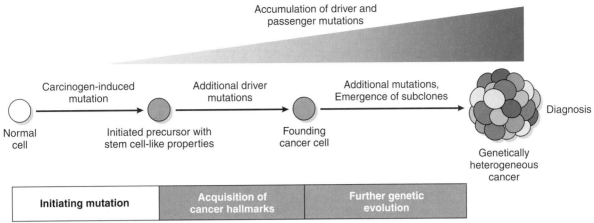

Fig. 5.14 Development of cancer through stepwise accumulation of complementary driver mutations. The order in which various driver mutations occur is usually unknown and may vary from tumor to tumor.

pernicious properties of cancers: the tendency for cancers over time to become more aggressive and less responsive to therapy.

Origin of Carcinogenic Mutations

Driver mutations that alter cancer gene function are most commonly acquired during life but may also be inherited.

Factors that contribute to the occurrence of oncogenic somatic mutations that are acquired during life include the following:

- *Age.* In general, the frequency of cancer increases with age, with most cancer deaths occurring between ages 55 and 75. The rising incidence with age is likely explained in large part by the accumulation of somatic mutations. Some mutations are explained by factors described below, but most of the mutational burden associated with aging is the result of spontaneous chemical reactions, such as the deamination of cytosine and methyl-cytosine residues to create uracil and thymine residues, respectively.
- *Exposure to mutagenic agents.* Agents that damage DNA are associated with an increased risk of a variety of cancers, including tobacco smoking, ultraviolet light (in lightly pigmented individuals), chemotherapy drugs (many of which damage DNA), radiation (often given as part of cancer therapy), and a variety of environmental chemicals. Some important carcinogenic agents are listed in Table 5.2. Chemical carcinogens have highly reactive electrophile groups that damage DNA, causing mutations. These fall into two classes: direct-acting agents (e.g., alkylating agents), which do not require metabolic conversion to become carcinogenic, and indirect-acting agents (e.g., benzo(a)pyrene, azo dyes, aflatoxin), which are not active until converted

to an ultimate carcinogen by endogenous metabolic pathways. Hence, polymorphisms of endogenous enzymes such as cytochrome P-450 may influence carcinogenesis by altering the conversion of indirect-acting agents to active carcinogens.

- *Increased cellular proliferation.* Mutations are more likely to occur during DNA replication and cellular division, which may be increased by several factors. Chronic inflammation is associated with increased cellular proliferation as part of the repair process. This may explain, at least in part, the increased incidence of carcinoma seen in the setting of many chronic inflammatory disorders (Table 5.3). Increased exposure to mitogenic hormones also is associated with an elevated risk of carcinoma in hormone-responsive tissues. For example, women exposed to high levels of estrogen (a potent mitogen for mammary and endometrial epithelium) over sustained periods of time have an increased risk of breast and endometrial carcinoma.
- *Regulated DNA rearrangement and mutagenesis.* B and T lymphocytes use regulated DNA breakage and rejoining to assemble a vast array of antigen-receptor genes (immunoglobulin and T-cell receptors) and (in the case of B cells) regulated mutagenesis to improve the affinity of immunoglobulins for antigens. Errors in these processes can create oncogenes and are important contributors to the pathogenesis of B-cell and T-cell tumors.

Another important source of driver mutations is germline (inherited) aberrations.

These inherited mutations are present in every cell in the body, placing the affected individual at a high risk for developing cancer. In

Table 5.2 Major Carcinogens and Associated Cancers

Agent	Associated Human Cancers	Mechanism
Tobacco	Lung, bladder, head and neck, pancreatic, and renal carcinomas	DNA damage caused by carcinogens and procarcinogens in tobacco smoke (e.g., benzo[a]pyrene)
Ultraviolet light	Skin cancer (melanoma, squamous cell carcinoma, basal cell carcinoma)	DNA damage
Asbestos	Lung, esophageal, gastric, and colon carcinoma; mesothelioma	Uncertain. Activates the inflammasome, leading to local inflammation.
Alkylating chemotherapy agents	Acute myeloid leukemia	DNA damage
Ionizing radiation	Many cancers	DNA damage
Aflatoxin B_1	Liver cancer	DNA damage
Nitrosamine and nitrosamides	Gastric cancer, esophageal cancer	DNA damage

Table 5.3   Chronic Inflammatory Disorders and Cancer

Pathologic Condition	Associated Neoplasm(s)	Etiologic Agent
Asbestosis, silicosis	Mesothelioma, lung carcinoma	Asbestos fibers, silica particles
Inflammatory bowel disease	Colorectal carcinoma	
Lichen sclerosis	Vulvar squamous cell carcinoma	
Pancreatitis	Pancreatic carcinoma	Alcoholism, germline mutations
Chronic cholecystitis	Gallbladder cancer	Gallbladder stones
Barrett esophagus	Esophageal carcinoma	Gastric acid
Sjögren syndrome, Hashimoto thyroiditis	Extranodal marginal zone lymphoma	
Opisthorchis, cholangitis	Cholangiocarcinoma, colon carcinoma	Liver flukes
Gastritis/ulcers	Gastric adenocarcinoma, MALT lymphoma	*Helicobacter pylori*
Hepatitis	Hepatocellular carcinoma	Hepatitis B and/or C virus
Osteomyelitis	Carcinoma in draining sinuses	Bacterial infection
Chronic cystitis	Bladder carcinoma	Schistosomiasis

Adapted from Tlsty TD, Coussens LM: Tumor stroma and regulation of cancer development. *Ann Rev Pathol Mech Dis* 1:119, 2006.

families with these mutations, cancer risk usually acts like an autosomal dominant inherited trait. The cause in most instances is a germline mutation in a gene encoding a tumor suppressor, a protein with one or more activities that prevent cellular transformation. Tumor suppressor genes typically provide adequate function in the heterozygous state; thus, affected individuals are perfectly normal until cancer arises (and, in some instances, multiple cancers arise), often early in life. The transformed cells typically contain a second, sporadic mutation in the normal allele that completely eliminates the function of the tumor suppressor. The need for a second hit (the *two-hit hypothesis*) to create a "procancer" phenotype was predicted from the autosomal dominant inheritance of one such cancer syndrome, familial retinoblastoma (described later), and has largely been borne out by subsequent molecular studies.

Important familial cancer syndromes and associated genes and cancers are summarized in Table 5.4. Sequencing of genomes has also revealed that a high fraction of cancers occurring in children are associated with germline mutations in cancer genes, even in children without any family history. Presumably, many of these are new mutations that arose in the germ cells of the parents or occurred in the fetus during early embryogenesis.

Role of Infectious Agents in Cancer

Infectious agents cause up to 25% of cancers worldwide; because of this, some cancers can be prevented through vaccination against causative agents or by effective treatment of established infections.

Epidemiologic and mechanistic studies have firmly implicated a number of infectious agents in the etiology of various cancers (Table 5.5). Infectious agents appear to increase the risk of cancer through two major mechanisms:

- *By inducing chronic inflammation and tissue repair,* thereby increasing the rate of acquisition of driver mutations, as described earlier. Examples include hepatitis B virus and hepatitis C virus, both of which induce chronic liver damage and are strongly associated with hepatocellular carcinoma (liver cancer), and *Helicobacter pylori,* a bacterium that colonizes and damages the gastric mucosa, which has been linked to the development of gastric carcinoma and gastric lymphoma.

Table 5.4   Inherited Predisposition to Cancer

Autosomal Dominant Cancer Syndromes		
Inherited Disorder	Gene(s)	Functional Defect
Retinoblastoma	*RB*	Loss of cell cycle control
Li-Fraumeni syndrome (various tumors)	*TP53*	Increased genomic instability
Melanoma	*p16-INK4A*	Loss of cell cycle control
Familial adenomatous polyposis/colon cancer	*APC*	Increased signaling in the Wnt pathway
Neurofibromatosis 1 and 2	*NF1, NF2*	Increased progrowth signaling
Breast and ovarian tumors	*BRCA1, BRCA2*	Increased genomic instability
Hereditary nonpolyposis colon cancer	*MSH2, MLH1, MSH6*	Increased genomic instability
Nevoid basal cell carcinoma syndrome	*PTCH1*	Increased signaling in the Hedgehog pathway
Autosomal Recessive Syndromes of Defective DNA Repair		
Xeroderma pigmentosum	Diverse genes involved in nucleotide excision repair	Increased genomic instability
Ataxia-telangiectasia	*ATM*	Increased genomic instability
Bloom syndrome	*BLM*	Increased genomic instability
Fanconi anemia	Diverse genes involved in repair of DNA cross-links	Increased genomic instability

Table 5.5 Infectious Agents Linked to Cancer

Agent	Cancers	Mechanism
DNA Viruses		
Human papillomavirus (HPV)	Squamous cell carcinomas of the cervix, tonsil, vulva, and penis	Virus encodes oncoproteins that inactivate p53 and RB
Epstein-Barr virus (EBV)	B cell lymphomas, nasopharyngeal carcinoma	Uncertain. Virus encodes proteins that activate oncogenic signaling pathways
Human herpesvirus 8 (HHV8)	Kaposi sarcoma, B cell lymphomas	Uncertain. Virus encodes proteins that activate oncogenic signaling pathways
Hepatitis B virus	Hepatocellular carcinoma	Uncertain. Causes chronic liver inflammation and associated repair
RNA Viruses		
Hepatitis C virus	Hepatocellular carcinoma	Uncertain. Causes chronic liver inflammation and associated repair
Retroviruses		
Human T-cell lymphotrophic virus 1 (HTLV1)	Adult T-cell leukemia	Uncertain. Virus encodes proteins that causes expansion of infected T cells
Bacteria		
Helicobacter pylori	Gastric carcinoma, gastric B cell lymphoma	Uncertain. Causes chronic gastritis and associated repair and stimulates a chronic immune response.
Parasites		
Schistosoma haematobium	Bladder carcinoma	Uncertain. Causes chronic cystitis and associated repair
Liver flukes	Cholangiocarcinoma	Uncertain. Causes chronic bile duct inflammation and associated repair

- *By altering the function of proteins made by cancer genes or by stimulating cellular proliferation.* The most important and best understood example of this mechanism is human papillomavirus (HPV), which is the etiologic agent in most cases of cervical carcinoma and many cases of head and neck squamous cell carcinoma. As will be discussed later, HPV encodes two proteins, E6 and E7, that bind and inactivate two of the most important tumor suppressor proteins, p53 and RB, respectively.

Significance of Passenger Mutations

Passenger mutations create variants that do not alter growth properties but influence host response to the tumor.

They greatly outnumber driver mutations, particularly in cancers caused by exposure to mutagens, such as most melanomas and smoking-related lung cancer. Despite their apparently innocuous nature, passenger mutations are important in several ways:

- *Passenger mutations may create genetic variants that confer resistance to therapeutic agents.* Under the selective pressure of therapy, rare cells harboring resistance mutations gain an advantage and eventually come to dominate the tumor cell population.
- *Passenger mutations may create tumor neoantigens* (protein sequences that differ from those of normal cells). Such antigens may be seen as "foreign" by cells of the immune system, potentially leading to a host antitumor response. Neoantigens and host immunity will be discussed later.

HALLMARKS OF CANCER

All cancers display fundamental changes in cell physiology, which are considered the hallmarks of cancer.

As has already been mentioned, cancer genes numbering at least in the hundreds can be considered in the context of the common phenotypic properties of cancer cells. These properties are illustrated in Fig. 5.15 and consist of the following:

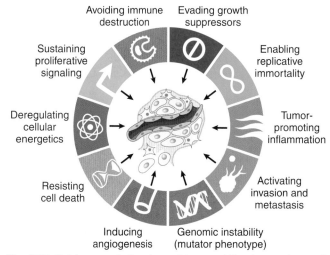

Fig. 5.15 Eight cancer hallmarks and two enabling factors (genomic instability and tumor-promoting inflammation). Most cancer cells acquire these properties during their development, typically owing to mutations in critical genes. (From Hanahan D, Weinberg RA: Hallmarks of cancer: the next generation. *Cell* 144:646, 2011.)

- Self-sufficiency in growth signals
- Insensitivity to growth-inhibitory signals
- Altered cellular metabolism
- Evasion of cell death
- Limitless replicative potential (immortality)
- Sustained angiogenesis
- Invasion and metastasis
- Evasion of immune surveillance

In addition, the acquisition of the genetic and epigenetic alterations that confer these properties may be accelerated by cancer-promoting

Table 5.6 Important Cancer Genes

Cancer Gene	Gene Class	Function	Effect of Mutations	Associated Cancers
TP53	Tumor suppressor	Sensor of cell stress, DNA repair	Loss of function leads to genomic instability, resistance to proapoptotic stresses	Diverse cancers
RB	Tumor suppressor	Negative regulator of cell cycle	Loss of function leads to increased growth, failure to differentiate	Mutated in retinoblastoma, osteosarcoma; dysregulated in diverse cancers
HER2	Oncogene	Growth factor receptor	Gain of function leads to growth factor–independent signaling	Amplified in a subset of breast cancers and other carcinomas
ABL	Oncogene	Nonreceptor tyrosine kinase	Gain of function leads to growth factor–independent signaling	Activated by translocations in several leukemias
RAS	Oncogene	Signaling molecule	Gain of function leads to growth factor–independent signaling	Diverse cancers
BRAF	Oncogene	Signaling molecule	Gain of function leads to growth factor–independent signaling	Commonly mutated in melanoma
Cyclin D	Oncogene	Cell cycle regulator	Gain of function opposes the action of RB, leads to increased proliferation	Overexpressed due to translocation or amplification in lymphoma, breast cancer
MYC, NMYC	Oncogene	Transcription factors	Overexpression leads to reprogramming of metabolism	Translocated in Burkitt lymphoma, amplified in neuroblastoma; dysregulated in diverse cancers
IDH1, IDH2	Oncogene	Metabolic enzyme	Mutation leads to new enzyme activity that produces an oncometabolite	Acute myeloid leukemia, glioma, chondrosarcoma, cholangiocarcinoma
BCL2	Anti-apoptosis	Opposes the activity of proapoptotic factors	Overexpression leads to resistance to apoptosis	Translocated in follicular lymphoma; dysregulated in diverse cancers
PDL1, PDL2	Host/cancer cell interactions	Activates immune checkpoint pathways in T cells	Overexpression leads to immunoevasion	Amplified in Hodgkin lymphoma, overexpressed in diverse cancers

inflammation and by genomic instability, which are enabling characteristics because they promote cellular transformation and subsequent tumor progression.

Mutations in genes that regulate some or all of these cellular traits are seen in every cancer; accordingly, these traits form the basis of the following discussion of the molecular origins of cancer, during which we will also discuss a subset of cancer genes with frequent or well-defined roles in cancer (summarized in Table 5.6). Throughout the discussion (by convention) gene symbols are *italicized* and their protein products are not (e.g., *RB* gene and RB protein).

Self-Sufficiency in Growth Signals

The self-sufficiency in growth that characterizes cancer cells most often stems from gain-of-function mutations in signaling proteins that reduce or eliminate growth factor dependency.

These mutations convert protooncogenes into oncogenes, which encode constitutively active proteins (oncoproteins) that transmit pro-growth signals even in the absence of growth factors. To appreciate how oncogenes drive inappropriate cell growth, recall that growth factor–induced signaling can be resolved into the following steps:

- *Binding of a growth factor to its specific receptor* on the cell membrane
- *Transient activation of the growth factor receptor,* which in turn activates signal-transducing proteins
- *Transmission of the transduced signal across the cytosol to the nucleus* by second messengers or a cascade of signal transduction molecules
- *Activation of transcription factors* that increase the expression of genes that regulate DNA replication and the biosynthesis of other

cellular components (e.g., organelles, membrane components, and ribosomes) needed for cell division
- *Progression of the cell through the cell cycle,* resulting ultimately in cell division and the "birth" of two daughter cells; this process is normally regulated on multiple levels by a balance between proteins that promote cell cycle progression (growth factors, growth factor receptors, signaling molecules, and cyclin/cyclin-dependent kinase complexes) and those that oppose it (RB, p53, and cyclin-dependent kinase inhibitors, described later)

Each step above is susceptible to corruption in cancer cells. The most frequently mutated oncoproteins that impart growth factor independence on cancer cells are various growth factor receptors, RAS proteins, and certain signaling factors that act downstream of RAS. Some of these same proteins are targets of effective therapeutic drugs.

- *Growth factor receptors and related proteins.* **One common type of oncogenic mutation causes growth factor receptors or related proteins to deliver mitogenic signals to cells continuously, even in the absence of growth factor.** Many growth factor receptors have an intrinsic tyrosine kinase activity that is activated by growth factors and stimulates downstream signaling cascades. Other proteins with tyrosine kinase activity are not surface receptors but still have the capacity to stimulate the same pathways when activated. Oncogenic mutations involving the genes that encode such proteins either create a constitutively activated tyrosine kinase or cause the overexpression of structurally normal receptors, allowing signaling to occur even when growth factor levels are very low. An example of a nonreceptor tyrosine kinase gene that is converted to an oncogene by chromosomal translocations is *ABL*,

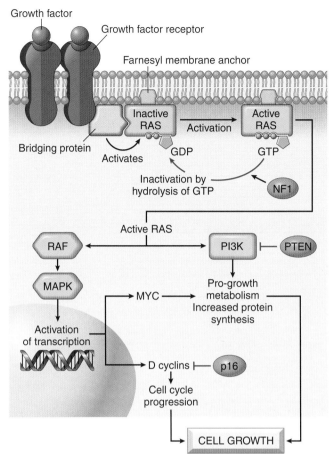

Fig. 5.16 Oncogenic growth factor signaling. When a normal cell is stimulated through a growth factor receptor with intrinsic tyrosine kinase activity (a so-called receptor tyrosine kinase), inactive (GDP-bound) RAS is activated to a GTP-bound state. Activated RAS transduces proliferative signals to the nucleus along two pathways: the so-called RAF/ERK/MAP kinase pathway and the PI3 kinase/AKT pathway, which upregulate the expression of D cyclins and MYC. The activity of RAS is normally held in check by GAPs (GTPase-activating proteins) such as NF1, whereas the activity of PI3 kinase is antagonized by PTEN. Factors shown in *green* are oncoproteins that are activated by gain-of-function mutations in various cancers, whereas factors shown in *red* are tumor suppressors that are often missing due to loss-of-function mutations. GDP, Guanosine diphosphate; GTP, guanosine triphosphate; MAP, mitogen-activated protein; PI3K, phosphatidylinositol-3 kinase.

which is rearranged in certain leukemias. In contrast, the *HER2* gene, which encodes a receptor tyrosine kinase, is often amplified in breast cancer. The net effect of both types of alterations is the same: overactivation of a signaling cascade involving RAS and factors downstream of RAS.

- *RAS.* **RAS genes are the most commonly mutated oncogenes in human tumors.** Approximately 30% of all human tumors have *RAS* mutations. RAS proteins are members of a family of G proteins that bind guanosine nucleotides (guanosine triphosphate [GTP] and guanosine diphosphate [GDP]). Normally, RAS flips back and forth between an excited (GTP-bound) signal-transmitting state and a quiescent (GDP-bound) state (Fig. 5.16). Activation of growth factor receptors (either by growth factors or, as in cancers, by mutation of the receptor) leads to the exchange of GDP for GTP and subsequent conformational changes that generate active RAS. This excited signal-emitting state is normally short lived because

RAS has an intrinsic guanosine triphosphatase (GTPase) activity that hydrolyzes GTP to GDP, returning the protein to its quiescent GDP-bound state. In cancers, this safeguard is often abrogated by point mutations, leading to amino acid substitutions that interfere with the GTPase activity: RAS is thus trapped in its activated, GTP-bound form and signals incessantly.

- *Signaling factors and transcription factors downstream of RAS.* Activated RAS stimulates downstream regulators of proliferation by several interconnected pathways. Mutation of some of these downstream factors mimics the growth-promoting effects of activated RAS (e.g., mutations of BRAF in melanomas and of PI3-kinase in multiple tumors). These signals converge on the nucleus and upregulate the expression of genes that support cell growth, including cyclin D, a factor required for cell cycle progression, and MYC, a transcription factor with wide-ranging effects on anabolic metabolism and cell growth, both of which are discussed later.

Insensitivity to Growth-Inhibitory Signals

Mutation of oncogenes is not sufficient to produce the unbridled proliferation that is characteristic of cancer cells; excessive growth also requires complementary mutations that inhibit the function of tumor suppressor genes, which in normal cells apply "brakes" to cellular proliferation.

Many tumor suppressor genes have been described, but two are particularly important in carcinogenesis: *RB*, a key regulator of the cell cycle, and *TP53*, which helps maintain the genomic integrity of cells. As discussed below, a high fraction of cancers contain genetic alterations that directly or indirectly disrupt the function of these two critical tumor suppressors.

RB: Governor of Cellular Proliferation

RB regulates the G1/S checkpoint, the portal through which cells must pass before DNA replication commences.

Normal cellular proliferation and differentiation are orchestrated by members of the retinoblastoma (RB) family of proteins, referred to here simply as RB. *RB* was the first tumor suppressor gene to be discovered and is a prototypical representative. Approximately 40% of retinoblastomas are familial, with the predisposition to develop tumors being transmitted as an autosomal dominant trait that is caused by the presence of one defective copy of the *RB* gene in the germline of affected individuals.

Retinoblastomas, whether familial or sporadic, always show complete loss of RB function due to inactivation of both *RB* alleles, an event that is much more likely in individuals who inherit one defective copy and acquire a somatic mutation of the other allele. *RB* mutations occur sporadically in a spectrum of different cancers, and many cancers have other alterations, such as epigenetic modifications, that impinge on *RB* indirectly. As a result, most (and perhaps all) cancers have one or more acquired defects that lead to loss of RB function.

To understand RB function, a brief review of the cell cycle is required. The successive phases of the cell cycle in growing cells are G_1, a phase of variable length; S, a phase during which cells replicate their DNA; G_2, a second phase of variable length; and M, during which cells enter into and complete mitosis, generating two daughter cells that return to G_1. The progression of cells through the cell cycle is controlled by three major sets of factors: cyclins, proteins whose levels oscillate up and down depending on the cell cycle phase; cyclin-dependent kinases (CDKs), proteins whose enzymatic activities depend on the binding of specific cyclins; and CDK inhibitors (CDKIs), proteins that act as negative regulators of cyclin/CDK complexes (Fig. 5.17). The transition from the G_1 phase to the S phase constitutes an important

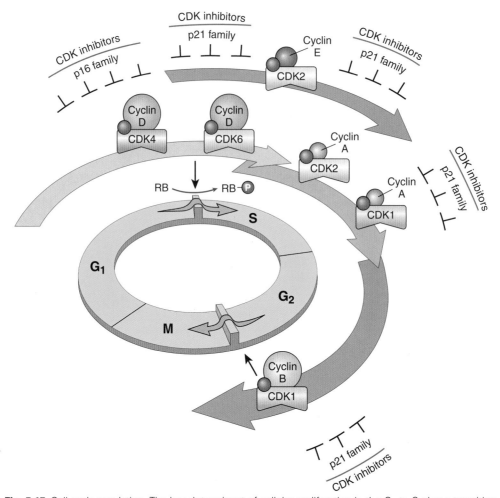

Fig. 5.17 Cell cycle regulation. The key determinant of cellular proliferation is the G_1 to S phase transition, which is inhibited by RB. This block is released by phosphorylation of RB by cyclin D/CDK4 and cyclin D/CDK6 complexes. CDK inhibitors of the p16 family provide another level of control by inhibiting cyclin D/CDK4 complexes, whereas CDK inhibitors of the p21 family negatively regulate multiple cyclin/CDK complexes throughout various cell cycle phases.

cell cycle checkpoint, because once cells move into the S phase they are committed to completing the cell cycle and dividing. The activity of RB "governs" G_1-S phase transition as follows (Fig. 5.18):
• Early in G_1, RB is in a hypophosphorylated active form that binds and inhibits transcription factors of the E2F family, preventing the expression of genes that are required for progression into S phase.
• Signals that are normally created by activated growth factor receptors upregulate the expression of D cyclins, which form complexes with CDK4 and CDK6 that phosphorylate and inactivate RB. This releases RB from E2F factors, permitting cells to express genes that are needed for entry into S phase.
• Subsequently, cellular phosphatases remove the phosphate groups from RB during M phase, regenerating the hypophosphorylated form of RB as the newly divided cells move back into the G_1 phase.
In cancers with normal RB genes, mutations in other genes that control RB phosphorylation are commonly found; as a result, virtually all cancer cells show dysregulation of the G1-S check point.

For the most part, these abnormalities increase the activation of cyclin D/CDK4 complexes, leading to inactivation of RB. The most common examples of such alternative mechanisms are mutations that result in constitutive activation of growth factor receptors or RAS.

The importance of RB in the control of cell growth and in cancer was recognized in part through the discovery that certain oncogenic

viruses (e.g., HPV) encode oncoproteins that inactivate RB. In HPV, the HPV E7 protein binds to the hypophosphorylated form of RB and prevents E2F inhibition. Persistent viral infection and sustained hyperproliferation over years sow the seeds for acquisition of additional mutations and the development of squamous cell carcinomas at sites that are susceptible to HPV infection (e.g., the cervix and the crypts of the oropharyngeal tonsils).

TP53: Guardian of the Genome

The TP53 tumor suppressor gene, the most commonly mutated gene in human cancers, functions to protect cells from stress-induced damage.

If RB is a "sensor" of external signals, the protein encoded by *TP53*, p53, can be viewed as a central monitor of internal stress. p53 is a transcription factor, and its effects are mediated through increased expression of genes that control cell growth and cell survival. Stresses that activate p53 include DNA damage, inappropriate progrowth stimuli (e.g., unbridled RAS activity), and hypoxia. In nonstressed, healthy cells, p53 has a short half-life because of its association with MDM2, a protein that targets p53 for destruction. In contrast, when the cell is stressed (e.g., due to DNA damage), "sensor" proteins modify and stabilize p53, enhancing its ability to drive the transcription of target genes. The products of these target genes act to prevent stressed cells from undergoing malignant transformation.

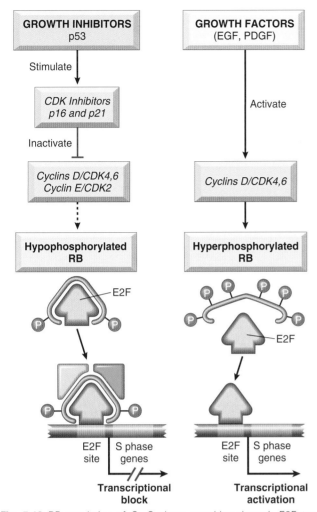

Fig. 5.18 RB regulation of G_1–S phase transition through E2F transcription factors. Hypophosphorylated RB in complex with the E2F transcription factors binds to DNA and inhibits transcription of genes whose products are required for the S phase of the cell cycle. When RB is phosphorylated by the cyclin D–CDK4 and cyclin D–CDK6 complexes, it releases E2F, which activates transcription of S-phase genes. The phosphorylation of RB is inhibited by CDKIs such as p16, which inactivate cyclin–CDK complexes. Virtually all cancer cells show dysregulation of the G_1–S checkpoint as a result of a mutation in at least one of four genes; *RB, CDK4, cyclin D,* and/or *CDKN2A [p16]*. EGF, Epidermal growth factor; PDGF, platelet-derived growth factor.

- *Triggering cell cycle arrest.* p53-mediated cell cycle arrest is a primordial response to DNA damage (Fig. 5.19). It occurs late in the G_1 phase and is caused mainly by p53-dependent expression of the CDKI p21. By inhibiting cyclin D–CDK4 complexes, p21 prevents RB phosphorylation and thereby arrests cells in the G_1 phase. This pause in cell cycling provides time to repair DNA damage (p53 also induces the expression of DNA damage repair genes). If DNA damage is repaired successfully, the cell is allowed to proceed through the cell cycle.
- *Inducing cellular senescence.* If the DNA damage cannot be repaired, cells with active p53 may undergo senescence, a form of permanent cell cycle arrest. The mechanisms of senescence are unclear but seem to involve p21 and epigenetic changes that permanently alter the expression of genes that are required for growth.
- *Killing stressed cells through apoptosis.* p53 induces apoptosis of cells with irreversible DNA damage by upregulating several proapoptotic genes.

The factors that determine whether a cell repairs its DNA, becomes senescent, or undergoes apoptosis are uncertain; both the duration and the level of p53 activation may be deciding factors. There is still much to be learned about the nuances of p53 function.

The importance of *TP53* dysregulation in cancer is highlighted by the following considerations:
- *More than 70% of human cancers have defects in* TP53, and other cancers often have defects in genes upstream or downstream of *TP53.* Biallelic abnormalities of the *TP53* gene are found in virtually every type of cancer, including carcinomas of the lung, colon, and breast, the three leading causes of cancer deaths.
- *The heritable cancer syndrome Li-Fraumeni syndrome is due to a germline mutation in one TP53 allele.* Patients with this syndrome have a 25-fold greater chance of developing a wide spectrum of malignant tumors by age 50 compared with the general population. The most common types of cancers seen are sarcomas, carcinomas of the breast, and certain leukemias and brain tumors; these cancers often occur at a young age, and many patients develop multiple tumors of different types.
- *The p53 protein is the target of viral oncoproteins.* As with RB, normal p53 is rendered nonfunctional by the binding of certain DNA viruses. The best characterized of these is E6, a viral oncoprotein encoded by HPV, discussed earlier as an important cause of cervical and tonsillar squamous cell carcinoma.

Cell Lineage–Specific Tumor Suppressor Genes

Unlike *RB* and *TP53*, which are commonly lost in many different human cancers, other tumor suppressor genes are strongly linked to only a few cancer types.

A classic example is the *APC* gene, which encodes a component of the Wnt signaling pathway. APC is a cytoplasmic protein whose dominant function is to promote the degradation of β-catenin. β-catenin is a transcriptional activator, and with loss of APC, β-catenin becomes hyperactive. In colonic epithelium (unlike most cells of other lineages), hyperactivity of β-catenin leads to increased transcription of growth-promoting genes, such as cyclin D and *MYC*. Individuals who inherit one defective copy of *APC* develop *adenomatous polyposis coli* (from which *APC* takes its name), a disease characterized by the appearance of hundreds of colonic polyps by early adulthood and the development of colon carcinoma by age 50. These tumors have somatic deletions or mutations that eliminate the function of the remaining normal copy of *APC.* Similar biallelic loss of APC is also seen in a subset of sporadic colon cancers. Other examples of lineage-specific tumor suppressor genes (and oncogenes) are discussed in later chapters.

Altered Cellular Metabolism

Even in the presence of ample oxygen, cancer cells demonstrate a distinctive form of cellular metabolism characterized by high levels of glucose uptake and increased conversion of glucose to lactose (fermentation) via the glycolytic pathway.

This phenomenon, called the *Warburg effect* and also known as *aerobic glycolysis,* is a characteristic of many rapidly proliferating cells, including fetal tissue, activated lymphocytes, and tumor cells. The "glucose hunger" of tumors is used to visualize tumors via positron emission tomography (PET) scanning, in which patients are injected with ^{18}F-fluorodeoxyglucose, a glucose derivative that is preferentially taken up into tumor cells (as well as normal, actively dividing tissues such as the bone marrow). Most tumors are PET-positive, and rapidly growing ones are markedly so.

Why do cancer cells rely on inefficient glycolysis (which generates two molecules of ATP per molecule of glucose) instead of oxidative phosphorylation (which generates up to 36 molecules of ATP per molecule of glucose)? The answer is that aerobic glycolysis provides rapidly

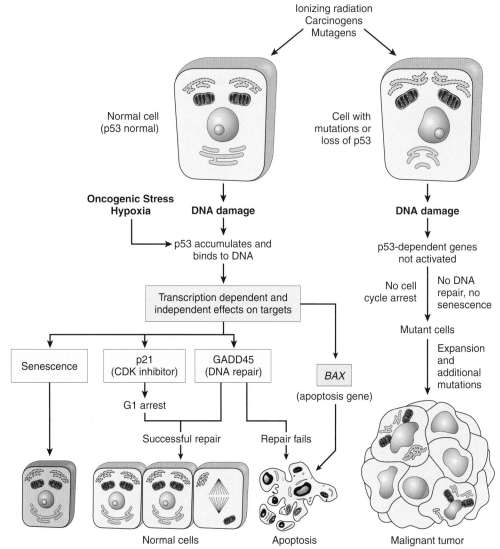

Fig. 5.19 The role of p53 in maintaining the integrity of the genome. Activation of normal p53 by DNA-damaging agents or by hypoxia leads to cell cycle arrest in G_1 and induction of DNA repair, by transcriptional upregulation of the cyclin-dependent kinase inhibitor *CDKN1A* (p21) and the *GADD45* genes. Successful repair of DNA allows cells to proceed with the cell cycle; if DNA repair fails, p53 triggers either apoptosis or senescence. In cells with loss or mutations of *TP53*, DNA damage does not induce cell cycle arrest or DNA repair, and genetically damaged cells proliferate, giving rise eventually to malignant neoplasms.

dividing tumor cells with metabolic intermediates that are needed for the synthesis of cellular components, whereas mitochondrial oxidative phosphorylation does not. During oxidative phosphorylation, a molecule of glucose combines with O_2 to produce H_2O and CO_2, which is lost through respiration. This yields abundant ATP, but it does not yield any of the carbon moieties needed to build the cellular components for growth (proteins, lipids, and nucleic acids). In contrast, aerobic glycolysis yields metabolic intermediates that are useful as cellular building blocks.

Metabolic reprogramming is produced by signaling cascades downstream of growth factor receptors, the same pathways that are deregulated by mutations in oncogenes and tumor suppressor genes in cancers.

In cancer cells, this reprogramming persists because of the actions of mutated oncoproteins and the loss of tumor suppressor function. Several important points of crosstalk between progrowth signaling factors and cellular metabolism have been discovered (Fig. 5.20).

Beyond the Warburg effect, two other links between metabolism and cancer are sufficiently important to merit brief mention: autophagy and "oncometabolism."

- *Autophagy* is a state of severe nutrient deficiency in which cells cannibalize their own organelles, proteins, and membranes to survive (see Chapter 1). Tumor cells often grow under marginal environmental conditions without triggering autophagy, suggesting that the pathways that induce autophagy are deranged. In keeping with this, several genes that promote autophagy are tumor suppressors.
- *Oncometabolism*. A surprising group of oncogenic alterations seen in certain neoplasms consists of mutations in enzymes that participate in the Krebs cycle. Some of these mutations lead to the loss of enzyme function, whereas in other cases the affected enzymes acquire new activities altogether and generate products that have been called oncometabolites. In each instance, it appears that the net effect of the mutations is to cause changes in metabolism that affect the expression or activity of currently unknown cancer genes.

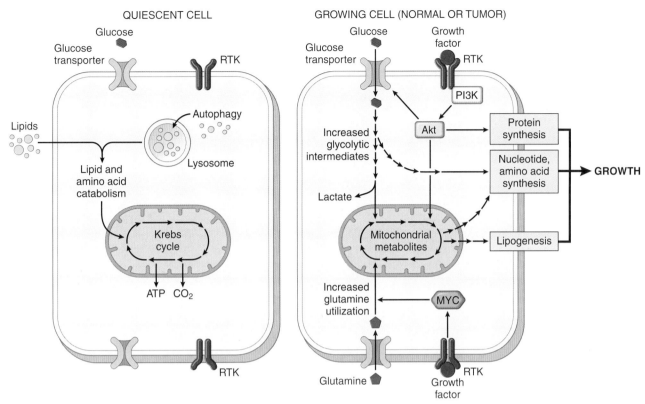

Fig. 5.20 Metabolism and cell growth. Quiescent cells rely mainly on the Krebs cycle for ATP production; if starved, autophagy (self-eating) is induced to provide a source of fuel. When stimulated by growth factors, normal cells markedly upregulate glucose and glutamine uptake, which provides carbon sources for the synthesis of nucleotides, proteins, and lipids. In cancers, oncogenic mutations involving growth factor signaling pathways and other key factors such as MYC deregulate these metabolic pathways, an alteration known as the Warburg effect.

Evasion of Cell Death

In certain cancers, the accumulation of neoplastic cells results from mutations that provide resistance to regulated cell death (apoptosis).

As discussed in Chapter 1, apoptosis is the orderly dismantling of cells into component pieces, a process that may be triggered by the intrinsic or extrinsic pathway that ultimately activates a proteolytic cascade involving caspases; these in turn are responsible for orderly disassembly of the cell. The sequence of events that lead to apoptosis can be triggered by stress-inducing cellular injuries or growth factor deficiency (the intrinsic pathway), or by activation of members of the TNF receptor family (the extrinsic pathway).

Of these two pathways of apoptosis, it is the intrinsic pathway (also known as the mitochondrial pathway) that is most frequently disabled in cancer (Fig. 5.21). A delicate balance between proapoptotic and antiapoptotic members of the BCL2 protein family determines whether or not a cell undergoes apoptosis. The release of cytochrome c by mitochondrial permeabilization promotes apoptosis via the proapoptotic proteins BAX and BAK, which are held in check by antiapoptotic members of the family (e.g., BCL2). A third set of proteins, the so-called BH3-only proteins, appears to shift the balance between the proapoptotic and antiapoptotic family members.

Within this framework, it is possible to illustrate the multiple ways in which apoptosis mediated by the intrinsic pathway is frustrated by cancer cells (Fig. 5.21).

- *Overexpression of BCL2* is a well-characterized mechanism that protects tumor cells from apoptosis. Approximately 85% of follicular lymphomas carry a chromosomal translocation that drives the overexpression of BCL2, and many other cancers are associated with high levels of expression of BCL2 or other antiapoptotic members of the BCL2 family.
- *Inactivation of sensors and effectors of cell stress that would normally trigger apoptosis* is another mechanism by which cancer cells escape death. As mentioned previously, p53 is the downstream effector of several pathways that sense cell stress. When activated, p53 changes gene expression to promote apoptosis in severely stressed cells. Loss of p53 function (due to mutation of *TP53* or p53 inactivation through indirect mechanisms) allows cells to survive stresses that would ordinarily kill them.

BCL2 protein expression and TP53 mutation status have important implications for treatment and prognosis.

Drugs that bind BCL2 and block its function are used to treat cancers associated with BCL2 overexpression. Conversely, the presence of *TP53* mutations is associated with a worse outcome in virtually all forms of cancer, likely because loss of p53 makes cells resistant to forms of therapy (e.g., radiation therapy and certain types of chemotherapy) that cause DNA damage, a potent inducer of apoptosis in cells with intact p53. Cancers that recur following treatment with agents that cause DNA damage are likely to be defective in *TP53* function, because these cells have a selective advantage that allows them to survive these types of therapies.

Limitless Replicative Potential (Immortality)

Loss of growth restraints is not enough for tumors to achieve immortality: tumor cells also must develop ways to avoid cellular senescence and mitotic catastrophe.

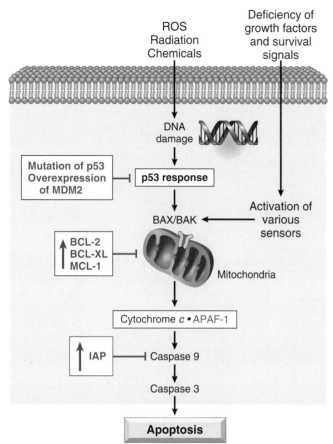

Fig. 5.21 Intrinsic pathway of apoptosis and mechanisms used by tumor cells to evade cell death. Evasion mechanisms in tumor cells are in red and include: (1) Loss of p53, leading to reduced function of proapoptotic factors such as BAX. (2) Reduced egress of cytochrome c from mitochondria as a result of upregulation of antiapoptotic factors such as BCL2, BCL-XL, and MCL-1. (3) Loss of apoptotic peptidase-activating factor 1 (APAF1). (4) Upregulation of inhibitors of apoptosis (IAP).

As discussed previously in the context of cellular aging (see Chapter 1), most normal human cells can double 60 to 70 times, after which the cells lose the ability to divide and enter senescence. This phenomenon is due to progressive shortening of *telomeres* at the ends of chromosomes.

The consequences of telomere shortening, when pronounced, are drastic. Short telomeres are recognized as double-stranded DNA breaks by the cell's DNA damage "sensors," leading to p53-mediated cell cycle arrest and apoptosis or senescence. Even in cells with *TP53* mutations, attempts to repair the damage through other DNA repair pathways leads to chromosome instability, which eventually leads to cell death. If, however, the cell reactivates the enzyme telomerase (a specialized RNA-protein complex that uses its own RNA as a template for adding nucleotides to the ends of chromosomes), cell death may be averted.

Telomerase is active in normal stem cells and is absent from, or present at very low levels in, most somatic cells. In 85% to 95% of cancers, telomere maintenance is due to upregulation of telomerase. The remaining tumors fail to express telomerase and use another mechanism termed *alternative lengthening of telomeres* that depends on DNA recombination to maintain telomeres.

Sustained Angiogenesis

In order to grow, solid tumors develop their own blood supply by inducing angiogenesis.

Like normal tissues, tumors require delivery of oxygen and nutrients and removal of waste products. Tumors are only able to grow to a size of 1 to 2 mm in the absence of angiogenesis, presumably because this size represents the maximal distance across which oxygen, nutrients, and waste can diffuse from preexisting blood vessels. For neoplasms to grow beyond this size limit, they have to stimulate neoangiogenesis, in which vessels sprout from previously existing capillaries. Neovascularization has a dual effect on tumor growth: Perfusion supplies needed nutrients and oxygen, and newly formed endothelial cells stimulate the growth of adjacent tumor cells by secreting growth factors. Although the resulting tumor vasculature is effective at delivering nutrients and removing wastes, it is not normal: The vessels are leaky and dilated with a haphazard pattern of connection. Invasive tumor cells may readily penetrate these vessels, contributing to metastasis.

Tumor angiogenesis may be stimulated by proangiogenic factors that are produced by the tumor cells, inflammatory cells (e.g., macrophages), and other resident stromal cells (e.g., tumor-associated fibroblasts). Proteases elaborated by the tumor cells or by stromal cells may also release peptides with angiogenic activity from the extracellular matrix. In full-blown cancers, the proangiogenic state is further reinforced by several other alterations that increase levels of vascular endothelial growth factor (VEGF), a key proangiogenic cytokine. Most notably, tissue hypoxia stabilizes hypoxia-induced factor (HIF), an oxygen-sensitive transcription factor that directly upregulates VEGF expression. This creates an angiogenic gradient that stimulates the proliferation of endothelial cells and guides the growth of new vessels toward the tumor. Mutations involving tumor suppressors often tilt the balance to favor angiogenesis. For example, p53 represses the expression of VEGF and stimulates the expression of antiangiogenic molecules. Thus, loss of p53 in tumor cells provides a more permissive environment for angiogenesis. Growth factor–receptor signaling and MYC also stimulate the expression of VEGF.

The dependence of tumors on angiogeneisis can be exploited therapeutically. The prototype antiangiogenesis drug, bevacizumab, is an antibody that neutralizes VEGF and is approved for the treatment of multiple cancers. However, angiogenesis inhibitors have not been as effective as originally hoped; presumably, subclones of tumor cells with greater invasive capacity and the ability to migrate to existing blood vessels emerge, thereby sidestepping the need for neoangiogenesis.

Invasion and Metastasis

Invasion and metastasis result from complex interactions involving cancer cells, stromal cells, and the extracellular matrix.

Most studies pertain to carcinomas, which are our focus here. For the purpose of discussion, invasion and metastasis can be broken down into a successive sequence of events, discussed next.

Invasion of the Extracellular Matrix

Tissues are organized into compartments separated from each other by two types of extracellular matrix (ECM), basement membranes and interstitial connective tissue, each composed of collagens, glycoproteins, and proteoglycans (see Chapter 2). Tumor cells interact with the ECM at several stages in the metastatic cascade (Fig. 5.22). A carcinoma cell must first breach the underlying basement membrane, then traverse the interstitial connective tissue, and ultimately gain access to the circulation by penetrating the vascular basement membrane. This process is repeated in reverse when tumor cells extravasate at distant sites. Invasion of the ECM initiates the metastatic cascade and is an active process that can be resolved into several sequential steps, as follows:

metalloproteases (MMPs) produced by tumor cells or stromal cells (e.g., fibroblasts and inflammatory cells) reacting to the tumor. The levels of metalloprotease inhibitors also are reduced in carcinomas, further tilting the balance toward tissue degradation.

- *Locomotion,* the final step of invasion, propels tumor cells through the degraded basement membranes and zones of matrix proteolysis. Such movement may be potentiated and directed by tumor cell–derived chemokines. In addition, cleavage products of matrix components (e.g., collagen, laminin) and some growth factors have chemotactic activity for tumor cells, and stromal cells also produce paracrine effectors of cell motility.

Vascular Dissemination and Homing of Tumor Cells

Tumor cells frequently escape their sites of origin and enter the circulation through blood vessels or lymphatics. Millions of tumor cells are shed daily from even small cancers. Several factors seem to limit the metastatic potential of circulating tumor cells: While in the circulation, tumor cells are vulnerable to destruction by host immune cells, and the process of adhesion to vascular beds and invasion of normal tissues may be more difficult than the initial invasion. Even following extravasation, tumor cells that grow well in their primary site may lack critical stromal support or be suppressed by resident immune cells. Despite these limiting factors, if neglected, virtually all malignant tumors will eventually produce macroscopic metastases.

The sites of metastases are related to two factors: the anatomic location and vascular or lymphatic drainage of the primary tumor, and the tropism of particular tumors for specific tissues.

Most metastases arise in the first capillary bed available to the tumor, but natural pathways of drainage cannot wholly explain the distribution of metastases. As mentioned earlier, for example, lung carcinoma has a high proclivity for spread to the adrenal glands and the brain, and melanoma of the eye almost always spreads to the liver. Such organ tropism may be related to the expression of tissue-selective adhesion molecules, the production of specific chemokines in different tissues for which tumor cells express receptors, and the presence of stromal cells that support the growth of tumors. All of these factors make different tissues favorable or unfavorable "soil" for different tumors.

Metastasis

Tumors vary greatly in their ability to metastasize, in part because of inherent differences in behavior. In general, large tumors are more likely to metastasize than small tumors, presumably because large tumors are typically present in the patient for longer periods of time, providing additional chances for metastasis to occur. However, tumor size and type cannot adequately explain the behavior of individual cancers, and it is still open to question whether metastasis is probabilistic (a matter of chance multiplied by tumor cell number and time) or deterministic (reflecting inherent differences in metastatic potential from tumor to tumor).

Evasion of Immune Surveillance

The host immune system is capable of destroying tumors, but cancers evolve to evade or inhibit immune responses.

Tumor cells can be recognized as "foreign" and eliminated by the immune system; *immune surveillance* refers to the role of the immune system in constantly "scanning" the body for emerging malignant cells and destroying them. Tumor-specific T cells and antibodies are found in many patients, and the extent and quality of immune infiltrates in cancers is often correlated with the clinical outcome (e.g., colon cancer). There is an increased incidence of certain cancers in immunodeficiency states. Recently, therapeutic agents that act by stimulating latent host T-cell responses (described later) have shown effectiveness in some advanced cancers.

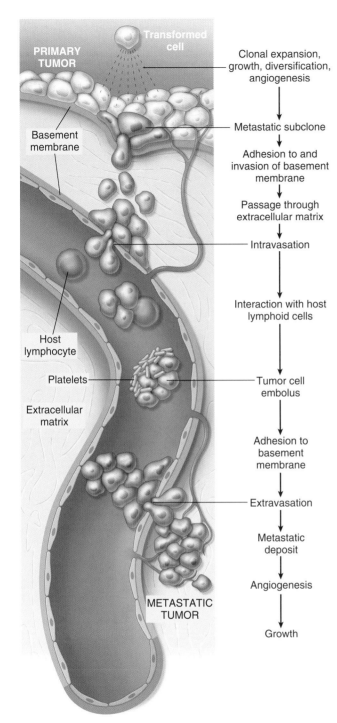

Fig. 5.22 The metastatic cascade: The sequential steps involved in the hematogenous spread of a tumor.

- *Loosening of intercellular connections between tumor cells.* Carcinoma cells are normally held together by adhesion proteins, such as E-cadherin. E-cadherin function is often lost in metastatic carcinomas due to either deleterious mutations in E-cadherin or silencing of E-cadherin expression. Loss of E-cadherin is associated with changes in cell shape, increased cell motility, and upregulation of genes that are more typical of mesenchymal cells (e.g., fibroblasts). These changes are referred to as epithelial-mesenchymal transition (EMT).
- *Local degradation of the basement membrane and interstitial connective tissue* by proteolytic enzymes, particularly *matrix*

Because the immune system is capable of recognizing and eliminating nascent cancers, cancer survival requires that the tumor cells be invisible to the host immune system or actively suppress host immunity. This understanding has led to a modern revolution in cancer immunotherapy.

Tumor Antigens

The major antigens of tumors that elicit immune responses are the products of mutated genes that produce neoantigens with MHC-binding mutated sequences.

Because these antigens are novel and are not present normally, they are seen as foreign by the host's immune system. Like all cytosolic proteins, these antigens are processed and displayed as class I MHC-associated peptides to CD8+ T cells. Some tumor antigens are not the products of mutated genes but are expressed in cancer cells at much higher levels than in normal cells (e.g., tyrosinase in melanomas), and others are normally expressed early in development, repressed in mature cells, and derepressed in cancer cells (e.g., the so-called cancer–testis antigens). Many other antigens have been identified in tumors because of their recognition by antibodies, but most of these are also present in normal cells and they are neither inducers nor targets of antitumor immunity.

Immune Mechanisms of Tumor Destruction

The most important mechanism of tumor elimination is the killing of tumor cells by CD8+ cytotoxic T lymphocytes (CTLs) specific for tumor antigens. The presence of functional CD8+ T cells is predictive of the outcome of many cancers, and quantification of the immune cell infiltrate (the *immunoscore*) has some predictive value. The significance of other killing mechanisms (e.g., macrophages and NK cells) is unclear.

Immune Escape

Tumor cells evade the immune system either by being invisible to lymphoid cells or by hijacking inhibitory pathways designed for regulation of immunity.

Several mechanisms of immune evasion have been described and have therapeutic value (Fig. 5.23):

- *Antigen loss variants.* As tumor subclones evolve, they tend to either lose expression of the antigens that are targets of host immunity or, more often, lose expression of class I MHC molecules or components of antigen-processing pathways, preventing the presentation of antigens to T cells.
- *Inhibition of T cells using checkpoint receptors.* The two best-known receptors that impose "checkpoints" in T-cell activation are PD-1 and CTLA-4. When PD-1 and CTLA-4 expressed on CD8+ T cells engage their ligands, the activation and function of these cells are inhibited. These checkpoints evolved to prevent immune responses against self-antigens and are "hijacked" by tumor cells to silence CD8+ T cells. PD-1 is engaged in tumors because tumor cells often express the ligands for these receptors (PDL-1 and PDL-2) or induce expression of PDL-1 and PDL-2 on other cells in the immune infiltrate. Blocking either PD-1 or CTLA-4 with antibodies leads to

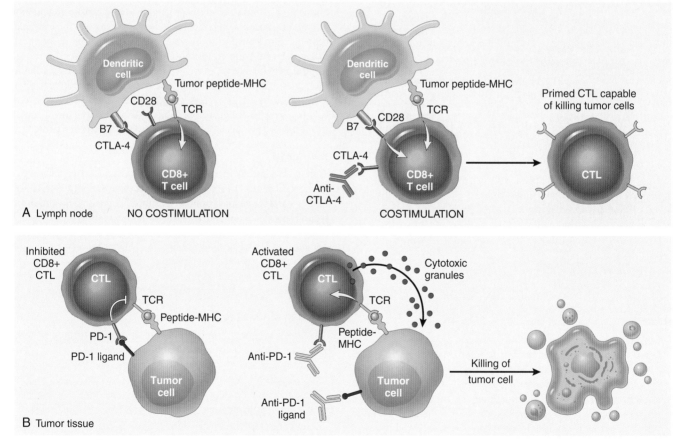

Fig. 5.23 Activation of host antitumor immunity by checkpoint inhibitors. (A) Blockade of the CTLA-4 surface molecule with inhibitory antibody allows cytolytic CD8+ T cells (CTLs) to engage B7 family co-receptors, leading to T cell activation. (B) Blockade of PD-1 receptor or PD-1 ligand abrogates inhibitory signals transmitted by PD-1, again leading to activation of CTLs. (Reprinted from Abbas AK, Lichtman AH, Pillai S: *Cellular and molecular immunology,* ed 7, Philadelphia, 2012, Saunders.)

the regression of many tumors, including melanoma, non–small cell lung cancer, bladder cancer, Hodgkin lymphoma, and others. This approach, called checkpoint blockade, is now an important component of anticancer therapy. Because the checkpoints evolved normally to prevent autoimmunity, patients given these treatments often develop autoimmune inflammation, including colitis, as well as inflammation of the endocrine organs, heart, and other tissues.

- *Other mechanisms* by which tumors inhibit immune responses include induction of regulatory T cells and the local production of immunosuppressive cytokines such as TGF-β.

Genomic Instability as an Enabler of Malignancy

Defects in DNA repair pathways enable tumor growth by allowing accumulation of mutations in cancer genes.

The preceding section identified the eight defining features of malignancy, all of which appear to be produced by genetic alterations involving cancer genes. Although humans are awash in environmental mutagens, cancers are relatively rare outcomes of these encounters because normal cells are able to sense and repair DNA damage. The importance of DNA repair in maintaining the integrity of the genome is highlighted by persons born with inherited defects in three types of DNA repair systems (mismatch repair, nucleotide excision repair, and recombination repair), all of which are associated with an increased risk for developing cancer. Although the discussion below focuses on these inherited syndromes, sporadic cancers often incur mutations in DNA repair genes, as well. Presumably, as in individuals with inherited DNA repair defects, these somatic mutations speed the accumulation of driver mutations in cancer genes and thereby the development of cancer.

Hereditary Nonpolyposis Colon Cancer Syndrome

The role of DNA mismatch repair genes in the predisposition to cancer is illustrated by the *hereditary nonpolyposis colon cancer (HNPCC) syndrome,* a disorder characterized by familial carcinoma of the colon. When a strand of DNA is being repaired, the proteins encoded by these genes act as "spell checkers." For example, if there is an erroneous pairing of G with T, rather than the normal A with T, the mismatch repair proteins correct the defect. Without these "proofreaders," errors accumulate at an increased rate. Mutations in at least four mismatch repair genes have been found in patients with HNPCC. One defective copy of a DNA mismatch repair gene is inherited, and a second "hit" in the other allele of the same gene occurs in colonic epithelial cells. In this respect, they resemble tumor suppressor genes. DNA repair genes affect cell growth indirectly by allowing mutations in other genes during the process of normal cell division. A characteristic finding in the genome of patients with mismatch repair defects is microsatellite instability (MSI). Microsatellites are tandem repeats of one to six nucleotides found throughout the genome. Usually, the length of these microsatellites remains constant. However, in patients with HNPCC, these satellites are unstable and increase or decrease in length. HNPCC syndrome accounts for only 2% to 4% of all colonic cancers, but MSI can be detected in about 15% of sporadic cancers. MSI-associated tumors tend to be more responsive to immune checkpoint inhibitor therapies, presumably because the defect in mismatch repair leads to a high burden of mutations producing tumor neoantigens. In fact, this type of immunotherapy is now approved for all recurrent tumors with mismatch repair defects regardless of the tumor type—the first time a treatment has been approved based only on a mutational signature.

Xeroderma Pigmentosum

Patients with the autosomal recessive disorder *xeroderma pigmentosum* are at increased risk for cancers arising in sun-exposed skin. Ultraviolet (UV) rays in sunlight cause cross-linking of pyrimidine residues, preventing normal DNA replication. Such DNA damage is repaired by the nucleotide excision repair system, which is defective in patients with this disease. The rate of somatic mutation in sun-exposed skin is greatly accelerated, resulting in an extraordinarily high incidence of skin cancers such as basal cell carcinoma and squamous cell carcinoma in these patients.

Diseases with Defects in DNA Repair by Homologous Recombination

The autosomal recessive disorders *Bloom syndrome, ataxia-telangiectasia,* and *Fanconi anemia* are characterized by hypersensitivity to DNA-damaging agents, such as ionizing radiation (in Bloom syndrome and ataxia-telangiectasia) or DNA cross-linking agents such as nitrogen mustard (in Fanconi anemia). Each is caused by defects in genes that are required for DNA repair by homologous recombination, in which a "good" strand of DNA is used to repair a damaged piece of DNA that has been broken or covalently cross-linked. The phenotypes of these diseases are complex and include, in addition to a predisposition to cancer, neural symptoms (in ataxia-telangiectasia), anemia (in Fanconi anemia), and developmental defects (in Bloom syndrome).

Evidence of the oncogenic role of defective homologous recombination also comes from the study of hereditary breast cancer. Germline mutations in two genes that also function in homologous recombination, *BRCA1* and *BRCA2,* are found in 50% of familial breast cancers. In addition to breast cancer, women with *BRCA1* mutations have a substantially higher risk of ovarian carcinoma and men have a slightly higher risk of prostate cancer; germline mutations in *BRCA2* increase the risk of breast cancer in both men and women, as well as other carcinomas, melanoma, and lymphomas. Similar to other tumor suppressor genes, both copies of *BRCA1* and *BRCA2* must be inactivated for cancer to develop.

Tumor-Promoting Inflammation as an Enabler of Malignancy

Inflammatory cells can facilitate tumor cell growth and survival by producing soluble factors that influence the hallmarks of cancer.

Infiltrating cancers provoke a chronic inflammatory reaction. In patients with advanced cancers, this inflammatory reaction can be so extensive as to cause systemic signs and symptoms, such as anemia (the anemia of chronic inflammation), fatigue, and cachexia. Animal models suggest that inflammatory cells also modify the tumor microenvironment to enable many of the hallmarks of cancer. These effects may stem from direct interactions between inflammatory cells and tumor cells, or indirect effects of inflammatory cells on other resident stromal cells, particularly cancer-associated fibroblasts and endothelial cells. Inflammatory cells and resident stromal cells may promote cancer development by producing growth factors that act on the neoplastic cells, promoting angiogenesis, activating cell survival pathways in tumors, producing enzymes that enhance local tumor invasion and metastasis, and suppressing effective antitumor immune responses. In this respect, they resemble tumor suppressor genes.

These pathophysiologic concepts have provided a road map for the development of new therapeutic agents for the treatment of cancer (Fig. 5.24). As our understanding of cancer pathogenesis expands, there is reason to hope that the next few years will see the development of many more effective targeted therapies.

CLINICAL ASPECTS OF NEOPLASIA

Ultimately, the importance of cancer is its impact on patients. The following discussion considers the effects of tumors on their hosts, the grading and clinical staging of cancer, and the laboratory diagnosis of neoplasms.

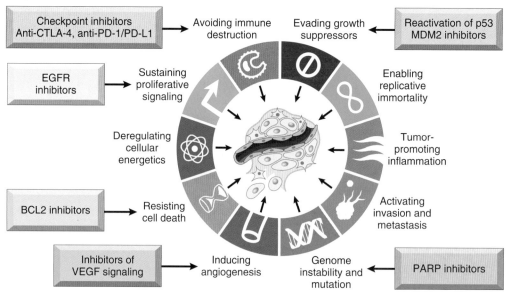

Fig. 5.24 Therapeutic targeting of hallmarks of cancer. Therapies approved for use or in advanced clinical trials are listed. (From Hanahan D, Weiberg RA: The hallmarks of cancer: the next generation. *Cell* 144:646, 2011.)

Clinical Effects of Tumors

Benign and malignant tumors may cause local and systemic problems through a variety of direct and indirect effects.

Anatomic location is a crucial determinant of the local, "space-filling" effects of both benign and malignant tumors. A small (1-cm) pituitary adenoma can compress and destroy the surrounding normal gland, giving rise to hypopituitarism, and a comparably small carcinoma within the common bile duct may induce fatal biliary tract obstruction. Other important local complications include spinal cord compression and pathologic fractures due to structural compromise of bones by malignant tumors.

Locally invasive cancers may ulcerate through a surface, with consequent bleeding or secondary infection. Erosion into major vessels or the heart can lead to catastrophic bleeding, a fortunately rare event. More commonly, secondary infection of nonhealing wounds may be due to interference of normal repair mechanisms by malignant cells.

Signs and symptoms related to hormone production are common with benign and malignant neoplasms arising in endocrine glands. Tumors arising in the β cells of the pancreatic islets of Langerhans can produce hyperinsulinism, and tumors of the adrenal cortex may elaborate a variety of steroid hormones (e.g., aldosterone, leading to sodium retention, hypertension, and hypokalemia).

Many cancer patients suffer from *tumor cachexia*, which is marked by progressive loss of body fat and skeletal muscle accompanied by profound weakness and anorexia. Tumor cachexia is caused not by the nutritional demands of the tumor but by an increase in circulating factors that suppress the appetite and cause changes in the metabolism of tissues, such as fat and skeletal muscle. Calorie expenditure remains high and the basal metabolic rate is increased, despite reduced food intake. These metabolic abnormalities are partly attributed to the actions of the cytokine tumor necrosis factor (TNF), produced by activated macrophages or by tumor cells themselves, which suppresses the appetite and inhibits the action of lipoprotein lipase, preventing the release of free fatty acids from lipoproteins.

Paraneoplastic syndromes are symptom complexes that occur in patients with cancer that cannot be explained by local or distant spread

of the tumor or by the elaboration of hormones indigenous to the tissue of origin of the tumor. They appear in 10% to 15% of cancer patients, and their clinical recognition is important for several reasons:

- They may be the earliest manifestation of an occult neoplasm
- They may be severe and, in some instances, may even be lethal
- They may mimic metastatic disease, thereby confounding treatment planning

Paraneoplastic syndromes are diverse and are associated with many different tumors (Table 5.7). One tumor may induce several syndromes concurrently: Bronchogenic carcinomas may elaborate products identical to or having the effects of ACTH, antidiuretic hormone, parathyroid hormone, serotonin, human chorionic gonadotropin, and other bioactive substances. The following are the most common paraneoplastic syndromes:

- *Hypercalcemia* in cancer patients is most often caused by the synthesis of a parathyroid hormone–related protein (PTHrP) by tumor cells.
- *Cushing syndrome,* usually related to production of ACTH or ACTH-like hormones by cancer cells, is most commonly seen with small cell carcinoma of the lung.
- *Hypercoagulability,* leading to venous thrombosis and nonbacterial thrombotic endocarditis, is primarily related to changes that enhance the activity of coagulation factors (rather than platelets). Suspected contributors include changes in endothelial function related to the proinflammatory effects of cancer, and substances released from tumor cells (such as mucins) that directly activate the coagulation cascade.

Grading and Staging of Cancer

Grading and staging are used to estimate the probable clinical aggressiveness of a given neoplasm and to provide a standard that is used when comparing the outcomes of different treatment protocols.

The stage of the cancer (how extensive it is in the patient) is assessed mainly by clinical and radiologic studies, whereas grading is done by pathologic examination using features that are described below. In general, although both are useful, the tumor stage is of greater prognostic value than the tumor grade.

Table 5.7 Paraneoplastic Syndromes

Clinical Syndrome	Associated Neoplasms	Causal Mechanism(s)/Agent(s)
Endocrinopathies		
Cushing syndrome	Small cell lung carcinoma Pancreatic carcinoma Neural tumors	ACTH or ACTH-like substance
Syndrome of inappropriate antidiuretic hormone secretion (SIADH)	Small cell lung carcinoma Intracranial neoplasms	Antidiuretic hormone or atrial natriuretic hormones
Hypercalcemia	Squamous cell lung carcinoma Breast carcinoma Renal cell carcinoma Adult T-cell leukemia/lymphoma	Parathyroid hormone–related protein, TGF-α, TNF, IL-1
Hypoglycemia	Fibrosarcoma Other mesenchymal sarcomas Ovarian carcinoma	Insulin or insulin-like substances
Nerve and Muscle Syndromes		
Myasthenia	Lung carcinoma Thymoma	Immunologic
Disorders of the central and peripheral nervous systems	Breast carcinoma Teratoma	Immunologic
Dermatologic Disorders		
Acanthosis nigricans	Gastric carcinoma Lung carcinoma Uterine carcinoma	Immunologic; secretion of epidermal growth factor
Dermatomyositis	Lung carcinoma Breast carcinoma	Immunologic
Osseous, Articular, and Soft Tissue Changes		
Hypertrophic osteoarthropathy and clubbing of the fingers	Lung carcinoma	Unknown
Vascular and Hematologic Changes		
Venous thrombosis (Trousseau phenomenon)	Pancreatic carcinoma Lung carcinoma Other cancers	Hypercoagulability due to secreted tumor products (e.g., mucins) that activate clotting factors
Red cell aplasia	Thymoma	Immunologic
Polycythemia	Renal carcinoma Cerebellar hemangioma Hepatocellular carcinoma	Erythropoietin secretion by tumor cells
Renal Dysfunction		
Nephrotic syndrome	Various cancers	Immune complexes

ACTH, Adrenocorticotropic hormone; IL-1, interleukin-1; TGF-α, transforming growth factor-α; TNF, tumor necrosis factor.

- *Grading.* Grading is based on the degree of differentiation of the tumor cells and, in some cancers, the number of mitoses and the presence of certain architectural features. Grading schemes differ for each type of malignancy and range from two categories (low grade and high grade) to four categories. Criteria for grading of specific tumors are described in later chapters, but all attempt, in essence, to judge the aggressiveness of the tumor cells, often based on the extent to which the tumor cells resemble (or fail to resemble) their normal counterparts. Although histologic grading has prognostic value, the correlation between histologic appearance and biologic behavior is far from perfect.
- *Staging.* The staging of solid cancers is based on the size of the primary lesion, the extent of its spread to regional lymph nodes, and the presence or absence of blood-borne metastases. The major staging system in current use is the American Joint Committee on Cancer Staging. This system uses a classification called the TNM system: T for primary tumor, N for regional lymph node

involvement, and M for metastases. TNM staging varies for specific forms of cancer, but there are general principles. The primary lesion is characterized as T1 to T4 based on increasing size; T0 is used to indicate an in situ lesion. N0 indicates no nodal involvement, whereas N1 to N3 denotes involvement of an increasing number and range of nodes. M0 signifies no distant metastases, whereas M1 or sometimes M2 reflects the presence and estimated number of metastases.

Cancer Diagnosis

No matter how strongly cancer is suspected on clinical grounds, diagnosis requires sampling of tissues and histologic identification of cancer cells.

Every year the approach to the laboratory diagnosis of cancer becomes more complex, more sophisticated, and more specialized. Each of the following sections attempts to present the state of the art, avoiding details of technologies.

Morphologic Methods

In most instances, is not difficult to diagnose cancer based on the appearance of the malignant cells under the microscope. However, in many cases with equivocal morphologic changes, clinical and radiologic features are essential to arrive at the diagnosis. Sampling of the tumor for morphologic analysis can be achieved through the following procedures:

- *Open (surgical) biopsy.* This affords the opportunity to select tissue for sampling based on its gross appearance. The biopsy can be examined by the routine hematoxylin-and-eosin stains after fixation. In some cases, the biopsy is sent for rapid evaluation by *frozen section.* This method, in which a sample is quick-frozen, sectioned, stained, and examined under the microscope, permits histologic evaluation within several minutes. In the vast majority of cases, frozen-section diagnosis has high accuracy and can be useful in distinguishing between benign and malignant tumors and identifying some nonneoplastic processes (e.g., infection).
- *Fine-needle aspiration* (FNA) is another widely used method for evaluating suspicious masses. Cells withdrawn by aspiration are spread out on a slide, stained, and examined. It is used most frequently to evaluate palpable lesions, but with image guidance can also be used to examine masses involving virtually any body site. FNA is less invasive than surgical biopsy, and in experienced hands provides a rapid, sensitive, and specific means to identify (or exclude) the presence of cancerous lesions.
- *Cytologic (Papanicolaou) preparations* from tissue scrapes, FNAs, or fluids provide another morphologic method for the detection of cancer. Initially developed to identify precancerous lesions of the cervix (Fig. 5.25), this technique is now used to evaluate suspected malignancy in many other sites; to identify tumor cells in abdominal, pleural, pericardial, and cerebrospinal fluids; and, less commonly, for evaluation of other forms of neoplasia.

Protein Markers

Identification of proteins or other molecules expressed by tumor cells has a broad role in establishing the diagnosis of specific cancer subtypes. Several complementary methods are used:

- *Immunohistochemistry* is a powerful adjunct to routine histology. Tissue sections are stained using a method that employs antibodies specific for proteins of interest. This method is useful in determining the cell of origin of poorly differentiated cancers and distinguishing among cancers with similar morphologic appearances. For example, detection of keratin in a poorly differentiated tumor establishes the diagnosis of carcinoma. It also can be used to demonstrate the presence of protein targets of therapeutic drugs and antibodies.
- *Flow cytometry* is used in the classification of leukemias and lymphomas. In this method, various combinations of fluorescent antibodies against cell surface molecules and differentiation antigens are bound to cells in suspension, which are then analyzed for staining to obtain the phenotype of malignant cells.
- *Circulating tumor markers.* Biochemical assays for tumor-associated enzymes, hormones, and other tumor markers are used with varying success as screening tests for certain cancers; however, they are most useful in assessing the response to therapy and in detecting early disease recurrence in patients with a known cancer diagnosis. Markers that are in current use are listed in Table 5.9.

Cytogenetic Markers

Many subtypes of cancer are highly associated with particular chromosomal aberrations; a few salient examples of such associations are given in Table 5.8, along with nucleic acid markers discussed later. Cytogenetic methods commonly used to identify chromosomal aberrations include:

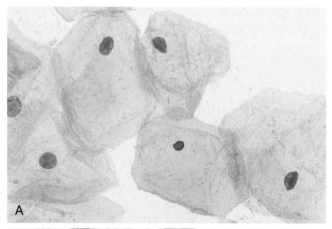

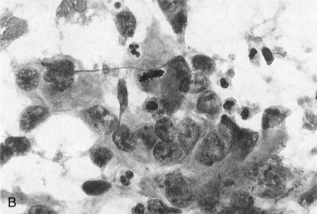

Fig. 5.25 Papanicolaou smears from the uterine cervix. (A) In normal smears, large, flat cells with small nuclei are typical. (B) Abnormal smear containing a sheet of malignant cells with large hyperchromatic nuclei. Nuclear pleomorphism is evident, and one cell is in mitosis. A few interspersed neutrophils, much smaller in size and with compact, lobate nuclei, are seen. (Courtesy of Dr. Richard M. DeMay, Department of Pathology, University of Chicago.)

- *Conventional karyotyping* of metaphase chromosomes is frequently used to support the diagnosis of hematopoietic cancers such as leukemias and lymphomas.
- *Fluorescence in situ hybridization (FISH)* is a method performed on fresh samples or paraffin-embedded sections in which fluorescently labeled nucleic acid probes bind with specific target regions of the genome. This technique can be used to subtype hematologic malignancies and to identify particular chromosomal aberrations in any tumor type.
- *Hybridization of tumor DNA to arrays of DNA probes* that span the genome permits the identification of small deletions and other changes in copy number that are below the resolution of karyotypic analysis. This method is used to diagnose and subtype certain kinds of brain tumors.

Nucleic Acid Markers

A number of techniques used to diagnose tumors and follow their response to therapy involve the identification of specific DNA and RNA sequences or fragments. Clinically relevant examples of such markers are listed in Table 5.8. Among the types of abnormalities for which testing is done most frequently are the following:

- *Chimeric nucleic acid sequences.* Chromosomal rearrangements often create fusion genes encoding chimeric mRNAs and proteins. These sequences are tumor-specific and can be detected even if

Table 5.8 Examples of Cytogenetic/Molecular Markers of Importance in Specific Cancers

Affected Gene/ Chromosomal Region	Event	Detection	Clinical Importance
Chromosomal Translocations/Fusion Genes			
ABL	Fusion with *BCR* gene through 9;22 translocation	Karyotype, FISH, RT-PCR	Diagnosis of chronic myeloid leukemia; target of therapy; marker used to follow therapeutic response and diagnose minimal residual disease
Gene Amplification			
NMYC	Gene amplification	FISH	Marker of poor prognosis in neuroblastoma
HER2	Gene amplification	FISH, IHC	Target of therapy in "HER2-positive" breast cancer
Chromosomal Deletion(s)			
1p	Segmental deletion	FISH, DNA array	Diagnosis of oligodendroglioma; marker of good prognosis
Point Substitution			
JAK2	Valine for phenylalanine substitution in codon 617	DNA sequencing	Diagnosis of polycythemia vera (a type of blood cancer)

Table 5.9 Circulating Tumor Markers

Marker	Tumor	Use
Prostate-specific antigen (PSA)	Prostatic carcinoma	Screening test (controversial); following response to therapy
Human chorionic gonadotropin (HCG)	Choriocarcinoma Some mixed germ cell tumors	Following response to therapy
Alphafetoprotein (AFP)	Germ cell tumors Hepatocellular carcinoma	Following response to therapy
Carcinoembryonic antigen (CEA)	Colonic carcinoma	Following response to therapy
CA-125	Ovarian carcinoma	Following response to therapy

present in very low abundance using sensitive polymerase chain reaction (PCR) methods. Many hematopoietic neoplasms, as well as a few solid tumors, are defined by the presence of particular fusion genes. In other instances, the products of fusion genes are targets of drugs and so are important to detect for purposes of selecting therapy. Finally, sensitive PCR-based tests for chimeric sequences can be used to detect small numbers of residual cancer cells in otherwise asymptomatic patients.

- *Single-nucleotide variants and small "indels."* As with chimeric gene products, single-nucleotide variants (point substitutions) and indels (small insertions and deletions) are specific for some cancer types and therefore diagnostically important, and in other cases generate oncoproteins that are drug targets and therefore are important to detect for purposes of guiding therapy.
- *Antigen-receptor gene rearrangements.* Because each T and B cell exhibits unique rearrangements of its antigen-receptor genes, PCR-based detection of T-cell receptor or immunoglobulin genes allows distinction between monoclonal (neoplastic) and polyclonal (reactive) proliferations of lymphocytes.

- *Molecular profiling of cancers.* Diverse technologies have been developed to analyze a single gene, sequence an entire genome, assess epigenetic modifications genome-wide, quantify all of the RNAs expressed in a cell population, measure many proteins simultaneously, and take a snapshot of all of the cell's metabolites. These advances have enabled the systematic sequencing and cataloging of alterations in various human cancers. The main impact has been in research; however, many centers are seeking to identify therapeutically "actionable" genetic lesions in a timely fashion at a reasonable cost. For example, most academic centers now routinely perform next generation sequencing on tumor specimens, usually with gene panels that cover commonly mutated protooncogenes and tumor suppressor genes. These new techniques complement information obtained from conventional histology and in situ biomarker tests performed on tissue sections. For the foreseeable future, the most accurate diagnosis and assessment of prognosis in cancer patients will be arrived at by a combination of morphologic and new molecular techniques.

6

Genetic Diseases

OUTLINE

Mendelian Disorders: Diseases Caused
  by Single-Gene Defects, 88
    Transmission Patterns of Single-Gene Disorders, 88
    Diseases Caused by Mutations in Genes Encoding Structural
      Proteins, 90
    Diseases Caused by Mutations in Genes Encoding Receptor
      Proteins or Channels, 90
    Diseases Caused by Mutations in Genes Encoding Enzyme
      Proteins, 93
Complex Multigenic Disorders, 96
Cytogenetic Disorders, 97
  Numerical Abnormalities, 97

Structural Abnormalities, 97
Cytogenetic Disorders Involving Autosomes, 98
Cytogenetic Disorders Involving Sex Chromosomes, 100
Single-Gene Disorders with Atypical Patterns of Inheritance, 101
  Trinucleotide Repeat Mutation Diseases, 101
  Diseases Caused by Mutations in Mitochondrial Genes, 102
  Diseases Caused by Alterations of Imprinted Regions:
    Prader-Willi and Angelman Syndromes, 102
Diagnosis of Genetic Disorders, 102
  Genetic Test Modalities and Applications, 102
  Indications for Genetic Analysis, 104

Genetic abnormalities that cause cellular dysfunction are one of the principal causes of disease. Some genetic diseases are inherited (familial) due to the presence of germline mutations, whereas others stem from acquired somatic mutations (e.g., cancer) and are not transmitted from one generation to the next. It is important to distinguish between congenital and genetic disorders. Congenital means "born with"; some genetic diseases are congenital (e.g., phenylketonuria), whereas others are manifest later in life (e.g., Huntington disease). Conversely, not all congenital diseases are genetic in origin (e.g., congenital syphilis). In this chapter, we discuss some of the more common or pathogenically interesting genetic diseases. We conclude the chapter by reviewing current technologies that are used to diagnose genetic disease.

MENDELIAN DISORDERS: DISEASES CAUSED BY SINGLE-GENE DEFECTS

Diseases caused by single-gene defects (mutations) follow one of three patterns of Mendelian inheritance: autosomal dominant, autosomal recessive, or X-linked.

Although rare individually (Table 6.1), taken together mendelian disorders account for approximately 1% of all adult hospital admissions and 6% to 8% of all pediatric hospital admissions. Most single-gene diseases follow simple patterns of inheritance, but genotype–phenotype associations are sometimes complex, reflecting the diverse functions of various affected gene products (Table 6.2). Several caveats must be kept in mind when considering mendelian disorders:
- *Phenotypic effects of specific single-gene mutations vary widely.* Some produce many phenotypic effects (*pleiotropy*) that may differ among individuals, a phenomenon called *variable expressivity.* In other instances, some persons with a disease-associated genotype are phenotypically normal; in this situation, the trait is said to have *low penetrance.* Why phenotypes fail to correlate with genotypes in such cases is not well understood. In some cases, it may be explained by coinheritance of variants in other genes that impact the phenotype; these are called *modifier genes.*
- *Mutations in different genes may cause similar or identical phenotypes.* This phenomenon, termed *genetic heterogeneity,* is often produced by mutations in genes belonging to the same metabolic or signaling pathways.

Transmission Patterns of Single-Gene Disorders
Autosomal Dominant Disorders
Autosomal dominant disorders affect both sexes and are manifested in the heterozygous state, so the inheritance of one abnormal allele (out of the two for autosomal genes) is sufficient to cause the disease.

When one parent is affected and the other is not, on average each child has a 50% chance of having the disease. The following additional features also pertain to autosomal dominant diseases:
- *Reduced penetrance and variable expressivity are common.* Not all individuals who inherit the defective gene develop the disease, or the same kind of disease, even within one family.
- *A 50% reduction in the normal gene product is sufficient to produce clinical signs and symptoms.* Because a 50% loss of enzyme activity usually can be compensated for, the genes that are affected in autosomal dominant disorders usually encode proteins other than enzymes, such as structural proteins, transport proteins, or proteins that function within higher-order complexes, which may be disrupted by the presence of a "bad component" that interferes with the formation of the functional multiprotein or multimeric assemblies. A protein that "poisons" the activity of its normal counterpart is called a *dominant negative.*
- *In many autosomal dominant conditions, the age at onset is delayed, with symptoms and signs first appearing in adulthood.*
- *Not all affected patients have affected parents.* Assuming the absence of nonpaternity, in such patients the disorder is usually attributable to new mutations involving the egg or the sperm from which they were derived. Their siblings are unaffected and not at risk.

Disorders of Autosomal Recessive Inheritance
Autosomal recessive diseases, which are the largest group of mendelian disorders, are caused by genetic defects that alter both alleles of a gene.

As a general rule, autosomal recessive disorders are characterized by the following:
- *The trait does not usually affect the parents, whereas each sibling has a 25% chance of being affected.*
- *If the mutant gene is rare in the population, there is a strong likelihood that the affected patient (the proband) is the product of a consanguineous marriage.*

Table 6.1 Prevalence of Selected Mendelian Disorders

Disorder	Estimated Prevalence
Autosomal Dominant Inheritance	
Familial hypercholesterolemia	1 in 500
Polycystic kidney disease	1 in 1000
Hereditary spherocytosis	1 in 5000 (Northern Europe)
Marfan syndrome	1 in 5000
Huntington disease	1 in 10,000
Autosomal Recessive Inheritance	
Sickle cell anemia	1 in 400 (U.S. African-Americans)
Cystic fibrosis	1 in 3200 (U.S. Caucasians)
Tay-Sachs disease	1 in 3500 (U.S. Ashkenazi Jewish; French Canadians)
Phenylketonuria	1 in 10,000
Mucopolysaccharidoses—all types	1 in 25,000
Glycogen storage diseases—all types	1 in 50,000
X-Linked Inheritance	
Duchenne muscular dystrophy	1 in 3500 males (U.S.)
Hemophilia	1 in 5000 males (U.S.)
G6PD[a] deficiency	1 in 10 males (U.S. African-Americans)

[a]Glucose-6-phosphate dehydrogenase.

- *Reduced penetrance and variable expressivity are less common than in autosomal dominant disorders.*
- *Onset is frequently early in life.*
- *Most autosomal recessive diseases are inherited from parents who are carriers of the mutant gene, or at least one may be affected.* Although new mutations for recessive disorders do occur, they rarely produce phenotypes because of the likelihood that the other allele will be normal.
- *Diseases resulting from enzyme deficiencies are usually autosomal recessive* because enzymes are normally present in large excess and only severe deficiencies, resulting from defects in both alleles, are sufficient to produce phenotypes.

X-Linked Disorders

Most X-linked disorders are X-linked recessive and therefore affect males much more frequently than females.

X-linked disorders are characterized by the following:
- *The disease is transmitted by asymptomatic heterozygous female carriers to male offspring,* who have only one X chromosome (a state referred to as *hemizygosity*). Sons of heterozygous women have one chance in two of receiving the mutant gene.
- *An affected male does not transmit the disorder to sons, but all daughters of affected males are carriers.*
- *Because males have only one "dose" of most X-linked genes, defects in X-linked genes are likely to produce disease in males.*
- *Heterozygous females rarely have the full-blown disease because they have a normal allele.* However, genotype–phenotype associations in females are complicated by the phenomenon of *X-inactivation (lyonization),* through which most of the genes on one of the two X chromosomes are silenced early in development. The X chromosome that is inactivated is "chosen" at random; hence, on average, half of cells express the mutated allele and half of cells express the normal allele. In most instances, this is sufficient to blunt or completely suppress the disease phenotype, but on occasion there is pronounced skewing toward silencing of the normal allele (unfavorable lyonization). Under such circumstances,

Table 6.2 Biochemical Basis and Inheritance Pattern of Selected Mendelian Disorders

Disease	Abnormal Protein	Protein Function
Autosomal Dominant Inheritance		
Familial hypercholesterolemia	Low-density lipoprotein receptor	Cholesterol transport
Marfan syndrome	Fibrillin	Extracellular matrix protein
Ehlers-Danlos syndrome[a]	Collagen	Extracellular matrix protein
Hereditary spherocytosis	Spectrin, ankyrin, or protein 4.1	Cell membrane stabilizer
Neurofibromatosis, type 1	Neurofibromin-1 (NF-1)	Regulator of RAS signaling
Adult polycystic kidney disease	Polycystin-1 (PKD-1)	Cell:cell, cell:matrix interactions
Autosomal Recessive Inheritance		
Cystic fibrosis (CF)	CF transmembrane regulator	Ion channel
Phenylketonuria	Phenylalanine hydroxylase	Enzyme
Tay-Sachs disease	Hexosaminidase	Enzyme
α- and β-Thalassemias	Hemoglobin	Oxygen transport
Sickle cell anemia	Hemoglobin	Oxygen transport
X-linked Recessive Inheritance		
Hemophilia A	Factor VIII	Coagulation factor
Duchenne muscular dystrophy	Dystrophin	Cell membrane stabilizer
Fragile X syndrome	FMRP	RNA translation regulator

[a]Some forms are autosomal recessive disorders.

females may exhibit features of the disease, though usually to a lesser degree than affected males.

Diseases Caused by Mutations in Genes Encoding Structural Proteins

Marfan Syndrome

Marfan syndrome, a connective tissue disorder of autosomal dominant inheritance, is caused by mutations affecting fibrillin-1.

Pathogenesis. Fibrillin-1 is encoded by the *FBN1* gene, which maps to chromosome 15q21. It is a glycoprotein secreted by fibroblasts that is the major component of microfibrils found in the extracellular matrix of many tissues. Microfibrils provide a scaffold that enables the proper assembly of elastic fibers and are particularly abundant in the aorta, the ligaments, and the ciliary zonules of the ocular lens, predictably the tissues that are most prominently affected in Marfan syndrome.

Many abnormalities in Marfan syndrome are attributable to a structural failure of connective tissues. However, others, such as bone overgrowth, appear to be related to excessive transforming growth factor-β (TGF-β) activity. Normal microfibrils sequester TGF-β, and loss of microfibrils therefore increases the bioavailability of this cytokine. Excessive TGF-β signaling has deleterious effects on vascular smooth muscle development and the integrity of the extracellular matrix. Of note, angiotensin receptor blockers, which lower blood pressure and inhibit the activity of TGF-β, improve aortic and cardiac function in mouse models of Marfan syndrome.

> *Morphology.* Abnormalities are most prominent in the skeleton, the eye, and the cardiovascular system, as follows:
> - *Skeletal abnormalities* are the most obvious feature of Marfan syndrome. Patients have a slender, elongated habitus; abnormally long legs, arms, and fingers *(arachnodactyly)*; a high-arched palate; and hyperextensible joints. Spinal deformities such as *kyphoscoliosis* may be present. The chest is deformed, exhibiting *pectus excavatum* (a deeply depressed sternum) or a pigeon-breast deformity.
> - *Bilateral dislocation (subluxation) of the lens* due to weakness of the suspensory ligaments *(ectopia lentis)* is the most characteristic ocular change. This abnormality is so specific that its presence is highly suggestive of a diagnosis of Marfan syndrome.
> - *Cardiovascular system abnormalities constitute a serious threat to life.* Fragmentation of the elastic fibers in the media of the aorta predisposes to aneurysmal dilation and aortic dissection (see Chapter 8). These changes, called *cystic medionecrosis*, also occur in hypertension and with aging. Loss of medial support causes dilation of the aortic valve ring, giving rise to aortic incompetence. The cardiac valves, especially the mitral valve, may be excessively distensible and regurgitant *(floppy valve syndrome)*, giving rise to mitral valve prolapse and congestive cardiac failure (see Chapter 8). Death from aortic rupture may occur at any age and is the most common cause of death. Less commonly, cardiac failure is the terminal event.

Clinical Features. The prevalence of Marfan syndrome is estimated to be 1 in 5000. Approximately 70% to 85% of cases are familial and the rest are sporadic, arising from de novo *FBN1* mutations in the germ cells of parents. Molecular diagnosis is not routine, because there are more than 600 distinct causative mutations in the large *FBN1* gene; most patients are diagnosed based on clinical features. The disease exhibits wide phenotypic variation that is believed to stem, at least in part, from differing effects of specific *FBN1* mutations.

Ehlers-Danlos Syndromes

Ehlers-Danlos syndromes (EDS) are a heterogeneous group of disorders caused by defects in collagen genes or genes that regulate collagen assembly.

Pathogenesis. EDSs are single-gene disorders that may have autosomal dominant or recessive modes of inheritance. At least six clinical and genetic variants are recognized.

The molecular bases of the more common variants are as follows:
- *Deficiency of the enzyme lysyl hydroxylase.* In this variant called the kyphoscoliosis type, decreased hydroxylation of lysine residues in types I and III collagen interferes with the covalent cross-linking of collagen molecules. As with other enzyme deficiencies, this disease is inherited as an autosomal recessive disorder.
- *Deficient synthesis of type III collagen.* This variant, the vascular type, is inherited as an autosomal dominant disorder and is characterized by weakness of tissues rich in type III collagen (e.g., blood vessels, bowel wall), predisposing them to rupture. The causative mutations often lead to the expression of a defective collagen III monomer that interferes with assembly of normal collagen, a classic example of a "dominant negative" mutant.
- *Deficient synthesis of type V collagen.* This variant is also inherited as an autosomal dominant disorder and results in classic EDS. More than 90% of affected patients carry mutations in the genes that encode type V collagen.

Clinical Features. Tissues rich in collagen, such as skin, ligaments, and joints, are involved in most variants of EDS. Because the abnormal collagen fibers lack adequate tensile strength, the skin is hyperextensible and joints are hypermobile. The skin also is fragile and vulnerable to trauma. Minor injuries produce gaping defects, and surgical repair or intervention is accomplished only with great difficulty because connective tissues lack normal tensile strength. The defect in connective tissue also may lead to other serious injuries in the absence of trauma, including rupture of the colon and large arteries; rupture of the cornea and retinal detachment; and diaphragmatic hernia.

Diseases Caused by Mutations in Genes Encoding Receptor Proteins or Channels

Familial Hypercholesterolemia

Familial hypercholesterolemia is caused most commonly by mutations in the gene that encodes the receptor for low-density lipoprotein (LDL) and is characterized by high serum cholesterol levels and early-onset atherosclerosis.

Pathogenesis. Familial hypercholesterolemia is an autosomal dominant disorder with a frequency of 1 in 500 in the general population, making it one of the most common mendelian disorders. Understanding its pathogenesis requires a working knowledge of normal cholesterol metabolism.

Cholesterol may be derived from the diet or from endogenous synthesis. Dietary cholesterol is incorporated in the intestinal mucosa into chylomicrons, which are delivered to the liver and taken up by hepatocytes. Some of this cholesterol enters the metabolic pool (see later), and some is excreted into the biliary tract as free cholesterol or bile acids. Cholesterol also is synthesized by hepatocytes and released into the circulation (Fig. 6.1). The first step in this process is the secretion of triglyceride-rich very-low-density lipoprotein (VLDL) into the blood. While in the circulation, the VLDL particle loses triglycerides through the action of lipases expressed by endothelial cells and is converted to intermediate-density lipoprotein (IDL) and low-density lipoprotein (LDL).

The LDL receptor pathway takes up two thirds of circulating LDL particles, as well as IDL particles, whereas the rest of the LDL particles are taken

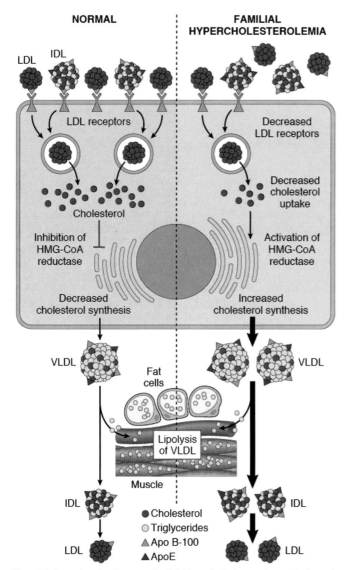

NORMAL

FAMILIAL HYPERCHOLESTEROLEMIA

Fig. 6.1 Low-density lipoprotein (LDL) and cholesterol metabolism in normal individuals and in familial hypercholesterolemia. In individuals with normal levels of LDL receptors *(left)*, receptor-mediated clearance of low-density lipoproteins (LDL) and intermediate-density lipoproteins (IDL) bearing Apo B-100 delivers cholesterol to hepatocytes, where its uptake inhibits HMG-CoA reductase, the rate-limiting step in cholesterol synthesis. Some hepatocyte cholesterol is packaged for export into very low-density lipoproteins (VLDL) bearing Apo B-100 and Apo E proteins. Lipolysis of VLDL by lipoprotein lipase in capillaries releases triglycerides, which are then stored in fat cells and used as a source of energy in skeletal muscle. Lipolysis converts VLDL into IDL and some LDL, completing the cycle. In individuals with familial hypercholesterolemia, a deficiency or dysfunction of LDL receptors leads to decreased LDL and IDL clearance and increased cholesterol synthesis, which together produce elevated levels of blood LDL (the "bad" form of cholesterol). Mutations affecting Apo B-100 prevent LDL and IDL binding to the LDL receptors, creating a functional deficiency of LDL receptors, thereby causing hypercholesterolemia.

up by a scavenger receptor for oxidized LDL. Although LDL receptors are widely distributed, approximately 75% are located on hepatocytes, so the liver has a central role in LDL metabolism. The pathway involves binding of LDL to the LDL receptor, endocytosis, and enzymatic degradation of the LDL particle within lysosomes, releasing the cholesterol load. The free cholesterol not only is used for membrane synthesis, but also controls cholesterol homeostasis through a sophisticated feedback control system that (1) suppresses cholesterol synthesis by inhibiting the activity of the enzyme 3-hydroxy-3-methylglutaryl–coenzyme A reductase (*HMG-CoA reductase*),

which is the rate-limiting enzyme in the synthetic pathway; (2) stimulates the formation of cholesterol esters, a storage form of cholesterol; and (3) inhibits the synthesis and down-regulates the number of LDL receptors on the cell surface, protecting cells from the excessive accumulation of cholesterol.

In most instances, familial hypercholesterolemia is caused by mutations in the LDL receptor protein that impair LDL metabolism, resulting in accumulation of LDL cholesterol in the plasma. Overall, LDL receptor mutations account for 90% of cases.

The paucity of LDL receptors on liver cells also impairs the transport of IDL into the liver, so a greater proportion of plasma IDL is converted into LDL. Patients with familial hypercholesterolemia thus have high serum levels of cholesterol as a result of both reduced catabolism and excessive biosynthesis. Hypercholesterolemia leads to an increase in cholesterol uptake into macrophages and vascular walls mediated by the LDL scavenger receptor, resulting in premature atherosclerosis and cholesterol-rich deposits in soft tissues called *xanthomas*. Most of the remaining cases of familial hypercholesterolemia are caused by mutations in the gene encoding Apo B-100 protein (6%–10% of cases) or mutations in *PCSK9* gene, which controls degradation of LDL receptor (2% of cases). Patients with these mutations are clinically indistinguishable from those with familial hypercholesterolemia caused by LDL receptor mutations.

Clinical Features. Heterozygotes with familial hypercholesterolemia caused by LDL receptor mutations have a two- to three-fold elevation of plasma cholesterol levels, whereas homozygotes may have in excess of a five-fold elevation. Although their cholesterol levels are elevated from birth, heterozygotes remain asymptomatic until adult life, when they develop cholesterol deposits (xanthomas) along tendon sheaths and premature atherosclerosis resulting in coronary artery disease. Homozygotes are more severely affected, developing cutaneous xanthomas in childhood and often dying of myocardial infarction before the age of 20 years.

Recognition of the critical role of LDL receptors in cholesterol homeostasis led to the design of the statin family of drugs that is now widely used to lower plasma cholesterol. They inhibit the activity of HMG-CoA reductase, increasing the level of LDL receptors on hepatocytes (see Fig. 6.1). Similarly, recognition that pathogenic *PCSK9* mutations cause increased PCSK9 function led to the development of PCSK9 inhibitors, which also are now approved for treatment of hypercholesterolemia.

Cystic Fibrosis

Cystic fibrosis is an autosomal recessive disorder of epithelial ion transport that leads to secretion of abnormally viscid mucus from exocrine glands and the linings of the respiratory, gastrointestinal, and reproductive tracts.

Pathogenesis. Cystic fibrosis (CF) is the most common life-shortening genetic disease in Caucasian populations, with an incidence of approximately 1 in 2500 births. It is caused by mutations in an epithelial ion channel protein encoded by the *CF transmembrane conductance regulator (CFTR)* gene located at chromosome 7q31.2. Phenotypes vary widely depending on the underlying causative mutations. The most common *CFTR* mutation is a deletion of three nucleotides coding for phenylalanine at amino acid position 508 (ΔF508) that causes misfolding of CFTR, leading to its degradation and loss of function. The small amount of the mutated ΔF508 protein that reaches the cell surface also is dysfunctional.

Mutations in *CFTR* render epithelial membranes relatively impermeable to chloride ions (Fig. 6.2); however, the consequences of this defect are tissue-specific. In sweat ducts, the major function of CFTR is to reabsorb luminal chloride ions and augment sodium reabsorption. Therefore, loss of CFTR function leads to decreased reabsorption of sodium chloride and production of hypertonic ("salty") sweat (see Fig. 6.2, *top*). In contrast to sweat glands, in respiratory and intestinal epithelium, CFTR is important for luminal secretion of chloride, and as a result of *CFTR* mutations reduce chloride secretion into the lumen

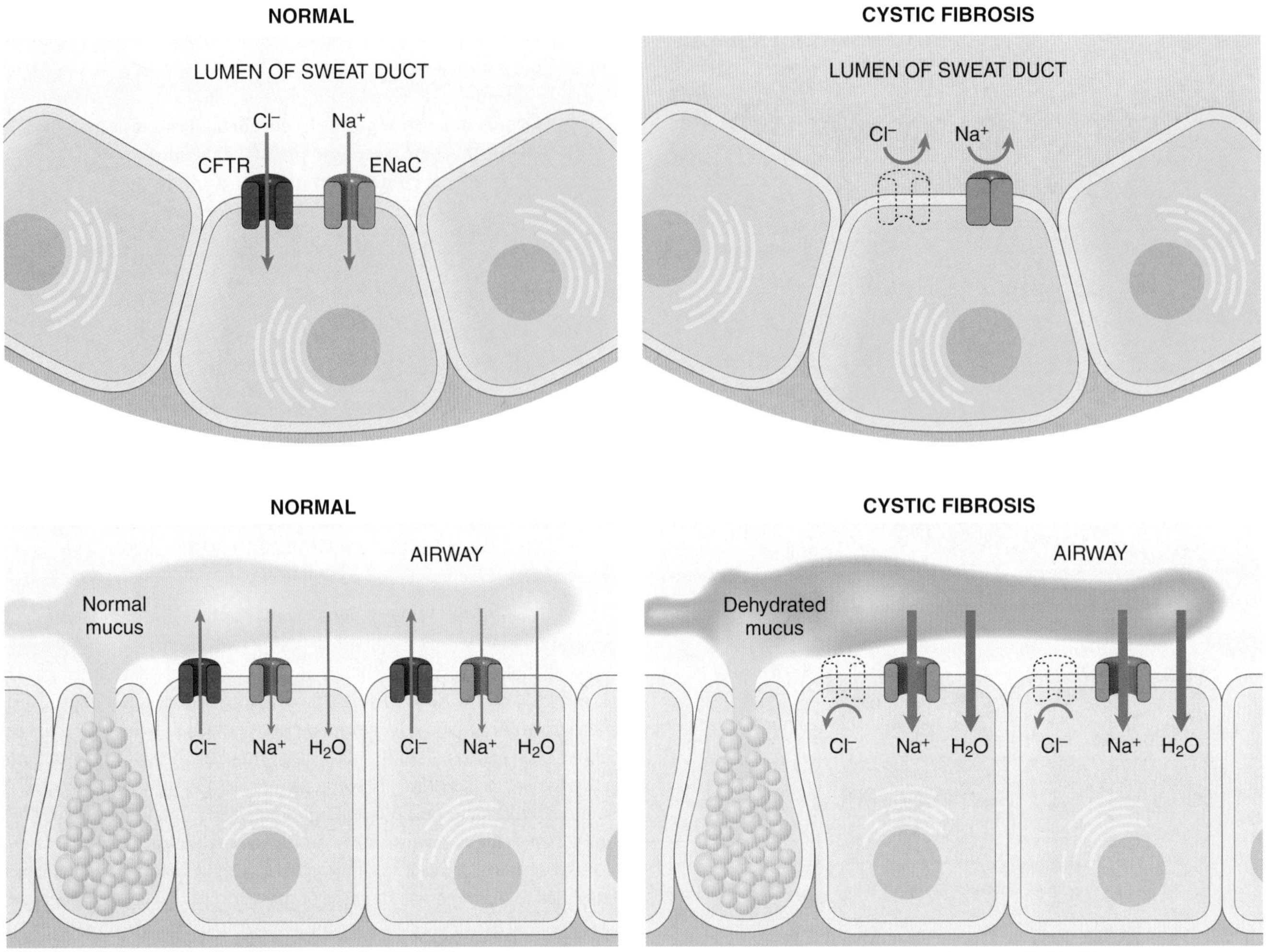

NORMAL

LUMEN OF SWEAT DUCT

CYSTIC FIBROSIS

LUMEN OF SWEAT DUCT

NORMAL

AIRWAY

CYSTIC FIBROSIS

AIRWAY

Fig. 6.2 Top, In cystic fibrosis (CF), a chloride channel defect in the sweat duct causes increased chloride and sodium concentration in sweat. **Bottom,** Patients with CF have decreased chloride secretion and increased sodium and water reabsorption in the airways, leading to dehydration of the mucous layer coating epithelial cells, defective mucociliary action, and mucous plugging. *CFTR,* Cystic fibrosis transmembrane conductance regulator; *ENaC,* epithelial sodium channel responsible for intracellular sodium conduction.

(see Fig. 6.2, *bottom*). This causes increased luminal sodium absorption through epithelial sodium channels. Increased intracellular sodium and chloride drives water reabsorption from the lumen, dehydrating the layer of mucus coating the underlying epithelial cells. In the lungs, this dehydration leads to defective mucociliary action and the accumulation of viscid secretions that obstruct air passages and predispose to recurrent pulmonary infections. Viscid secretions also may obstruct pancreatic ducts and the vas deferens, leading to pancreatic insufficiency and male infertility, respectively. In addition, CFTR regulates the transport of bicarbonate ions in the epithelial cells of the exocrine pancreas, and its dysfunction causes the acidification of pancreatic secretions. This results in precipitation of mucin and impairs the activity of digestive enzymes such as trypsin that function best under alkaline conditions, both of which exacerbate pancreatic insufficiency.

Morphology. Lesions vary in distribution and severity depending on genotype.
- *Pulmonary disease* stemming from obstruction and infection of the air passages is the most serious feature (Fig. 6.3). The bronchioles often are distended with thick mucus associated with marked hyperplasia and hypertrophy of the mucus-secreting cells. Superimposed infections give rise to severe

chronic bronchitis and bronchiectasis. Development of lung abscesses is common.
- *Pancreatic abnormalities* are present in 85% to 90% of patients. In severe cases, the pancreatic ducts are obstructed by mucous plugs, causing atrophy of the exocrine glands and progressive fibrosis (Fig. 6.4). The loss of pancreatic exocrine secretion impairs fat absorption, leading to vitamin A deficiency, which may contribute to squamous metaplasia of the pancreatic duct epithelium.
- *Meconium ileus,* a type of bowel obstruction, may occur in the small intestine of infants because of the presence of thick plugs of mucus.
- *Liver involvement* may lead to mucus plugging of bile canaliculi, accompanied by ductular proliferation and portal inflammation. Hepatic steatosis is common. Over time, cirrhosis may develop, resulting in diffuse hepatic nodularity. Such severe hepatic involvement is encountered in fewer than 10% of patients.
- *Azoospermia and infertility* are found in 95% of the affected males who survive to adulthood; bilateral *absence of the vas deferens* is a frequent finding.

Clinical Features. The clinical manifestations of CF are protean. Signs and symptoms vary from mild to severe, may present at birth or years

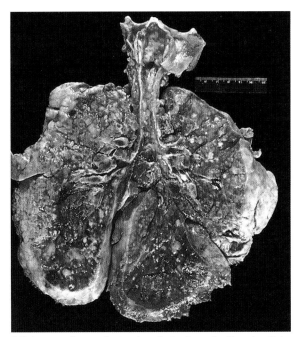

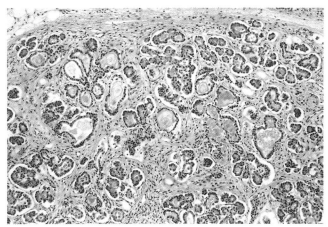

Fig. 6.4 Pathologic changes of cystic fibrosis in the pancreas. The ducts are dilated and plugged with eosinophilic mucin, and the parenchymal glands are atrophic and replaced by fibrous tissue.

Fig. 6.3 Lungs of a patient who died of cystic fibrosis. Extensive mucous plugging and dilation of the tracheobronchial tree are apparent. The pulmonary parenchyma is consolidated by a combination of both secretions and pneumonia; the *greenish* discoloration is the product of *Pseudomonas* infection. (Courtesy of Dr. Eduardo Yunis, Children's Hospital of Pittsburgh, PA.)

later, and may be related to the involvement of one organ or many. Approximately 5% to 10% of the cases come to attention at birth or soon after because of meconium ileus. Exocrine pancreatic insufficiency occurs in a majority (85% to 90%) of patients with CF and is associated with inheritance of two "severe" *CFTR* mutations (e.g., ΔF508/ΔF508), whereas patients carrying at least one "mild" *CFTR* mutation often retain pancreatic exocrine function. Pancreatic insufficiency is associated with malabsorption of protein and fat. The faulty fat absorption may induce deficiency states of the fat-soluble vitamins A, D, and K. Hypoproteinemia may be severe enough to cause generalized edema. Persistent diarrhea results in rectal prolapse in as many as 10% of children with CF.

The pancreas-sufficient phenotype usually is not associated with other gastrointestinal complications and, in general, these patients demonstrate excellent growth and development.

Cardiorespiratory complications, such as persistent lung infections, obstructive pulmonary disease, and cor pulmonale, are the most common cause of death (approximately 80% of fatalities in the United States). By 18 years of age, patients with severe CF often are colonized with pathogens such as *Pseudomonas aeruginosa* and *Burkholderia cepacia*. Significant liver disease occurs late in the course and is foreshadowed by pulmonary and pancreatic involvement; with improved survival, liver disease is now the third most common cause of death in patients with CF (after cardiopulmonary and transplant-related complications).

The diagnosis is usually suspected based on persistently elevated sweat electrolyte concentrations, characteristic clinical findings (pulmonary disease and gastrointestinal manifestations), and family history, and is established by sequencing the *CFTR* gene. The use of antibiotics and pancreatic enzyme replacement therapy, as well as bilateral lung transplantation, has improved outcomes in patients with severe CF. New drug therapies also are now available that improve the folding, membrane expression, and function of mutated CFTR molecules. These advances have extended the median life expectancy to 40 years, changing a lethal disease of childhood into a chronic disease of adults.

Diseases Caused by Mutations in Genes Encoding Enzyme Proteins

Phenylketonuria

Phenylketonuria is caused by mutations that disable the enzyme phenylalanine hydroxylase.

Pathogenesis. Phenylketonuria (PKU) is an inborn error of metabolism that affects 1 in 10,000 live-born Caucasian infants. The most common (classic) form is relatively common in persons of Scandinavian descent and uncommon in Jewish populations and in persons of African descent. This autosomal recessive disorder is caused by a severe deficiency of *phenylalanine hydroxylase* (PAH), which blocks the conversion of phenylalanine to tyrosine and leads to hyperphenylalaninemia. Affected infants are normal at birth but within a few weeks exhibit a rising plasma phenylalanine level, which impairs brain development. As phenylalanine levels rise, normally minor metabolic pathways become more active, yielding intermediates that are excreted in large amounts in the urine and in the sweat, imparting a strong musty or "mousy" odor to affected infants. Affected infants' pale coloration is due to the defective synthesis of tyrosine, which is required for melanin synthesis.

Clinical Features. If untreated, by 6 months of life PKU produces severe mental disability (intelligence quotient less than 60). About one third of these children never walk and two thirds cannot talk. Seizures, other neurologic abnormalities, decreased pigmentation of hair and skin, and eczema are also seen. These complications can be avoided by limiting phenylalanine intake early in life; therefore, infants are screened for PKU immediately after birth. Dietary treatment is discontinued after adulthood; however, women of childbearing age who have PKU must go on a low phenylalanine diet prior to conception because of the teratogenic effects of phenylalanine and its metabolites on the fetus.

Lysosomal Storage Diseases

Lysosomal storage diseases stem from mutations that lead to deficiencies of enzymes required for the degradation of various metabolites and certain organelles.

Pathogenesis. Lysosomes, the digestive system of cells, contain a number of hydrolytic enzymes that are involved in the breakdown of complex substrates into soluble end products. These substrates may be derived from intracellular organelles that are undergoing autophagy or may be taken up into the cell by phagocytosis. If an enzyme required for the catabolism of a substrate is missing, partially degraded insoluble metabolites accumulate within the lysosomes (Fig. 6.5). In addition,

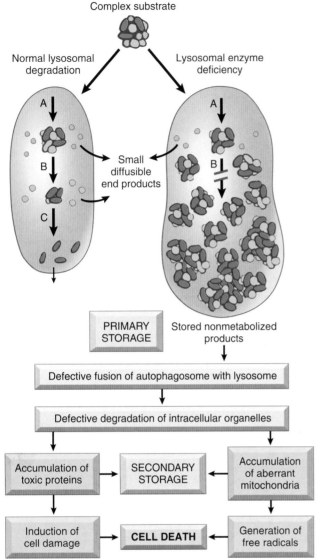

Fig. 6.5 Pathogenesis of lysosomal storage diseases. In this example, a complex substrate is normally degraded by a series of lysosomal enzymes (*A, B,* and *C*) into soluble end products. If there is a deficiency or malfunction of one of the enzymes (e.g., *B*), catabolism is incomplete, and insoluble intermediates accumulate in the lysosomes. In addition to this primary storage defect, secondary storage and toxic effects result from defective autophagy, leading to the accumulation of dysfunctional mitochondria and accumulation of toxic wastes.

lysosome dysfunction interferes with clearance of defective organelles such as mitochondria, which may generate destructive free radicals. This combination of defects ultimately leads to cell death.

Lysosomal storage disorders are subdivided based on the biochemical nature of the substrates and the accumulated metabolites (Table 6.3). Certain features are common to most diseases in this group:

- *Autosomal recessive transmission*
- *Onset of disease in infancy or early childhood*
- *Hepatosplenomegaly*, due to accumulation of partially digested metabolites in phagocytes
- *Frequent CNS involvement* with associated neuronal damage
- *Cellular dysfunction*, caused not only by accumulation of undigested material but also by a cascade of secondary events triggered, for example, by macrophage activation and release of cytokines

Most lysosome storage disorders are very rare; only a few of the more common conditions are considered here.

Tay-Sachs Disease (G_{M2} Gangliosidosis: Deficiency in Hexosaminidase A)

Tay-Sachs disease, the most common gangliosidosis, is caused by loss of function mutations affecting expression of the enzyme hexosaminidase A.

Pathogenesis. In Tay-Sachs disease, glycolipids called *gangliosides* accumulate in many tissues, but damage is mostly confined to neurons and glial cells throughout the CNS. The molecular basis for neuronal injury is not understood. In many cases the mutant protein misfolds, and this may induce the unfolded protein response (see Chapter 1), which can lead to apoptotic cell death.

Morphology. Affected cells appear swollen and sometimes foamy. Electron microscopy reveals whorled, onion skin–like layers of membranes within the lysosomes (Fig. 6.6). These changes are found throughout the CNS, peripheral nerves, and autonomic nervous system. The retina usually is involved, where the pallor produced by swollen ganglion cells in the peripheral retina results in a contrasting "cherry red" spot in the relatively unaffected central macula.

Clinical Features. In the most common variant of Tay-Sachs disease, infants appear normal at birth, but motor weakness begins at 3 to 6 months of age, followed by neurologic impairment, blindness, and progressively more severe neurologic dysfunctions. Death occurs within 2 or 3 years. Tay-Sachs disease, like other lipidoses, is most common among Ashkenazi Jews, among whom the frequency of heterozygous carriers is estimated to be 1 in 30.

Niemann-Pick Disease Types A and B

Type A and type B Niemann-Pick disease is caused by loss of function mutations that affect the enzyme acid sphingomyelinase.

Pathogenesis. The disease is caused by a deficiency of *sphingomyelinase*, more severe in type A than in type B, resulting in impaired breakdown of sphingomyelin into ceramide and phosphorylcholine.

Morphology. In type A, excess sphingomyelin accumulates in phagocytes and neurons. The macrophages become stuffed with droplets or particles of the complex lipid, imparting a fine vacuolation or foaminess to the cytoplasm (Supplemental eFig. 6.1). When

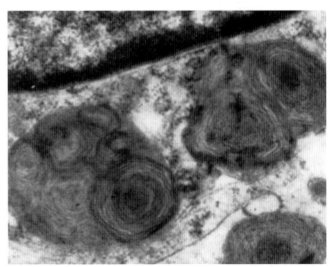

Fig. 6.6 Ganglion cells in Tay-Sachs disease. A portion of a neuron under the electron microscope shows prominent lysosomes with whorled configurations. Part of the nucleus is shown above. (Courtesy Dr. Joe Rutledge, Children's Regional Medical Center, Seattle.)

Table 6.3 Selected Lysosomal Storage Disorders

Disease	Deficient Enzyme or Protein	Accumulating Metabolite(s)	Clinical Features
Tay-Sachs disease	Hexosaminidase	GM2 ganglioside	CNS disease
Gaucher disease	Glucocerebrosidase	Glucocerebroside	Mild forms: organomegaly, bone marrow failure Severe forms: CNS disease
Niemann-Pick disease, types A and B	Sphingomyelinase	Sphingomyelin	Type A: early-onset CNS disease, organomegaly Type B: early-onset organomegaly, late-onset CNS disease
Niemann-Pick disease, type C	NPC1 or NPC2; part of a lipid transport complex	Cholesterol, gangliosides	Neurologic symptoms, including ataxia, dementia; variable organomegaly
MPS Type I (Hurler syndrome)	α-L-Iduronidase	Heparin and dermatan sulfate	Organomegaly, cardiovascular disease, CNS disease
MPS Type II (Hunter syndrome)	L-iduronate sulfatase	Heparin and dermatan sulfate	Similar to Hurler syndrome, but milder phenotype
Glycogenosis type 2, Pompe disease	Lysosomal glucosidase (acid maltase)	Glycogen	Cardiac failure

viewed by electron microscopy, the vacuoles are engorged secondary lysosomes that often contain membranous cytoplasmic bodies resembling concentric lamellated myelin figures. Because of their high content of phagocytes, the most severely affected organs are the spleen, liver, bone marrow, lymph nodes, and lungs. The splenic enlargement may be striking. Neurons throughout the CNS also accumulate sphingomyelin, which results in neuronal enlargement and vacuolization. Type B is associated with less severe sphingomyelinase deficiency and the manifestations are milder.

Clinical Features. Type A presents in infancy with massive organomegaly and severe neurologic deterioration. Death usually occurs within the first 3 years of life. In comparison, patients with the type B variant have organomegaly but no neurologic manifestations.

Niemann-Pick Disease Type C

Type C Niemann-Pick disease is caused by defects in lipid transport, leading to lipid accumulation in cells.

Niemann-Pick disease type C results from mutations in two related genes, *NPC1* and *NPC2*, which encode proteins that form a complex that is involved in intracellular trafficking of cholesterol and other lipids. Defective lipid transport results in the intracellular accumulation of cholesterol and gangliosides such as GM1 and GM2. Affected children exhibit ataxia, visual disturbances, dystonia, dysarthria, and psychomotor regression.

Gaucher Disease

Gaucher disease is caused by loss of function mutations in glucocerebrosidase that result in the accumulation of glucocerebrosides in phagocytes and more variable accumulations in neurons.

Pathogenesis. Gaucher disease is an autosomal recessive disorder with variable expressivity due to mutations of differing severity. *Glucocerebrosidase* normally cleaves a glucose residue from ceramide. Its deficit leads to an accumulation of glucocerebroside in macrophages, particularly in the spleen, liver, and bone marrow. This is because much of the glucocerebroside is derived from senescent red cells, which are normally removed from the circulation by macrophages in these tissues. The macrophages are activated while attempting to digest the glucocerebroside and release a number of cytokines. These are suspected of altering bone metabolism and may explain the association of Gaucher disease with variable degrees of osteopenia, osteoporosis, osteolytic lesions, and occasionally osteonecrosis.

Morphology. Phagocytes stuffed with glucocerebroside—so-called *Gaucher cells*—become markedly enlarged and acquire a pathognomonic cytoplasmic appearance characterized as "wrinkled tissue paper" (Fig. 6.7). Splenomegaly may be massive, and the marrow may be largely replaced by sheets of Gaucher cells.

Clinical Features. One variant, type 1, accounts for 99% of cases of Gaucher disease. It is associated with bone lesions, hepatosplenomegaly, and the absence of CNS involvement. Type 1 is most common in Ashkenazi Jews and is compatible with long life. Types 2 and 3 are characterized by neurologic signs and symptoms, which may appear during infancy (type 2) or later in life (type 3). Although the liver and spleen also are involved, the clinical features in types 2 and 3 are dominated by neurologic disturbances, including convulsions and progressive mental deterioration. Of interest, heterozygous carriers of Gaucher disease are at increased risk of Parkinson disease, for reasons that are uncertain.

Current therapy is aimed at reducing the burden of glucocerebrosides by infusion of recombinant glucocerebrosidase and with drugs that inhibit glucocerebroside synthase.

Mucopolysaccharidoses

Mucopolysaccharidoses are characterized by defective degradation and excessive accumulation of mucopolysaccharides in various tissues.

Pathogenesis. Mucopolysaccharides are synthesized by connective tissue fibroblasts and are part of the extracellular matrix. Turnover or remodeling of mucopolysaccharide is mediated by uptake into phagocytes and enzymatic degradation within lysosomes. If any of these enzymes are defective, mucopolysaccharides, mainly heparan sulfate and dermatan sulfate, accumulate within the lysosomes of phagocytes and other cells.

Clinical and Morphologic Features. Hepatosplenomegaly, skeletal deformities, subendothelial arterial deposits (particularly in the coronary arteries), and lesions in heart valves and in the brain are common to all of the mucopolysaccharidoses (MPSs). Coronary subendothelial lesions often lead to myocardial ischemia, and myocardial infarction and cardiac decompensation are important causes of death. Most cases are associated with coarse facial features, clouding of the cornea, joint stiffness, and mental disability. Urinary excretion of mucopolysaccharides often is increased.

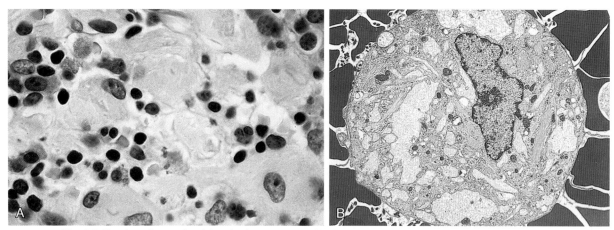

Fig. 6.7 Gaucher disease involving the bone marrow. (A) Gaucher cells with abundant lipid-laden granular cytoplasm. (B) Electron micrograph of Gaucher cells with elongated distended lysosomes. (Courtesy Dr. Matthew Fries, Department of Pathology, University of Texas Southwestern Medical Center, Dallas.)

Several clinical variants of MPS exist, each resulting from the deficiency of a different enzyme. Only two well-characterized syndromes merit brief discussion.

- *MPS type I,* also known as *Hurler syndrome,* is an autosomal recessive disorder caused by a deficiency of α-L-iduronidase. Affected children have a life expectancy of 6 to 10 years, and death is often due to cardiac complications. Mucopolysaccharides accumulate in macrophages, fibroblasts, endothelium and smooth muscle cells of the vascular wall, and other cells. The affected cells are swollen and have clear cytoplasm, resulting from the accumulation of engorged, vacuolated lysosomes. Accumulation in neurons accounts for the mental disability.

- *MPS type II,* or *Hunter syndrome,* differs from Hurler syndrome in its mode of inheritance (X-linked) and the absence of corneal clouding. It also often has a more prolonged, milder clinical course. Unlike Hurler syndrome, it results from a deficiency of L-iduronate sulfatase (a different enzyme than α-L-iduronidase). Despite the different enzyme deficiency, identical substrates accumulate because breakdown of heparan sulfate and dermatan sulfate requires the function of both enzymes.

Glycogen Storage Diseases (Glycogenoses)

The various glycogen storage diseases are caused by inherited deficiencies of enzymes involved in glycogen metabolism and result in excessive accumulation of glycogen or some abnormal form of glycogen in tissues.

Pathogenesis. In glycogen storage diseases, the specific enzyme deficiency dictates the type of glycogen that accumulates, its intracellular location, and its tissue distribution. Glycogen may accumulate within the cytoplasm and sometimes within the nuclei of affected cells. Most glycogenoses are inherited as autosomal recessive diseases.

Approximately a dozen glycogenoses have been described. On the basis of pathophysiologic findings, they fall into three groups (Table 6.4):

- *Hepatic type.* The liver synthesizes glycogen and also breaks it down into free glucose. Glycogenoses caused by defects in hepatic enzymes involved in glycogen metabolism have two major effects: liver enlargement due to accumulation of normal or abnormal forms of glycogen, and hypoglycemia due to a failure of glucose production (Fig. 6.8). *Von Gierke disease* (type I glycogenosis), resulting from a lack of glucose-6-phosphatase, is the most important hepatic form of glycogenosis.

- *Myopathic type.* Glycogen is an important energy source in striated muscle. Glycogen storage diseases caused by defects in enzymes that are required for glycogen breakdown lead to the accumulation of glycogen in muscles and muscle weakness due to impaired energy production. Myopathic forms of glycogen storage diseases are marked by muscle cramps after exercise, muscle injury leading to myoglobinuria, and failure of exercise to induce an elevation in blood lactate levels because of a block in glycolysis. *McArdle disease* (type V glycogenosis), resulting from a deficiency of muscle phosphorylase, is the prototype of myopathic glycogenoses.

- *Pompe disease* (type II glycogenosis) is caused by a deficiency of lysosomal glucosidase (acid maltase), which is required for glycogen breakdown throughout the body (Supplemental eFig. 6.2). However, the most affected cell type is the cardiac myocyte. Cardiomegaly is prominent, and most patients die within 2 years of disease onset owing to cardiorespiratory failure. Therapy with the missing enzyme can reverse cardiac muscle damage and increase longevity.

COMPLEX MULTIGENIC DISORDERS

Complex multigenic disorders are caused by interactions between multiple gene variants and environmental factors.

Genetic variants are referred to as polymorphisms if they have an allele frequency in the population of at least 1%. According to the common disease–common variant hypothesis, complex multigenic disorders occur when several polymorphisms, each with a modest effect and low penetrance, are coinherited. Many common diseases are thought to fall in this group, including autoimmune and allergic diseases, diabetes, hypertension, and ischemic heart disease, but it is often not possible to pinpoint a specific causative polymorphism. When considering complex multigenic disorders, several other principles should be kept in mind:

- Although complex disorders result from the collective inheritance of several polymorphisms, certain polymorphisms may have a dominant influence. For example, although variants in 20 to 30 genes are implicated in type 1 diabetes, a few HLA alleles contribute more than 50% of the risk.

- Some polymorphisms are associated with multiple diseases, usually of the same type (e.g., autoimmune disorders), whereas others are disease-specific.

- Many genetic variants linked to disease fall in the noncoding regulatory regions of the genome and thus are likely associated with a quantitative variation in gene expression, rather than a structural change in the encoded protein.

- Environmental factors play a significant role in the expression of complex multigenic disorders. Type 2 diabetes is an example of a

Table 6.4   Subgroups of Glycogenoses

Clinicopathologic Category	Specific Type	Enzyme Deficiency	Organs Affected
Hepatic	von Gierke disease (type I)	Glucose-6-phosphatase	Liver, kidney
Myopathic	McArdle syndrome (type V)	Muscle phosphorylase	Skeletal muscle
Miscellaneous	Pompe disease (type II)	Lysosomal glucosidase (acid maltase)	Cardiac and skeletal muscle, liver

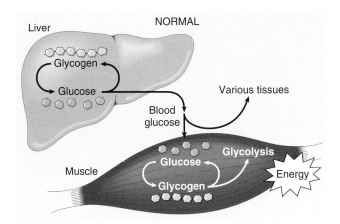

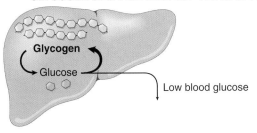

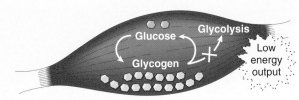

Fig. 6.8 Top, A simplified scheme of normal glycogen metabolism in the liver and skeletal muscles. **Middle,** The effects of an inherited deficiency of hepatic enzymes involved in glycogen metabolism. **Bottom,** The consequences of a genetic deficiency in the enzymes that metabolize glycogen in skeletal muscles.

complex multigenic disease that has important interactions with other factors, because affected persons often exhibit clinical manifestations of disease only after weight gain. In this instance, the genetic risk for diabetes is "unmasked" by obesity.

CYTOGENETIC DISORDERS

It is estimated that 50% of first-trimester spontaneous abortions are caused by chromosome abnormalities and that 1 in every 200 newborns has a chromosome aberration.

Cytogenetic disorders are defined by the presence of numerical or structural alterations of autosomes or sex chromosomes.

Numerical Abnormalities

In humans, the normal chromosome count is 46 (i.e., 2n = 46). Any exact multiple of the haploid number (n) is called *euploid.* Any

number that is not an exact multiple of n is called *aneuploid.* The chief cause of aneuploidy is nondisjunction of a homologous pair of chromosomes at the first meiotic division or a failure of sister chromatids to separate during the second meiotic division. The latter also may occur during mitosis in somatic cells, leading to the production of two aneuploid cells. Failure of pairing of homologous chromosomes followed by random assortment (anaphase lag) also can lead to aneuploidy. When nondisjunction occurs at the time of meiosis, the gametes formed have either an extra chromosome (n + 1) or one less chromosome (n − 1). Fertilization of such gametes by normal gametes may result in two types of zygotes, trisomic, with an extra chromosome (2n + 1), or monosomic (2n − 1). Monosomy involving an autosome is fatal during fetal development, whereas trisomies of certain autosomes and a monosomy involving sex chromosomes are compatible with life. *Mosaicism* is a term used to describe the presence of two or more populations of cells with different complements of chromosomes in the same individual. One type of mosaicism is caused by mitotic nondisjunction during early embryogenesis, resulting in the production of trisomic and monosomic daughter cells, whose descendants then produce a mosaic. Mosaicism affecting sex chromosomes is common, whereas autosomal mosaicism is not.

Structural Abnormalities

Structural changes in the chromosomes typically result from chromosomal breakage followed by loss or rearrangement of material. Such changes usually are designated using a cytogenetic shorthand in which p denotes the short arm of a chromosome and q the long arm. Each arm is then divided into numbered regions (1, 2, 3, and so on) from the centromere outward, and within each region the bands are numerically ordered.

The main types of structural chromosomal abnormalities (Fig. 6.9) are the following:
- *Translocation* implies transfer of a part of one chromosome to another chromosome. The process is usually reciprocal (i.e., fragments are exchanged between two chromosomes). In genetic shorthand, translocations are indicated by t followed by the involved chromosomes in numerical order, for example, 46,XX,t(2;5)(q31;p14). This notation indicates a reciprocal translocation involving the long arm (q) of chromosome 2 at region 3, band 1, and the short arm of chromosome 5, region 1, band 4. When the broken fragments are evenly exchanged, the resulting *balanced reciprocal translocation* is not harmful to the carrier, who has the normal number of chromosomes and the full complement of genetic material. However, during gametogenesis, abnormal (unbalanced) gametes are formed, resulting in abnormal zygotes. A special pattern of translocation involving two acrocentric chromosomes is called *centric fusion type,* or *robertsonian, translocation.* The breaks typically occur close to the centromere, affecting the short arms of both chromosomes. Transfer of the segments leads to one very large chromosome and one extremely small one. The short fragments are lost, and the affected individual has 45 chromosomes. Because the short arms of all acrocentric chromosomes carry highly redundant genes (e.g., ribosomal RNA genes), such loss is compatible with survival. However, difficulties again arise during gametogenesis,

resulting in the formation of unbalanced gametes that may lead to abnormal zygotes.

- *Isochromosomes* are formed when the centromere divides horizontally rather than vertically. One of the two arms of the chromosome is then lost, and the remaining arm is duplicated, resulting in a chromosome with only two short arms or two long arms. The most common isochromosome present in live births involves the long arm of the X chromosome and is designated i(Xq). When fertilization occurs by a gamete that contains a normal X chromosome, the result is monosomy for genes on Xp and trisomy for genes on Xq.
- *Deletion* involves loss of a portion of a chromosome. A single break may delete a terminal segment. Two interstitial breaks, with reunion of the proximal and distal segments, results in the removal of an internal segment. The removed fragment, which lacks a centromere, is almost never retained, and the genes encoded by this region are lost.
- *Inversions* occur when there are two interstitial breaks in a chromosome and the involved segment reunites after flipping around.
- A *ring chromosome* is a variant of a deletion. After loss of segments from each end of the chromosome, the arms unite to form a ring.

Cytogenetic Disorders Involving Autosomes

Three autosomal trisomies (13, 18, and 21; Fig. 6.10) and two deletion syndromes (*cri du chat syndrome,* caused by deletion of chromosome 5p, and *22q11 deletion syndrome*) are relatively common in live births and have characteristic clinical features. Only trisomy 21 and 22q11 deletion syndrome occur with sufficient frequency to merit brief consideration.

Trisomy 21 (Down Syndrome)

Down syndrome is the most common chromosome disorder and is most frequently caused by meiotic nondisjunction in the ova of older mothers.

Pathogenesis. Down syndrome has two major causes, trisomy 21 and robertsonian translocation.

- *About 95% of patients with Down syndrome have trisomy 21;* their parents have a normal karyotype. This form of Down syndrome is strongly linked to maternal age: Its incidence is 1 in 1550 live births in women younger than 20 years but rises to 1 in 25 live births in women older than 45 years. In 95% of cases, the extra chromosome is of maternal origin. The reason for the increased susceptibility of the aging ovum to nondisjunction is not understood.
- *About 4% of persons with Down syndrome carry a robertsonian translocation* that involves the long arm of chromosome 21 and chromosome 22 or chromosome 14. The translocated segment of chromosome 21 provides the extra chromosomal material. The parental carrier is phenotypically normal. Other siblings are at increased risk for having Down syndrome.
- *Rarely, persons with a Down syndrome phenotype are mosaic for trisomy 21.* These cases result from mitotic nondisjunction of chromosome 21 during an early stage of embryogenesis. Clinical manifestations are variable and milder, depending on the proportion of abnormal cells.

Although the chromosomal abnormality in Down syndrome has been known for many years, the pathogenesis of the disease remains elusive. Mouse models suggest a gain of a particular region on chromosome 21 bearing loci encoding multiple proteins and several microRNAs is responsible for the observed phenotype, but how these gene products give rise to the clinical features remain to be determined.

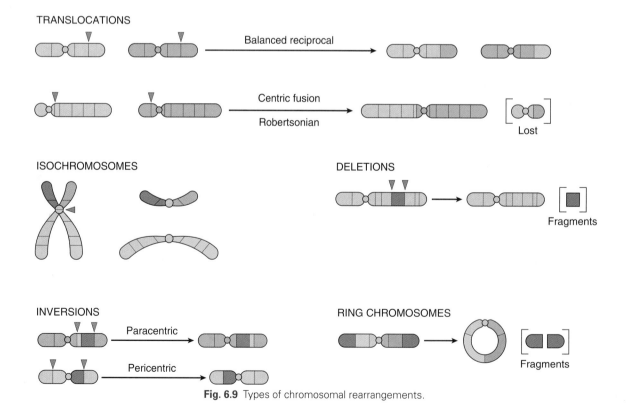

Fig. 6.9 Types of chromosomal rearrangements.

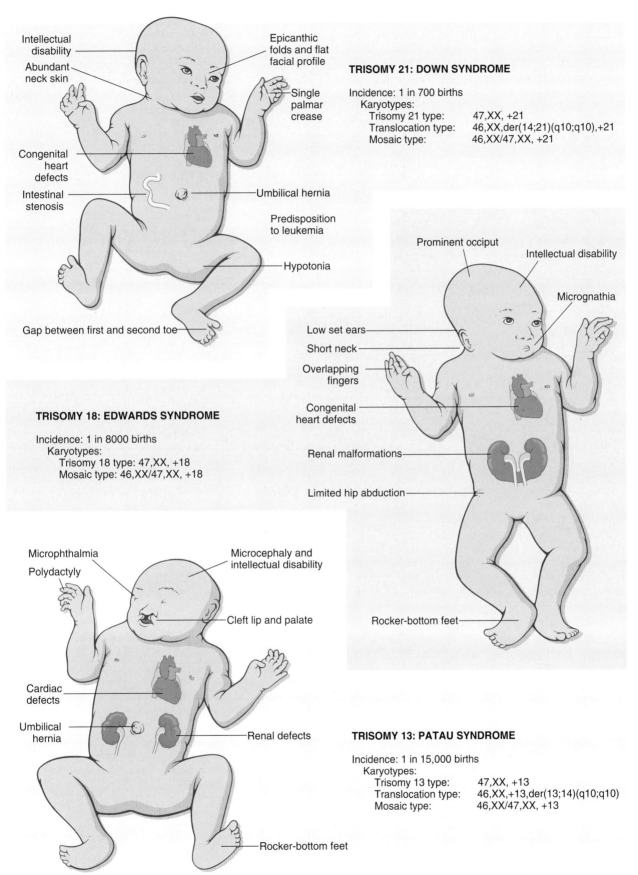

TRISOMY 21: DOWN SYNDROME

Incidence: 1 in 700 births
Karyotypes:
Trisomy 21 type: 47,XX, +21
Translocation type: 46,XX,der(14;21)(q10;q10),+21
Mosaic type: 46,XX/47,XX, +21

TRISOMY 18: EDWARDS SYNDROME

Incidence: 1 in 8000 births
Karyotypes:
Trisomy 18 type: 47,XX, +18
Mosaic type: 46,XX/47,XX, +18

TRISOMY 13: PATAU SYNDROME

Incidence: 1 in 15,000 births
Karyotypes:
Trisomy 13 type: 47,XX, +13
Translocation type: 46,XX,+13,der(13;14)(q10;q10)
Mosaic type: 46,XX/47,XX, +13

Fig. 6.10 Clinical features and karyotypes of the three most common autosomal trisomies: trisomy 21, Down syndrome; trisomy 18, Edwards syndrome; and trisomy 13, Patau syndrome.

Clinical Features. The facial appearance of the infant—flat facial profile, oblique palpebral fissures, and epicanthic folds (see Fig. 6.11)—is characteristic and immediately suggests the diagnosis. Severe intellectual disability is common; approximately 80% of those afflicted have an IQ of 25 to 50. Mosaics with Down syndrome have a milder phenotype and may have normal or near-normal intelligence. Down syndrome also carries a high risk of other developmental and acquired disorders:

- *Congenital heart disease* occurs in approximately 40% of patients, most commonly atrial septal defects, atrioventricular valve malformations, and ventricular septal defects (see Chapter 8). Cardiac problems are responsible for a majority of the deaths in infancy and early childhood. Atresias of the esophagus and small bowel also are common.
- *Childhood acute leukemia* (see Chapter 9) occurs at rates 10- to 20-fold higher than those in unaffected children.
- *Neuropathologic changes* characteristic of Alzheimer disease, a neurodegenerative disease (see Chapter 17), occur in virtually all patients older than age 40.
- *Abnormal immune function* that predisposes to infections, particularly of the lungs, and to thyroid autoimmunity, is common. The basis for this immunologic disturbance is unclear.

Improved medical care has increased the life span of persons with trisomy 21, and the current median age at death is around 50 years. The prenatal diagnosis of Down syndrome and other trisomies is possible using screening tests that rely on the analysis of cell-free fetal DNA found in maternal blood, imaging studies, and (most directly) karyotyping of cells obtained from the conceptus by amniocentesis or chorionic villus sampling.

22q11 Deletion Syndrome

22q11 deletion syndrome encompasses a spectrum of phenotypes that result from interstitial deletions of band 11 on the long arm of chromosome 22 (del22q11). These phenotypes include:

- *Congenital heart disease* affecting the outflow tracts
- *Abnormalities of the palate, facial dysmorphism, developmental delay*
- *Thymic hypoplasia and impaired T-cell immunity*
- *Parathyroid hypoplasia* resulting in hypocalcemia
- *Schizophrenia and bipolar disorder*

Variation in the size and position of the deletions is thought to be responsible for differing phenotypes. When T-cell immunodeficiency and hypocalcemia dominate, patients are said to have *DiGeorge syndrome,* whereas those with the so-called *velocardiofacial syndrome* have mild immunodeficiency and pronounced dysmorphology and cardiac defects. Patients also are at high risk for psychoses such as bipolar disorder and schizophrenia, which develops in up to 25% of cases. The pathogenesis of 22q11 deletion syndrome is not fully understood, because the deleted region encodes many genes. The diagnosis may be suspected on clinical grounds and is established by detection of the deletion by fluorescence in situ hybridization (FISH) (described later).

Cytogenetic Disorders Involving Sex Chromosomes

Numerical abnormalities involving the sex chromosomes, ranging from 45,X to 49,XXXXY, are compatible with life and observed in patients who often exhibit infertility and certain other abnormalities.

Phenotypically normal males with two and even three Y chromosomes have been identified. In contrast, numerical abnormalities of X chromosomes produce atypical phenotypes in both males and females, albeit ones that are mild compared with those observed with numerical abnormalities involving autosomal chromosomes. In large part, the lack of a phenotype related to abnormalities of sex chromosomes relates to two factors: (1) the small amount of genetic information carried by the Y chromosome (including the gene *SRY* that specifies male sex) and (2) X inactivation (lyonization), which tends to balance gene expression in males and females. X inactivation occurs early in fetal life, about 16 days after conception. During this process, either the paternal or the maternal X chromosome is randomly inactivated in each cell of the developing embryo and remains genetically silent in the progeny of these cells throughout life. Moreover, if extra X chromosomes are present (e.g., in 48,XXXX females), all but one is inactivated. As a result, females do not have an "extra dose" of most of the genes found on the X chromosome. Note that because of lyonization, normal females are mosaics composed of two cell populations, one with an active maternal X and the other with an active paternal X.

Phenotypic changes associated with loss of an X chromosome, as occurs in Turner syndrome, appear because several regions on the X chromosome escape inactivation. Thus, loss of one X chromosome results in monosomy of those genes that are active on both X chromosomes. The two disorders resulting from gains or losses of X chromosomes are Klinefelter syndrome and Turner syndrome, respectively.

Klinefelter Syndrome

Klinefelter syndrome is the most common cause of hypogonadism in males and results from the presence of at least one extra X chromosome.

Most patients with Klinefelter syndrome have a 47,XXY karyotype that stems from nondisjunction of sex chromosomes during meiosis. The extra X chromosome may be of either maternal or paternal origin. Approximately 15% of the patients are mosaics, such as 46,XY/47,XXY, 47,XXY/48,XXXY. The presence of a 46,XY line in mosaics usually is associated with a milder clinical condition.

The range of manifestations is wide, and they often include the following:

- *Hypogonadism, testicular atrophy, and infertility.* Sterility is due to impaired spermatogenesis. Histologic examination reveals hyalinization of tubules, which may lack spermatogonia entirely. Leydig cells are prominent, as a result of hyperplasia or an apparent increase related to loss of tubules. The diagnosis is often made during the evaluation of infertility.
- *Increase in length between the soles and the pubic bone,* which creates the appearance of an elongated body
- *Eunuchoid body habitus,* marked by reduced facial, body, and pubic hair and gynecomastia
- *Mental impairment.* The degree of intellectual impairment typically is mild, and in some cases, no deficit is detectable. The reduction in intelligence correlates with the number of extra X chromosomes.

Serum testosterone levels are lower than normal, and urinary gonadotropin levels are elevated. Patients are rarely fertile, and such persons may be mosaics with a large proportion of 46,XY cells. Klinefelter syndrome is associated with a higher frequency of several disorders, including breast cancer (20 times more common than in normal males), extragonadal germ cell tumors, and autoimmune diseases such as systemic lupus erythematosus.

Turner Syndrome

Turner syndrome, characterized by primary hypogonadism in females, results from partial or complete monosomy of the short arm of the X chromosome.

Pathogenesis. Normal oogenesis occurs before lyonization and requires both X chromosomes to be active. In Turner syndrome, fetal ovaries initially develop normally early in embryogenesis, but the absence of the second X chromosome leads to an accelerated loss of oocytes, which is complete by age 2 years. The ovaries are reduced to atrophic fibrous strands, devoid of ova and follicles *(streak ovaries).* Because Turner syndrome also causes nongonadal abnormalities, genes required for the growth and development of somatic tissues also must reside on the X chromosome. An example is the short stature homeobox gene *(SHOX)*. This is one of the genes that are active on both X chromosomes.

Clinical Features. The majority of patients have complete loss of one X chromosome and a 45,X karyotype. These patients are the most severely affected and are diagnosed at birth or early in childhood. Typical features associated with 45,X Turner syndrome are shown in Fig. 6.11 and include:

- *Growth retardation* and short stature (below the third percentile)
- Swelling of the nape of the neck due to distended lymphatic channels (in infancy) that is seen as *webbing of the neck* in older children
- *Low posterior hairline*
- *Cubitus valgus* (an increase in the carrying angle of the arms)
- *Shield-like chest* with widely spaced nipples
- *High-arched palate*
- *Lymphedema* of the hands and feet
- *Malformations* such as horseshoe kidney, bicuspid aortic valve, and coarctation of the aorta

Cardiovascular abnormalities are the most common cause of death in childhood. Because of ovarian atrophy, affected adolescent girls fail to develop secondary sex characteristics: the genitalia remain infantile, breast development is minimal, and little pubic hair appears. Most patients have primary amenorrhea. Hypothyroidism caused by autoantibodies occurs in as many as 50% of patients.

In a significant minority of patients, Turner syndrome is caused by mosaicism (in which the individual is made up of a mixture of 45,X and 46,XX cells) or by structural abnormalities of the X chromosome. The most common is deletion of the short arm, resulting in partial monosomy of the X chromosome. Combinations of deletions and mosaicism are reported and account for significant variations in the phenotype. Some patients with mosaicism or partial deletions have an almost normal appearance and may present only with primary amenorrhea. In adult patients, a combination of short stature and primary amenorrhea should prompt strong suspicion for Turner syndrome. The diagnosis is usually established by karyotyping.

SINGLE-GENE DISORDERS WITH ATYPICAL PATTERNS OF INHERITANCE

Three groups of genetic diseases resulting from single-gene mutations do not follow mendelian rules of inheritance:

- Diseases caused by trinucleotide repeat mutations
- Diseases caused by mutations in mitochondrial genes
- Diseases associated with alterations of imprinted regions of the genome

Trinucleotide Repeat Mutation Diseases

Trinucleotide repeat diseases are caused by mutations that amplify a DNA sequence consisting of three base pair (trinucleotide) repeats.

Pathogenesis. Fragile X syndrome, Huntington disease, and myotonic dystrophy, all associated with neurodegeneration, are among the more prominent examples of genetic diseases caused by trinucleotide repeat expansions. The expansions may involve the promoter, untranslated portions of the encoded mRNA (as in fragile X syndrome), or coding regions (as in Huntington disease, described in Chapter 16) of the affected gene. When mutations affect noncoding regions, RNA translation is suppressed and there is "loss of function." By contrast, mutations involving coding sequences of the gene often give rise to misfolded proteins that both interfere with the function of the protein and have a toxic "gain-of-function" activity. This property is conferred by mutations involving CAG repeats that encode polyglutamine tracts, which cause protein misfolding and aggregation within the cytoplasm, a common feature of diseases such as Huntington disease.

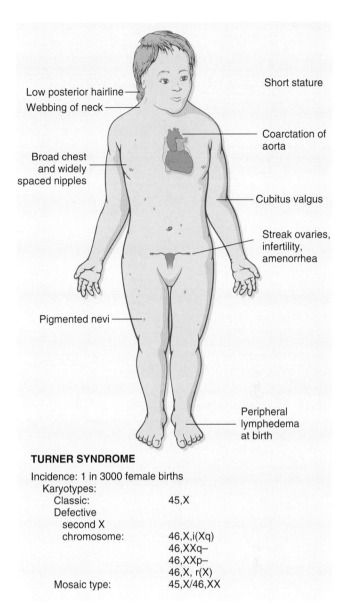

TURNER SYNDROME

Incidence: 1 in 3000 female births
Karyotypes:

Classic:	45,X
Defective second X chromosome:	46,X,i(Xq)
	46,XXq–
	46,XXp–
	46,X, r(X)
Mosaic type:	45,X/46,XX

Fig. 6.11 Clinical features and karyotypes of Turner syndrome.

A unique feature of diseases caused by trinucleotide repeat mutations is a phenomenon called *anticipation,* in which the disease becomes more severe with each successive generation. This unusual feature is related to the dynamic nature of trinucleotide repeat mutations. An example can be found in Huntington disease, in which expansion of a CAG repeat sequence within the Huntingtin gene *(HTT)* gene is responsible for the disease. Once these repeats reach a certain number, they are prone to further expansions during spermatogenesis, an alteration that results in disease that is more severe and occurs earlier in life in affected offspring compared to the disease in the parent. Since CAG repeats encode polyglutamine tracts in the affected proteins, CAG repeat diseases are often called **polyglutamine** diseases. For unclear reasons, in other trinucleotide repeat diseases, such as fragile X disease, triple mutation repeat instability is more pronounced in developing oocytes, and hence anticipation is seen when the abnormal alleles are passed down through the mother.

***Fragile X syndrome* is the prototypic trinucleotide repeat mutation disease. It is the second most common genetic cause of mental disability (after Down syndrome).**

It results from a triplet repeat mutation affecting the *FMR1* gene, which encodes the familial mental retardation protein (FMRP). As with all X-linked diseases, fragile X syndrome affects predominantly males. Affected males have a long face and large mandible. Large testicles are present in 90% of cases. In unaffected males, there are around 30 CGG repeats in the *FMR1* gene, whereas in affected males there are 200 to 4000 repeats. These "full" mutations arise from permutations with 52 to 200 repeats. The permutations are converted to full mutations by further amplification during oogenesis. FMRP regulates the translation of synaptic proteins, and its absence in affected males causes marked mental disability.

Diseases Caused by Mutations in Mitochondrial Genes

Mitochondria in the fertilized zygote are entirely derived from the ovum; thus, only mothers transmit mitochondrial genes and their defects to their offspring.

This unusual pattern of transmittance is referred to as *maternal inheritance*. Diseases caused by mutations in mitochondrial genes are rare. One class of mitochondrial genes that is mutated in mitochondrial disorders encode enzymes involved in oxidative phosphorylation, and as might be expected, the tissues that are most affected in these disorders are those that are most dependent on oxidative phosphorylation, that is, skeletal muscle, the heart, and the brain.

Diseases Caused by Alterations of Imprinted Regions: Prader-Willi and Angelman Syndromes

Certain genes are normally subject to differential "silencing" through epigenetic modifications in male and female gametes, and disturbances in this process (termed imprinting) can lead to abnormal gene expression and developmental abnormalities.

Pathogenesis. Although all humans inherit two copies of each autosomal gene, carried on homologous maternal and paternal chromosomes, the activities of the male and female alleles of some genes differ. These differences arise from an epigenetic process called genomic imprinting. Maternal imprinting refers to transcriptional silencing of the maternal allele in the ovum, whereas paternal imprinting refers to transcriptional silencing of the paternal allele in the sperm. Imprinting occurs in the ovum or sperm and is then stably transmitted to all somatic cells derived from the zygote.

Two uncommon genetic disorders are caused by defects involving an imprinted genomic region, Prader-Willi syndrome and Angelman syndrome (Fig. 6.12).

- *Prader-Willi syndrome* is characterized by intellectual disability, short stature, hypotonia, obesity, small hands and feet, and hypogonadism. Affected patients have deletions of band q12 in the long arm of chromosome 15 (15q12), and in all cases the deletion is found in the paternally derived chromosome 15.
- *Angelman syndrome* is associated with intellectual disability, as well as ataxic gait, seizures, and inappropriate laughter, a phenotype quite distinct from Prader-Willi syndrome. Affected patients also have deletions involving chromosome 15q12, but the deletion occurs in the maternally derived chromosome 15 rather than the paternally derived chromosome.

The molecular basis of these two syndromes is complex but can be understood in the context of imprinting. A set of genes on maternal chromosome 15q12 is imprinted (and hence silenced), such that all gene function depends on the paternal allele. If the paternal genes are deleted, gene function is completely lost and the patient develops Prader-Willi syndrome. A different gene that also maps to chromosome 15q12 is imprinted on the paternal chromosome, such that the function of this gene depends on the maternal allele. If this gene is deleted from the maternal allele, gene function again is completely lost

and the patient develops Angelman syndrome. The precise way that the affected genes contribute to these syndromes is not understood.

DIAGNOSIS OF GENETIC DISORDERS

Once a phenotype is recognized that suggests a particular genetic disorder, pedigree analysis may be used to further evaluate the possibility that a genetic disease is segregating within a family. The absence of other affected family members, however, does not exclude a genetic disorder, as many mutations arise *de novo*. An additional confounding factor is nonpaternity, estimated to involve 2% to 5% of births. Confirmation of a suspected genetic disorder relies on specific tests, which also have important roles in evaluating fetuses that are deemed to be at increased risk for genetic disorders.

The field of testing for genetic disorders is evolving at a rapidly accelerating pace. A brief review of current testing modalities and their use for the diagnosis of genetic disorders is offered below and is summarized in Table 6.5.

Genetic Test Modalities and Applications

Tests that are used to confirm the diagnosis of various genetic disorders are designed to identify the causative genetic abnormality or, in some instances, the effect of the abnormality on proteins encoded by mutated genes. These tests can be broadly divided into several categories:

1. *Tests that detect structural abnormalities of chromosomes.* Historically, these were identified solely by *karyotype analysis*, in which metaphase chromosomes prepared from cultured cells (usually peripheral blood lymphocytes) are stained with a dye that produces a unique pattern of alternating light and dark bands on each chromosome. Increasingly, karyotyping is being replaced by array-based *comparative genomic hybridization* (CGH), in which DNA from a patient and a normal control are labeled with two different fluorescent dyes. The DNAs are mixed and hybridized to an array of probes displayed as distinct spots on a slide that span the genome. Over- or underrepresentation of patient DNA corresponding to a particular genomic region is scored as a change in the ratio of fluorescent tag 1 to fluorescent tag 2. Array CGH has several advantages over karyotyping: It does not require cell culture, is easy to interpret, and also has much greater resolution, which is limited only by the number of discrete probes that are present in the array. *Fluorescence in situ hybridization* (FISH) is used to identify chromosomal abnormalities affecting specific genomic regions. Fluorescent probes containing DNA sequences of interest are applied to metaphase spreads or interphase nuclei. The probe hybridizes to its complementary sequence on the chromosome, which is then visualized with a fluorescence microscope. FISH can detect chromosomal gains, losses, or translocations of particular genomic regions (Fig. 6.13). Molecular tests also have been developed that use cell free fetal DNA found in maternal blood (a so-called *liquid biopsy*) to assess whole-chromosome numbers in the developing fetus. Current applications include identification of fetal sex and the detection of copy number changes in sex chromosomes and autosomes, including trisomies 13, 18, and 21.
2. *Tests that detect mutations in single genes.* If a mutation in a particular gene is suspected, that region can be amplified by *polymerase chain reaction* (PCR), sequenced, and compared with a normal reference sequence. It is becoming easier to sequence many genes, even the entire genome, by capturing DNA regions by hybridizing to a known set of nucleotide sequences and sequencing all of these. This method, called *next generation sequencing* (NGS), is becoming increasingly affordable and is being used widely, but interpretation of the results is complex and requires specially trained individuals.
3. *Tests that detect biochemical abnormalities associated with particular genotypes.* In many instances involving single-gene disorders, it is

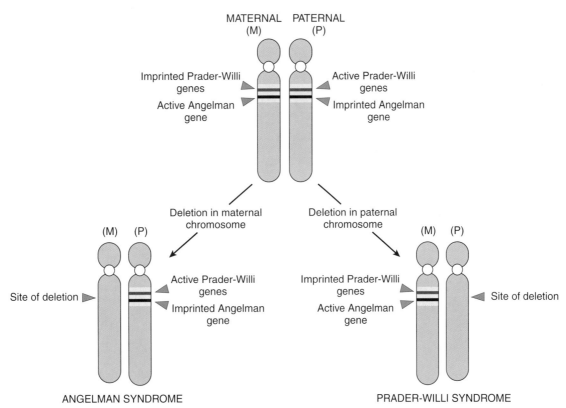

Fig. 6.12 Genetics of Angelman and Prader-Willi syndromes.

Table 6.5 Testing Modalities for Genetic Disorders

Test Type	Applications and Examples
Biochemical Assays	
Quantitative assays for metabolites or electrolytes	Detection of abnormal metabolite levels in metabolic disorders (e.g., phenylketonuria); detection of high sodium levels in sweat (cystic fibrosis)
Assay of enzyme activity	Detection of enzyme deficiencies (e.g., acid maltose in Pompe disease; G6PD deficiency)
Hemoglobin electrophoresis	Detection of abnormal hemoglobins (e.g., sickle hemoglobin)
Cytogenetic Assays	
Karyotyping	Grossly evident structural changes in chromosomes (e.g., trisomy 21 in Down syndrome)
Fluorescence in situ hybridization (FISH)	Subtle/submicroscopic structural changes in chromosomes (e.g., del(5) in cri du chat syndrome)
"Molecular" Cytogenetic Assays	
Multiplex ligation-dependent probe amplification	Small deletions and insertions (e.g., partial deletion of *BRCA1* in familial breast cancer)
Array-based genomic hybridization	Copy number changes (e.g., trisomy 21 in Down syndrome)
NextGeneration sequencing	Copy number changes, translocations (mainly used clinically to identify somatic copy number changes and translocations in cancer cells)
Genetic Assays	
Allele-specific PCR and related techniques	Specific base pair changes (single, e.g., sickle hemoglobin mutation, or multiple, e.g., *CFTR* mutations in cystic fibrosis)
Sanger DNA sequencing	Mutations in individual genes (e.g., glucose-6-phosphatase mutations in von Gierke disease)
NextGeneration sequencing	Mutations in many genes and/or in noncoding regions (used clinically to identify somatic mutations in cancer cells and in research to discover mutations responsible for unusual phenotypes)

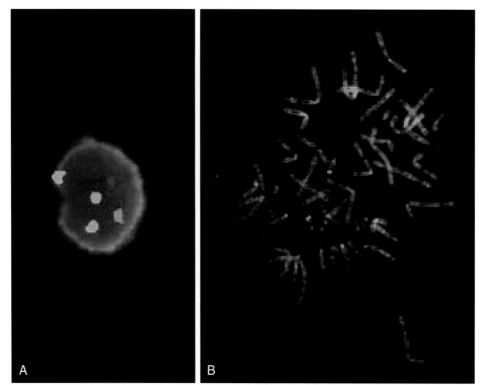

Fig. 6.13 Fluorescence in situ hybridization (FISH). (A) Interphase nucleus from a male patient with suspected trisomy 18. Three different fluorescent probes have been used: a green probe specific for the X chromosome centromere (one copy), a red probe specific for the Y chromosome centromere (one copy), and an aqua probe specific for the centromere of chromosome 18 (three copies). (B) A metaphase spread in which two fluorescent probes have been used, one hybridizing to chromosome region 22q13 *(green)* and the other hybridizing to chromosome region 22q11.2 *(red)*. There are two 22q13 signals. One of the two chromosomes does not stain with the probe for 22q11.2, indicating a microdeletion in this region. This abnormality gives rise to the deletion 22q11.2 syndrome. (Courtesy Dr. Nancy R. Schneider and Jeff Doolittle, Cytogenetics Laboratory, University of Texas Southwestern Medical Center, Dallas.)

easier, cheaper, or faster to test for alterations in mutated proteins or their functions than to identify the underlying DNA mutation directly. Examples abound and include sweat testing in cystic fibrosis; identification of high serum phenylalanine levels in phenylketonuria; identification of sickle hemoglobin in red cells in sickle cell disease; and identification of enzyme deficiencies in a wide variety of disorders.

Indications for Genetic Analysis

The preceding discussion described some of the techniques available for the diagnosis of genetic diseases. For judicious application of these methods, it is important to recognize which persons require genetic testing and the best technique for detection of the suspected genetic disorder. Genetic testing can be divided into prenatal and postnatal testing, each with its own set of indications.

Prenatal genetic analysis should be offered to all patients who are at risk of having cytogenetically abnormal progeny. It may be performed on cells obtained by amniocentesis, on chorionic villus biopsy material, or cell free fetal DNA obtained from maternal blood. Indications include the following:

- *Advanced maternal age* (beyond 34 years), which is associated with greater risk of trisomies
- *Confirmed carrier status* for a balanced reciprocal translocation, robertsonian translocation, or inversion
- *A chromosomal abnormality* affecting a previous child
- *Determination of fetal sex* when the patient or partner is a confirmed carrier of an X-linked genetic disorder

Postnatal genetic analysis usually is performed on peripheral blood lymphocytes because of ease of sampling. Indications are as follows:

- *Multiple congenital anomalies*
- *Unexplained intellectual disability* and/or developmental delay
- *Suspected aneuploidy* (e.g., features of Down syndrome)
- *Suspected unbalanced autosome* (e.g., Prader-Willi syndrome)
- *Suspected sex chromosome abnormality* (e.g., Turner syndrome)
- *Suspected fragile X syndrome*
- *Infertility* (to rule out a sex chromosome abnormality)
- *Multiple spontaneous abortions* (to rule out a balanced translocation in a parent)

7

Diseases of Blood Vessels

O U T L I N E

Mechanisms of Vascular Diseases, 105
Congenital Vascular Anomalies, 105
Hypertension, 106
Atherosclerosis, 107
Aneurysms and Dissections, 110
    Aortic Aneurysms, 110
    Aortic Dissections, 111
Vasculitis, 112
    Giant Cell (Temporal) Arteritis, 112
    Takayasu Arteritis, 113
    Polyarteritis Nodosa, 113

Kawasaki Disease, 114
Thromboangiitis Obliterans (Buerger Disease), 114
Small-Vessel Vasculitides, 114
Infectious Vasculitis, 114
Disorders of Veins, 114
    Varicose Veins, 114
    Thrombophlebitis, 115
Tumors of Blood Vessels and Lymphatics, 115
    Hemangiomas, 115
    Kaposi Sarcoma, 115
    Angiosarcomas, 116

Despite advances in medical and surgical interventions, vascular disease remains a leading cause of mortality in the United States. The largest toll is taken by complications related to atherosclerosis, mainly because it compromises blood flow and has serious deleterious effects on the heart, brain, and other vital organs. In addition, hypertension and venous thrombosis also are common causes of clinically significant disease. Although the following discussion separates diseases of vessels from diseases of the heart, the circulatory system and the heart function as a unit, and it should be recognized that primary defects in one component often have important impacts on another. These interactions will be highlighted throughout the following chapter and in Chapter 8.

MECHANISMS OF VASCULAR DISEASES

Common forms of vascular disease develop through two principal mechanisms:
- *Narrowing* or *complete obstruction of* vessel lumens, occurring either progressively (e.g., by atherosclerosis) or acutely (e.g., by thrombosis or embolism)
- *Weakening* of vessel walls, causing dilation and/or rupture
    Anatomically, the vasculature can be subdivided into high-pressure arterial vessels, which supply blood; capillary beds, where diffusion of gases (O_2 and CO_2) and solutes happens; and low-pressure venous vessels, which return blood to the heart. Arterial vessels have thick muscular walls rich in smooth muscle cells and play a key role in blood pressure regulation, whereas venous vessels have thinner walls and high blood volume capacity, owing to their distensibility. The luminal surface of all vessels is covered by a layer of endothelial cells, which under normal circumstances inhibits coagulation and inflammation and maintains fluid balances between the vasculature and the

interstitium (see Chapter 3). As we will discuss, disturbances of endothelial function are common in vascular disease. Also important are disturbances of blood flow, because a transition from normal laminar flow to stasis or to turbulent flow can alter endothelial function and set the stage for several types of vascular disease.

With this as a brief primer, we now turn to specific diseases of blood vessels.

CONGENITAL VASCULAR ANOMALIES

Anatomic variants of blood vessels are common but are largely of concern only to surgeons and interventional cardiologists, for whom they present clinical challenges. Several may cause disease, however, and deserve brief mention:
- *Berry aneurysms* are thin-walled arterial outpouchings in cerebral vessels, most commonly found at branch points around the circle of Willis; they may rupture spontaneously, causing fatal intracerebral hemorrhage (see Chapter 17).
- *Arteriovenous fistulas* are abnormal connections between arteries and veins without an intervening capillary bed. They may be developmental defects or may form after rupture of arterial aneurysms into adjacent veins, following injuries that pierce arteries and veins, or from inflammatory necrosis of adjacent vessels, as may occur with infections and other forms of vasculitis. Arteriovenous fistulas can cause high-output cardiac failure by shunting large volumes of blood from the arterial to the venous circulation.
- *Fibromuscular dysplasia* is a focal irregular thickening of the walls of medium- and large-sized muscular arteries. The wall thickening produces luminal stenosis or can be associated with abnormal vessel spasm that reduces vascular flow. In the renal arteries, it can lead to *renovascular hypertension*.

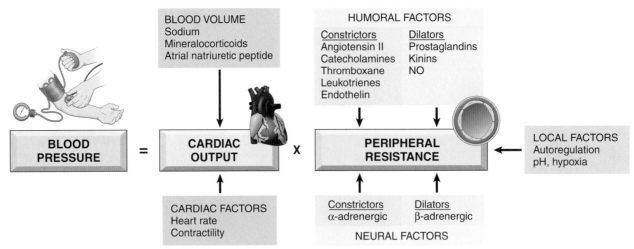

Fig. 7.1 Blood pressure regulation. *NO,* nitric oxide.

HYPERTENSION

Sustained high blood pressure (hypertension) causes vessel and end-organ damage and is a major risk factor for atherosclerosis.

Blood pressure must be maintained within a narrow range to ensure delivery of O_2 and nutrients to tissues and removal of CO_2 and metabolic wastes. Low pressure *(hypotension)* results in inadequate perfusion, organ dysfunction, and if severe and systemic, shock and sometimes death (see Chapter 3). Much more common is *hypertension,* an insidious but important cause of morbidity and mortality.

Pathogenesis. Resting blood pressure is a function of cardiac output and resistance to flow, which is dictated by the muscular tone of arterioles (Fig. 7.1). All of these factors are subject to regulation and counterregulation by hormones produced by the kidney and the heart (Fig. 7.2), as well as by neural inputs from the sympathetic nervous system, as follows:

- *Renin* is a hormone that is produced in the kidney by cells that sense renal perfusion. Decreased perfusion stimulates production of renin, a protease that cleaves circulating angiotensinogen to angiotensin I.
- The active form of *angiotensin* is a hormone with two important activities: (1) it increases vascular smooth muscle tone and resistance to flow and (2) it stimulates the release of *aldosterone* from the adrenal gland, leading to increased retention of sodium by the kidney and increased blood volume, which in turn enhances cardiac filling, stroke volume, and cardiac output. Both of these alterations raise blood pressure. The active form of angiotensin is created by successive cleavages of angiotensinogen by renin followed by angiotensin-converting enzyme, an important target of drugs used to treat hypertension.
- The heart contains cells that respond to increased stretch due to atrial dilation by releasing *atrial natriuretic hormone,* which increases renal excretion of sodium and water and thereby lowers blood volume and blood pressure.
- Superimposed on these hormonal regulators are inputs from the *sympathetic nervous system,* which act to increase vascular tone and cardiac output.

Hypertension is defined, somewhat arbitrarily, as a resting systolic pressure of 130 mm Hg or greater or a diastolic pressure of 80 mm Hg or greater. Both genetic and environmental factors (stress, obesity, smoking, physical inactivity, and high salt consumption)

have been implicated in the risk of developing hypertension, but in 95% of cases the specific cause is unknown (hence it is called *essential hypertension).* Most of the remaining cases of hypertension occur secondary to renal disease or hormone-secreting adrenal tumors (e.g., tumors secreting aldosterone, norepinephrine, or epinephrine). Rarely, hypertension is caused by mutations in individual genes that increase aldosterone production or reabsorption of sodium by the kidney, emphasizing the importance of these mechanisms of blood pressure control.

Morphology. Hypertension accelerates atherogenesis and causes degenerative changes in the walls of large- and medium-sized arteries that can lead to aortic dissection and cerebrovascular hemorrhage (described later and in Chapter 17). Arterioles can also be affected by these changes.

- *Hyaline arteriolosclerosis* is marked by thickening of the arteriolar walls by pink, amorphous, hyaline material and narrowing of vessel lumens (Fig. 7.3A). The thickening is caused by plasma proteins and lipids that leak across injured endothelial cells into vessel walls and by increased production of extracellular matrix proteins by smooth muscle cells.
- *Hyperplastic arteriolosclerosis* is more typical of severe hypertension. Vessels exhibit "onion skin," concentric, laminated thickening of arteriolar walls due to proliferation of smooth muscle cells and deposition of basement membrane material, leading to luminal narrowing (Fig. 7.3B). In very severe hypertension, fibrinoid necrosis of vessel walls may occur.

Clinical Features. Unless severe, hypertension may be asymptomatic for many years until cardiovascular complications (e.g., stroke, myocardial infarction, aortic aneurysm) develop. Less dramatic presentations include slowly progressive renal failure due to narrowing of renal arterioles. These complications can be prevented by medications that enhance renal sodium excretion or inhibit angiotensin production (e.g., angiotensin-converting enzyme inhibitors). Therefore, screening patients for hypertension is one of the most effective and important facets of preventive medicine. Severe hypertension (systolic pressures > 200 mm Hg) occurs less commonly and is associated with headache and altered sensorium. This variant, termed *malignant hypertension,* can lead to retinal hemorrhages, renal failure, cerebral edema, and death and is a medical emergency that requires immediate treatment.

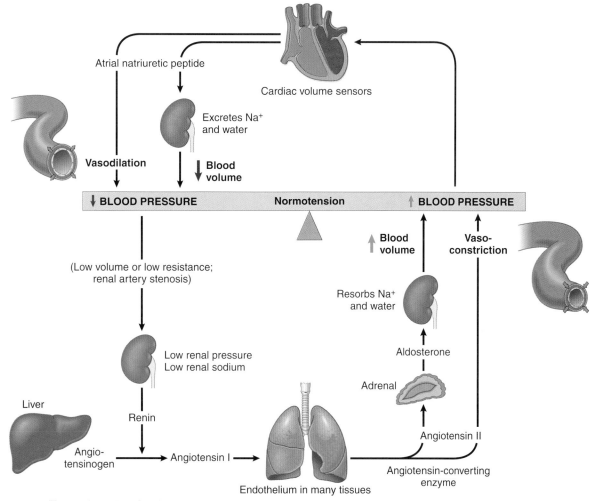

Fig. 7.2 Interplay of renin, angiotensin, aldosterone, and atrial natriuretic peptide in blood pressure regulation.

ATHEROSCLEROSIS

Atherosclerosis underlies the pathogenesis of coronary, cerebral, and peripheral vascular disease, and causes more morbidity and mortality in the western world than any other disorder.

Originally confined mainly to higher-income countries, atherosclerosis is increasingly prevalent in lower-income countries as Western diets and lifestyles spread. Lesions in the intima called *atheromas* or *atheromatous plaques* impinge on vessel lumens and restrict blood flow. More importantly, atheromatous plaques can bleed or fracture; the latter often provokes thrombosis, causing rapid occlusion of vessels and ischemia and infarction of downstream tissues. Inflammation secondary to atheromas can weaken vessel walls, leading to aneurysmal dilation and significant clinical consequences.

Pathogenesis. **Atherosclerosis appears to be the consequence of chronic, repetitive endothelial injury leading to inflammation and vessel wall damage**.

The events that culminate in formation of an atheroma play out over decades (Fig. 7.4) and are not entirely understood, but the following scenario is favored:

- *Endothelial injury* leads to increased vascular permeability and leukocyte adhesion, and alters endothelial gene expression, favoring inflammation and thrombosis.
- *Accumulation of lipoproteins and associated lipids* occurs in the vessel wall because of endothelial damage. The most important

of these are oxidized low-density lipoprotein (LDL) and cholesterol crystals. Since these are not normally present, they are recognized as foreign substances (so-called "danger signals") by cells such as macrophages, triggering an inflammatory response.

- *Vessel wall inflammation* results in the accumulation of inflammatory cells, including macrophages and T cells, which release cytokines that induce smooth muscle cell proliferation and the synthesis and deposition of extracellular matrix components such as collagen. This inflammation contributes to the initiation, progression, and complications of atherosclerotic lesions.

Hypercholesterolemia and hemodynamic factors (hypertension and turbulent blood flow) are believed to be the major initiators of endothelial damage. In general, all conditions associated with high LDL levels or other forms of dyslipidemia are also associated with an increased risk of clinically significant atherosclerosis. Risk factors are multiplicative. Factors associated with increased risk include the following:

- *Hypercholesterolemia.* The central role of cholesterol, and more specifically LDL, is highlighted by the accelerated atherosclerosis seen in *familial hypercholesterolemia* (see Chapter 6), which is characterized by elevated serum LDL levels due to inherited defects in the LDL receptor. LDL ("bad" cholesterol) delivers cholesterol to peripheral tissues including the vessel wall, whereas high-density lipoprotein (HDL) cholesterol ("good" cholesterol) mobilizes cholesterol from the periphery and transports it to the

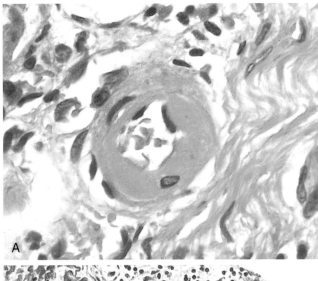

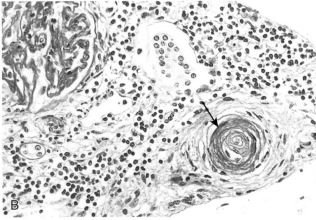

Fig. 7.3 Hypertensive vascular disease. (A) Hyaline arteriolosclerosis. The arteriolar wall is thickened with the deposition of amorphous proteinaceous material (hyalinized), and the lumen is markedly narrowed. (B) Hyperplastic arteriolosclerosis (onion-skinning) *(arrow)* causing luminal obliteration (periodic acid–Schiff stain). (B, Courtesy Helmut Rennke, MD, Brigham and Women's Hospital, Boston.)

liver for biliary excretion. Consequently, higher levels of HDL correlate with a reduced risk. Several other factors associated with an increased risk of atherosclerosis (diet, sedentary lifestyle, obesity, smoking, diabetes) lower HDL levels or elevate LDL levels. Statin drugs, which inhibit cholesterol synthesis and suppress LDL levels, also lower the risk of atherosclerosis-related cardiovascular disease.

- *Hemodynamic factors.* Atheromas tend to occur at sites of turbulent blood flow: the ostia of exiting vessels, at major arterial branch points, and along the posterior wall of the abdominal aorta. The role of hypertension in the development of atherosclerosis is presumably due to hemodynamic effects on endothelial function.
- *Genetics.* Family history is an important risk factor for atherosclerosis. Familial hypercholesterolemia, an autosomal dominant disease, and multigenic diseases such as hypertension and type 2 diabetes, also are associated with increased risk.
- *Age.* Symptoms from advanced lesions appear in middle age or later. The incidence of myocardial infarction increases five-fold between 40 and 60 years of age, and death rates from ischemic heart disease rise with each successive decade.

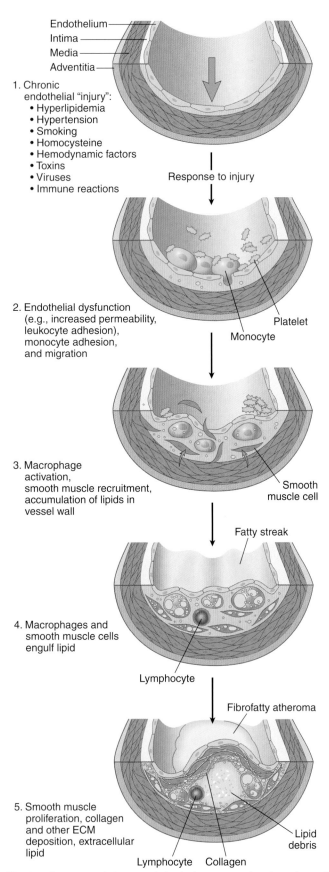

Endothelium
Intima
Media
Adventitia

1. Chronic endothelial "injury":
   • Hyperlipidemia
   • Hypertension
   • Smoking
   • Homocysteine
   • Hemodynamic factors
   • Toxins
   • Viruses
   • Immune reactions

Response to injury

2. Endothelial dysfunction (e.g., increased permeability, leukocyte adhesion), monocyte adhesion, and migration

Platelet
Monocyte

3. Macrophage activation, smooth muscle recruitment, accumulation of lipids in vessel wall

Smooth muscle cell

Fatty streak

4. Macrophages and smooth muscle cells engulf lipid

Lymphocyte

Fibrofatty atheroma

5. Smooth muscle proliferation, collagen and other ECM deposition, extracellular lipid

Lipid debris

Lymphocyte   Collagen

Fig. 7.4 Summary of the morphologic features and main pathogenic events of atherosclerosis.

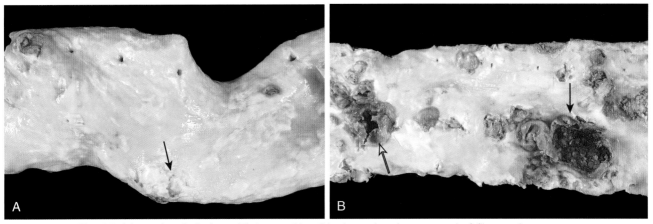

Fig. 7.5 Atherosclerotic lesions. (A) Aorta with mild atherosclerosis composed of fibrous plaques, one denoted by the *arrow*. (B) Aorta with severe, diffuse complicated lesions, including an ulcerated plaque *(open arrow)*, and a lesion with overlying thrombus *(closed arrow)*.

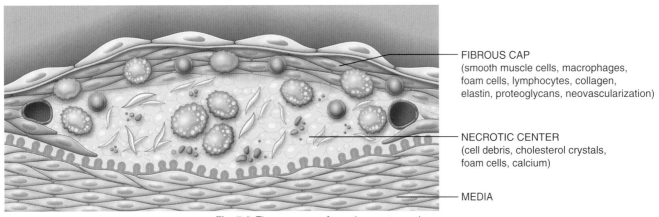

FIBROUS CAP
(smooth muscle cells, macrophages, foam cells, lymphocytes, collagen, elastin, proteoglycans, neovascularization)

NECROTIC CENTER
(cell debris, cholesterol crystals, foam cells, calcium)

MEDIA

Fig. 7.6 The structure of an atheromatous plaque.

- *Gender.* Premenopausal women are relatively protected against atherosclerosis compared with age-matched men, possibly because of the beneficial effects of estrogen and progesterone on lipid profiles.
- *Clonal hematopoiesis.* The peripheral blood cells of over 10% of adults over the age of 70 years with normal blood counts have clonal mutations in genes that are associated with various types of myeloid neoplasms, such as acute myeloid leukemia (see Chapter 9). Individuals with clonal hematopoiesis have a two-fold elevated risk of dying from cardiovascular disease, possibly because these mutations dysregulate the function of macrophages and thereby enhance local inflammation within atheromas.

Morphology. In descending order, atherosclerosis most often involves the infrarenal abdominal aorta, the coronary arteries, the popliteal arteries, the internal carotid arteries, and the vessels of the circle of Willis. Lesions at various stages of severity often coexist (Fig. 7.5). Atheromatous plaques are white to yellow raised lesions with soft lipid cores covered by fibrous caps containing smooth muscle cells and collagen, associated with macrophage and T-lymphocyte infiltrates and variable degrees of neoangiogenesis (Fig. 7.6 and Supplemental eFig. 7.1). Macrophages stuffed with lipid, so-called foam cells, may be prominent. Extracellular cholesterol is often present, frequently in the form of crystalline aggregates (cholesterol clefts). The media beneath the plaque may be attenuated and fibrotic, with smooth muscle atrophy. Plaques progressively enlarge through synthesis and degradation of the extracellular matrix (remodeling) and thrombus organization, and often undergo calcification, which can be seen radiographically.

Acute and chronic changes in atheromas can have serious consequences:
- *Rupture or ulceration* exposes thrombogenic substances, inducing thrombus formation (Fig. 7.7).
- *Hemorrhage,* caused by damage to fragile capillaries in the atheroma, leads to rapid plaque expansion or plaque rupture.
- *Embolism* of small fragments of atheroma during plaque rupture may cause ischemia in downstream organs.
- *Aneurysm formation* is caused by loss of elastic fibers and other supporting structures from the medial layer of the vessel wall.

Clinical Features. **Myocardial infarction (heart attack), cerebral infarction (stroke), aortic aneurysm, and peripheral vascular disease (gangrene of extremities) are the major clinical consequences of atherosclerosis.**

These complications may stem from slow progression of atherosclerotic lesions or from dramatic acute events, as follows:
- *Atherosclerotic stenosis.* Slowly advancing stenosis may present with symptoms of ischemia in tissues supplied by the affected vessels. The occlusion is described as a *critical stenosis* when it blocks 70% of the lumen, because at this point and beyond, the tissue demand often outpaces the blood supply. Presentations include *angina pectoris,* which typically appears with exertion and remits with rest; *chronic ischemic heart disease,* with symptoms related to heart failure; and *intermittent claudication,* due to leg ischemia with exertion.

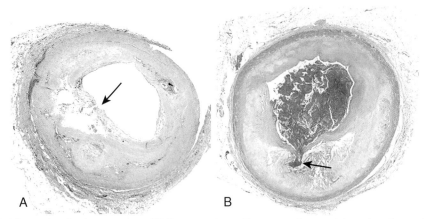

Fig. 7.7 Atherosclerotic plaque rupture. (A) Plaque rupture without superimposed thrombus, in a patient who died suddenly. (B) Acute coronary thrombosis superimposed on an atherosclerotic plaque with focal disruption of the fibrous cap, triggering fatal myocardial infarction. In both (A) and (B), an *arrow* points to the site of plaque rupture. (B, Reproduced from Schoen FJ: *Interventional and Surgical Cardiovascular Pathology: Clinical Correlations and Basic Principles,* Philadelphia, Saunders, 1989, p. 61.)

- *Acute plaque change.* Acute plaque changes, such as rupture, intraplaque hemorrhage, or weakening of the fibrous cap by proteases released from inflammatory cells, often have serious consequences. Superimposed thrombosis and rapid, complete occlusion may lead to myocardial infarction and stroke, medical emergencies that must be diagnosed rapidly and treated with anticoagulants (particularly antiplatelet drugs) and thrombolytic agents or endovascular stents. Other times, plaque ruptures lead to increased ischemia, particularly in the heart, without infarction, a change marked by increasingly severe "unstable" angina, which may strike even when the patient is at rest.

ANEURYSMS AND DISSECTIONS

Aneurysms and dissections are caused by congenital or acquired defects in the walls of blood vessels or the heart.

Aneurysms are outpouchings that involve all three layers of an artery (intima, media, and adventitia) or the attenuated wall of the heart, and may stem from inherited defects, hypertension, atherosclerosis, or transmural myocardial infarctions. Dissections occur when high-pressure arterial blood gains entry to the arterial wall through a surface defect and pushes apart the underlying layers. Aneurysms and dissections cause stasis and thrombosis and have a propensity to rupture—often with catastrophic results.

The most common and important vascular aneurysms and dissections involve the aorta and are described next.

Aortic Aneurysms

Aortic aneurysms most often occur in the abdomen and are prone to catastrophic ruptures, which often prove fatal.

Aneurysms in the thorax and abdomen have different risk factors: Thoracic aortic aneurysms are relatively uncommon and are associated with inherited defects in the extracellular matrix, as in Ehlers-Danlos syndrome, Marfan syndrome, and cardiovascular syphilis (see Chapter 6), whereas abdominal aortic aneurysms (AAAs) are much more common, particularly in males and in adults over the age of 60 years who smoke. Atherosclerosis and hypertension are important predisposing conditions. It is estimated that approximately 1,000,000 individuals in the United States have an AAA and that between 0.5% and 1% of these lesions will rupture each year. The discussion that follows is focused on AAAs.

Pathogenesis. The pressure wave produced during systole produces maximal wall stress and turbulence in the infrarenal aorta, the most common site of AAAs. These wall stresses are exacerbated by hypertension, which enhances the rate of expansion of AAAs once they form. There is a strong association with smoking that is not well understood, but it may be related to an elevated risk of hypertension and atherosclerosis, as well as the effects of toxins in tobacco smoke. Aneurysmal dilations often coincide with areas of atherosclerosis, which, as already discussed, can contribute to medial scarring. These factors, alone or in combination, may lead to loss of smooth muscle and extracellular matrix components, weakening the vessel wall and setting the stage for aneurysmal dilation.

Morphology. Abdominal aortic aneurysms typically occur between the renal arteries and the aortic bifurcation; they can be saccular or fusiform in shape and up to 15 cm in diameter and 25 cm in length (Fig. 7.8). In most cases, extensive atherosclerosis is present, with thinning and focal destruction of the underlying media. The aneurysm sac usually contains bland, laminated, poorly organized mural thrombus, which can fill much of the dilated segment.

Clinical Features. Most AAAs are asymptomatic until an acute complication develops. Physical examination may reveal a pulsating abdominal mass. They are diagnosed and sized by imaging studies, most often abdominal ultrasound. Acute complications of AAAs include the following:

- *Obstruction of a branching vessel* (e.g., the renal, iliac, vertebral, or mesenteric arteries) due to expansion, extension, and often superimposed thrombosis, resulting in distal ischemia of the kidneys, legs, spinal cord, or gastrointestinal tract
- *Embolism* from a ruptured atheroma or a mural thrombus
- *Impingement on adjacent structures* (e.g., compression of a ureter or erosion of vertebrae by the expanding aneurysm)
- *Rupture* into the peritoneal cavity or retroperitoneal tissues, leading to massive, often fatal hemorrhage

Women are less likely to have AAAs, but those that occur in women are more likely to rupture. The risk for rupture is determined by size: Aneurysms 5 cm in diameter or larger are considered high risk and require surgery. Timely intervention is critical: the mortality rate for elective procedures is approximately 5%, whereas the rate for emergency surgery after rupture is roughly 50%.

Aortic Dissections

Aortic dissection occurs when arterial blood penetrates the intima and splays apart the media to form a blood-filled channel within the aortic wall.

Aortic dissection may produce fatal hemorrhage if the blood ruptures through the adventitia and escapes into adjacent tissues.

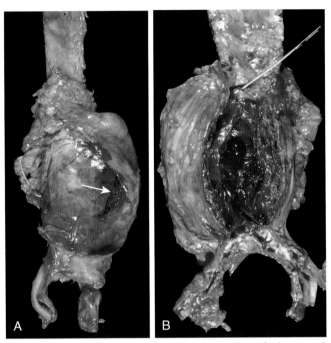

Fig. 7.8 Abdominal aortic aneurysm. (A) External view of a large aortic aneurysm that ruptured at the site is indicated by the *arrow*. (B) Opened view, with the location of the rupture tract indicated by a *probe*. The wall of the aneurysm is attenuated, and the lumen is filled by a large, layered thrombus.

Pathogenesis. Aortic dissection mainly occurs in two settings: (1) men 40 to 60 years of age with antecedent hypertension (>90% of cases) and (2) younger patients with genetic diseases of connective tissue, such as Marfan syndrome and Ehlers-Danlos syndrome (see Chapter 6). The aortas of aging hypertensive patients show medial hypertrophy of the vasa vasorum (the small vessels that supply the vessel wall); this may diminish perfusion of the media, leading to loss of smooth muscle cells and degenerative changes in the extracellular matrix. What initiates the intimal tearing is unknown, but once blood gains access to the vessel wall it tunnels through the media along the path of least resistance.

Morphology. The intimal tear marking the origin usually is found in the ascending aorta within 10 cm of the aortic valve (Fig. 7.9A). The dissection plane within the media can extend retrograde toward the heart or distally, occasionally as far as the iliac and femoral arteries (see Fig. 7.9B). External rupture causes massive hemorrhage, or results in cardiac tamponade if it occurs into the pericardial sac. In some instances, the dissecting blood reenters the lumen of the aorta through a second distal intimal tear, creating a vascular channel within the media *(double-barreled aorta)*. Histologically, *cystic medial degeneration,* characterized by loss of smooth muscle cells, elastic tissue fragmentation, and accumulation of abnormal proteoglycan-rich extracellular matrix, may be seen (Supplemental eFig. 7.2). In most instances, no specific defect is identified.

Clinical Features. Patients typically present with the sudden onset of excruciating tearing or stabbing pain, beginning in the anterior chest and radiating to the middle of the back. Retrograde dissection into the aortic root may disrupt aortic valve function, cause myocardial infarction by compressing the coronary arteries, or lead to massive hemorrhage into the pericardial space. Other complications are related to extension of the dissection to the great arteries of the neck or to the renal, mesenteric, iliac, or spinal arteries, any of which may become obstructed. Rapid diagnosis, antihypertensive

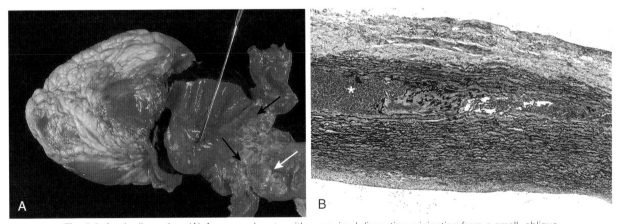

Fig. 7.9 Aortic dissection. (A) An opened aorta with a proximal dissection originating from a small, oblique intimal tear *(identified by the probe)* associated with an intramural hematoma. Note that the intimal tear occurred in a region largely free of atherosclerotic plaque. The distal edge of the intramural hematoma *(black arrows)* lies at the edge of a large area of atherosclerosis *(white arrow),* which arrested the propagation of the dissection. (B) Histologic preparation showing the dissection and intramural hematoma *(asterisk).* Aortic elastic layers are *black,* and blood is *red* in this section, stained with Movat stain.

therapy, and surgical repair of the aortic intimal tear can save 65% to 85% of the patients with dissection involving the aortic arch. Dissections that do not involve the aortic arch can be repaired surgically or managed conservatively with antihypertensive drugs and have somewhat better outcomes.

VASCULITIS

Vasculitis encompasses a group of disorders with highly varied pathophysiology and clinical features that are defined by the presence of vessel wall inflammation.

Clinical manifestations depend on the specific vascular bed that is affected and sometimes include signs and symptoms of systemic inflammation. Many forms of vasculitis are recognized, some with overlapping features. Etiology is diverse and includes immune-mediated inflammation, infections, drugs and chemicals, radiation exposure, and trauma. It is critical to distinguish infectious from immune-mediated forms because immunosuppressive therapy is appropriate for the latter but could exacerbate infectious vasculitis. We will restrict our discussion to forms of vasculitis that are most common or of greatest pathogenic interest, starting with those that primarily affect large vessels.

Giant Cell (Temporal) Arteritis

Giant cell (temporal) arteritis is a chronic granulomatous disorder that principally affects large-sized arteries in the head.

The temporal, vertebral, and ophthalmic arteries and the aorta can be involved. Ophthalmic artery involvement can cause sudden and permanent blindness; therefore, prompt diagnosis and treatment are essential.

Pathogenesis. The characteristic granulomatous inflammation, an association with certain HLA class II haplotypes, and the excellent therapeutic response to steroids all support an immune etiology. Giant cell arteritis likely occurs as a result of a chronic Th1 cell–mediated immune response, presumably to antigens present in the vessel wall. The identity of these antigens and the basis for the predilection for vessels of the head are unknown.

Morphology. Granulomatous inflammation occurs in a patchy distribution along the length of affected vessels. Involved arterial segments exhibit nodular intimal thickening (and occasional thromboses) that impinge on the lumen and cause distal ischemia. Fully developed lesions consist of nonnecrotizing granulomas with multinucleated giant cells centered on the internal elastic membrane, which is often fragmented (Fig. 7.10). Healing of the injury is associated with intimal thickening, thinning and scarring of the media, and adventitial fibrosis.

Clinical Features. Giant cell arteritis is the most common form of vasculitis among older adults in higher-income countries. It is rare before 50 years of age. Signs and symptoms may reflect systemic inflammation (fever, malaise, weight loss) or take the form of facial pain or headache, most intense along the temporal artery, which is painful to palpation. Ocular symptoms appear abruptly in about 50% of patients and range from diplopia to complete vision loss. Diagnosis requires biopsy, typically of the temporal artery; however, because the arteritis is patchy, a negative biopsy result does not exclude the diagnosis. Corticosteroid or anti–tumor necrosis factor (TNF) therapies are effective treatments.

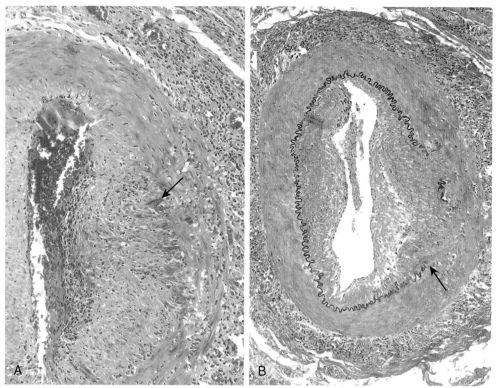

Fig. 7.10 Giant cell arteritis. (A) Hematoxylin-and-eosin (H&E)–stained section of a temporal artery showing giant cells near the fragmented internal elastic membrane *(arrow)*, along with medial and adventitial inflammation. (B) Elastic tissue staining demonstrating focal destruction of the internal elastic membrane *(arrow)* and associated medial attenuation and scarring.

Takayasu Arteritis

Takayasu arteritis is a granulomatous vasculitis of large-sized arteries characterized by ocular disturbances and weakened pulses in the upper extremities.

Takayasu arteritis manifests with transmural scarring and thickening of the aorta—particularly the aortic arch and great vessels—and luminal narrowing of the major branch vessels. Its features overlap with those of giant cell arteritis the distinction between the two entities is made largely on the basis of a patient's age, with those younger than 50 years of age being designated as having Takayasu arteritis. Like giant cell arteritis, Takayasu arteritis appears to be caused by a chronic granulomatous T-cell–mediated immune response to an unknown vessel antigen.

Morphology. The aorta, the aortic arch, and its branches, as well as the pulmonary, renal, and coronary arteries, may be affected. The takeoffs of the great vessels may be narrowed or obliterated (Fig. 7.11), leading to upper extremity weakness and faint carotid pulses. Inflammatory infiltrates in vessel walls range from nonspecific accumulations of T cells and macrophages to granulomatous inflammation, both of which may be associated with wall thickening and fibrosis.

Clinical Features. Involvement of the aortic arch and major branches produces reduced upper-extremity blood pressure and pulse strength, neurologic deficits, visual field defects, and blindness. Symptoms related to involvement of the distal aorta (leg claudication), the pulmonary artery (pulmonary hypertension), the heart (myocardial infarction), and the renal arteries (systemic hypertension) also may appear. The disease has a variable course. Some cases rapidly progress, but others become quiescent after 1 to 2 years and are compatible with long-term survival, albeit with visual or neurologic deficits.

Polyarteritis Nodosa

Polyarteritis nodosa is a systemic vasculitis of medium-sized muscular arteries that commonly involves renal and visceral vessels and usually spares the lung.

Pathogenesis. The cause of polyarteritis nodosa is unknown, but the disease responds well to immunosuppressive agents and therefore is believed to have an immunologic basis. One third of patients have chronic hepatitis B infection and may have circulating immune complexes composed of viral antigens and specific antibodies, which deposit in vessel walls and provoke an inflammatory response. Why immune complexes localize in medium-sized arteries and not in other vessels is unknown.

Morphology. Vessels of the kidney, heart, liver, and gastrointestinal tract vessels are affected in descending order of frequency. Fully developed lesions are composed of segmental transmural necrotizing inflammation of medium-sized or, occasionally, small arteries, often with superimposed thrombosis. Acute lesions have fibrinoid necrosis of the vessel wall and infiltrating neutrophils (Fig. 7.12), whereas older lesions are fibrotic and associated with chronic inflammation. Acute and chronic lesions coexist, suggesting ongoing recurrent inflammatory damage. The vascular injury may impair the perfusion of downstream tissues, leading to ulcerations, infarcts, and ischemic atrophy, or may provoke aneurysm formation and the attendant risk of hemorrhage.

Clinical Features. Polyarteritis nodosa is more common in young adults but can occur at any age. The clinical course typically is episodic, with long symptom-free intervals. Initial symptoms—malaise, fever, and weight loss—are related to inflammation and are nonspecific, and the vascular involvement is varied and may be widely distributed, leading to puzzling, protean manifestations such as hypertension due to renal artery involvement and abdominal pain and bloody stools caused by gastrointestinal lesions; diffuse muscular aches and pains; and peripheral neuritis, predominantly affecting motor nerves. Renal involvement is a major cause of death. Untreated, polyarteritis nodosa is usually fatal,

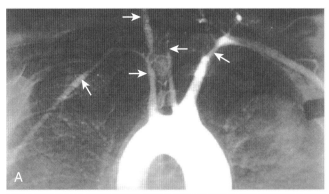

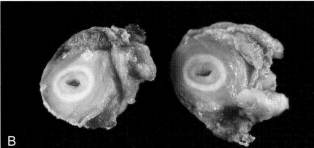

Fig. 7.11 Takayasu arteritis. (A) Aortic arch angiogram showing reduced flow of contrast material into the great vessels and narrowing of the brachiocephalic, carotid, and subclavian arteries *(arrows)*. (B) Cross sections of the right carotid artery from the patient shown in (A) demonstrating marked intimal thickening and luminal narrowing. The white circles correspond to the original vessel wall; the inner core of tan tissue is the area of intimal hyperplasia.

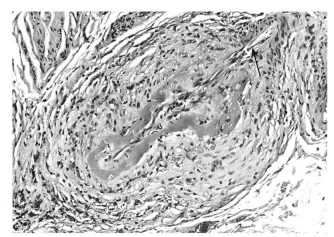

Fig. 7.12 Polyarteritis nodosa, associated with segmental fibrinoid necrosis and thrombotic occlusion of a small artery. Note that part of the vessel *(upper-right, arrow)* is uninvolved. (Courtesy Sidney Murphree, MD, Department of Pathology, University of Texas Southwestern Medical School, Dallas.)

but with immunosuppressive therapy remission or cure is achieved in 90% of cases.

Kawasaki Disease

Kawasaki disease is an acute, febrile, self-limited illness of infancy and childhood associated with an arteritis of large- to medium-sized vessels.

Its clinical significance stems from frequent involvement of coronary arteries.

Pathogenesis. The cause of Kawasaki disease is unknown. The disease shows a seasonal variation in incidence, suggesting that a viral infection triggers an immune response that injures arteries secondarily.

> *Morphology.* The vasculitis resembles that seen in polyarteritis nodosa, although fibrinoid necrosis is usually not as prominent. Affected vessels have a dense transmural inflammatory infiltrate that includes neutrophils and mononuclear cells. If left untreated, damage caused by the inflammation may lead to aneurysm formation.

Clinical Features. Kawasaki disease typically manifests with conjunctival and oral erythema accompanied by blistering, erythema and edema of the hands and feet, a desquamative rash, and cervical lymph node enlargement. Approximately 20% of untreated patients have cardiovascular complications, most notably the development of coronary artery aneurysms, which may rupture or thrombose, leading to myocardial infarction and/or sudden death. The disease responds well to antiinflammatory agents (specifically, intravenous immunoglobulin and aspirin), which sharply reduce the incidence of symptomatic coronary artery disease.

Thromboangiitis Obliterans (Buerger Disease)

Thromboangiitis obliterans is a severe form of vasculitis that is strongly associated with tobacco smoking.

It primarily affects small and middle-sized arteries of the arms and legs, and often produces severe ischemia, ulcerations, and gangrene and amputation of affected tissues.

Pathogenesis. Both the initiation and progression of thromboangiitis obliterans depend on exposure to tobacco smoke, but the precise role of smoking is unclear. One idea is that some component of tobacco smoke directly damages the endothelium and that the vascular changes are due to direct toxicity. Alternatively, a reactive compound in tobacco smoke may modify vessel wall components and induce an immune response. Certain HLA-types are more susceptible, consistent with a role for immune injury. Certain ethnic groups (Israeli, Indian subcontinent, Japanese) are also at greater risk, pointing to one or more genetic factors.

> *Morphology.* Characteristically, there is segmental acute and chronic transmural vasculitis of medium- and small-sized arteries, predominantly in the extremities. In the early stages, mixed inflammatory infiltrates, which may give rise to microabscesses, are accompanied by luminal thrombosis. The inflammation often extends into contiguous veins and nerves (a feature rarely seen in other forms of vasculitis). With time, thrombi organize and eventually the artery and adjacent structures become encased in fibrous tissue.

Clinical Features. Patients are usually younger than 45 and have a smoking history of more than 20 pack-years. Thromboangiitis obliterans may present with Raynaud phenomenon, instep foot pain induced by exercise, or superficial nodular phlebitis (venous inflammation). The vascular insufficiency tends to be accompanied by severe pain—even at rest—probably due to involvement of nerves. If the patient continues to smoke, chronic ulcerations may develop and progress over time to gangrene. Smoking abstinence can halt progression, but once established, the vascular lesions do not remit with smoking abstinence.

Small-Vessel Vasculitides

Many other forms of vasculitis primarily affect small vessels. Although their pathogenesis is incompletely understood, two groups have emerged:
- *Antineutrophil cytoplasmic antibody (ANCA)–associated vasculitides.* These vasculitides are defined by the presence of autoantibodies against various components of neutrophil granules. There are two forms of ANCA: (1) anti-proteinase-3 ANCA (formerly referred to as c-ANCA), directed against PR-3, a neutrophil azurophilic granule constituent (PR3-ANCA); and (2) anti–myeloperoxidase ANCA (formerly referred to as p-ANCA), directed against a neutrophil lysosomal enzyme, myeloperoxidase (MPO-ANCA). Several forms of ANCA-associated vasculitides are recognized with partially overlapping features. They include PR3-ANCA positive granulomatosis with polyangiitis and MPO-ANCA positive microscopic polyangitis. Both are associated with glomerulonephritis and pulmonary disease, frequently leading to hemoptysis. It is unclear if the ANCAs have a direct pathogenic role, but these antibodies are present in a high fraction of affected patients and therefore are of diagnostic value. Treatment is with immunosuppressive agents.
- *Immune-complex, small-vessel vasculitides.* These vasculitides are characterized by immunoglobulin and complement deposition at the sites of vascular injury. Antibodies may bind directly to components of the vessel wall or be deposited as part of immune complexes, for example in association with systemic lupus erythematosus. The distribution of vascular injury and the resultant clinical findings differ depending on the nature of the autoantibodies or immune complexes. In systemic lupus erythematosus and Goodpasture syndrome, the kidney is severely affected (see Chapter 11).

Infectious Vasculitis

Direct vascular invasion by infectious agents, usually bacteria or fungi, particularly *Pseudomonas, Aspergillus,* and *Mucor* spp, may cause localized arteritis. Vascular invasion can be part of a tissue infection (e.g., bacterial pneumonia or adjacent to abscesses), or, less commonly, may arise from hematogenous spread of bacteria during septicemia or embolization from infective endocarditis. Vascular infections can weaken arterial walls sufficiently to cause aneurysms (*mycotic aneurysm*) or can induce thrombosis and infarction.

DISORDERS OF VEINS

Varicose veins and thrombophlebitis account for at least 90% of clinically relevant venous diseases.

Varicose Veins

Varicose veins are abnormally dilated tortuous veins produced by chronically increased intraluminal pressures and weakened vessel wall support.

Venous dilation can occur at multiple sites:
- *Varicose veins* of the extremities occur in up to 20% of men and one third of women; obesity and pregnancy increase the risk. They most commonly affect the superficial veins of the legs. Varicose dilation renders the venous valves incompetent and leads to lower-extremity stasis, congestion, edema, pain, and thrombosis. Persistent edema and secondary ischemic skin changes may lead to stasis dermatitis and ulcerations, which often heal poorly and are prone to superimposed infection.

- *Esophageal varices* may arise in the setting of portal hypertension secondary to liver cirrhosis and (less frequently) portal vein obstruction or hepatic vein thrombosis (see Chapter 13). Esophageal varices are one of several types of portosystemic shunts that may appear with portal hypertension; other common sites of shunting include the rectal veins (*hemorrhoids,* described below) and the periumbilical veins (producing what is known as *caput medusa,* a fanciful term for the imagined resemblance of the dilated snake-like veins to the head of Medusa). Esophageal varices are clinically significant because they are prone to rupture, leading to massive, sometimes fatal upper gastrointestinal hemorrhages.
- *Hemorrhoids* are varicose dilations of the venous plexus at the anorectal junction. They result from prolonged pelvic vascular congestion, most commonly due to pregnancy or straining to defecate. Hemorrhoids are a source of bleeding and are prone to thrombosis and painful ulceration.

Thrombophlebitis

Thrombosis of deep leg veins accounts for more than 90% of cases of thrombophlebitis and is the source of most pulmonary emboli.

Other sites where deep venous thrombi may form are the periprostatic venous plexus in males and the pelvic venous plexus in females, as well as the large veins in the skull and the dural sinuses (especially in the setting of infection or inflammation). Peritoneal infections and certain conditions associated with hypercoagulability (e.g., polycythemia vera; see Chapter 9) may lead to portal vein thrombosis.

Pathogenesis. Thrombosis is related to one or more components of the Virchow triad: flow abnormalities, endothelial injury or dysfunction, and hypercoagulability (see Chapter 3). Prolonged immobilization that results in venous stasis (e.g., extended bed rest in the postsurgical state, or long plane or automobile trips) increases the risk of deep venous thrombosis (DVT) of the leg veins, as do factors causing hypercoagulability (e.g., malignancy and inherited defects, such as factor V Leiden; see Chapter 3). Male sex and age older than 50 years also are associated with increased risk.

Clinical Features. DVTs produce few reliable signs or symptoms. Local manifestations include edema, redness, swelling, and pain. In some cases, pain can be elicited by pressure over affected veins, squeezing the calf muscles, or forced dorsiflexion of the foot *(Homan sign).* However, symptoms often are absent, especially in bedridden patients, and the absence of findings does not exclude DVT. In many cases, the first manifestation of DVT is a pulmonary embolism (see Chapter 3). To prevent recurrent DVT, anticoagulant treatment is given, which may be temporary or lifelong, depending on the etiology of the DVT.

TUMORS OF BLOOD VESSELS AND LYMPHATICS

Tumors of blood vessels and lymphatics include benign hemangiomas (extremely common), locally aggressive neoplasms that metastasize infrequently, and rare, highly malignant angiosarcomas. Vascular neoplasms may arise from the endothelium or cells that support or surround blood vessels. Primary tumors of large vessels (aorta, pulmonary artery, and vena cava) occur infrequently and are mostly sarcomas.

Hemangiomas

Hemangiomas are common benign tumors composed of blood-filled vessels.

Several varieties of hemangiomas are recognized, including types that occur preferentially in newborns:

- *Capillary hemangiomas* are the most common type; these occur in the skin, subcutaneous tissues, and mucous membranes of the oral cavities and lips, as well as in the liver, spleen, and kidneys (Fig. 7.13A). Histologically, they are composed of thin-walled capillaries with scant stroma (Fig. 7.13B).
- *Juvenile hemangiomas* (so-called *strawberry hemangiomas*) of the newborn are common (1 in 200 births), involve the skin, and may be multiple. They grow rapidly, but most regress completely.
- *Pyogenic granulomas* manifest as rapidly growing, red pedunculated lesions on the skin or gingival or oral mucosa that bleed easily and are often ulcerated. Microscopically, they resemble exuberant granulation tissue (Fig. 7.13C).
- *Cavernous hemangiomas* are composed of large, dilated vascular channels (Fig. 7.13D). Compared with capillary hemangiomas, cavernous hemangiomas are more infiltrative, frequently involve deep structures, and do not spontaneously regress. They may be locally destructive; surgical excision may be required in some cases. Cavernous hemangiomas are one component of *von Hippel-Lindau disease* (Chapter 17), in which vascular lesions are commonly found in the cerebellum, brain stem, retina, pancreas, and liver.

Kaposi Sarcoma

Kaposi sarcoma is a vascular neoplasm caused by human herpesvirus-8 (HHV-8, also known as Kaposi sarcoma herpesvirus [KSHV]).

Kaposi sarcoma (KS) is most common in individuals with impaired T-cell function. Four forms of KS, based on population demographics and risks, are recognized:

- *Classic KS* occurs in older men of Mediterranean, Middle Eastern, or Eastern European descent (especially Ashkenazi Jews). Altered immunity is suspected in affected individuals, but overt T-cell immunodeficiency is not present. It manifests as red-purple skin plaques or nodules, usually on the lower extremities. With time the lesions may increase in size and number, but they usually remain confined to the skin and subcutaneous tissue.
- *Endemic African KS* typically occurs in HIV-negative children and young adults and can follow an indolent or aggressive course. It often involves lymph nodes. A severe form, with prominent visceral involvement, occurs in children and is virtually always fatal.
- *Transplantation-associated KS* occurs in solid-organ transplant recipients in the setting of T-cell immunosuppression. It pursues an aggressive course and often involves the lymph nodes, mucosa, and viscera. Lesions often regress with attenuation of immunosuppression, but at the risk of organ rejection.
- *AIDS-associated (epidemic) KS* is an AIDS-defining illness and remains the most common HIV-related malignancy worldwide. The incidence has fallen more than 80% in populations with access to antiretroviral therapy, but KS still occurs in HIV-infected individuals with an incidence that is 1000-fold higher than in the general population. AIDS-associated KS often involves lymph nodes and disseminates widely to viscera early in its course.

Pathogenesis. KS is an unusual neoplasm that likely begins as a reactive proliferation stimulated by factors produced by HHV-8 infected stromal cells. These include viral homologs of cytokines such as interleukin 6, as well as viral factors that enhance cell cycle progression and interfere with the function of tumor suppressors such as RB. In the absence of an effective T-cell response, this proliferation persists; with time and clonal evolution, it may progress to a full-fledged malignancy.

Morphology. Cutaneous lesions progress through three sequential stages: *patch, plaque,* and *nodule.* Patches are pink, red, or purple macules composed of dilated, irregular, and angulated blood vessels associated with an infiltrate of chronic inflammatory cells. Plaques (Fig. 7.14A) are elevated lesions composed of dilated dermal vascular channels lined and surrounded by plump spindle cells. Nodular lesions are overtly neoplastic and contain increased numbers of plump, proliferating spindle cells, often with interspersed slit-like spaces (Fig. 7.14B). The nodular stage often is accompanied by nodal and visceral involvement, particularly in the African and AIDS-associated variants.

Clinical Features. The course of KS varies widely according to the clinical setting. Classic KS is largely restricted to the surface of the body, and surgical resection usually is adequate treatment. In KS associated with immunosuppression, restoration of T-cell function by reducing immunosuppression often is effective. Similarly, for AIDS-associated KS, antiretroviral therapy generally is beneficial.

Angiosarcomas

Angiosarcoma is a malignant neoplasm defined by evidence of endothelial differentiation.

Pathogenesis. Angiosarcomas can arise in the setting of lymphedema (e.g., following lymph node resection for breast cancer), radiation, and, rarely, indwelling of foreign bodies (e.g., shrapnel). Historically, polyvinyl chloride has been associated with angiosarcoma of the liver.

Morphology. In the skin, angiosarcomas first appear as small, sharply demarcated, red nodules. Advanced lesions are large, fleshy red-tan to gray-white masses (Fig. 7.15A) with ill-defined margins that blend imperceptibly with surrounding structures. The extent of differentiation is variable, ranging from tumors that form vascular channels (Fig. 7.15B) to undifferentiated spindle cell tumors without discernible blood vessels.

Clinical Features. Older adults are more commonly affected, and lesions most often involve the skin, soft tissue, breast, and liver. Angiosarcomas are aggressive tumors that invade locally and metastasize. Complete resection often is not possible, and current 5-year survival rates are only about 30%.

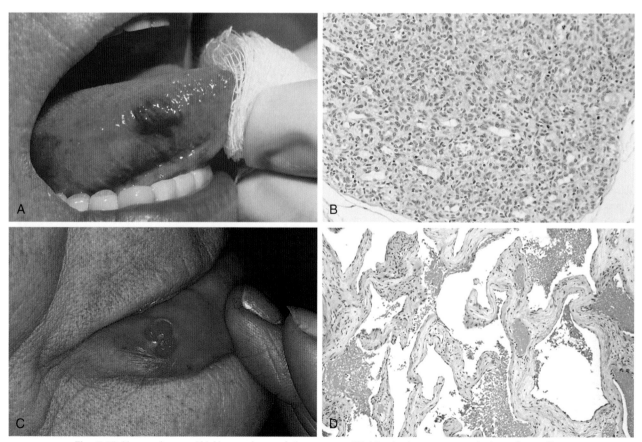

Fig. 7.13 Hemangiomas. (A) Hemangioma of the tongue. (B) Histologic appearance in juvenile capillary hemangioma. (C) Pyogenic granuloma of the lip. (D) Histologic appearance in cavernous hemangioma. (A and D, Courtesy John Sexton, MD, Beth Israel Hospital, Boston. B, Courtesy Christopher D.M. Fletcher, MD, Brigham and Women's Hospital, Boston. C, Courtesy Thomas Rogers, MD, University of Texas Southwestern Medical School, Dallas.)

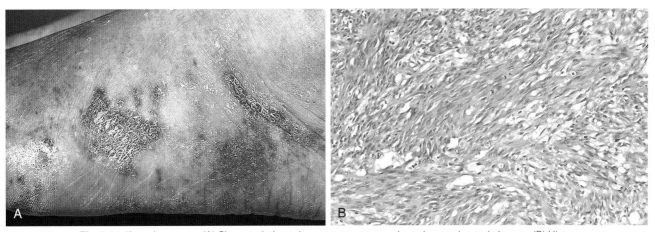

Fig. 7.14 Kaposi sarcoma. (A) Characteristic coalescent cutaneous red-purple macules and plaques. (B) Histologic view of the nodular stage, demonstrating sheets of plump, proliferating spindle cells and slit-like vascular spaces. (Courtesy Christopher D.M. Fletcher, MD, Brigham and Women's Hospital, Boston.)

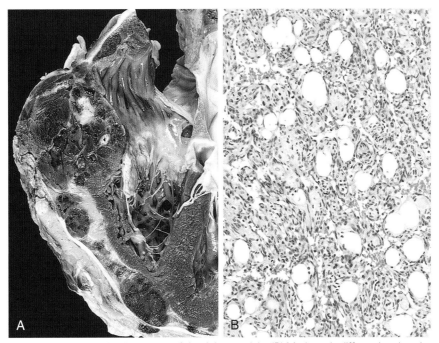

Fig. 7.15 Angiosarcoma. (A) Angiosarcoma of the right ventricle. (B) Moderately differentiated angiosarcoma with dense clumps of atypical cells lining distinct vascular lumina.

8

Heart

OUTLINE

Congenital Heart Disease, 118
   Malformations Associated with Left-to-Right Shunts, 119
   Malformations Associated with Right-to-Left Shunts, 120
   Malformations Leading to Obstruction, 120
Ischemic Heart Disease, 121
   Angina Pectoris, 121
   Myocardial Infarction, 121
   Chronic Ischemic Heart Disease, 125
Arrhythmia, 125
Hypertensive Heart Disease, 126
   Systemic (Left-Sided) Hypertensive Heart Disease, 126
   Right-Sided (Pulmonary) Hypertensive Heart Disease, 126
Valvular Heart Disease, 126
   Degenerative Valve Disease, 127

Rheumatic Valvular Disease, 128
Infective Endocarditis, 130
Nonbacterial Thrombotic Endocarditis, 131
Cardiomyopathies and Myocarditis, 131
   Dilated Cardiomyopathy, 131
   Hypertrophic Cardiomyopathy, 132
   Restrictive Cardiomyopathy, 133
   Myocarditis, 133
   Other Causes of Myocardial Disease, 134
Congestive Heart Failure, 135
   Left-Sided Heart Failure, 135
   Right-Sided Heart Failure, 136
Cardiac Tumors, 136

The heart is a remarkably resilient organ, beating more than 40 million times per year and pumping more than 7500 L of blood a day. Given this workload and the importance of the circulatory system for the function of every organ in the body, it is not surprising that the consequences of heart disease may be severe: Cardiovascular disease is the leading cause of mortality worldwide and accounts for one in four deaths in the United States.

In this chapter, we focus on the most common forms of heart disease, including congenital and acquired forms, and then finish our discussion with heart failure.

CONGENITAL HEART DISEASE

Both genetic and environmental factors contribute to congenital abnormalities of the heart or great vessels, which account for 20% to 30% of all birth defects.

Congenital heart disease affects nearly 1% of births (roughly 40,000 infants per year), with a higher incidence in premature infants and stillborns. Defects compatible with live birth usually involve only single chambers or regions of the heart. Twelve entities account for 85% of cases of congenital heart disease; their frequencies are shown in Table 8.1.

Pathogenesis. Congenital heart disease usually arises from faulty embryogenesis during gestational weeks 3 through 8, when major cardiovascular structures develop. The cause is unknown in almost 90% of cases. Known etiologic factors include acquired conditions such as congenital rubella infection, teratogen exposure, maternal diabetes, and genetic factors such as trisomies 13, 15, 18, and 21 and Turner syndrome.

Most single-gene defects that disrupt cardiac development are autosomal dominant mutations, some of which affect transcription factors that serve as "master regulators" of cardiac development. The function of the same genes may also be impaired by transient environmental stresses at critical early stages of cardiac development, giving rise to lesions similar to those caused by genetic factors.

Clinical Features. Structural anomalies in congenital heart disease can be categorized as (1) malformations causing a *left-to-right shunt;* (2) malformations causing a *right-to-left shunt* (cyanotic congenital heart diseases); and (3) malformations causing *obstruction.*

A *shunt* is an abnormal communication between chambers or blood vessels that permits blood to flow from the left to the right side of the heart (or vice versa).
- *Left-to-right shunts* increase blood flow into the pulmonary circulation and expose the low-pressure, low-resistance pulmonary circulation to increased pressures and volumes, resulting in right ventricular hypertrophy and, eventually, right-sided heart failure *(cor pulmonale).* With time, increased pulmonary resistance may lead to shunt reversal (right to left) and late-onset cyanosis *(Eisenmenger syndrome).*
- *With right-to-left shunts,* a dusky blueness of the skin (cyanosis) results because the pulmonary circulation is bypassed and poorly oxygenated blood enters the systemic circulation.
- *Some congenital anomalies* obstruct vascular flow, by narrowing the chambers, valves, or major blood vessels. A malformation characterized by complete obstruction is called an *atresia.*

Table 8.1 Frequency of Congenital Cardiac Malformations[a]

Malformation	Incidence per 1 Million Live Births	Percentage
Ventricular septal defect	4482	42
Atrial septal defect	1043	10
Pulmonary stenosis	836	8
Patent ductus arteriosus	781	7
Tetralogy of Fallot	577	5
Coarctation of aorta	492	5
Atrioventricular septal defect	396	4
Aortic stenosis	388	4
Transposition of great arteries	388	4
Truncus arteriosus	136	1
Total anomalous pulmonary venous connection	120	1
Tricuspid atresia	118	1
TOTAL	9757	

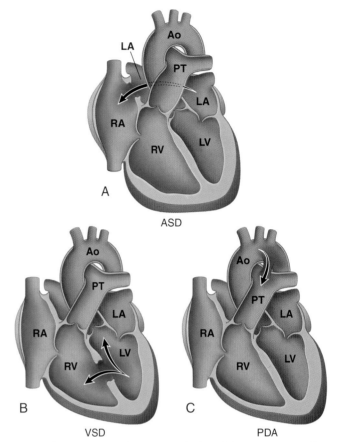

Fig. 8.1 Common congenital causes of left-to-right shunts (*arrows* indicate direction of blood flow). (A) Atrial septal defect *(ASD)*. (B) Ventricular septal defect *(VSD)*. (C) Patent ductus arteriosus *(PDA)*. Ao, aorta; LA, left atrium; LV, left ventricle; PT, pulmonary trunk; RA, right atrium; RV, right ventricle.

Malformations Associated with Left-to-Right Shunts

Left-to-right shunts are associated with atrial septal defects, ventricular septal defects, and patent ductus arteriosus and are the most common type of congenital cardiac malformation (Fig. 8.1). Atrial septal defects typically increase only right ventricular and pulmonary outflow volumes, whereas ventricular septal defects and patent ductus arteriosus cause increases in pulmonary blood flow and blood pressure. Cyanosis is not an early feature of these defects, but reversal of the shunt due to pulmonary hypertension can cause cyanosis and irreparable cardiac dysfunction. Thus, left-to-right shunts must be repaired before shunt reversal occurs, usually with surgery.

Atrial Septal Defects and Patent Foramen Ovale

Atrial septal defects and patent foramen ovale are the most common congenital cardiac anomalies diagnosed in adults.

During cardiac development, patency is maintained between the right and left atria by the *foramen ovale,* which is later closed by tissue flaps. In 80% of people, these septa eventually fuse. In the remaining cases, a *patent foramen ovale* may allow *transient* right-to-left blood flow, as may occur with sneezing or straining during bowel movements. Such right-to-left flow of blood puts patients at risk for a paradoxical embolism: a venous embolus (e.g., from deep leg veins) that enters the arterial circulation via an atrial defect due to increased right-sided atrial pressures. This may give rise to stroke due to lodging of paradoxical emboli in vessels of the central nervous system. In contrast, an atrial septal defect is a fixed opening in the atrial septum that allows unrestricted blood flow from left to right atrium.

Atrial septal defects usually are asymptomatic until adulthood, when long-standing chronic right-sided volume and pressure overloads may eventually produce pulmonary hypertension and shunt reversal. These complications do not occur with patent foramen ovale.

Ventricular Septal Defects

Defects in the ventricular septum allow left-to-right shunting and are the most common congenital cardiac anomalies at birth, but most close spontaneously and do not come to clinical attention.

Most are associated with other cardiac malformations. The ventricular septum is formed by the fusion of a muscular ridge that grows upward from the heart apex and a thinner membranous partition that grows downward to meet it (Supplemental eFig. 8.1). The membranous portion is the site of approximately 70% of ventricular septal defects.

Small defects may be asymptomatic, and defects in the muscular wall of the septum may close spontaneously during infancy or early childhood. Larger defects, however, result in chronic left-to-right shunting complicated by pulmonary hypertension and congestive heart failure. Early surgical correction is imperative for such lesions.

Patent Ductus Arteriosus

The ductus arteriosus is a connecting link between pulmonary artery and aorta that normally closes after birth.

It arises from the left pulmonary artery and joins the aorta just distal to the origin of the left subclavian artery. During intrauterine life, it permits blood flow from the pulmonary artery to the aorta, bypassing the unoxygenated lungs. Within 1 to 2 days of birth, the ductus normally constricts and closes in response to increased arterial oxygenation, decreased pulmonary vascular resistance, and declining levels of prostaglandin E_2 derived from the placenta. Known causes of persistent patent ductus arteriosus include hypoxia (e.g., due to right to left shunts) and certain autosomal dominant gene defects, but 90% of cases are of uncertain pathogenesis.

Small ductal shunts generally cause no symptoms, but larger defects eventually lead to shunt reversal, cyanosis, and heart failure. Patent ductus arteriosus creates a high-pressure left-to-right shunt that produces a harsh, "machinery-like" murmur. Isolated patent ductus requires surgical intervention as early in life as possible to prevent these complications.

Malformations Associated with Right-to-Left Shunts

Cardiac malformations resulting in right-to-left shunts give rise to cyanosis due to admixture of venous blood with the arterial circulation. The most common conditions associated with cyanotic congenital heart disease are tetralogy of Fallot and transposition of the great vessels (Fig. 8.2).

Tetralogy of Fallot

Tetralogy of Fallot is the most common cause of cyanotic congenital heart disease (~5% of congenital cardiac malformations).

The tetralogy consists of the following four abnormalities:

- Ventricular septal defect
- Overriding of the ventricular septal defect by the aorta
- Right ventricular outflow tract obstruction (subpulmonic stenosis)
- Right ventricular hypertrophy

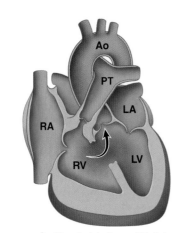

A Classic tetralogy of Fallot

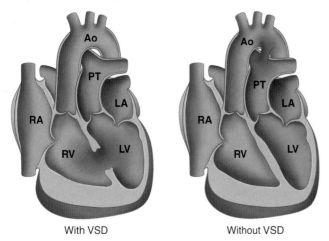

With VSD   Without VSD

B Complete transposition

Fig. 8.2 Common congenital right-to-left shunts (cyanotic congenital heart disease). (A) Tetralogy of Fallot (*arrow* indicates direction of blood flow). (B) Transposition of the great vessels with and without ventricular septal defect. *Ao,* aorta; *LA,* left atrium; *LV,* left ventricle; *PT,* pulmonary trunk; *RA,* right atrium; *RV,* right ventricle; *VSD,* ventricular septal defect.

Morphology. Tetralogy of Fallot results from anterosuperior displacement of the muscular septum that separates the pulmonary trunk and the aortic root (Fig. 8.2A). The heart is enlarged and boot-shaped due to right ventricular hypertrophy; the proximal aorta is dilated; and the pulmonary trunk is hypoplastic. The ventricular septal defect usually is large and is overridden by the aortic valve, which receives most of the output from both ventricles. Obstruction of right ventricular outflow may be due to narrowing just below the pulmonary valve (most common) or pulmonary valve stenosis or atresia. In such cases, a patent ductus arteriosus or dilated bronchial arteries provide the only route for blood to reach the lungs.

Clinical Features. The clinical severity depends on the degree of pulmonary outflow obstruction. In most cases, pulmonic obstruction is severe enough to cause right-to-left shunting and cyanosis, which worsens with time because the malformed pulmonic orifice does not expand as the rest of the heart grows. If the pulmonic obstruction is mild, the condition resembles an isolated ventricular septal defect, because shunting occurs from left to right. The pulmonic stenosis provides protection from pulmonary hypertension, but other sequelae of cyanotic heart disease are seen, such as polycythemia (due to hypoxia). Right-to-left shunting also increases the risk for infective endocarditis and paradoxical embolization. Complete surgical repair is possible but is more complicated if pulmonary atresia is present.

Transposition of the Great Vessels

In transposition of the great vessels, the aorta arises from the right ventricle and the pulmonary artery emanates from the left ventricle.

It is incompatible with postnatal life unless a shunt exists that delivers oxygenated blood to the aorta such as a ventricular septal defect (one third of cases) (Fig. 8.2B; Supplemental eFig. 8.2). In these cases, the right ventricle is hypertrophied because it is the pump for the high-pressure systemic circulation, and the left ventricle is hypoplastic because it provides blood to the low-pressure pulmonary circulation. In other instances, shunts are provided by a patent foramen ovale or ductus arteriosus; these tend to close soon after birth, and such infants require emergent surgical intervention. The dominant feature is cyanosis. Improved surgical techniques now permit repair, and patients often survive into adulthood.

Malformations Leading to Obstruction

Congenital obstructions to blood flow can occur proximal to the heart valves, at the level of the valves, or distally within a great vessel. The latter most commonly involve the aorta and merit a brief discussion.

Aortic Coarctation

Coarctation (narrowing, or constriction) of the aorta is a common form of obstructive congenital heart disease. Males are affected twice as often as females. Coarctation may be a solitary defect or may be associated with other defects, of which the most common is a bicuspid aortic valve. There are two forms of coarctation (Fig. 8.3):

- *An "infantile" form* featuring circumferential narrowing of the aortic segment between the left subclavian artery and a patent ductus arteriosus (referred to as preductal). In this circumstance, the ductus is the main source of (unoxygenated) blood delivered to the distal aorta. The pulmonary trunk is dilated due to increased blood flow, and because the right side of the heart perfuses the body distal to the narrowed segment, the right ventricle is hypertrophied.
- *An "adult" form* consisting of ridge-like infolding of the aorta adjacent to the ligamentum arteriosum, a remnant of the ductus arteriosus (referred to as postductal) (Fig. 8.4). Proximal to the

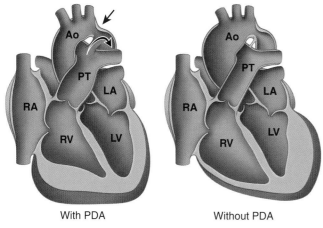

With PDA   Without PDA

Coarctation of aorta

Fig. 8.3 Coarctation of the aorta with ("infantile" or preductal form) and without a patent ductus arteriosus (PDA) ("adult" or postductal form); *arrow* indicates direction of blood flow. Ao, aorta; LA, left atrium; LV, left ventricle; PT, pulmonary trunk; RA, right atrium; RV, right ventricle.

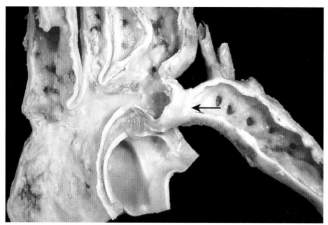

Fig. 8.4 Coarctation of the aorta, postductal type. The coarctation is a segmental narrowing of the aorta *(arrow)*. Such lesions typically manifest later in life than preductal coarctations. The dilated ascending aorta and major branch vessels are to the left of the coarctation. The lower extremities are perfused predominantly by way of dilated, tortuous collateral channels. (Courtesy of Sid Murphree, MD, Department of Pathology, University of Texas Southwestern Medical School, Dallas.)

coarctation, the aortic arch and its branch vessels are dilated and the left ventricle is hypertrophied.

Clinical Features. These depend on the position and severity of the narrowing and the patency of the ductus arteriosus:
- *Preductal coarctation with a patent ductus* usually presents early in life with cyanosis in the lower half of the body. Without intervention, most affected infants do not survive the neonatal period.
- *Postductal coarctation without a patent ductus* usually is asymptomatic early in life and may remain unrecognized into adulthood. There often is upper-extremity hypertension and relative hypotension in the lower extremities associated with claudication. Collateral circulation often develops through the intercostal and internal mammary arteries, and increased blood flow and dilation of these vessels can produce visible "notching" of the ribs on radiologic studies. Treatment with balloon dilation or surgical resection generally yields excellent outcomes.

ISCHEMIC HEART DISEASE

Ischemic heart disease encompasses several related syndromes caused by insufficient delivery of oxygen and nutrients to meet myocardial demand.

It is most often due to coronary artery disease, the chief cause of mortality in the United States and other high income nations. Encouragingly, mortality related to ischemic heart disease in the United States has declined by 50% since 1963. This improvement is largely due to interventions that have reduced coronary artery atherosclerosis, including smoking cessation programs, better treatments for hypertension and diabetes, and use of cholesterol-lowering drugs. Therapeutic advances such as more effective arrhythmia control, improvements in coronary care units, angioplasty, and endovascular stenting have also contributed.

Pathogenesis. In a large majority of cases, ischemic heart disease stems from reduced blood flow caused by atherosclerosis of the coronary arteries, often referred to simply as coronary artery disease. Atherosclerosis (see Chapter 7) can affect any of the main coronary arteries, singly or in any combination.

Angina Pectoris

Angina pectoris is intermittent chest pain caused by reversible myocardial ischemia.

Three variants are recognized.
- *Stable angina* is predictable episodic chest pain associated with particular levels of exertion or increased demand (e.g., tachycardia). It is usually associated with stable atherosclerotic plaques that narrow the lumen of a coronary artery by 70% or more (*critical stenosis*). The pain is a crushing or squeezing substernal sensation that may radiate to the left arm or the left jaw. It is relieved by rest or by nitroglycerin, a vasodilator that increases coronary perfusion.
- *Prinzmetal* or *variant angina* occurs at rest and is caused by coronary artery spasm, typically near atherosclerotic plaques. It also responds to vasodilators such as nitroglycerin and calcium channel blockers.
- *Unstable angina* (crescendo angina) is characterized by increasingly frequent pain that is precipitated by progressively less exertion or even occurs at rest. It may be associated with severe narrowing of a coronary artery (obstruction of > 90% of the vessel lumen) or by plaque rupture and superimposed thrombosis. Unstable angina can be a harbinger of myocardial infarction.

Myocardial Infarction

Myocardial infarction is necrosis of the heart muscle resulting from ischemia.

The incidence of myocardial infarction rises progressively with age and the presence of increasing numbers of risk factors for atherosclerosis. Men are affected significantly more often than women, but this gender gap narrows with age.

Pathogenesis. **Most myocardial infarctions are caused by acute thrombotic obstruction of a coronary artery due to rupture of an atherosclerotic plaque** (Fig. 8.5).

The initiating plaque disruption of myocardial infarction (MI) is typically sudden. Plaques that contain large lipid-rich cores or have thin overlying fibrous caps are particularly vulnerable to rupture. Hemorrhage into the plaque can cause rapid plaque expansion and rupture, or an occlusive thrombus can form because of exposure of collagen,

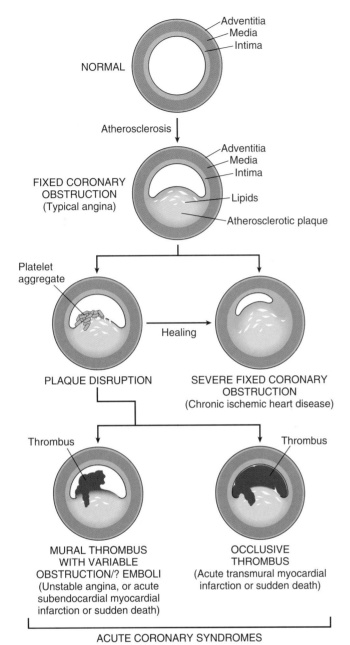

NORMAL

Adventitia
Media
Intima

↓ Atherosclerosis

FIXED CORONARY
OBSTRUCTION
(Typical angina)

Adventitia
Media
Intima
Lipids
Atherosclerotic plaque

Platelet
aggregate

PLAQUE DISRUPTION

→ Healing →

SEVERE FIXED CORONARY
OBSTRUCTION
(Chronic ischemic heart disease)

Thrombus

MURAL THROMBUS
WITH VARIABLE
OBSTRUCTION/? EMBOLI
(Unstable angina, or acute
subendocardial myocardial
infarction or sudden death)

Thrombus

OCCLUSIVE
THROMBUS
(Acute transmural myocardial
infarction or sudden death)

ACUTE CORONARY SYNDROMES

Fig. 8.5 Diagram of sequential progression of coronary artery lesions leading to various acute coronary syndromes. (Modified and redrawn from Schoen FJ: *Interventional and surgical cardiovascular pathology: clinical correlations and basic principles*, Philadelphia, Saunders, 1989, p. 63.)

von Willebrand factor, and tissue factor, leading to platelet adhesion and aggregation and activation of coagulation factors (see Fig. 8.5). Platelets are central to thrombus formation in the high shear stress environment in arteries. Therefore, antiplatelet agents (e.g., aspirin) are useful in both the prevention and treatment of myocardial infarction.

Within seconds of vascular obstruction, aerobic glycolysis ceases in the myocardium, adenosine triphosphate levels fall, and noxious metabolites (e.g., lactic acid) accumulate. Loss of contractility occurs within a minute or so of the onset of ischemia. Ischemia lasting 20 to 40 minutes causes irreversible damage and myocyte death in the form of coagulative necrosis (see Chapter 1). The location, size, and morphologic features of a myocardial infarct depend on the size and distribution of the involved vessel (Fig. 8.6), the rate of development

and the duration of the occlusion, the metabolic demands of the myocardium, and the existence of collateral vessels. Most infarcts involve the left ventricle, because the right ventricle is relatively protected by lower blood pressure (and thus lower metabolic demands) and perfusion during both diastole and systole (due to lower wall pressures). An infarct usually achieves its full extent within 3 to 6 hours. Clinical intervention within this critical window of time can lessen the size of the infarct within the "territory at risk."

Depending on the position and degree of coronary artery obstruction, two patterns of infarction are seen:

- *Transmural infarcts* result in the death of myocytes across the full thickness of the myocardium, except for a thin layer of subendocardial myocytes that receive their oxygen and nutrient supply directly from blood in the ventricles. These infarcts are generally caused by complete obstruction of an epicardial coronary vessel. Because such infarcts usually produce elevated ST segments in electrocardiograms (ECGs), they are also called ST-segment elevated MI (STEMI).
- *Endocardial infarcts* result in the death of myocytes in the inner portion of the myocardium. This type of infarct may be caused by obstruction of more distal coronary vessels or by severe, but incomplete, obstructions. The latter may preferentially kill endocardium because it is in the distal distribution of the coronary arteries and also is exposed to high ventricular pressures, which impede delivery of blood. On the basis of common ECG findings, these infarcts are called non-ST-segment elevated MI (NSTEMI).

Myocardial ischemia also disturbs electrical conductance in the heart, increasing the risk of arrhythmias. Indeed, although myocardial ischemia and infarction can result in death due to pump failure, in 80% to 90% of cases death is caused by ventricular fibrillation, a particularly lethal arrhythmia.

Morphology. The gross and microscopic appearance of a myocardial infarction depends on the age of the injury. There is a highly characteristic sequence of morphologic changes: (1) coagulative necrosis; (2) acute and then chronic inflammation; and (3) fibrosis. Myocardial infarcts less than 12 hours old usually are not grossly apparent, but infarcts more than 3 hours old can be visualized by exposing myocardium to vital stains (Fig. 8.7). Microscopically, typical features of coagulative necrosis become detectable within 4 to 12 hours of infarction (Fig. 8.8). By 12 to 24 hours, an infarct usually can be grossly identified by red-blue discoloration caused by trapped blood. Necrotic myocardium elicits acute inflammation (which typically peaks 1 to 3 days after infarction) followed by an influx of macrophages, which remove necrotic myocytes and neutrophil fragments, and is most pronounced 5 to 10 days after infarction. During this time, infarcts become progressively better delineated as soft, yellow-tan areas that by 10 to 14 days become rimmed by highly vascularized granulation tissue. Healing requires the migration of inflammatory cells and ingrowth of new vessels from the infarct margins, and large infarcts take longer to heal than small ones. Eventually, over a period of weeks, fibrous scar replaces the infarcted tissue.

Clinical Features. The classic myocardial infarction is heralded by severe, crushing substernal chest pain or pressure that radiates to the neck, jaw, epigastrium, or left arm. In contrast to angina pectoris, the associated pain is persistent and is not relieved by nitroglycerin or rest. In a minority of patients, myocardial infarction may be asymptomatic. Such "silent" infarcts are relatively common in older patients and diabetics (due to autonomic neuropathies that blunt the perception of pain).

TRANSMURAL INFARCTS   NON-TRANSMURAL INFARCTS

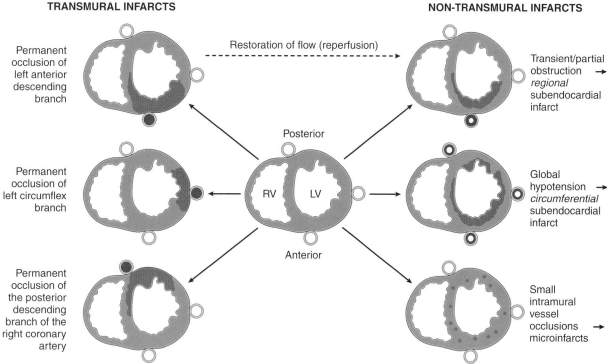

Fig. 8.6 Dependence of myocardial infarction on the location and nature of the diminished perfusion. *Left,* Patterns of transmural infarction resulting from major coronary artery occlusion. The right ventricle may be involved with occlusion of the right main coronary artery *(not depicted). Right,* Patterns of infarction resulting from partial or transient occlusion *(top),* global hypotension superimposed on fixed three-vessel disease *(middle),* or occlusion of small intramyocardial vessels *(bottom).*

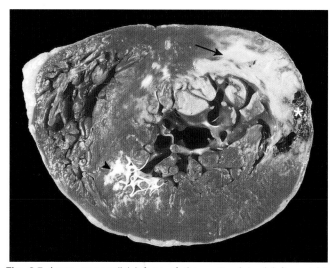

Fig. 8.7 Acute myocardial infarct of the posterolateral left ventricle demonstrated by a lack of triphenyltetrazolium chloride staining in areas of necrosis *(arrow);* the absence of staining is due to enzyme leakage after cell death. Note the anterior scar *(arrowhead),* indicative of remote infarction. The myocardial hemorrhage at the right edge of the infarct *(asterisk)* is due to ventricular rupture, and was the acute cause of death in this patient (specimen is oriented with the posterior wall at the *top).*

The pulse usually is rapid and weak and patients are often diaphoretic and nauseated. Dyspnea is common, due to impaired myocardial contractility and dysfunction of the mitral valve apparatus, with resultant acute pulmonary congestion and edema. With massive myocardial infarction, cardiogenic shock develops due to pump failure.

Characteristic electrocardiographic abnormalities are usually present and can help to determine the type of infarction (STEMI or NSTEMI)

and its location in the heart. Serum levels of proteins that leak from injured myocardial cells are useful in diagnosis. Cardiac troponins T and I have high specificity and sensitivity for myocardial damage (Fig. 8.9).

More than 90% of patients who make it to a hospital survive the acute event, but nearly three fourths experience one or more of the following complications (Fig. 8.10):

- *Contractile dysfunction.* Infarcts impair left ventricular pump function in proportion to the volume of damaged myocardium. Severe "pump failure" *(cardiogenic shock)* occurs in roughly 10% of patients with transmural infarcts, typically those that damage 40% or more of the left ventricle.
- *Papillary muscle dysfunction.* Although papillary muscles rupture infrequently after infarction, they often are dysfunctional, leading to postinfarct mitral regurgitation.
- *Myocardial rupture.* Rupture complicates only 1% to 5% of infarctions but is frequently fatal when it occurs. It is more common in those who receive thrombolytic therapy. Left ventricular free wall rupture is most common, usually resulting in rapidly fatal hemopericardium and cardiac tamponade (see Figs. 8.7 and 8.10A). Ventricular septal rupture may create a left-to-right shunt (see Fig. 8.10B), and papillary muscle rupture may lead to severe mitral regurgitation (Fig. 8.10C). Rupture usually occurs within the first 5 days in 50% of cases and within the first two weeks in 90% of cases, the time during the healing process when much of the infarct consists of soft, friable granulation tissue.
- *Arrhythmia.* Approximately 90% of patients develop some form of rhythm disturbance. The risk for serious arrhythmia (e.g., ventricular fibrillation) is greatest in the first hour and declines thereafter. It is responsible for the majority of deaths occurring prior to hospitalization.
- *Pericarditis.* Transmural infarction can elicit a painful fibrinohemorrhagic pericarditis due to underlying myocardial inflammation

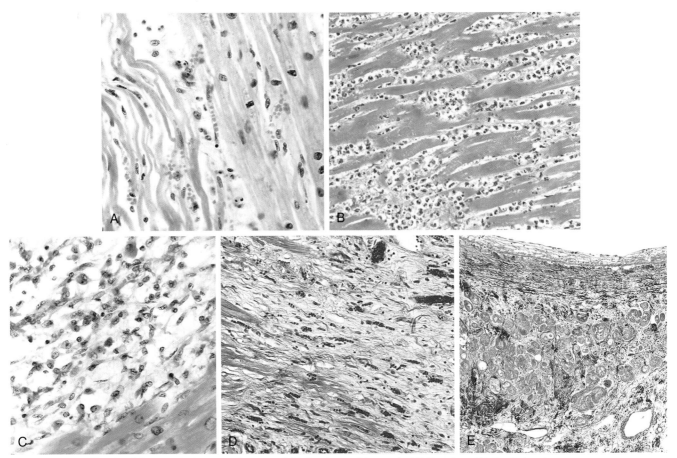

Fig. 8.8 Microscopic features of myocardial infarction and its repair. (A) One-day-old infarct showing coagulative necrosis and wavy fibers, compared with adjacent normal fibers *(right)*. Necrotic cells are separated by edema fluid. (B) Dense neutrophilic infiltrate in the area of a 2- to 3-day-old infarct. (C) Nearly complete removal of necrotic myocytes by phagocytic macrophages (7 to 10 days). (D) Granulation tissue characterized by loose connective tissue and abundant capillaries. (E) Healed myocardial infarct consisting of a dense collagenous scar. A few residual cardiac muscle cells are present. (D) and (E) are Masson's trichrome stain, which stains collagen blue.

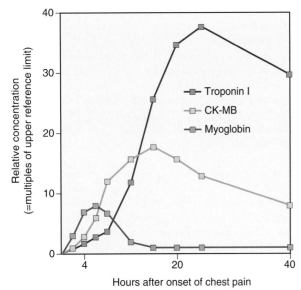

Fig. 8.9 Increases in myocardium-derived troponin I, myocardial creatine kinase (CK-MB), and myoglobin following myocardial infarction. Troponins are particularly sensitive and specific markers of myocardial injury.

(see Fig. 8.10D). Pericarditis typically appears 2 to 3 days after infarction and resolves over the next few days.

- *Ventricular dilation and aneurysm formation.* Because necrotic muscle is weak, there may be disproportionate stretching, thinning, and dilation of the infarcted region (especially with anteroseptal infarcts). In some large transmural infarctions, this leads to ventricular aneurysms (see Fig. 8.10F), which are prone to mural thrombosis and are associated with arrhythmia and heart failure. Rupture is uncommon.
- *Mural thrombus.* Stasis due to diminished myocardial contractility and endocardial damage fosters mural thrombosis (see Fig. 8.10E), with risk for left-sided thromboembolism.
- *Reperfusion injury.* As discussed in Chapter 2, restoration of blood flow to ischemic muscle may paradoxically cause the death of viable "at-risk" myocardium. The precise mechanism is uncertain: increased production of reactive oxygen species from cells with damaged mitochondria, increased uptake of calcium into cells with damaged membranes, and deleterious effects of inflammatory cells have all been proposed to contribute.

The long-term prognosis after myocardial infarction depends on many factors, the most important of which are left ventricular function and the severity of atherosclerotic coronary artery disease. The overall mortality rate within the first year is about 30%, including deaths occurring before the patient reaches the hospital. Thereafter,

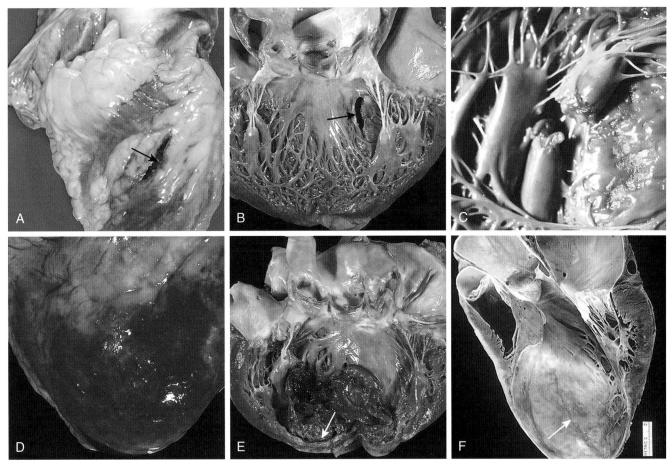

Fig. 8.10 Complications of myocardial infarction. (A to C) Cardiac rupture. (A) Anterior free wall myocardial rupture *(arrow).* (B) Ventricular septal rupture *(arrow).* (C) Papillary muscle rupture. (D) Fibrinous pericarditis, with a hemorrhagic, roughened epicardial surface overlying an acute infarct. (E) Recent expansion of an anteroapical infarct with wall stretching and thinning *(arrow)* and mural thrombus. (F) Large apical left ventricular aneurysm *(arrow).* (A to E, Reproduced by permission from Schoen FJ: *Interventional and surgical cardiovascular pathology: clinical correlations and basic principles,* Philadelphia, Saunders, 1989; F, Courtesy of William D. Edwards, MD, Mayo Clinic, Rochester, Minnesota.)

the annual mortality rate for patients who have suffered a myocardial infarction is 3% to 4%.

Chronic Ischemic Heart Disease

Chronic ischemic heart disease, also called ischemic cardiomyopathy, is characterized by progressive heart failure due to cumulative myocardial damage.

Pathogenesis. Usually, there is a history of one or more myocardial infarctions: Chronic ischemic heart disease occurs when compensatory mechanisms of the residual myocardium can no longer maintain cardiac function. In other cases, severe coronary artery disease and chronic ischemia cause widespread myocardial dysfunction without overt myocardial infarction.

> *Morphology.* Chronic ischemic heart disease typically results in left ventricular dilation and hypertrophy, often with discrete areas of scarring from previous healed infarcts. Invariably, there is moderate to severe atherosclerosis of the coronary arteries. The endocardium generally shows patchy, fibrous thickening, and mural thrombi may be present. Microscopic findings include myocyte hypertrophy and fibrosis at sites of prior infarction.

Clinical Features. Chronic ischemic heart disease is associated with severe, progressive heart failure, occasionally punctuated by new episodes of angina or infarction. Arrhythmia, heart failure, and intercurrent myocardial infarction account for most of the associated morbidity and mortality.

ARRHYTHMIA

Aberrant heart rhythm (arrhythmia) frequently arises in the setting of myocardial ischemia or scarring and is a major cause of sudden death.

The electrical signals that coordinate myocardial contraction are transmitted from cell to cell through gap junctions in a wave that propagates from the sinoatrial node (the cardiac pacemaker) through the atrioventricular node to the base of the ventricles. Aberrant rhythms may start anywhere in the conduction system and are subdivided based on the site of origin, either the supraventricular (atrial) or ventricular myocardium. Arrhythmias may be sustained or sporadic, and can manifest as rhythms that are too slow *(bradycardia),* too fast *(tachycardia),* irregular, or that preclude effective cardiac pumping *(ventricular fibrillation* and *asystole).* Atrial fibrillation occurs when atrial myocytes become "irritable" and depolarize independently and sporadically (as occurs with atrial dilation); the signals are variably transmitted through the atrioventricular node, leading to the "irregularly irregular" heart rate and rhythm of atrial fibrillation. If the atrioventricular node is dysfunctional, varying degrees of heart block occur.

Pathogenesis. **Acquired myocardial diseases and inherited disorders of ion transport are important causes of rhythm disorders.**

Acquired factors that disturb myocardial signal conduction include ischemia, inflammation or scarring, and deposition of extracellular material between myocytes (e.g., cardiac amyloidosis). The most important risk factor is coronary artery disease and associated ischemic injury. In most cases, there is no associated myocardial infarction, and arrhythmia thus appears to be triggered by the electrical "irritability" of abnormal myocardium. Inherited forms of arrhythmias are less common and are usually due to mutations in genes that encode cardiac ion channels (so-called channelopathies). The prototypical channelopathy is the *long QT syndrome,* caused most often by a mutation affecting a potassium channel. Many commonly used medications can trigger arrhythmias in patients with long QT syndrome. Channelopathies are diagnosed by genetic testing, typically performed in patients with a family history or an unexplained nonlethal arrhythmia.

Clinical Features. Arrhythmia may be asymptomatic, be sensed as abnormal beats *(palpitations)* or a rapid heart rate, or cause symptoms related to inadequate cardiac output, such as fainting *(syncope).* Sudden death caused by ventricular fibrillation or asystole occurs in roughly 400,000 people each year in the United States. It is due to coronary artery disease in 80% to 90% of cases and may be the first manifestation of coronary artery disease. In younger patients, nonatherosclerotic causes are more common, including channelopathies, congenital abnormalities in valves or coronary arteries, myocarditis and inflammatory disorders, cardiomyopathies, and myocardial hypertrophy secondary to hypertension and other factors.

HYPERTENSIVE HEART DISEASE

Hypertension increases the cardiac workload and also has deleterious effects on arterial vessels (see Chapter 7). The cardiac complications include congestive heart failure and fatal arrhythmia. Although the left side of the heart is most commonly affected due to the frequency of systemic hypertension, right-sided hypertensive changes *(cor pulmonale)* also occur in some disease settings.

Systemic (Left-Sided) Hypertensive Heart Disease

Systemic hypertensive heart disease is defined by left ventricular hypertrophy secondary to documented hypertension in the absence of other cardiovascular pathology (e.g., valvular stenosis).

Pathogenesis. Even mild hypertension (>140/90 mm Hg), if prolonged, induces left ventricular hypertrophy as an adaptation to the increased workload against resistance (Fig. 8.11A). If the hypertensive stress is prolonged or severe, the heart may no longer be able to adapt effectively and may begin to fail.

Morphology. The heart is heavy and the left ventricular wall is thickened. Microscopically, myocytes and myocyte nuclei are increased in size (boxcar nuclei). With failure, degenerative changes appear, including fragmentation and loss of myocyte contractile fibers. There often are scattered foci of intercellular fibrosis, representing sites of myocyte dropout due to ischemia. Initially the thickened left ventricular wall becomes stiff, impairing diastolic filling and leading to left atrial dilation, but with progression to congestive heart failure ventricular dilation appears.

Clinical Features. Early hypertensive heart disease is asymptomatic and is suspected only from the discovery of elevated blood pressure or incidentally discovered left ventricular hypertrophy. Poorly controlled hypertension increases the risk for ischemic heart disease (by potentiating coronary atherosclerosis), renal damage, cerebrovascular stroke, atrial fibrillation, heart failure, and sudden death. Effective hypertension control greatly lessens the risk of all of these complications.

Right-Sided (Pulmonary) Hypertensive Heart Disease

Right-sided hypertensive heart disease may be caused by primary disorders of the lung parenchyma or vasculature, or may occur secondary to left-sided ventricular failure or congenital heart disease associated with left-to-right shunts.

Causes of isolated right-sided hypertensive heart disease (also known as *cor pulmonale*) include diverse disorders affecting pulmonary air exchange or the pulmonary vasculature (Chapter 10). All produce increased pulmonary vascular resistance, leading to hypertension, right ventricular hypertrophy (Fig. 8.11B), and eventually right-sided heart failure. The most common such disorders are:

- *Diseases of pulmonary parenchyma,* such as chronic obstructive pulmonary disease and diffuse interstitial fibrosis
- *Diseases of pulmonary vessels,* such as recurrent thromboembolism and primary pulmonary hypertension
- *Diseases affecting chest movement,* such as kyphoscoliosis and obesity
- *Diseases causing pulmonary vascular constriction,* such as obstructive sleep apnea

Right-sided heart failure may be acute in onset (e.g., with pulmonary embolism) or may appear slowly and insidiously because of prolonged pressure overload in the setting of chronic pulmonary disease.

VALVULAR HEART DISEASE

Valvular disease results in cardiac dysfunction by causing stenosis and/or insufficiency (regurgitation or incompetence).

Stenosis is the failure of a valve to open completely, obstructing forward flow, almost always due to a chronic process (e.g., calcification or valve scarring) that affects one or more valve cusps. *Insufficiency* results from failure of a valve to close completely, allowing blood to regurgitate (backflow). Valvular insufficiency can result from disease of the valve cusps (e.g., endocarditis) or of the supporting structures (e.g., the tendinous cords or papillary muscles). Insufficiency may appear abruptly (e.g., from chordal rupture) or insidiously due to leaflet scarring and retraction. Valvular disease is much more common on the left side of the heart and is usually acquired. Causes of acquired valvular disease are summarized in Table 8.2.

Abnormal flow through diseased valves produces abnormal heart sounds called *murmurs;* severe flow abnormalities may be externally palpated as *thrills.* The location, quality, and timing of the murmur are determined by the valve affected, the effect of the lesion (regurgitation versus stenosis), and the severity of the defect.

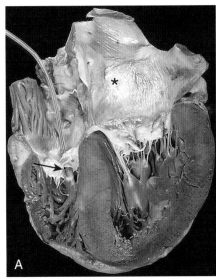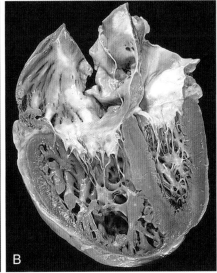

Fig. 8.11 Hypertensive heart disease. (A) Systemic (left-sided) hypertensive heart disease. There is marked concentric thickening of the left ventricular wall, causing a reduction in lumen size. The left ventricle and left atrium are shown on the *right* in this four-chamber view of the heart. A pacemaker is present incidentally in the right ventricle *(arrow)*. Note also the left atrial dilation *(asterisk)* due to stiffening of the left ventricle and impaired diastolic relaxation, leading to atrial volume overload. (B) Chronic cor pulmonale. The right ventricle *(shown on the left)* is markedly dilated and hypertrophied with a thickened free wall and hypertrophied trabeculae. The shape and volume of the left ventricle have been distorted by the enlarged right ventricle.

Table 8.2 Etiology of Acquired Heart Valve Disease

Mitral Valve Disease	Aortic Valve Disease
Mitral Stenosis	**Aortic Stenosis**
Postinflammatory scarring (rheumatic heart disease)	Postinflammatory scarring (rheumatic heart disease)
Calcification of mitral ring	Senile calcific aortic stenosis
	Calcification of congenitally deformed valve
Mitral Regurgitation	**Aortic Regurgitation**
Abnormalities of leaflets and commissures	Intrinsic valvular disease
Postinflammatory scarring	Postinflammatory scarring (rheumatic heart disease)
Infective endocarditis	Infective endocarditis
Mitral valve prolapse	Aortic disease
"Fen-phen"–induced valvular fibrosis	Degenerative aortic dilation
Abnormalities of tensor apparatus	Syphilitic aortitis
Rupture of papillary muscle	Ankylosing spondylitis
Papillary muscle dysfunction (fibrosis)	Rheumatoid arthritis
Rupture of chordae tendineae	Marfan syndrome
Abnormalities of left ventricular cavity and/or annulus	
Left ventricular enlargement (myocarditis, dilated cardiomyopathy)	
Calcification of mitral ring	

Fen-phen, Fenfluramine-phentermine.
Data from Schoen FJ: Surgical pathology of removed natural and prosthetic valves, *Hum Pathol* 18:558, 1987.

Degenerative Valve Disease

Degenerative valve disease is an umbrella term that describes changes in the valvular extracellular matrix that negatively affect valve function.

Degenerative changes in cardiac valves are related to repetitive mechanical stresses that require substantial valve deformation with each normal opening. The most common degenerative changes are:

- *Calcifications,* which can be cuspal (in the aortic valve) (Fig. 8.12A and B) or annular (in the mitral valve) (Fig. 8.12C and D).
- *Alterations in the extracellular matrix.* There can be increased proteoglycan and diminished fibrillar collagen and elastin *(myxomatous degeneration)* or fibrosis and scarring.

Calcific Aortic Degeneration

Calcific aortic degeneration is the most common cause of aortic stenosis.

Calcific degeneration usually is asymptomatic, but it may be severe enough to cause stenosis, necessitating surgical intervention. The incidence increases with age, and most patients present at the age of 70 years or greater. An important risk factor is *bicuspid aortic valve,* a congenital disorder in which the valve contains two functional cusps instead of three. Bicuspid aortic valve occurs in 1% to 2% of all live births. It is generally asymptomatic early in life but is prone to calcification leading to aortic stenosis 1 to 2 decades earlier than normal tricuspid valves.

Pathogenesis. Risk factors for aortic valve degeneration and calcification include male sex, high low-density lipoprotein cholesterol, hypertension, and smoking, all of which are also associated with atherosclerosis. The accumulation of lipoproteins induces local inflammation, which may be exacerbated by flow abnormalities (e.g., bicuspid valve, hypertension) that alter endothelial cell function. The resulting injury predisposes the valve for calcification.

Morphology. Heaped-up calcified masses on the outflow side of the cusps protrude and mechanically impede valve opening, causing stenosis (Fig. 8.12A and B). The cusps often show thickening due to fibrosis.

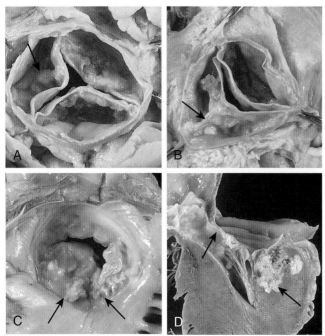

Fig. 8.12 Calcific valvular degeneration. (A) Calcific aortic stenosis of a previously normal valve (viewed from above the valve). Nodular masses of calcium are heaped up within the sinuses of Valsalva *(arrow)*. Note that the commissures are not fused, as in rheumatic aortic valve stenosis (see Fig. 11.19C). (B) Calcific aortic stenosis occurring on a congenitally bicuspid valve. One cusp has a partial fusion at its center, called a raphe *(arrow)*. (C and D) Mitral calcification, with calcific nodules within the annulus (attachment margin) of the mitral leaflets *(arrows)*. (C) Left atrial view. (D) Cut section demonstrating the extension of the calcification into the underlying myocardium. Such involvement of adjacent structures near the interventricular septum can impinge on the conduction system.

Clinical Features. In severe disease (aortic valve orifice reduced to 20% to 30% of normal), chronic outflow obstruction may raise left ventricular pressures to 200 mm Hg or more, causing left ventricular hypertrophy. The hypertrophied myocardium is prone to ischemia and systolic and diastolic dysfunction, leading to congestive heart failure. Once angina, congestive heart failure, or syncope appears, the prognosis is poor, with death usually occurring within 5 years. The treatment is surgical replacement of the diseased valve.

Myxomatous Mitral Valve Disease

In myxomatous degeneration of the mitral valve, one or both mitral leaflets are "floppy" and prolapse, ballooning back into the left atrium during systole.

Primary *mitral valve prolapse* is a form of myxomatous degeneration affecting 0.5% to 2.4% of adults. It is one of the most common forms of valvular heart disease; women are affected almost seven times more often than men.

Pathogenesis. The etiology is usually unknown (idiopathic). Rarely, it is a manifestation of a connective tissue disorder, particularly Marfan syndrome. As discussed in Chapter 6, Marfan syndrome is most commonly caused by mutation in the gene encoding fibrillin.

> *Morphology.* There is ballooning (hooding) of the affected mitral leaflets (Fig. 8.13), which are enlarged, redundant, thick, and rubbery. The tendinous cords are elongated and thinned, and may rupture. On histologic examination, the valve shows deposition of myxomatous (mucoid) material.

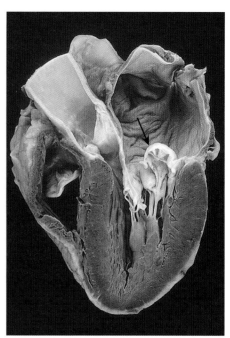

Fig. 8.13 Myxomatous degeneration of the mitral valve. There is prominent hooding with prolapse of the posterior mitral leaflet *(arrow)* into the left atrium; the atrium also is dilated, reflecting long-standing valvular insufficiency and volume overload. The left ventricle is shown on the *right* in this four-chamber view. (Courtesy of William D. Edwards, MD, Mayo Clinic, Rochester, Minnesota.)

Clinical Features. Most patients are asymptomatic; the valvular abnormality is discovered incidentally on physical examination. A minority of patients has palpitations, dyspnea, or atypical chest pain. Auscultation discloses a midsystolic click, sometimes with a regurgitant murmur. The clinical course is usually benign, though there is an increased risk of infective endocarditis (see later) and approximately 3% of patients develop hemodynamically significant mitral regurgitation and congestive heart failure, usually following rupture of the chordae or valve leaflets. Treatment requires repair or replacement of the mitral valve.

Rheumatic Valvular Disease

Rheumatic heart disease is the cardiac manifestation of rheumatic fever, an acute immunologically mediated multisystem inflammatory disease that occurs after group A β-hemolytic streptococcal infections.

The triggering infection typically involves the pharynx. Mitral stenosis, which is virtually always caused by rheumatic heart disease, is due to valvular inflammation and scarring. The incidence of rheumatic heart disease has declined in many parts of the Western world over the past several decades, due to improved socioeconomic conditions, rapid diagnosis and treatment of streptococcal pharyngitis, and a decline in the virulence of many strains of group A streptococci. However, in low income countries and economically depressed areas in the United States, rheumatic heart disease is an important public health problem, and it remains the most common cause of acquired valvular disease in the world.

Pathogenesis. Antibodies against the M proteins of certain streptococcal strains cross-react with proteins found in the myocardium and cardiac valves. These antibodies are thought to cause injury by activating complement and Fc receptor–bearing cells (e.g., macrophages). CD4+ T cells that recognize streptococcal peptides and host antigens also appear and may elicit cytokine-mediated inflammatory responses. Only about 3% of patients infected with streptococci develop rheumatic fever, suggesting that host genetic variants may influence susceptibility.

Morphology. In acute rheumatic fever, there are inflammatory foci affecting a variety of tissues, including all three layers of the heart. Acute cardiac involvement may lead to one or more of the following:

- *Pericarditis* associated with a fibrinous exudate
- *Myocarditis* in the form of scattered *Aschoff bodies* within the interstitial connective tissue; pathognomonic Aschoff bodies (Fig. 8.14A) consist of collections of lymphocytes (primarily T cells), scattered plasma cells, and plump, activated macrophages (Anitschkow cells) with associated fibrinoid necrosis
- *Valvulitis*, resulting in fibrinoid necrosis and fibrin deposition along the lines of closure, often associated with small thrombotic vegetations (Fig. 8.14B).

Pericarditis and myocarditis may lead to focal scarring but not persistent abnormalities. In contrast, valvulitis often leads to chronic rheumatic heart disease with valve dysfunction involving the mitral valve in 95% of cases; 25% of these cases also affect the aortic valve. Fibrosis of the mitral valve leaflets (Fig. 8.14C to E) leads to fusion of the commissures and severe mitral stenosis. Fibrosis and fusion of the chordae tendineae may also occur, further exacerbating valve dysfunction. With tight mitral stenosis, the left atrium progressively becomes dilated owing to pressure overload.

Clinical Features. Acute rheumatic fever is most common in children, but first attacks also occur in adults. Two to three weeks after the initial infection, there is one of two constellations of symptoms: (1) most commonly, a migratory arthritis in one or more joints often accompanied by carditis; or (2) in about 20% of patients, neurologic symptoms, most notably *Sydenham chorea* (St. Vitus dance), characterized by involuntary movements, muscle weakness, and emotional disturbances. Fever may also be seen in some cases. There is variable involvement of the skin (rash and subcutaneous nodules). Throat cultures are negative when symptoms begin, but serum titers

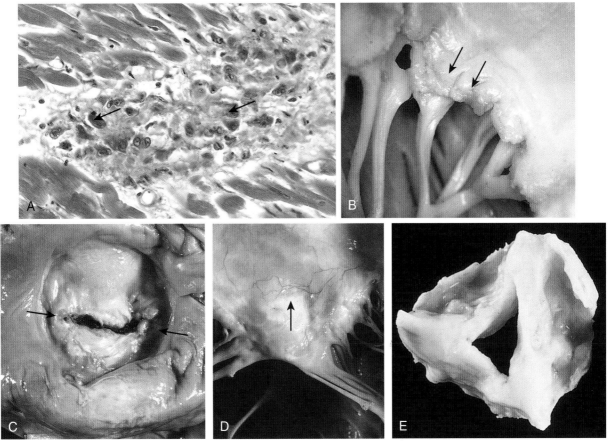

Fig. 8.14 Rheumatic heart disease. (A) Microscopic appearance of an Aschoff body in acute rheumatic carditis; there is central necrosis associated with a circumscribed collection of mononuclear inflammatory cells, including some activated macrophages with prominent nucleoli and central wavy (caterpillar) chromatin *(arrows)*. (B) Acute rheumatic mitral valvulitis superimposed on chronic rheumatic heart disease. Small vegetations (verrucae) are visible along the line of closure of the mitral valve leaflet *(arrows)*. Previous episodes of rheumatic valvulitis have caused fibrous thickening and fusion of the chordae tendineae. (C and D) Mitral stenosis with diffuse fibrous thickening and distortion of the valve leaflets, commissural fusion *(arrows)*, and thickening and shortening of the chordae tendineae. There is marked left atrial dilation as seen from above the valve (C). (D) Anterior leaflet of an opened rheumatic mitral valve; note the inflammatory neovascularization *(arrow)*. (E) Surgically removed specimen of rheumatic aortic stenosis, demonstrating thickening and distortion of the cusps with commissural fusion. (E, From Schoen FJ, St John-Sutton M: Contemporary issues in the pathology of valvular heart disease, *Hum Pathol* 18:568, 1967.)

of antibodies against streptococcal antigens (e.g., streptolysin O or DNase) usually are elevated. Clinical signs of carditis include pericardial friction rubs, cardiac dilation, mitral insufficiency, and congestive heart failure, but less than 1% of patients die of acute rheumatic fever. The diagnosis is made based on evidence of prior streptococcal infection in conjunction with the typical clinical features described earlier.

After acute disease subsides, reactivation may occur with subsequent streptococcal infections, causing additional injury to the heart (carditis) and mitral valve (mitral stenosis). With mitral stenosis, atrial dilation often leads to atrial fibrillation, increasing the risk of mural thrombi in the left atrium and thromboembolism. Chronic pulmonary venous congestion produces the pulmonary vascular and parenchymal changes of left-sided heart failure; with time, right ventricular hypertrophy and right-sided heart failure may ensue. In addition, scarred and deformed valves are more susceptible to infective endocarditis. Mitral valvuloplasty or surgical repair or replacement of diseased valves can forestall many of these complications and has greatly improved the outlook for these patients.

Infective Endocarditis

Infective endocarditis is a microbial infection of the heart valves or the endocardium marked by the presence of vegetations composed of thrombus and organisms that lead to varying degrees of damage to underlying cardiac tissues.

The aorta, aneurysmal sacs, other blood vessels, and prosthetic devices may also become infected. Most cases are caused by bacterial infections. Infective endocarditis is classified as acute or subacute based on the tempo and severity of the clinical course.

- *Acute endocarditis* refers to destructive infections by highly virulent organisms that may involve previously normal valves. Morbidity and mortality are significant, even with appropriate antibiotic therapy and/or surgery.
- *Subacute endocarditis* refers to infections by organisms of low virulence in a previously abnormal heart, usually involving scarred or deformed valves. The onset is insidious and even when untreated the course is protracted over weeks to months. Most patients recover after appropriate antibiotic therapy.

Pathogenesis. Acquired structural abnormalities of heart valves (such as rheumatic mitral stenosis, mitral valve prolapse, and aortic stenosis) as well as prosthetic heart valves predispose to infective endocarditis.

Small thrombi that form at sites of pacemaker lines, indwelling vascular catheters, or damaged endocardium provide a fertile soil for bacterial seeding and ensuing endocarditis. Increased susceptibility to bacterial infections (e.g., secondary to neutropenia and intravenous drug abuse) also increases the risk and adversely affects outcomes.

The causative organisms vary depending on the underlying risk factors. From 50% to 60% of cases of endocarditis of damaged or deformed valves are caused by *Streptococcus viridans,* a component of the normal oral flora. By contrast, the more virulent *Staphylococcus aureus* (common to the skin) can attack healthy as well as deformed valves and is responsible for 10% to 20% of cases overall; it also is the major offender in infections occurring in intravenous drug users. Many other bacterial species, often commensal in the oral cavity, and even fungi on occasion prove to be the culprit. In about 10% of cases, no organism is isolated from the blood, probably because organisms embedded within vegetations are released into the blood in very small numbers.

Seeding of the blood with microbes is the proximate cause. This may occur due to an obvious or occult infection, a dental or surgical procedure, injection of contaminated material into the bloodstream by intravenous drug users, or trivial injuries. Antibiotic prophylaxis is critical in patients with predisposing factors (e.g., prosthetic heart valves) undergoing dental or surgical procedures.

Morphology. In acute endocarditis, bulky and potentially destructive vegetations containing fibrin, neutrophils, and microorganisms are present on the heart valves (Fig. 8.15). The aortic and mitral valves are the most common sites of infection except in intravenous drug users, in which the tricuspid valve is frequently involved. Vegetations sometimes erode into the underlying myocardium to produce an abscess *(ring abscess)* (see Fig. 8.15B). Septic emboli are shed from the friable vegetations, leading to septic infarcts and abscess formation where they lodge. Seeding to the vessel walls may lead to the development of *mycotic aneurysms* (see Chapter 7). Subacute endocarditis elicits less valvular destruction and is associated with formation of vegetations, chronic inflammatory infiltrates, and valvular fibrosis and calcification.

Clinical Features. Fever is the most consistent sign of infective endocarditis, but it may be absent in subacute disease (particularly in older adults), in which only vague symptoms such as fatigue,

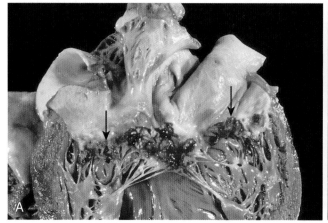
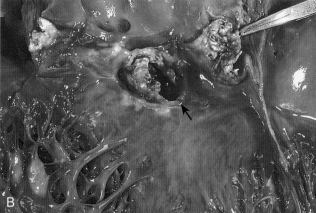

Fig. 8.15 Infective endocarditis. (A) Subacute endocarditis caused by *Streptococcus viridans* on a previously myxomatous mitral valve. The large, friable vegetations are denoted by *arrows.* (B) Acute endocarditis caused by *Staphylococcus aureus* on a congenitally bicuspid aortic valve with extensive cuspal destruction and ring abscess *(arrow).*

weight loss, and a flulike syndrome are found. By contrast, acute endocarditis often has a stormy onset with rapidly developing fever, chills, and weakness. Murmurs are present in 90% of patients with left-sided lesions. Microemboli can give rise to petechiae, nail bed and retinal hemorrhages, painless erythematous palm or sole lesions, or painful fingertip nodules. The diagnosis is confirmed by positive blood cultures and the identification of vegetations by echocardiography.

The prognosis depends on the infecting organism and the extent of complications. Adverse sequelae include glomerulonephritis due to trapping of antigen–antibody complexes in glomeruli (see Chapter 11), septicemia, arrhythmia (from invasion into the underlying myocardium and conduction system), and systemic embolization. Left untreated, infective endocarditis generally is fatal. Appropriate long-term (6 weeks or more) antibiotic therapy and/or valve replacement reduce mortality rates. For infections involving low-virulence organisms (e.g., S. viridans), the cure rate is 98%, and for S. aureus infections, cure rates range from 60% to 90%; however, with infections due to aerobic gram-negative bacilli or fungi, half of patients ultimately succumb.

Nonbacterial Thrombotic Endocarditis

Nonbacterial thrombotic endocarditis (NBTE) is characterized by the deposition of small (1 to 5 mm), sterile, nondestructive thrombotic masses on cardiac valves (Supplemental eFig. 8.3).

Previous valvular damage is not a prerequisite. Indeed, it typically occurs on previously normal valves. Diseases associated with general debility or wasting are associated with an increased risk for NBTE, as are hypercoagulable states (e.g., chronic disseminated intravascular coagulation, hyperestrogenic states, and underlying malignancies, particularly mucinous adenocarcinomas) and endocardial trauma (e.g., indwelling catheter). The local effect on the valve is usually trivial, but emboli from NBTE lesions can cause infarcts in the brain, heart, and other organs. NBTE lesions also increase the risk of infective endocarditis.

CARDIOMYOPATHIES AND MYOCARDITIS

These diseases are characterized by cardiac myocyte dysfunction that may be confined to the myocardium (primary) or may be a cardiac manifestation of a systemic disorder (secondary).

Included among the diverse diseases that lead to myocyte dysfunction are infectious, immunologic, metabolic, and genetic disorders. Those that are inflammatory in nature are generally considered forms of myocarditis, whereas those that are noninflammatory fall into the category of cardiomyopathies, which can be further subdivided into three more or less distinct functional and pathologic patterns (Fig. 8.16 and Table 8.3):
- Dilated cardiomyopathy
- Hypertrophic cardiomyopathy
- Restrictive cardiomyopathy

Of these patterns, dilated cardiomyopathy is most common and restrictive cardiomyopathy least common.

Dilated Cardiomyopathy

Dilated cardiomyopathy is characterized by progressive cardiac dilation and contractile (systolic) dysfunction.

Pathogenesis. At diagnosis, dilated cardiomyopathy has usually progressed to end-stage disease marked by heart failure secondary to poor myocardial contractility. The damage that culminates in end-stage dilated cardiomyopathy can be initiated by inherited abnormalities or by environmental exposures, as follows:

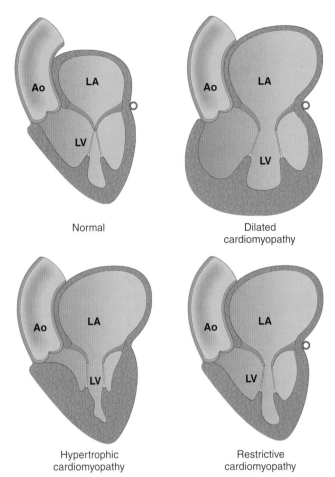

Fig. 8.16 The three major forms of cardiomyopathy. Dilated cardiomyopathy leads primarily to systolic dysfunction, whereas restrictive and hypertrophic cardiomyopathies result in diastolic dysfunction. Note the changes in atrial and/or ventricular dilation and in ventricular wall thickness. Ao, aorta; LA, left atrium; LV, left ventricle.

- *Inherited gene defects.* Dilated cardiomyopathy is hereditary in 20% to 50% of cases. Mutations in over 50 genes have been implicated, usually with autosomal dominant inheritance. Genes that encode cytoskeletal proteins or proteins that link the sarcomere to the cytoskeleton are most commonly involved, typically by mutations that result in loss-of-function.
- *Infection.* Coxsackievirus B and other enteroviruses are occasionally detected in the myocardium of end-stage dilated cardiomyopathy, and instances in which infectious myocarditis has progressed to dilated cardiomyopathy have been documented. By the time of diagnosis, inflammation is absent.
- *Alcohol and other toxins.* Rarely, alcohol abuse is associated with the development of dilated cardiomyopathy, by unknown mechanisms. Toxic agents, such as doxorubicin and related chemotherapeutic drugs, can also cause dilated cardiomyopathy.
- *Peripartum cardiomyopathy.* Dilated cardiomyopathy occurs late in gestation or several weeks to months postpartum. The etiology is uncertain and may be multifactorial. Approximately half of these patients spontaneously recover normal function.
- *Iron overload.* Dilated cardiomyopathy can be seen in the setting of hereditary hemochromatosis, chronic ineffective hematopoiesis, or multiple red cell transfusions due to injury caused by iron deposition in the heart and iron-mediated production of reactive oxygen species.

Table 8.3 Cardiomyopathies: Functional Patterns and Causes

Functional Pattern	Left Ventricular Ejection Fraction[a]	Mechanisms of Heart Failure	Causes	Secondary Myocardial Dysfunction (Mimicking Cardiomyopathy)
Dilated	<40%	Impairment of contractility (systolic dysfunction)	Genetic; alcohol; peripartum; myocarditis; hemochromatosis; chronic anemia; doxorubicin (Adriamycin); sarcoidosis; idiopathic	Ischemic heart disease; valvular heart disease; hypertensive heart disease; congenital heart disease
Hypertrophic	50% to 80%	Impairment of compliance (diastolic dysfunction)	Genetic; Friedreich ataxia; storage diseases; infants of diabetic mothers	Hypertensive heart disease; aortic stenosis
Restrictive	45% to 90%	Impairment of compliance (diastolic dysfunction)	Amyloidosis; radiation-induced fibrosis; idiopathic	Pericardial constriction

[a]Range of normal values is approximately 50% to 65%.

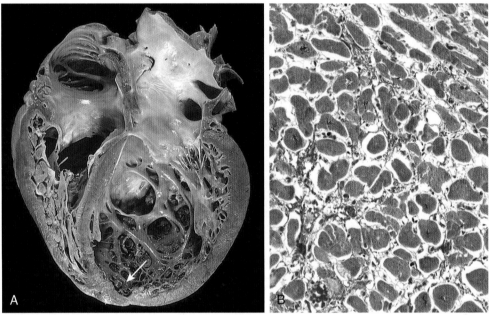

Fig. 8.17 Dilated cardiomyopathy (DCM). (A) Four-chamber dilation and hypertrophy are evident. A small mural thrombus can be seen at the apex of the left ventricle *(arrow)*. (B) The nonspecific histologic picture in typical DCM, with myocyte hypertrophy and interstitial fibrosis (collagen is *blue* in this Masson trichrome–stained preparation).

Morphology. The heart characteristically is enlarged (up to two to three times the normal weight) and flabby, with dilation of all chambers (Fig. 8.17A). Mural thrombi are often present and may be a source of thromboemboli. The histologic abnormalities are nonspecific (Fig. 8.17B) and consist of myocyte hypertrophy, enlargement of myocyte nuclei, and variable endocardial and interstitial fibrosis; the latter may correspond to small areas of myocyte necrosis and dropout caused by hypoperfusion.

Clinical Features. Patients are usually between 20 and 50 years of age and present with slowly progressive congestive heart failure and poor exercise capacity. In end-stage disease, the cardiac ejection fraction is less than 25% (normal, 50% to 65%) and mitral regurgitation and abnormal cardiac rhythms are common. One half of patients die within 2 years, and only 25% survive longer than 5 years. Death is usually due to progressive cardiac failure or arrhythmia. Cardiac transplantation is the only definitive treatment.

Hypertrophic Cardiomyopathy

Hypertrophic cardiomyopathy is characterized by ventricular hypertrophy leading to defective diastolic filling and obstruction of the ventricular outflow tract.

Pathogenesis. Most cases are caused by "gain-of-function" missense mutations in one of several genes encoding proteins that are part of the contractile apparatus. The net effect of these mutations is to increase myocyte contractility. The pattern of transmission usually is autosomal dominant, with variable expressivity.

Morphology. The heart is thick-walled and heavy without ventricular dilation (Fig. 8.18A). Usually, there is disproportionate thickening of the ventricular septum relative to the left ventricle free wall. Bulging of the enlarged septum during systole impinges on the anterior mitral leaflet, producing variable degrees of left ventricular outflow tract obstruction. The characteristic histologic features are marked myocyte hypertrophy, myocyte and myofiber disarray, and interstitial fibrosis (Fig. 8.18B).

Clinical Features. Hypertrophic cardiomyopathy typically manifests during the postpubertal growth spurt. Following systole, the myocardium does not fully relax, which limits ventricular filling during diastole. This, combined with functional obstruction of the ventricular outflow tract, decreases the effectiveness of cardiac pumping. The diastolic filling defect and variable outflow obstruction lead to a secondary increase in pulmonary venous pressure, causing

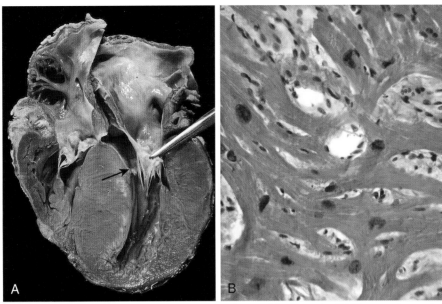

Fig. 8.18 Hypertrophic cardiomyopathy with asymmetric septal hypertrophy. (A) The septal muscle bulges into the left ventricular outflow tract, giving rise to a banana-shaped ventricular lumen, and the left atrium is enlarged. The anterior mitral leaflet has been moved away from the septum to reveal a fibrous endocardial plaque *(arrow)* (see text). (B) Histologic appearance demonstrating disarray, extreme hypertrophy, and characteristic branching of myocytes, as well as interstitial fibrosis.

exertional dyspnea. The outflow obstruction may produce a harsh systolic ejection murmur. Massive hypertrophy and high left-ventricular pressures that compromise the delivery of blood by intramural arteries frequently lead to myocardial ischemia and angina, even in the absence of coronary artery disease. Major complications include atrial fibrillation with mural thrombus formation, infective endocarditis of the mitral valve, congestive heart failure, and ventricular fibrillation leading to sudden cardiac death. Sudden death, particularly common in young athletes, is sometimes the first manifestation of the disease. Drugs that promote ventricular relaxation provide symptomatic relief, and outflow tract obstruction can be relieved by surgical excision or the controlled infarction of septal muscle induced by chemical injections.

Restrictive Cardiomyopathy

Restrictive cardiomyopathy is caused by disorders that increase the stiffness of the ventricular wall, resulting in impaired ventricular filling during diastole.

This type of cardiomyopathy is most commonly associated with systemic disorders that affect the myocardium. Three forms of restrictive cardiomyopathy merit brief mention:

- *Amyloidosis.* Cardiac amyloidosis (see Chapter 4) can occur in the setting of systemic amyloidosis or can be restricted to the heart (Supplemental eFig. 8.4). Amyloid in the latter is derived from normal or mutant forms of transthyretin (a liver-synthesized circulating protein that transports thyroxine and retinol) and usually occurs in older adults.
- *Endomyocardial fibrosis* is an idiopathic disease that affects children and young adults in Africa and other tropical areas. There is dense diffuse fibrosis of the ventricular endocardium and subendocardium, often involving the tricuspid and mitral valves. Worldwide, it is the most common form of restrictive cardiomyopathy.
- *Loeffler endomyocarditis* also exhibits endocardial fibrosis, typically associated with formation of large mural thrombi. It is characterized by eosinophilia and eosinophilic tissue infiltrates. The

eosinophilia can be primary (sometimes as part of a myeloid neoplasm) or secondary (e.g., to helminthic infection). Major basic protein release from eosinophil granules is thought to cause endocardial and myocardial necrosis, leading to scarring and mural thrombosis.

Morphology. In restrictive cardiomyopathy the ventricles are of normal size or only slightly enlarged, the cavities are not dilated, and the myocardium is firm. Both atria are typically dilated as a consequence of reduced ventricular filling and pressure overload. Microscopic findings vary according to the cause, and may include interstitial amyloid deposits; tissue eosinophilia; interstitial and endomyocardial fibrosis; and mural thrombosis.

Myocarditis

Myocarditis encompasses a diverse group of clinical entities in which infectious agents and/or inflammatory processes primarily target the myocardium.

Pathogenesis. In the United States, viral infections are the most common cause of myocarditis, with coxsackieviruses A and B and other enteroviruses accounting for a majority of the cases. Myocyte death may stem from direct cytopathic effects of the virus or may be caused by the immune response to virally infected cells. In some instances, it is suspected that viruses trigger a cross-reactive immune reaction against host proteins such as the myosin heavy chain.

Nonviral causes of myocarditis include Chagas disease, Lyme disease, and hypersensitivity reactions induced by drugs and autoimmune disorders. *Chagas disease* is caused by the protozoan *Trypanosoma cruzi* and affects up to one half of the population in endemic areas of South America, with myocardial involvement in the vast majority. About 10% of the patients die during an acute attack; in others, immunologically mediated injury leads to congestive heart failure and arrhythmias 10 to 20 years later. *Lyme disease,* a systemic illness caused by the spirochete *Borrelia burgdorferi,* causes myocarditis in approximately 5% of patients, which may result in self-limited conduction system dysfunction and arrhythmias that may necessitate temporary pacemaker insertion.

Morphology. In acute myocarditis, the heart may appear normal or may be dilated; in advanced stages, the myocardium typically is dilated and is often mottled by pale and hemorrhagic areas. Mural thrombi may be present. *Viral myocarditis* is characterized by edema, interstitial lymphocytic infiltrates, and myocyte injury (Fig. 8.19A). If the patient survives the acute phase of myocarditis, lesions can resolve without significant sequelae or heal by progressive fibrosis. In *hypersensitivity myocarditis,* interstitial and perivascular infiltrates include numerous eosinophils (Fig. 8.19B). *Giant cell myocarditis,* a distinctive entity thought to be mediated by autoreactive T cells, is characterized by widespread inflammatory cell infiltrates containing multinucleate giant cells (Fig. 8.19C) and carries a poor prognosis. In *Chagas myocarditis,* trypanosomes may be seen in scattered myofibers, particularly in acute disease, and there is an inflammatory infiltrate of neutrophils, lymphocytes, macrophages, and occasional eosinophils (Fig. 8.19D) that is centered on areas where there is histologic or molecular evidence of parasitic infection.

Clinical Features. The clinical spectrum of myocarditis is broad, ranging from a lack of symptoms and complete recovery to precipitous onset of heart failure or arrhythmia, sometimes causing sudden death. Between these extremes are modest levels of cardiac dysfunction with fatigue, pain, and fever. Patients may recover completely or develop dilated cardiomyopathy.

Other Causes of Myocardial Disease

Exposures to various drugs and certain hormones have been linked to myocyte injury and dysfunction:

- *Cardiotoxic drugs.* Cardiac complications of cancer therapy are important clinical problems. Agents associated with cardiotoxicity include conventional chemotherapeutic agents, targeted drugs (e.g., tyrosine kinase inhibitors), and immunotherapeutic agents (e.g., immune checkpoint inhibitors, which may induce severe myocarditis). Doxorubicin and daunorubicin are often associated with toxic myocardial injury and may cause heart failure. Recovery is the rule following the discontinuation of such agents, but dilated cardiomyopathy may occur.
- *Catecholamines.* High levels of catecholamines may injure myocytes, leading to focal myocardial necrosis. This type of injury may be seen in the setting of pheochromocytoma (a tumor that elaborates catecholamines; see Chapter 16), cocaine use, autonomic stimulation secondary to intracranial lesions, and administration of vasopressor agents such as dopamine. The

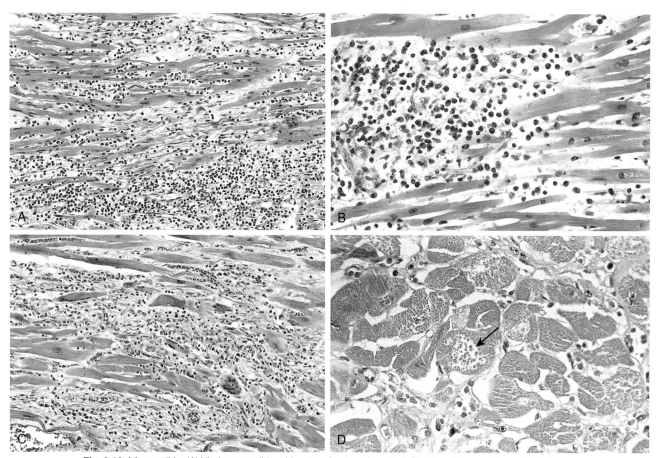

Fig. 8.19 Myocarditis. (A) Viral myocarditis with extensive lymphocytic infiltrate, edema, and associated myocyte injury. (B) Hypersensitivity myocarditis, characterized by perivascular eosinophil-rich inflammatory infiltrates. (C) Giant cell myocarditis, with lymphocyte and macrophage infiltrates, extensive myocyte damage, and multinucleate giant cells. (D) Chagas myocarditis. A myofiber distended with trypanosomes *(arrow)* is present, along with mononuclear inflammation and myofiber necrosis.

mechanism is uncertain but may be related to direct toxic effects of catecholamines on myocytes or to catecholamine-induced vasospasm and ischemia.

CONGESTIVE HEART FAILURE

Congestive heart failure is the common endpoint for many forms of cardiac disease, is usually progressive, and carries a poor prognosis.

In the United States alone, more than 5 million individuals are affected, with well over 1 million hospitalizations per year. Roughly one half of patients die within 5 years. Overall, heart failure is a contributory cause in 1 in 9 deaths in the United States.

Pathogenesis. Congestive heart failure usually occurs when cardiac damage limits the heart's ability to meet the metabolic demands of peripheral tissues at normal filling pressures. In a minority of cases, it is a consequence of increased tissue demands, as in hyperthyroidism, or a decreased oxygen-carrying capacity (so-called high-output failure, usually associated with severe chronic anemia). The onset can be abrupt, as in the setting of a myocardial infarct or acute valve dysfunction, but in most cases it develops insidiously owing to the cumulative effects of chronic work overload or progressive loss of myocardial function. It can be divided into several categories according to the underlying cause:
- *Systolic failure* results from inadequate myocardial contractility, most commonly as a consequence of ischemic heart disease or hypertension.
- *Diastolic failure* refers to an inability of the heart to adequately relax and fill, as in marked left ventricular hypertrophy, restrictive cardiomyopathies, or constrictive pericarditis. Approximately half of cases of congestive heart failure are attributable at least in part to diastolic dysfunction, with a greater frequency seen in obese individuals, older adults, diabetic patients, and women. Although we distinguish between systolic and diastolic heart failure, in most cases both coexist.
- *Valve dysfunction* (e.g., due to endocarditis or rheumatic heart disease) can lead to the failure of an otherwise normal heart. Depending on the affected valve and the consequence of the valve disease (insufficiency versus stenosis), failure secondary to valve disease may stem from pressure overload (e.g., aortic stenosis) or volume overload (e.g., mitral valve insufficiency).

Regardless of the mechanism, the failure of the heart to pump blood efficiently leads to increased end-diastolic ventricular volumes, increased end-diastolic pressures, and elevated venous pressures. Thus, inadequate cardiac output, called *forward failure*, is almost always accompanied by congestion of the venous circulation, that is, *backward failure*. Although the root problem is deficient cardiac function, virtually every other organ is eventually affected by some combination of forward and backward failure.

Once failure appears, compensatory mechanisms ensue:
- *The Frank-Starling mechanism.* Increased end-diastolic filling volumes dilate the heart, stretching cardiac myofibers; these lengthened fibers contract more forcibly, thereby increasing the cardiac output. If the dilated ventricle is able to maintain cardiac output by this means, the patient is said to be in *compensated heart failure.* However, ventricular dilation comes at the expense of increased wall tension and increased oxygen requirements. With time and disease progression, the patient develops *decompensated heart failure.*
- *Activation of neurohumoral feedback loops.* Lack of adequate perfusion of various tissues induces the release of norepinephrine by the autonomic nervous system and activates the renin–angiotensin–aldosterone system. This increases the heart rate and contractility,

increases the vascular tone, and spurs water and salt retention. The latter often is counterproductive, however, because it increases the blood volume and worsens the venous congestion.
- *Myocardial structural changes, including hypertrophy.* Cardiac myocytes adapt to increased workloads by assembling new sarcomeres, leading to myocyte hypertrophy. The increase in ventricular mass carries a risk of possible ischemic injury because the myocardial capillary bed does not expand sufficiently.

These compensatory mechanisms may be effective for a time, but the usual course is one of progressively worsening failure. Early in the course, heart failure often preferentially involves only one side of the heart, leading to isolated left- and right-sided heart failure (discussed next). In most cases of chronic heart failure, there is biventricular dysfunction with signs and symptoms of both right-sided and left-sided heart failure.

Left-Sided Heart Failure
The effects of left-sided heart failure stem from diminished systemic perfusion and elevated back pressures within the pulmonary circulation.

Pathogenesis. The most common causes of left-sided failure are ischemic heart disease, systemic hypertension, mitral or aortic valve disease, and primary diseases of the myocardium (e.g., amyloidosis).

Morphology. The principal morphologic findings are in the heart and the lungs, as follows:
- *Heart.* With the exception of failure due to mitral valve stenosis or restrictive cardiomyopathies, the left ventricle is hypertrophied and may be dilated, sometimes massively. Left ventricular dilation can result in mitral insufficiency and left atrial enlargement, often associated with atrial fibrillation and mural thrombosis.
- *Lungs.* In acute left heart failure, increased pulmonary vein pressures are transmitted back to the capillaries and arteries of the lungs, resulting in congestion, edema, and pleural effusions due to increased hydrostatic pressure in pleural venules. Microscopically, there are perivascular and interstitial transudates, alveolar septal edema, and intraalveolar edema fluid. In chronic left heart failure, red cells extravasate into alveoli, where they are phagocytosed by macrophages that become laden with hemosiderin *(heart failure cells).*

Clinical Features. Dyspnea (shortness of breath) on exertion is usually the earliest and most prominent symptom of left-sided heart failure. Cough occurs due to transudates in air spaces. As failure progresses, patients experience dyspnea when recumbent *(orthopnea)* because the supine position increases venous return from the lower extremities and elevates the diaphragm. Sitting relieves orthopnea, and patients usually sleep in a semiseated position. *Paroxysmal nocturnal dyspnea* is a dramatic form of breathlessness, awakening patients from sleep with a feeling of suffocation. Other manifestations include heart enlargement (cardiomegaly), tachycardia, and fine rales at the lung bases, caused by the opening of edematous pulmonary alveoli. With progressive ventricular dilation, the papillary muscles are displaced, causing mitral regurgitation and a systolic murmur. Subsequent chronic dilation of the left atrium can cause *atrial fibrillation,* reducing the atrial contribution to ventricular filling, further reducing the ventricular stroke volume, and causing stasis, with its attendant risk of thrombosis (particularly in the atrial appendage) and embolism.

Systemically, diminished cardiac output activates the renin–angiotensin–aldosterone axis, increasing the intravascular volume and pressures and exacerbating pulmonary edema. Reduced renal perfusion may lead to *renal failure,* and with severe congestive heart failure, diminished cerebral perfusion can manifest as *hypoxic encephalopathy,* with irritability, diminished cognition, and restlessness that can progress to stupor and coma.

Right-Sided Heart Failure

Right-sided heart failure is usually the consequence of left-sided heart failure, because any pressure increase in the pulmonary circulation inevitably produces an increased burden on the right side of the heart.

Pathogenesis. Causes of right-sided heart failure include all of those that induce left-sided heart failure. Isolated right-sided heart failure *(cor pulmonale)* is infrequent and typically is due to disorders that cause pulmonary hypertension (e.g., parenchymal lung diseases, primary pulmonary hypertension, recurrent pulmonary thromboembolism, or conditions that cause pulmonary vasoconstriction such as obstructive sleep apnea). Pulmonary hypertension results in hypertrophy and dilation of the right side of the heart. In cor pulmonale, myocardial hypertrophy and dilation generally are confined to the right ventricle and atrium, although bulging of the ventricular septum can impede left ventricular output by causing outflow tract obstruction.

> *Morphology.* The major morphologic features of pure right-sided heart failure differ from those of left-sided heart failure in that engorgement of the systemic and portal venous systems typically is pronounced and pulmonary congestion is minimal. The liver usually is increased in size and weight *(congestive hepatomegaly).* A cut section displays prominent passive congestion of centrilobular areas, a pattern referred to as *nutmeg liver* (see Chapter 3). When left-sided heart failure is also present, severe central hypoxia produces *centrilobular necrosis,* and with long-standing severe right-sided heart failure, the central areas can become fibrotic, creating so-called *cardiac cirrhosis.* Right-sided heart failure may also lead to *portal hypertension, congestive splenomegaly,* and congestion and edema of the bowel wall, causing malabsorption. Elevated venous pressures cause pleural, pericardial, and peritoneal effusions and peripheral edema in the skin, particularly in dependent portions of the body.

Clinical Features. Pure right-sided heart failure typically is associated with few respiratory symptoms. Instead, its manifestations are related to systemic and portal venous congestion, as listed previously. In addition, venous congestion and hypoxia of the kidneys and brain due to right-sided heart failure can produce deficits comparable to those caused by hypoperfusion in left-sided heart failure.

CARDIAC TUMORS

Primary tumors of the heart are uncommon, and most are benign. Only *myxoma,* the most common primary tumor of the adult heart, is described here. The vast majority of myxomas occur in the left atrium. They usually are between 2 and 6 cm in diameter and may be sessile or pedunculated (Supplemental eFig. 8.5). The latter are sufficiently mobile to swing into the mitral or tricuspid valve during systole, causing intermittent obstruction and damage to valve leaflets over time (ball valve obstruction). Clinical symptoms arise from valvular obstruction, embolization of fragments, and, in some cases, a systemic syndrome of fever and malaise due to the elaboration of interleukin 6.

9

Hematopoietic and Lymphoid Systems

OUTLINE

Red Blood Cell Disorders, 137
Anemias, 137
    Hemolytic Anemias, 137
    Underproduction Anemias, 143
White Blood Cell Disorders, 146
Nonneoplastic Disorders of White Cells, 146
    Leukopenia, 146
    Reactive Leukocytosis, 146
Neoplastic Proliferations of White Cells, 147
    Acute Leukemias, 148
    Myelodysplastic Syndromes, 150
    Myeloproliferative Neoplasms, 150

Non-Hodgkin Lymphomas and Chronic Lymphoid Leukemias, 151
Hodgkin Lymphoma, 156
Plasma Cell Neoplasms and Related Entities, 157
Histiocytic Neoplasms, 158
Bleeding Disorders, 158
    Thrombocytopenia, 159
    Coagulation Disorders, 160
Disorders of Spleen and Thymus, 162
Splenomegaly, 162
Disorders of the Thymus, 162
    Thymic Follicular Hyperplasia, 162
    Thymoma, 162

The hematopoietic and lymphoid systems are affected by a wide spectrum of diseases, which can be subdivided based on whether they primarily affect red cells, white cells, or the hemostatic system (platelets and coagulation factors). We will organize our discussion accordingly, recognizing that disorders that primarily affect one component of the hematolymphoid system often secondarily impact others. In addition, we will briefly discuss disorders of the spleen and (because of their link to certain immunologic disorders) disorders of the thymus.

RED BLOOD CELL DISORDERS

ANEMIAS

Anemia, one of the most common disorders of humans, is a state of red cell deficiency that lowers the oxygen-carrying capacity of the blood.

Anemia may result from blood loss, increased red cell destruction (hemolysis), or decreased red cell production. Hemolytic anemias can be further subclassified based on whether they are caused by defects that are intrinsic or extrinsic to the red cell. These mechanisms provide one basis for classifying anemias (Table 9.1).

Clinical Features. Careful assessment of red cell morphology and red cell indices helps to narrow the diagnostic possibilities. The mean cell volume (MCV; the average volume per red cell) distinguishes the microcytic (low MCV), normocytic (normal MCV), and macrocytic (high MCV) anemias, which typically have distinct causes (Table 9.2). In isolated anemia, peripheral blood tests usually suffice to establish the cause. When anemia occurs in concert with thrombocytopenia and/or granulocytopenia, a marrow disorder (e.g., aplasia or infiltration by a neoplasm) is likely and a bone marrow examination is often warranted.

Pallor, fatigue, and lassitude are common to all forms of anemia. If the onset is slow, the deficit in oxygen-carrying capacity is partially compensated for by adaptive increases in plasma volume, cardiac output, respiratory rate, and other metabolic changes that increase oxygen delivery

to tissues. Other clinical consequences of anemia are determined by its severity, rapidity of onset, and underlying pathogenic mechanism, and will be discussed under the specific entities that follow.

Hemolytic Anemias

Hemolytic anemias are a diverse group of disorders that have as a common feature accelerated red cell destruction (hemolysis).

The red cell life span is shortened below its normal 120 days, leading to anemia and attendant tissue hypoxia. Oxygen-sensing cells in the kidney respond by increasing the production of erythropoietin, stimulating the proliferation of marrow erythroid elements and increasing red cell production. Thus, hyperplasia of marrow erythroid precursors and increased numbers of newly released red cells *(reticulocytes)* in the blood are hallmarks of hemolytic anemias.

Pathogenesis. Most hemolytic anemias are caused by intrinsic red cell defects or damage induced by extrinsic factors that increase red cell destruction by phagocytes, particularly in the spleen. Because the red cells are removed from the circulation by phagocytes, this is referred to as *extravascular hemolysis.* Findings that are relatively specific for extravascular hemolysis include the following:

- *Hyperbilirubinemia and jaundice,* due to degradation of hemoglobin in macrophages
- *Splenomegaly* due to "work hyperplasia" of phagocytes in the spleen
- *Bilirubin-rich gallstones* (pigment stones), because bilirubin is a breakdown product of hemoglobin, and an increased risk of cholecystitis secondary to bile duct obstruction

Intravascular hemolysis is caused by injuries that are so severe that red cells burst within the circulation. These may be caused by mechanical forces (e.g., turbulent blood flow) or biochemical or physical agents that damage the red cell membrane. Findings that distinguish intravascular hemolysis from extravascular hemolysis include:

- *Hemoglobinemia and hemoglobinuria.* Hemoglobin released into the circulation passes into the urinary space and is oxidized to methemoglobulin, leading to brownish discoloration of the urine.

Table 9.1 Classification of Anemia According to Underlying Mechanism

Blood Loss
Acute
Trauma
Chronic
Gastrointestinal tract lesions, gynecologic disturbances
Increased Destruction (Hemolytic Anemias)
Intrinsic (Intracorpuscular) Abnormalities
Hereditary   Membrane abnormalities (e.g., hereditary spherocytosis)
Enzyme deficiencies (e.g., glucose-6-phosphate dehydrogenase)
Disorders of hemoglobin synthesis
Structurally abnormal globin synthesis (hemoglobinopathies): sickle cell anemia
Deficient globin synthesis: thalassemia syndromes
Acquired   Membrane defect: paroxysmal nocturnal hemoglobinuria (rare)
Extrinsic (Extracorpuscular) Abnormalities
Antibody-mediated   Nonautoantibodies: transfusion reactions, hemolytic disease of the fetus and newborn
Autoantibodies
Mechanical trauma to red cells
Microangiopathic hemolytic anemias (e.g., disseminated intravascular coagulation)
Defective cardiac valves
Infections: malaria
Impaired Red Cell Production
Disturbed proliferation and differentiation of stem cells: aplastic anemia
Disturbed proliferation and maturation of erythroblasts
Defective DNA synthesis: vitamin B_{12} and folic acid deficiency (megaloblastic anemias)
Anemia of renal failure (erythropoietin deficiency)
Anemia of chronic inflammation (iron sequestration, relative erythropoietin deficiency)
Marrow replacement: primary hematopoietic neoplasms (acute leukemia, myelodysplastic syndromes)
Marrow infiltration (myelophthisic anemia): metastatic neoplasms, granulomatous disease

Table 9.2 Microcytic, Normocytic, and Macrocytic Anemias

Microcytic Anemia (Causes and Characteristic Laboratory Findings)	
Iron deficiency	Low serum iron, low serum ferritin, high serum transferrin
Thalassemia	High serum iron, high serum ferritin, normal serum transferrin
Normocytic Anemia (Causes and Characteristic Findings)	
Anemia of chronic inflammation	Elevated red cell sedimentation rate, low serum iron, high serum ferritin, normal or low serum transferrin
Anemia of renal failure	Elevated creatinine and blood urea nitrogen
Hereditary spherocytosis	Evidence of hemolysis, spherocytic red cells
Immunohemolytic anemia	Evidence of hemolysis, spherocytic red cells, direct Coombs test positive
Mechanical destruction of red cells	Evidence of hemolysis, red cell fragments (schistocytes) in peripheral blood
Sickle cell anemia	Evidence of hemolysis, sickled red cells in peripheral blood
Anemia of marrow infiltration	Teardrop-shaped red cells, nucleated red cells, early white cell progenitors in peripheral blood (leukoerythrocytosis)
Malaria, babesiosis	Evidence of hemolysis, organisms seen within red cells
G6PD deficiency	Evidence of hemolysis, red cells with "bites"
Macrocytic Anemia (Causes and Characteristic Laboratory Findings)	
Folate, Vitamin B_{12} deficiency	Macroovalocytic red cells, hypersegmented neutrophils, megaloblastic marrow progenitors
Myelodysplastic syndromes	Dysplastic marrow progenitors and peripheral blood elements
Aplastic anemia	Pancytopenia
Liver disease, alcoholism	Target red cells in peripheral blood smears

- *Hemosiderinuria and loss of iron.* Hemoglobin absorbed by renal tubular cells is processed into hemosiderin and lost when renal cells slough into the urine.

Laboratory findings shared by intravascular and extravascular hemolytic anemias include *reticulocytosis* (increased immature red cells, called reticulocytes, in the peripheral blood), *elevated serum lactate dehydrogenase* (an enzyme released from lysed red cells), and *decreased serum levels of haptoglobin* (a plasma protein that binds free hemoglobin).

Hemolytic anemias are less common than underproduction anemias (discussed later), but several are of pathogenic interest and merit consideration.

Hereditary Spherocytosis

Hereditary spherocytosis is caused by inherited defects in red cell membrane skeleton proteins that lead to membrane loss and the formation of spherocytes that lose deformability.

Pathogenesis. The inheritance of hereditary spherocytosis (HS) is usually autosomal dominant. In peripheral blood smears, spherocytes lack central pallor (Fig. 9.1). The cells cannot pass through the narrow slit-like openings that separate the splenic red pulp

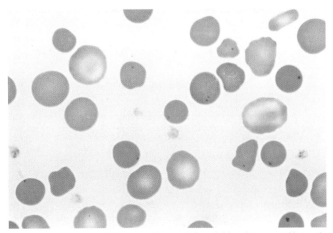

Fig. 9.1 Hereditary spherocytosis: peripheral blood smear. Note the anisocytosis and several hyperchromic spherocytes. Howell-Jolly bodies (small nuclear remnants) are also present in the red cells of this asplenic patient. (Courtesy of Dr. Robert W. McKenna, Department of Pathology, University of Texas Southwestern Medical School, Dallas.)

from the splenic venous circulation, resulting in extravascular hemolysis. Splenectomy improves the anemia, but not the underlying genetic defect, hence spherocytes remain in the blood.

Clinical Features. The diagnosis depends on the family history, the evidence of extravascular hemolysis, the presence of spherocytes in peripheral smears, and other tests. Following splenectomy, patients have an excellent prognosis but are at risk for sepsis with encapsulated bacteria due to the loss of splenic function. They also are prone to aplastic crises during infections by parvovirus B19, which infects and kills erythroid progenitors in the marrow. This infection is rapidly cleared by the immune system and has no consequences in normal individuals, but it leads to rapidly worsening anemia in HS and other hemolytic anemia patients in whom the red cell half-life is markedly decreased.

Sickle Cell Anemia

Sickle cell anemia, a prototypical hemoglobinopathy, is an autosomal recessive disorder caused by a single amino acid substitution in β-globin that creates sickle hemoglobin.

Sickle cell anemia is the most common familial hemolytic anemia. In parts of Africa, the gene frequency approaches 30%, apparently because of a protective effect of sickle hemoglobin (HbS) against malaria in heterozygotes. In the United States, approximately 8% of patients of African descent are heterozygous HbS carriers and about 1 in 600 has sickle cell anemia.

Pathogenesis. Sickle cell anemia is caused by a mutation in β-globin that leads to the polymerization of sickle hemoglobin (HbS) into long, stiff chains when it is deoxygenated. As a result, the cell assumes an elongated sickle shape but it returns to its normal shape when oxygenated (Fig. 9.2). The most important variable that determines whether HbS-containing red cells undergo sickling is the intracellular concentration of other hemoglobins. In heterozygotes, approximately 60% of hemoglobin is normal HbA, which interacts only weakly with deoxygenated HbS and retards HbS polymerization; as a result, heterozygotes with HbS are generally asymptomatic (they are said to have the sickle cell trait). Fetal hemoglobin (HbF) also interacts weakly with HbS; this explains why newborns with sickle cell anemia are asymptomatic until the HbF levels fall at 5 to 6 months of age.

Sickling of red cells in patients with sickle cell anemia has two major consequences: (1) chronic hemolytic anemia and (2) episodic pain crises associated with ischemic tissue damage (Fig. 9.3). Hemolysis stems from repeated sickling, which damages the red cell membrane, eventually

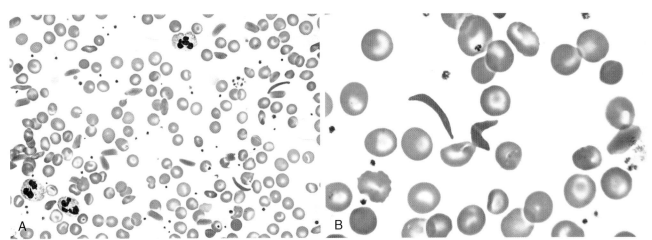

Fig. 9.2 Sickle cell anemia: peripheral blood smear. (A) Low magnification shows sickle cells, anisocytosis, poikilocytosis, and target cells. (B) Higher magnification shows an irreversibly sickled cell in the center. (Courtesy of Dr. Robert W. McKenna, Department of Pathology, University of Texas Southwestern Medical School, Dallas.)

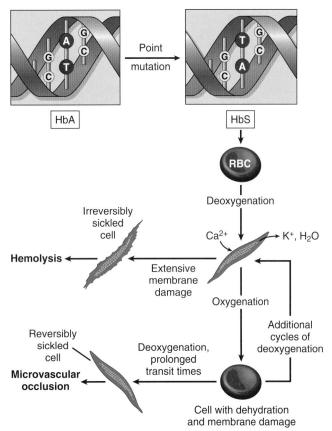

Fig. 9.3 Pathophysiology of sickle cell disease. HbA, hemoglobin A; HbS, sickled hemoglobin; RBC, red blood cell.

producing irreversibly sickled cells that are rapidly removed from the circulation. Pain crises are caused by localized obstruction of the microvasculature by sickled red cells. These obstructions are largely confined to tissues in which blood flow is sluggish, such as the spleen, the marrow, and inflamed tissues, where the transit time of red cells through capillaries exceeds the time required for sickling of cells following deoxygenation.

Clinical Features. In sickle cell disease, irreversibly sickled cells can be seen in peripheral blood smears. In heterozygotes, sickling is induced in vitro by exposing cells to hypoxic conditions. The presence of HbS is confirmed by hemoglobin electrophoresis.

Obstruction of blood flow in the spleen leads to splenic autoinfarction, markedly increasing the risk for sepsis with encapsulated bacteria. Additional complications include life-threatening sickling crises of the lung (acute chest syndrome) following pulmonary infections; stroke; and retinal damage that may lead to blindness. Hydroxyurea raises HbF levels and has antiinflammatory effects, both of which decrease the incidence of pain crises.

Thalassemias

Thalassemias are inherited disorders caused by mutations in globin genes that result in decreased synthesis of α- or β-globin. The associated anemia results from reduced hemoglobin synthesis and hemolysis due to an imbalance in globin chain synthesis.

Thalassemia is common in Mediterranean, African, and Asian regions in which malaria is endemic; the associated mutations may protect against falciparum malaria.

Pathogenesis. A diverse collection of α-globin and β-globin mutations causes severe forms of thalassemia, which is an autosomal codominant

condition. Adult hemoglobin, or HbA, is a tetramer composed of two α chains and two β chains. The α chains are encoded by two α-globin genes lying in tandem on chromosome 16, whereas the β chains are encoded by a single β-globin gene located on chromosome 11. Much of the variation in α- and β-thalassemias is due to the inheritance of different combinations of mutated alleles (Table 9.3).

- *β-Thalassemia.* There are two types of alleles, distinguished by different single-base mutations: (1) β^0 alleles, which produce no β-globin and (2) β^+ alleles, which produce reduced amounts of β-globin. Persons inheriting one abnormal allele have β-thalassemia minor (also known as β-thalassemia trait). Most people inheriting any two β^0 and β^+ alleles have β-thalassemia major, but occasionally persons inheriting at least one β^+ allele have a milder disease termed β-thalassemia intermedia.

  The defective synthesis of β-globin contributes to anemia in two ways: (1) the inadequate formation of HbA results in microcytic, poorly hemoglobinized red cells and (2) the excess unpaired α-globin chains form toxic precipitates that damage the membranes of erythroid precursors, most of which die by apoptosis (Fig. 9.4) (ineffective erythropoiesis). The red cells that are produced have membrane damage, leading to hemolysis. Factors released from erythroid progenitors indirectly increase the absorption of dietary iron, leading to iron overload (discussed later).

- *α-Thalassemia.* α-Thalassemia is caused by deletion of one or more of the α-globin genes; disease severity is proportional to the number of α-globin genes that are deleted (see Table 9.3). Excess β-globin and γ-globin chains form relatively stable β_4 and γ_4 tetramers known as HbH and Hb Barts, respectively, which cause less membrane damage than free α-globin chains. Ineffective erythropoiesis and hemolysis are less pronounced in HbH disease than in β-thalassemia. However, both HbH and Hb Barts deliver oxygen inefficiently to tissues.

Morphology. In β-thalassemia minor and α-thalassemia trait, abnormalities are confined to the peripheral blood. Red cells are small *(microcytic)* and pale *(hypochromic)* but normal in shape. β-thalassemia major red cells show marked *microcytosis, hypochromia, anisocytosis* (variation in cell size), and *poikilocytosis* (variation in cell shape). Nucleated red cells (normoblasts) also are seen in the peripheral blood. β-Thalassemia intermedia and HbH disease show features between these two extremes. In β-thalassemia major, hyperplastic erythroid progenitors fill the marrow, invade the bony cortex, impair bone growth, and produce skeletal deformities. *Extramedullary hematopoiesis* results in prominent splenomegaly, hepatomegaly, and lymphadenopathy. HbH disease and β-thalassemia intermedia are associated with a lesser degree of splenomegaly, erythroid hyperplasia, and growth retardation.

Clinical Features. The diagnosis is based on the family history, peripheral blood findings, and laboratory tests. Hemoglobin electrophoresis can detect abnormal hemoglobins such as HbH, as well as HbA_2, a minor hemoglobin that is often increased in β-thalassemia. Clinical features vary widely:

- *β-Thalassemia trait* and *α-thalassemia trait* patients are typically asymptomatic and have mild microcytic anemia.
- *β-Thalassemia major* manifests postnatally when HbF synthesis diminishes. Increased numbers of red cell precursors consume nutrients, causing growth retardation and cachexia. Survival into adulthood is possible with transfusions and treatment with an iron chelator, which prevents iron overload and associated cardiac dysfunction. Hematopoietic stem cell transplantation at an early age is the treatment of choice.
- *HbH disease* and *β-thalassemia intermedia* are not as severe as β-thalassemia major. Anemia is moderate and patients usually do not require transfusions.

Table 9.3 Clinical and Genetic Classification of Thalassemias

Clinical Syndrome	Genotype	Clinical Features	Molecular Genetics
β-Thalassemias			
β-Thalassemia major	Homozygous β-thalassemia (β^0/β^0, β^+/β^+, β^0/β^+)	Severe anemia; regular blood transfusions required	Mainly point mutations that lead to defects in the transcription, splicing, or translation of β-globin mRNA
β-Thalassemia intermedia	Variable (β^0/β^+, β^+/β^+, β^0/β, β^+/β)	Severe anemia, but regular blood transfusions not required	
β-Thalassemia minor	Heterozygous β-thalassemia (β^0/β, β^+/β)	Asymptomatic with mild or absent anemia; red cell abnormalities seen	
α-Thalassemias			
Silent carrier	$-/\alpha$, α/α	Asymptomatic; no red cell abnormality	Mainly gene deletions
α-Thalassemia trait	$-/-$, α/α (Asian) $-/\alpha$, $-/\alpha$ (black African, Asian)	Asymptomatic, like β-thalassemia minor	
HbH disease	$-/-$, $-/\alpha$	Severe; resembles β-thalassemia intermedia	
Hydrops fetalis	$-/-$, $-/-$	Lethal in utero without transfusions	

HbH, hemoglobin H; mRNA, messenger ribonucleic acid.

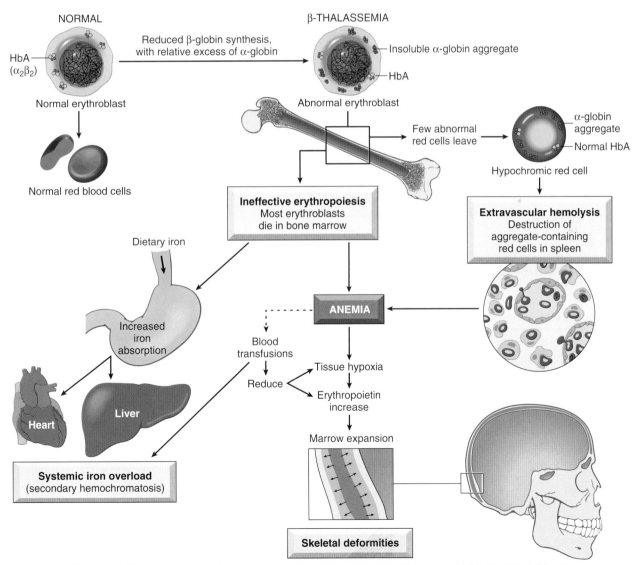

Fig. 9.4 Pathogenesis of β-thalassemia major. Note that aggregates of excess α-globin are not visible on routine blood smears. Blood transfusions constitute a double-edged sword, diminishing the anemia and its attendant complications but also adding to the systemic iron overload. HbA, hemoglobin A.

Glucose-6-Phosphate Dehydrogenase (G6PD) Deficiency

Mutations that cause G6PD deficiency decrease the half-life of G6PD protein, leaving older red cells at risk for oxidant damage and intravascular hemolysis.

G6PD deficiency is an X-linked disorder that affects approximately 10% of black males in the United States. G6PD is an enzyme needed for the synthesis of reduced glutathione (GSH), which participates in the elimination of potentially injurious reactive oxygen species. The enzyme deficiency results in cell damage caused by exposure to free radicals. All cells in the body express mutated G6PD, but the disorder manifests only in red cells because they lack the capacity to synthesize new proteins. Thus, the aging red cells of affected patients become severely G6PD deficient and are particularly susceptible to oxidant-induced damage and lysis.

Hemolysis in G6PD deficiency is episodic and follows exposures that increase the production of oxidants, particularly acute infections and exposure to certain drugs. A characteristic finding in peripheral smears is "bite" cells, red cells with severely damaged membranes that have portions "bitten off" by macrophages removing patches of membrane with associated hemoglobin precipitates known as Heinz bodies, leading to intravascular hemolysis (Supplemental eFig. 9.1). The hemolysis is often transient, even with persistent infection or drug exposure, because lysis of older cells leaves younger cells with higher levels of G6PD that are resistant to oxidant stress.

Immunohemolytic Anemia

Immunohemolytic anemia is caused by antibodies that bind to antigens found on red cell membranes.

The pathogenic antibodies may arise spontaneously or be induced by exogenous agents such as drugs or chemicals. Immunohemolytic anemia is classified on the basis of (1) the nature of the antibody and (2) the presence of predisposing conditions (summarized in Table 9.4). Thus, the anemia may be primary (idiopathic) or secondary to other disorders of the immune system. In most instances, the bound antibodies act as opsonins and the hemolysis is extravascular. The direct Coombs test detects antibodies and/or complement on red cells and is therefore positive. Depending on the cause and the severity of the hemolysis, treatment may involve immunosuppression, removal of suspected triggers, or treatment of underlying conditions.

Hemolytic Disease of the Fetus and Newborn

This disorder results from an antibody-induced hemolytic anemia caused by blood group incompatibility between the mother and the fetus.

Pathogenesis. Red cell incompatibility occurs when the fetus inherits red cell antigenic determinants from the father that are foreign to the mother. Fetal red cells often enter the maternal circulation during the last trimester of pregnancy or during childbirth (fetomaternal bleed), sensitizing the mother to paternal red cell antigens and leading to the production of anti–red cell

Table 9.4   Classification of Immunohemolytic Anemias

Warm Antibody Type (active at 37°C)
Primary (idiopathic)
Secondary: B-cell neoplasms (e.g., chronic lymphocytic leukemia), autoimmune disorders (e.g., systemic lupus erythematosus), drugs (e.g., α-methyldopa, penicillin, quinidine)

Cold Antibody Type (active at temperatures lower than core body temperature)
Acute: *Mycoplasma* infection, infectious mononucleosis
Chronic: idiopathic, B-cell lymphoid neoplasms (e.g., lymphoplasma-cytic lymphoma)

antibodies that cross the placenta and cause hemolysis of fetal red cells. Most cases of hemolytic disease of the fetus and newborn occur in pregnancies in which the fetus expresses RhD antigen and the mother is RhD antigen negative, or in which there is ABO antigen incompatibility between the fetus and the mother. Generally, the first antigen-incompatible pregnancy does not produce disease because the mother does not produce anti–red cell IgG antibodies (the type that crosses the placenta) before delivery. The risk rises with each subsequent incompatible pregnancy owing to memory B cells that respond rapidly when they are reexposed to antigen. IgG-mediated lysis of fetal red cells leads to progressive anemia, tissue ischemia, intrauterine cardiac failure, and peripheral edema, and may be fatal in severe cases.

Rh-negative mothers are treated with Rh immune globulin (RhIg) at 28 weeks and within 72 hours after delivery of an Rh-positive baby. The RhIg masks the antigenic sites on the fetal red cells and prevents sensitization to Rh antigens. As a result, ABO incompatibility is now the most common cause of hemolytic disease of the fetus and newborn. ABO incompatibility occurs in approximately 20% to 25% of pregnancies, but hemolysis develops in only a small fraction of subsequent pregnancies, primarily in certain group O women who make IgG antibodies directed against group A or B antigens (or both) that cross the placenta and reach the fetal circulation. In general, the disease is much milder than Rh incompatibility, in part because many cells other than red cells express A and B antigens and thus adsorb some of the transferred antibodies. There is no effective method of preventing hemolytic disease resulting from ABO incompatibility.

Mechanical Trauma to Red Cells

Intravascular hemolysis of red cells due to their exposure to abnormal mechanical forces occurs in two settings.

- *Traumatic hemolysis* due to defective cardiac valve prostheses, which may shear red cells (the blender effect), or an activity resulting in repeated physical pounding of one or more body parts (e.g., marathon racing, bongo drumming, karate).
- *Microangiopathic hemolytic anemia* occurs when small vessels become narrowed by thrombi. Most frequently, this is due to disseminated intravascular coagulation (DIC) (described later), in which vessels are narrowed by the intravascular deposition of fibrin, and thrombotic thrombocytopenic purpura and hemolytic-uremic syndrome, in which vessels are narrowed by platelet-rich thrombi. The clinical significance of microangiopathic hemolysis is that it often indicates a serious underlying condition.

Mechanically fragmented red cells (schistocytes) are easily recognized in peripheral blood smears, where they take on the appearance of burr cells, helmet cells, and triangle cells (Fig. 9.5).

Malaria

It is estimated that malaria affects 500 million and kills more than 400,000 people per year, making it one of the most widespread afflictions of humans.

Malaria is transmitted by the bite of *Anopheles* mosquitoes and is endemic in Asia and Africa; due to widespread jet travel, cases are seen worldwide. Of the five causative *Plasmodium* species, *Plasmodium falciparum* is the most important because it causes a serious disorder with a high fatality rate.

Pathogenesis. When mosquitoes feed on humans, sporozoite forms are introduced that infect liver cells, where they multiply as merozoites and are then released to infect red cells (Fig. 9.6). Intraerythrocytic parasites either continue asexual reproduction as trophozoites or give rise to gametocytes that are capable of infecting the next hungry mosquito. The asexual phase is complete when the trophozoites give rise to new merozoites, which escape by lysing the red cells.

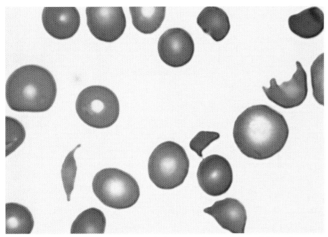

Fig. 9.5 Microangiopathic hemolytic anemia: peripheral blood smear. This specimen from a patient with hemolytic uremic syndrome contains several fragmented red cells. (Courtesy of Dr. Robert W. McKenna, Department of Pathology, University of Texas Southwestern Medical School, Dallas.)

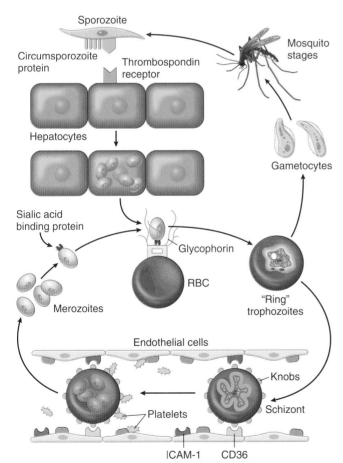

Fig. 9.6 Life cycle of *Plasmodium falciparum*. Entry of sporozoites into hepatocyes is mediated through binding to the thrombospondin receptor, whereas merozoites recognize and gain entry into red cells by binding glycophorin. Arrest of infected red cells in capillaries is mediated by interactions with CD36 and ICAM-1 expressed on endothelial cells. ICAM-1, intercellular adhesion molecule-1; RBC, red blood cell. (Drawn by Dr. Jeffrey Joseph, Department of Pathology, Beth Israel Deaconess Hospital, Boston.)

Infection of red cells with *P. falciparum* induces surface knobs containing parasite-encoded proteins that bind to adhesion molecules on activated endothelium, trapping infected red cells in postcapillary venules. In some patients, mainly children, this process involves cerebral vessels, which become engorged and occluded by the entrapped red cells.

Clinical Features. Clinical features commonly seen in falciparum malaria include hemolytic anemia, splenomegaly, and episodic shaking, chills, and fever, which occur during the release of organisms from lysed red cells. Intraerythrocytic trophozoites seen in peripheral blood smears are diagnostic. Cerebral malaria, seen in *P. falciparum* infection, may lead to coma and death and is a leading killer of children in some parts of Africa.

Underproduction Anemias

Like hemolytic anemias, anemias stemming from decreased red cell production have diverse etiologies, including inherited and acquired causes, and are commonly seen. They range in severity from laboratory abnormalities of minor clinical significance to life-threatening disorders that require rapid diagnosis and treatment. We will start our discussion with underproduction anemias related to inflammation, and then move to nutritional deficiencies, the most important of which are deficiencies of iron, folate, and vitamin B_{12} (cobalamin).

Anemia of Chronic Inflammation

Anemia associated with chronic inflammation is the most common form of anemia in hospitalized patients.

This type of anemia occurs in a variety of disorders associated with sustained inflammation, including:

- Chronic *bacterial infections*, such as osteomyelitis, bacterial endocarditis, disseminated tuberculosis, and lung abscess
- Chronic *immune disorders*, such as poorly controlled rheumatoid arthritis and inflammatory bowel disease
- *Cancer*, particularly when disseminated

Pathogenesis. The anemia of chronic inflammation is caused in large part by increases in circulating levels of hepcidin, a critical regulator of iron metabolism. Hepcidin is a small protein made by hepatocytes. It inhibits the activity of ferroportin, an iron transporter that is expressed on duodenal epithelial cells and on macrophages. Hepcidin production by the liver is normally inversely related to iron levels. In iron deficiency (discussed later), hepcidin levels fall, ferroportin activity rises, and iron uptake from the gut and iron mobilization from macrophage stores increases (Fig. 9.7). However, hepcidin expression is also increased by inflammatory mediators such as interleukin-6 (IL-6), independent of the iron status of the patient. Thus, inflammation decreases iron uptake and also prevents release of iron from macrophages, "starving" developing red blood cells of iron. Chronic inflammation also blunts erythropoietin synthesis by the kidney through different mechanisms, further lowering marrow red cell output.

Clinical Features. As in anemia of iron deficiency, serum iron levels usually are low and red cells may be slightly hypochromic and microcytic. Unlike iron deficiency anemia, however, storage iron in the marrow is increased, the serum ferritin concentration is elevated, and the total iron-binding capacity is normal or reduced. Administration of erythropoietin and iron can improve the anemia, but only effective treatment of the underlying condition is curative.

Iron Deficiency Anemia

Deficiency of iron is the most common nutritional deficiency in the world.

About 10% of people living in higher income countries and 25% to 50% of those in lower income countries are anemic, and in both settings

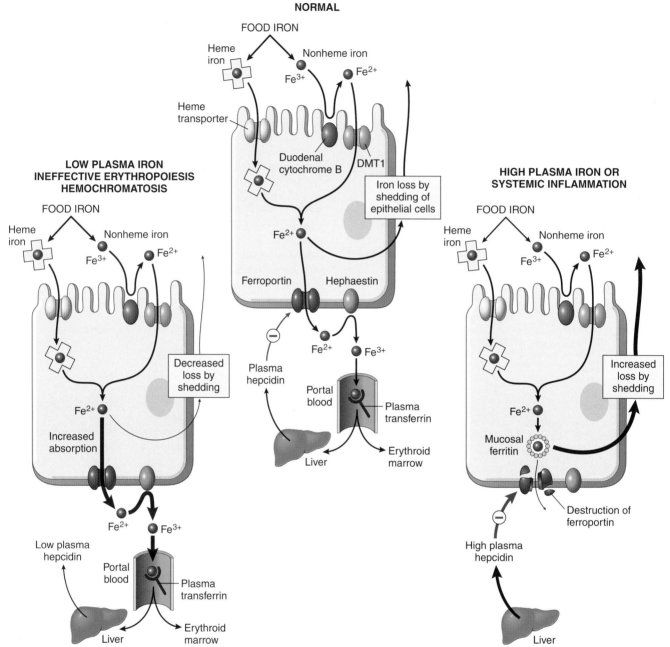

Fig. 9.7 Regulation of iron absorption. Duodenal epithelial cell uptake of heme and nonheme iron discussed in the text is depicted. When the storage sites of the body are replete with iron and erythropoietic activity is normal, plasma hepcidin balances iron uptake and loss to maintain iron hemostasis by downregulating ferroportin and limiting iron uptake *(middle panel)*. Hepcidin rise in the setting of systemic inflammation or when iron levels are high, decreasing iron uptake and increasing iron loss by shedding of duodenocytes *(right panel)*, and fall in the setting of low plasma iron or primary hemochromatosis, resulting in increased iron uptake. DMT1, divalent metal transporter-1.

the most frequent cause is iron deficiency, though the etiology differs. The normal Western diet is rich in heme from meat and poultry and contains sufficient iron to balance daily losses, which total about 2 mg/day. Thus, in the West, iron deficiency is mostly due to excessive bleeding (e.g., menorrhagia, occult gastrointestinal malignancy) or increased physiologic requirements (e.g., pregnancy). In contrast, in other parts of the world the dietary supply of iron is marginal at best and dietary iron deficiency is more common and more severe.

Pathogenesis. Iron is required for hemoglobin synthesis; iron deficiency impairs red cell maturation and diminishes red cell production. Accordingly, iron deficiency produces a microcytic hypochromic anemia.

Morphology. Peripheral smears reveal small (microcytic) red cells with increased central pallor (Fig. 9.8). Oblong, cylindrical red cells *(pencil cells)* are commonly seen and are characteristic of iron deficiency.

Clinical Features. Iron deficiency anemia is usually mild and asymptomatic; weakness, listlessness, and pallor are present in severe cases. With long-standing iron deficiency anemia, patients may demonstrate pica, a drive to consume non–foodstuffs such as dirt or clay. Laboratory studies reveal microcytic anemia, low serum ferritin and low serum iron levels, and elevated transferrin levels. When the cause of iron

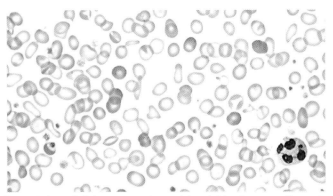

Fig. 9.8 Iron deficiency anemia: peripheral blood smear. Note the increased central pallor of most of the red cells. Scattered, fully hemoglobinized cells, from a recent blood transfusion, stand out in contrast. (Courtesy of Dr. Robert W. McKenna, Department of Pathology, University of Texas Southwestern Medical School, Dallas.)

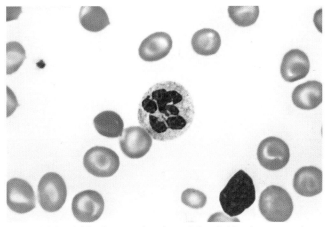

Fig. 9.9 Megaloblastic anemia. A peripheral blood smear shows a hypersegmented neutrophil with a six-lobed nucleus. (Courtesy of Dr. Robert W. McKenna, Department of Pathology, University of Texas Southwestern Medical School, Dallas.)

deficiency is not obvious, a thorough clinical evaluation is warranted to exclude an occult gastrointestinal malignancy or other sources of bleeding.

Folate and Vitamin B₁₂ Deficiency Anemias (Megaloblastic Anemias)

Deficiencies of folate and vitamin B_{12} result in anemias caused by metabolic defects in the biosynthesis of thymidine, one of the essential building blocks of DNA.

The net effects of the folate and vitamin B_{12} deficiencies on hematopoiesis are identical, but their causes and consequences differ in important ways. We will first review commonalities and then touch on distinctive features.

Pathogenesis. The functions of folate and vitamin B_{12} with respect to thymidine synthesis are intertwined. Folate exists in several forms that act as donors or acceptors of one-carbon units. For folate to participate in the synthesis of deoxythymidine monophosphate (dTMP), an essential building block for DNA, it needs to be converted from dihydrofolate to tetrahydrofolate. If intracellular stores of tetrahydrofolate fall due to folate deficiency, insufficient dTMP is synthesized and DNA replication is blocked. Vitamin B_{12} is required for the recycling of folate to tetrahydrofolate; thus its deficiency also leads to inadequate synthesis of dTMP.

Thymidine deficiency affects all rapidly dividing cells, but the hematopoietic marrow is most severely affected. The synthesis of RNA and cytoplasmic elements proceeds normally and outpaces that of the nucleus *(nuclear-cytoplasmic asynchrony)*. The defect in DNA synthesis contributes to anemia in two ways: (1) incomplete replication of DNA activates cell cycle checkpoints and induces apoptosis of marrow progenitors *(ineffective hematopoiesis)* and (2) cells that mature do so after fewer cell divisions, diminishing marrow output. Red cell precursors are most severely affected, but granulocytes and platelet precursors also show effects.

Morphology. In all forms of megaloblastic anemia, the marrow is hypercellular and contains numerous megaloblastic erythroid progenitors. Megaloblasts are larger than normal erythroid progenitors (normoblasts) and have delicate, fine nuclear chromatin. As megaloblasts differentiate and acquire hemoglobin, the nucleus retains its finely distributed chromatin and fails to undergo the chromatin clumping typical of normoblasts. Granulocyte and megakaryocyte

precursors also demonstrate nuclear-cytoplasmic asynchrony, yielding giant metamyelocytes and megakaryocytes with large, bizarre multilobed nuclei.

Characteristically, the peripheral blood contains *hypersegmented neutrophils* (**Fig. 9.9**). Normal neutrophils have three or four nuclear lobes, but in megaloblastic anemias they often have five or more. Red cells may appear as large, egg-shaped *macroovalocytes,* and the MCV is markedly elevated (*macrocytosis*). Megaloblastic morphologic changes are also seen in other rapidly growing cells, particularly cells of the gastrointestinal epithelium.

We now turn to specific features of folate and B_{12} deficiencies.

Folate Deficiency Anemia. Folate is present in nearly all foods but is destroyed by 10 to 15 minutes of cooking; as a result, folate stores are marginal in many healthy persons. The risk of deficiency is highest in those with a poor diet (the poor, indigent, and elderly) or with increased metabolic needs (pregnant women and those with chronic hemolytic anemia). Deficiency also may result from defects in folate absorption or metabolism. Food folates are predominantly in polyglutamate form and must be split into monoglutamates for absorption, a process that is inhibited by acidic foods and substances found in beans and other legumes. Some drugs also interfere with folate absorption, and others, such as methotrexate, inhibit folate metabolism. Malabsorptive disorders, such as celiac disease, that affect the upper third of the small intestine where folate is absorbed, also may impair folate uptake.

Clinical Features. The onset of the anemia of folate deficiency is insidious, being associated with nonspecific symptoms such as weakness and easy fatigability. The clinical picture may be complicated by the coexistence of other vitamin deficiencies, especially in alcoholics. Symptoms referable to the alimentary tract, such as sore tongue, also are common. The diagnosis is based on the recognition of the presence of megaloblastic anemia and the measurement of serum or red cell folate levels. The anemia responds rapidly (in 3 to 5 days) to treatment with folate.

Vitamin B_{12} (Cobalamin) Deficiency Anemia. Vitamin B_{12} is widely present in foods, is resistant to cooking and boiling, and is even synthesized by gut flora. Thus, unlike folate, vitamin B_{12} deficiency is not caused by inadequate intake except in vegetarians who scrupulously avoid milk and eggs. Instead, deficiencies typically arise from an abnormality of vitamin B_{12} absorption. Normally, vitamin B_{12} must bind to the *intrinsic factor* secreted by gastric parietal cells for absorption; the B_{12}–intrinsic factor complex then binds to a receptor for intrinsic factor in the distal ileum and enters ileal epithelial cells. Vitamin B_{12} is stored in the liver and hepatic reserves are usually sufficient to support bodily needs for 5 to 20 years. Because of these large liver stores, clinical manifestations usually follow years of unrecognized malabsorption.

Pathogenesis. The most frequent cause of vitamin B_{12} deficiency is *pernicious anemia*, due to an autoimmune attack on the gastric mucosa associated with the loss of parietal cells and intrinsic factor production. The serum of most affected patients contains several types of autoantibodies against intrinsic factor, but it is thought that an autoreactive T-cell response initiates gastric mucosal injury and triggers the formation of autoantibodies. Other causes of vitamin B_{12} malabsorption include gastrectomy, ileal resection, and disorders that disrupt the function of the distal ileum (such as Crohn disease). In addition, gastric atrophy and achlorhydria may interfere with the production of acid and pepsin, which help release vitamin B_{12} from its bound form in food.

Clinical Features. The hematopoietic manifestations of vitamin B_{12} deficiency are identical to those seen with folate deficiency. Unique to vitamin B_{12} deficiency are neurologic symptoms, which may be present even when anemia is absent, and include psychiatric disorders (such as depression) and demyelination of the lateral tracts of the spinal cord. Spinal cord disease begins with symmetric numbness, tingling, and burning in the feet or hands, followed by ataxia and loss of position sense. The diagnosis is based on the recognition of megaloblastic anemia and/or characteristic neurologic findings and the measurement of serum vitamin B_{12} levels. Treatment usually consists of parenteral vitamin B_{12} because the underlying defect in absorption (regardless of cause) is likely to persist. Although the anemia resolves rapidly following vitamin B_{12} therapy, the neurologic manifestations often fail to respond.

Aplastic Anemia

Aplastic anemia is a disorder caused by suppression of multipotent hematopoietic stem cells, leading to bone marrow hypocellularity and pancytopenia.

Pathogenesis. The marrow in aplastic anemia is often devoid of recognizable hematopoietic elements (Supplemental eFig. 9.2). There are two major etiologies: an extrinsic, immune-mediated suppression of marrow progenitors and an intrinsic abnormality of stem cells. In the former, it is thought that stem cells are antigenically altered by exposure to drugs, infectious agents, or other insults, provoking a cellular immune response in which activated T cells produce cytokines that suppress and kill hematopoietic progenitors. T-cell immunosuppressive therapy restores hematopoiesis in 60% to 70% of patients. Alternatively, a role for an intrinsic stem cell abnormality is supported by observations showing that 5% to 10% of patients with aplastic anemia have inherited defects in telomerase, which is needed for the maintenance and stability of chromosomes. The defect in telomerase may lead to premature senescence of hematopoietic stem cells and marrow failure. These two mechanisms are not mutually exclusive, because genetically altered stem cells (e.g., those with abnormal telomeres) also might express "neoantigens" that could serve as targets for a T-cell attack.

Clinical Features. Aplastic anemia affects persons of all ages and both sexes. The slowly progressive anemia causes the insidious development of weakness, pallor, and dyspnea. Thrombocytopenia often manifests with petechiae and ecchymoses, and neutropenia may result in serious infections. The prognosis is unpredictable. Withdrawal of an inciting drug only rarely leads to remission. Immunosuppression can restore hematopoiesis, but many patients develop a myeloid neoplasm

(discussed later), consistent with the idea that the marrow progenitors have genomic damage. Hematopoietic stem cell transplantation often is curative, particularly in younger patients.

Anemia due to Marrow Infiltration

Anemia due to marrow infiltration is caused by replacement of the marrow by tumors or other lesions.

Anemia due to marrow infiltration is most commonly associated with metastatic breast, lung, or prostate cancer, but can also be seen in advanced tuberculosis and lipid storage disorders. Misshapen red cells, some resembling teardrops, are seen in the peripheral blood. Immature granulocytic and erythrocytic precursors also may be present (*leukoerythroblastosis*), along with mild leukocytosis. The principal manifestations include anemia and thrombocytopenia; the white cell series is less affected. Treatment is directed at the underlying condition.

WHITE BLOOD CELL DISORDERS

Disorders of white cells include deficiencies (leukopenias) and proliferations, which may be reactive or neoplastic. Reactive proliferation in response to a primary, often infectious, disease is common. Neoplastic disorders, although less common, are more ominous. They cause approximately 9% of cancer deaths in adults and 40% in children younger than 15 years of age.

Presented next are descriptions of some nonneoplastic conditions, followed by more detailed considerations of neoplastic proliferations of white cells.

NONNEOPLASTIC DISORDERS OF WHITE CELLS

Leukopenia

Leukopenia usually reflects a decrease in granulocytes, the most numerous circulating white cells. Lymphopenia is much less common; it is associated with rare congenital immunodeficiency diseases, advanced human immunodeficiency virus (HIV) infection, and treatment with high doses of corticosteroids. Only the more common leukopenias of granulocytes are discussed here.

Pathogenesis. A reduction in the number of neutrophils in blood is known as *neutropenia* or, when severe, *agranulocytosis*. The mechanisms underlying neutropenia can be divided into two broad categories:

- *Decreased granulocyte production.* Causes include marrow hypoplasia (during cancer chemotherapy or due to aplastic anemia), extensive marrow replacement by tumor (e.g., leukemia), and idiosyncratic reactions to certain drugs.
- *Increased granulocyte destruction.* Causes include immune-mediated injury and overwhelming infections due to increased peripheral utilization. Splenomegaly also can lead to the sequestration and accelerated removal of neutrophils.

Clinical Features. Neutropenic patients are susceptible to severe, potentially fatal bacterial and fungal infections. The risk of infection rises as the neutrophil count falls below 500 cells/µL. Infection often begins at a superficial site (e.g., oropharynx) without signs and symptoms because of the inadequate innate immune response. Because of the danger of sepsis, neutropenic patients are treated with broad-spectrum antibiotics at the first sign of infection.

Reactive Leukocytosis

The finding of increased numbers of white cells in the blood is common in a variety of inflammatory states. Leukocytoses are relatively nonspecific and are classified according to the white cell series that is affected (Table 9.5). In some cases, reactive leukocytosis may be severe

Table 9.5 Causes of Leukocytosis

Neutrophilic Leukocytosis

Acute bacterial infections (especially those caused by pyogenic organisms)
Sterile inflammation caused by tissue damage (myocardial infarction, burns)

Eosinophilic Leukocytosis (Eosinophilia)

Allergic disorders (asthma, hay fever, pemphigus, dermatitis herpetiformis)
Parasitic infestations
Drug reactions
Neoplasms (e.g., Hodgkin lymphoma and some non-Hodgkin lymphomas)
Collagen-vascular disorders, vasculitides

Basophilic Leukocytosis (Basophilia)

Rare, often indicative of a myeloproliferative neoplasm (e.g., chronic myeloid leukemia)

Monocytosis

Chronic infections (e.g., tuberculosis), bacterial endocarditis, rickettsiosis, and malaria
Collagen vascular diseases (e.g., systemic lupus erythematosus)
Inflammatory bowel diseases (e.g., ulcerative colitis)

Lymphocytosis

Accompanies monocytosis in many disorders associated with chronic immunologic stimulation (tuberculosis, brucellosis)
Viral infections (hepatitis A, cytomegalovirus, Epstein-Barr virus)
Bordetella pertussis infection

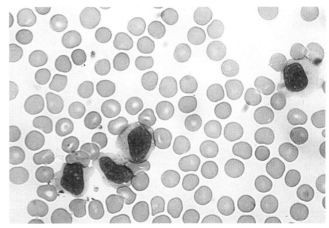

Fig. 9.10 Atypical lymphocytes in infectious mononucleosis.

latently infected cells is released from T-cell control and often gives rise to EBV-positive B-cell lymphoproliferative disease or even frank lymphomas.

Morphology. The major alterations involve the blood, lymph nodes, and spleen. There is peripheral blood leukocytosis of large *atypical cytotoxic T lymphocytes* with abundant cytoplasm containing a few azurophilic granules (Fig. 9.10). Lymphadenopathy is common and is most prominent in the posterior cervical, axillary, and groin regions. The enlarged nodes contain an expanded population of activated T cells that may mimic lymphoma. The *spleen* is usually enlarged and infiltrated by atypical lymphocytes.

Clinical Features. Mononucleosis classically manifests with fever, sore throat, and lymphadenitis, but atypical presentations (e.g., febrile rash, hepatitis) are not unusual. The diagnosis depends on the following features: (1) atypical lymphocytosis; (2) a positive heterophil antibody reaction (Monospot test); and (3) a rising titer of antibodies specific for EBV antigens. The rapid increase in spleen size increases the risk of splenic rupture, even with minor trauma, which can be fatal. In most patients, mononucleosis resolves within 4 to 6 weeks, but fatigue may last longer.

Reactive Lymphadenitis

Infections and nonmicrobial inflammatory stimuli (e.g., neoantigens from cancer cells) often activate immune cells in lymph nodes and can lead to lymph node enlargement (lymphadenopathy). Infections causing lymphadenitis may be acute or chronic. Usually, histologic changes in lymph nodes are nonspecific. The exception is granulomatous lymphadenitis, which can be seen in tuberculosis (marked by caseous necrosis), other infectious entities (cat-scratch disease, fungal infections), and sarcoidosis.

NEOPLASTIC PROLIFERATIONS OF WHITE CELLS

The most important disorders of white cells are neoplasms. All are malignant, but they have a wide range of clinical behaviors. Hematologic malignancies occur at all ages and as a group are quite common; in aggregate, there are about 150,000 new hematologic malignancies diagnosed each year in the United States.

Classification systems for white cell neoplasms rely on morphologic and molecular criteria, including identification of lineage-specific protein markers and specific genetic aberrations. The number of recognized entities is numerous (>70 at last count), reflecting the complexity of the normal hematopoietic and immune systems from which these tumors are derived. Here, we focus on relatively common

enough to mimic leukemia *(leukemoid reactions).* In particular, infectious mononucleosis, which gives rise to a distinctive syndrome associated with lymphocytosis, can simulate neoplasia.

Infectious Mononucleosis.

Infectious mononucleosis is an acute, self-limited disease caused by Epstein-Barr virus infection.

Epstein-Barr virus (EBV), a member of the herpesvirus family, is ubiquitous in human populations. In lower-income countries, EBV infection in early childhood is nearly universal. Infected children mount an immune response, but most remain asymptomatic and more than half continue to shed virus, usually for life. In contrast, in higher-income countries, infection typically is delayed until adolescence or young adulthood and symptomatic infection is much more common. For unclear reasons, in this setting only about 20% of those who are infected continue to shed the virus.

Pathogenesis. Transmission of EBV usually involves oral contact with saliva containing virus. EBV may first infect oropharyngeal epithelial cells, but it then spreads to underlying tonsils and adenoids, where B cells are infected. The infection of B cells takes one of two forms: In a minority of cells, the infection is lytic, leading to viral replication and release of virions, whereas in most B cells the infection is nonproductive and the virus persists in latent form. Several EBV-encoded proteins expressed in latently infected cells stimulate proliferation of the infected cells, which disseminate to lymphoid tissues and secrete various antibodies. Included among these are heterophil (cross-reactive with another species) anti–sheep red cell antibodies, which are detected in diagnostic tests for mononucleosis.

Host CD8+ cytotoxic T cells specific for viral antigens control the proliferation of EBV-infected B cells. However, a few latently infected EBV-positive B cells escape the immune response by downregulating the expression of viral proteins and persist for the life of the patient. In patients with defective T-cell immunity (e.g., AIDS patients or transplant recipients treated with immunosuppressive drugs), this persistent population of

Table 9.6   Acute Leukemias and Myeloid Neoplasms

Entity	Cell of Origin	Salient Pathologic Features	Commonly Mutated Genes
B-cell acute lymphoblastic leukemia	Immature B cell	Marrow replacement by lymphoid blasts, absence of Auer rods	Transcription factor genes, often by translocations; ABL tyrosine kinase, in the form of a *BCR-ABL* fusion gene (subset of cases)
T-cell acute lymphoblastic leukemia	Immature T cell	Marrow replacement by lymphoid blasts, absence of Auer rods, frequent mediastinal involvement	Transcription factor genes, often by translocations; signaling molecule genes
Acute myeloid leukemia	Hematopoietic stem cell or early myeloid progenitor	Marrow replacement by myeloid blasts, often with Auer rods	Transcription factor genes, often by translocations (e.g., *RARA*); signaling molecule genes
Myelodysplastic syndrome	Hematopoietic stem cell or early myeloid progenitor	Dysplastic marrow progenitors and peripheral blood elements	Genes encoding epigenetic regulators, RNA splicing factors, and transcription factors
Chronic myeloid leukemia	Hematopoietic stem cell	Increased marrow granulocytic precursors and megakaryocytes, leukocytosis, basophilia, thrombocytosis, splenomegaly	ABL tyrosine kinase, in the form of *BCR-ABL* fusion gene
Polycythemia vera	Early myeloid progenitor	Increase in all marrow elements, polycythemia, basophilia	Activating mutations in the *JAK2* tyrosine kinase gene
Primary myelofibrosis	Early myeloid progenitor	Increased and atypical megakaryocytes, marrow fibrosis, splenomegaly, leukoerythroblastosis	Activating mutations in the *JAK2* or *MPL* tyrosine kinase genes; mutations in the *CALR* gene

or clinicopathologically distinctive entities. We will first consider hematologic malignancies that originate in hematopoietic stem cells or early marrow progenitors, the acute leukemias and myeloid neoplasms, characteristics of which are summarized in Table 9.6.

Acute Leukemias

Acute leukemias are a diverse group of neoplastic proliferations of immature hematopoietic cells that often replace normal marrow elements, leading to symptoms related to marrow failure.

Acute leukemias are subclassified by immunophenotype into B-cell tumors (B-cell acute lymphoblastic leukemia, or B-ALL), T-cell tumors (T-cell acute lymphoblastic leukemia, or T-ALL), and myeloid tumors (acute myeloid leukemia, or AML). The immature neoplastic cells are referred to as blasts. Typically, in ALL there is a complete maturation arrest at early stages of B- or T- cell differentiation and blasts are the major tumor cell population in involved tissues. In contrast, in AML the block in differentiation is often incomplete and diagnosis is based on the presence of at least 20% blasts in the marrow or blood. Beyond their immunophenotypic differences, B-cell, T-cell, and myeloid acute leukemias also have somewhat distinct clinicopathologic features, as follows:

- *B-ALL* is the most common childhood leukemia, with a peak incidence between the ages of 2 and 10 years. It almost always arises within the marrow and replaces normal marrow elements, resulting in symptoms related to anemia (weakness, fatigue), thrombocytopenia (petechiae [small bleeds into the skin and mucosal membranes]), and neutropenia (infection). The blasts have scant basophilic cytoplasm and nuclei with delicate, finely stippled chromatin and small nucleoli (Fig. 9.11A).
- *T-ALL* most commonly presents during adolescence and often involves the thymus, as well as the bone marrow. In addition to marrow failure, more than half of T-ALLs present with mediastinal masses due to thymic involvement. Blasts are morphologically identical to those of B-ALL and can only be distinguished by immunophenotyping.
- *AML* occurs throughout life but is most common in individuals older than 60. Unlike ALL, AML often arises from a preexisting

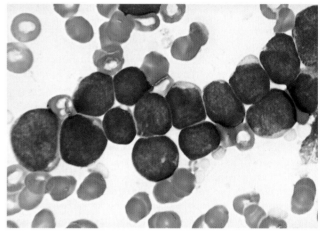

Fig. 9.11 Acute lymphoblastic leukemia (ALL). Lymphoblasts with condensed nuclear chromatin, small nucleoli, and scant agranular cytoplasm are shown. TdT, terminal deoxynucleotidyl transferase.

myeloid neoplasm (either a myeloproliferative neoplasm or a myelodysplastic syndrome, described later), sometimes after a prodrome lasting for years. Like ALL, most symptoms are related to marrow failure. Myeloid blasts tend to be larger than lymphoid blasts and have fine chromatin, distinct nucleoli, and moderate amounts of cytoplasm with variable numbers of granules (Fig. 9.12A). In a subset of cases, these granules take the form of *Auer rods*, needle-like inclusions that are pathognomonic for myeloid blasts (Fig. 9.13). In other instances, the blasts of AML are so immature that they are difficult to distinguish from lymphoid blasts morphologically and immunophenotyping is necessary for diagnosis.

Pathogenesis. Among the most common driver mutations in all types of acute leukemia are gene rearrangements and base pair substitutions that interfere with the function of transcription factors that regulate normal

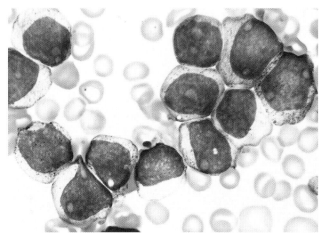

Fig. 9.12 Acute myeloid leukemia (AML). Myeloblasts with delicate nuclear chromatin, prominent nucleoli, and fine azurophilic cytoplasmic granules are shown.

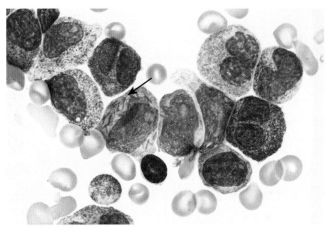

Fig. 9.13 Acute promyelocytic leukemia, a variant of AML. The neoplastic promyelocytes have abnormally coarse and numerous granules. A characteristic finding is a cell in the center of the field with multiple needle-like Auer rods *(arrow)*. (Courtesy of Dr. Robert W. McKenna, Department of Pathology, University of Texas Southwestern Medical School, Dallas.)

hematopoietic cell differentiation. These mutations typically involve factors that regulate the lineage to which the leukemia belongs. For example, B-ALL often contains mutations in transcription factors required for early stages of B-cell differentiation. These mutations cause maturation arrest and accumulation of immature blasts. Mutations in other genes lead to growth factor–independent signaling and proliferation. *RAS* and genes encoding signaling molecules that act upstream and downstream of RAS, including several growth factor receptors, are often mutated.

Pathology. The diagnosis and subtyping of acute leukemia requires a combination of complementary tests:
- *Morphology.* Blasts can be seen in the peripheral blood and bone marrow, although biopsy of a tissue mass may be required for diagnosis, particularly in T-ALL. The peripheral blood findings are highly variable. The white cell count may be markedly elevated

(>100,000 cells/μL) but is sometimes normal. Anemia is almost always present, and the platelet count usually is below 100,000/μL. Neutropenia is common.
- *Immunophenotyping.* Definitive diagnosis relies on stains performed with antibodies to lineage-specific antigens, usually by flow cytometry. For example, detection of terminal deoxyribose transferase (TdT) is useful for identifying earlier B and T cell progenitors. Histochemical stains may also be used, including myeloperoxidase, seen in acute myeloid leukemia.
- *Cytogenetics.* Specific translocations are associated with particular subtypes of acute leukemia, have prognostic importance, and may identify therapeutic targets.
- *Molecular Genetics.* Certain forms of acute leukemia are now defined by the presence of driver mutations in specific cancer genes. Most acute leukemias are currently evaluated by targeted DNA sequencing. Some of them are discussed later.

Clinical Features. Acute leukemia is an aggressive disease. In addition to symptoms related to marrow replacement and the attendant pancytopenia, there may be
- Bone pain resulting from marrow expansion and infiltration of the subperiosteum
- Lymphadenopathy, splenomegaly, and hepatomegaly, more common and more pronounced in ALL than AML
- Testicular enlargement due to leukemic infiltration
- Infiltration of the skin and gums, most characteristic of AML with monocytic differentiation
- In T-ALL with thymic involvement, compression of large vessels and airways in the mediastinum
- Central nervous system manifestations resulting from meningeal spread, such as headache, vomiting, and nerve palsies

Treatment of acute leukemia varies according to subtype. Most patients are treated with combination chemotherapy using regimens that differ for ALL and AML. More than 80% of children with B-ALL and T-ALL are cured. Highly effective targeted therapies are available for two molecular subtypes of acute leukemia: (1) *BCR-ABL–positive B-ALL*, defined by the presence of a *BCR-ABL* fusion gene (described in detail under chronic myeloid leukemia) and (2) *acute promyelocytic leukemia*, a distinctive subtype of AML characterized by the presence of a (15;17) translocation that creates a *PML-RARA* fusion gene encoding an aberrant form of the retinoic acid receptor that blocks terminal differentiation of promyelocytes. This form of acute leukemia is now almost always cured with targeted treatment consisting of all-*trans* retinoic acid, a vitamin A analog that binds the PML-RARA fusion protein, combined with arsenic salts, which cause the degradation of PML-RARA. This treatment induces the differentiation of immature cells presumably into neutrophils, which rapidly die, clearing the neoplastic clone. A recent development is treatment of B-ALL with cytotoxic T cells bearing chimeric antigen receptors (CARs) engineered to specifically recognize and kill cells expressing the B-cell antigen CD19. This therapy has produced dramatic responses in relapsed/refractory B-ALL in children and adults, but at the cost of permanent loss of normal B cells and sometimes severe or even fatal toxicity caused by production of cytokines by the massively activated injected T cells (cytokine storm).

Challenges remain. Infantile acute leukemias associated with rearrangements of the *KMT2A* gene (previously known as *MLL*), which encodes an epigenetic regulator, have a poor prognosis. The prognosis for adults with *BCR-ABL*–negative ALL is guarded, and the prognosis for patients with AML subtypes other than acute promyelocytic leukemia remains poor, particularly in adults older than age 60 years. A particularly challenging problem is the small subset of acute leukemias with *TP53* mutations, which have dismal outcomes even with hematopoietic stem cell transplantation.

Myelodysplastic Syndromes

There is a large group of myeloid neoplasms that lack the features that define AML (>20% blasts and specific AML-defining driver mutations). These neoplasms fall into two broad, overlapping groups, the myelodysplastic syndrome (MDS) and the myeloproliferative neoplasms (MPNs; discussed later). MDS is nearly as common as AML. It affects about 15,000 patients per year in the United States and is increasing in frequency as the population ages.

Pathogenesis. MDS is characterized by maturation defects associated with ineffective hematopoiesis and a high risk of transformation to AML. The marrow is partly or wholly replaced by the clonal progeny of a transformed multipotent stem cell that demonstrates ineffective and disordered multilineage differentiation. The marrow is hypercellular or normocellular, but the peripheral blood shows one or more cytopenias.

In children and young adults, MDS is often due to inheritance of a mutated cancer gene or exposure to mutagens (e.g., therapeutic alkylating agents or ionizing radiation). In adults over the age of 60 years, MDS appears to be caused by sporadic mutations in cancer genes. Transformation to AML is associated with additional mutations that drive cell growth, such as mutations in RAS and other signaling molecules. In addition, roughly 10% of MDS cases have loss-of-function mutations in *TP53*; these patients have particularly poor clinical outcomes.

Morphology. The marrow is populated by hematopoietic precursors that exhibit disordered differentiation (dysplasia), including "megaloblastoid" erythroid precursors resembling those seen in the megaloblastic anemias, erythroid forms with iron deposits within their mitochondria *(ring sideroblasts),* granulocyte precursors with abnormal granules or nuclear maturation, and small megakaryocytes with single small nuclei or multiple separate nuclei.

Clinical Features. Most patients are 50 to 70 years of age. As a result of cytopenias, infections, anemia, and bleeding are common. The diagnosis relies on the presence of cytopenias and characteristic morphologic and genetic findings. Cytogenetic studies often reveal clonal abnormalities; loss of all or a portion of chromosomes 5 and/or 7 is particularly common. DNA sequencing studies identify driver mutations in the majority of cases.

MDS is difficult to treat; it does not respond well to conventional chemotherapy, and most patients are too old to undergo stem cell transplantation. Transformation to AML occurs in 10% to 40% of cases. The median survival time ranges from 9 to 29 months and is worse in cases associated with increased marrow blasts, cytogenetic abnormalities, or *TP53* mutations.

Myeloproliferative Neoplasms

The common pathogenic feature of myeloproliferative neoplasms is the presence of mutated, constitutively activated tyrosine kinases or other acquired aberrations in signaling pathways that lead to growth factor independence.

These diverse myeloid malignancies are rare but are notable because of the remarkable response of chronic myeloid leukemia (CML) to targeted therapy. We will discuss CML and two other clinicopathologically distinct myeloproliferative neoplasms, polycythemia vera and primary myelofibrosis.

Chronic Myeloid Leukemia

Chronic myeloid leukemia is distinguished from other myeloproliferative neoplasms by the presence of a *BCR-ABL* fusion gene derived from portions of the *BCR* gene on chromosome 22 and the *ABL* gene on chromosome 9.

The positions of the DNA breakpoints in chronic myeloid leukemia (CML) and *BCR-ABL*–positive B-ALL (described earlier) differ in subtle ways but have similar downstream consequences.

Pathogenesis. The *BCR-ABL* gene found in CML encodes a chimeric protein in which the ABL tyrosine kinase becomes constitutively active because of fusion to part of the BCR protein and mimics signals produced by activated growth factor receptors. Because BCR-ABL does not inhibit differentiation, the early disease course is marked by excessive production of relatively normal blood cells, particularly granulocytes and platelets.

Morphology. The leukocyte count is elevated, often exceeding 100,000 cells/μL, due to the presence of increased numbers of neutrophils, eosinophils, and basophils, as well as earlier granulocytic forms such as metamyelocytes and myelocytes (Fig. 9.14). The platelet count is also frequently elevated. The marrow is hypercellular, and the spleen is markedly enlarged by extramedullary hematopoiesis. If the blood supply cannot keep up with the massive splenomegaly, the result may be splenic infarcts.

Clinical Features. The onset of CML is insidious and initial symptoms are nonspecific. Splenomegaly may be the earliest symptom. The natural history is variable, but untreated CML is eventually fatal due to transformation to acute leukemia (so-called blast crisis). In 70% of cases, the blast crisis resembles AML; in the remainder, it resembles B-ALL, which is consistent with the idea that CML originates from multipotent hematopoietic stem cells.

Targeted therapy has dramatically altered the disease course. Tyrosine kinase inhibitors that target the BCR-ABL fusion protein induce sustained remissions and prevent blast crisis, particularly in patients with early disease. The BCR-ABL–positive clone persists, and patients must be treated

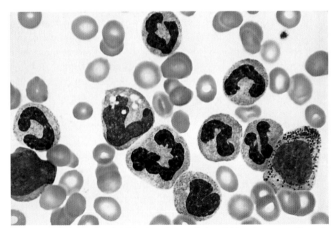

Fig. 9.14 Chronic myeloid leukemia: peripheral blood smear. Granulocytic forms at various stages of differentiation are present. (Courtesy of Dr. Robert W. McKenna, Department of Pathology, University of Texas Southwestern Medical School, Dallas.)

for life. Relapses sometimes occur, often due to outgrowth of clones with mutations in BCR-ABL that prevent inhibitors from binding. In some instances, remissions can be obtained by switching to different inhibitors that are active against particular mutated forms of BCR-ABL. For others, hematopoietic stem cell transplantation offers a chance of cure.

Polycythemia Vera

Polycythemia vera is a myeloproliferative disorder marked by increased production of all myeloid lineage cells and symptoms related to increased red cell mass (polycythemia).

Pathogenesis. Polycythemia vera (PCV) is associated with activating point mutations in the tyrosine kinase JAK2, a signaling molecule in pathways downstream of the erythropoietin receptor and other growth factor receptors. The JAK2 mutations reduce the dependence of hematopoietic cells on growth factors for growth and survival, leading to excessive proliferation of erythroid, granulocytic, and megakaryocytic elements.

> *Morphology.* The marrow is hypercellular due to increased numbers of erythroid, myeloid, and megakaryocytic forms. Marrow fibrosis is seen in 10% of patients at diagnosis. This can progress to a *spent phase,* where the marrow is replaced by fibroblasts and collagen. Increased blood volume and viscosity due to polycythemia cause congestion of many tissues. Platelets are often abnormally large and may be dysfunctional, leading to thrombosis and bleeding. Basophils are often increased in the peripheral blood.

Clinical Features. PCV appears insidiously, usually in late middle age. Symptoms include cyanosis, headache, dizziness, gastrointestinal symptoms, hematemesis, and melena. Thromboses may involve veins or arteries and can lead to stroke, myocardial infarction, and pulmonary embolism. Epistaxis is common, and life-threatening hemorrhages occur in 5% to 10% of patients. Because of the high cell turnover, gout is seen in 5% to 10% of patients.

Common laboratory findings include a hematocrit that is often 60% or greater, granulocytosis with basophilia, and thrombocytosis. Detection of *JAK2* mutations confirms the diagnosis.

Without treatment, death from vascular complications occurs within months; however, the median survival time is increased to about 10 years by lowering of the hematocrit to near normal by repeated phlebotomy. Prolonged survival has revealed a propensity for PCV to evolve to a spent phase resembling primary myelofibrosis (described later) after an average interval of 10 years. JAK2 inhibitors are used to treat the spent phase and lead to improvement in most patients. Transformation to a blast crisis identical to that of AML also occurs, but much less frequently than in CML.

Primary Myelofibrosis

The hallmark of primary myelofibrosis is the development of obliterative marrow fibrosis, which reduces marrow hematopoiesis and leads to cytopenias and extensive extramedullary hematopoiesis.

Pathogenesis. Primary myelofibrosis is caused by various mutations that increase JAK/STAT signaling, a pathway downstream of growth factor receptors. The most frequent of these are *JAK2* mutations, which are present in 50% to 60% of cases. It is not known why *JAK2* mutations are associated with PCV in some patients and primary myelofibrosis in others. Fibrosis is caused by pro-fibrogenic factors such as platelet-derived growth factor and TGF-β that are elaborated by neoplastic megakaryocytes. TGF-β promotes angiogenesis as well as collagen deposition, both of which are prominent in myelofibrotic marrows.

> *Morphology.* The marrow appearance is identical to the spent phase that is seen occasionally late in the course of other myeloproliferative neoplasms such as PCV. Initially, the marrow is hypercellular and mildly distorted by fibrosis. Megakaryocytes are larger than normal and present in clusters. In advanced cases, the marrow is hypocellular and diffusely fibrotic, and compensatory extramedullary hematopoiesis occurs. The peripheral blood smear is markedly abnormal (Fig. 9.15). Red cells exhibit bizarre shapes, and nucleated erythroid precursors are commonly seen, along with immature white cells (myelocytes and metamyelocytes), a combination of findings referred to as *leukoerythroblastosis.* Abnormally large platelets are often present. Marked *splenomegaly* due to extensive extramedullary hematopoiesis, often associated with *subcapsular infarcts,* is typical. The spleen may weigh up to 4000 g, roughly 20 times its normal weight. Moderate *hepatomegaly,* also due to extramedullary hematopoiesis, is commonplace.

Clinical Features. Primary myelofibrosis usually occurs in individuals older than 60 years who present with symptoms related to anemia and splenomegaly. Fatigue, weight loss, and night sweats are frequent complaints. Hyperuricemia and gout due to a high rate of cell turnover are often seen. Laboratory studies show a moderate to severe normocytic anemia accompanied by leukoerythroblastosis. The white cell count is usually normal or mildly reduced but can be elevated early in the course. The platelet count is usually normal or elevated at diagnosis, but thrombocytopenia often supervenes as the disease progresses.

Primary myelofibrosis is more difficult to treat than PCV and CML. The median survival is 4 to 5 years. Threats to life include infection, thrombosis and bleeding, and transformation to AML, which occurs in 5% to 20% of cases. JAK2 inhibitors are effective at decreasing the splenomegaly and constitutional symptoms. Hematopoietic stem cell transplantation may be curative.

Non-Hodgkin Lymphomas and Chronic Lymphoid Leukemias

These common hematologic malignancies include a wide variety of neoplasms that are derived from mature lymphoid cells. Hodgkin lymphomas and plasma cell neoplasms and related entities are also derived from mature lymphocytes, but have unique clinicopathologic features and are discussed later.

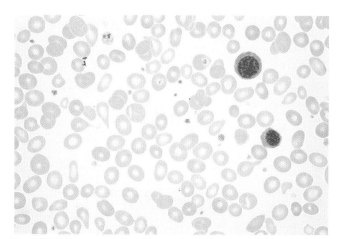

Fig. 9.15 Primary myelofibrosis: peripheral blood smear. Two nucleated erythroid precursors and several teardrop-shaped red cells are evident. Immature myeloid cells were present in other fields. An identical histologic picture can be seen in other diseases producing marrow distortion and fibrosis.

Some general aspects of malignancies of mature lymphoid cells bear emphasis:

- *The terms leukemia and lymphoma refer to the usual patterns of tissue involvement.* Leukemias typically arise in bone marrow and are apparent in peripheral blood, whereas lymphomas present as masses in lymph nodes and other tissues. However, these distinctions are not absolute: "lymphomas" occasionally have peripheral blood involvement and "leukemias" may present as masses, without peripheral blood involvement. The diagnosis is based on the morphologic and molecular characteristics of the tumor cells, regardless of their location in the body.
- *Mature lymphoid neoplasms often disrupt the function of the adaptive immune system;* immunodeficiency and autoimmunity coexist in some instances.
- *Patients with inherited or acquired immunodeficiencies are at higher risk for lymphoid neoplasms,* particularly those associated with EBV infection.
- *Although lymphoma often appears to be localized, neoplastic lymphocytes recirculate like normal lymphocytes and tumors are usually widespread at diagnosis.* Therefore, with few exceptions, only systemic therapies are curative.
- *B-cell tumors are much more common than T-cell tumors,* probably because translocations and mutations related to double-strand DNA breaks in immunoglobulin genes (during somatic hypermutation and class-switching) increase the risk for oncogene activation. Many driver mutations in B-cell malignancies consist of translocations that fuse immunoglobulin genes to protooncogenes.

The classification of non-Hodgkin lymphomas and chronic lymphoid leukemias considers the morphology, cell of origin (determined by immunophenotyping), clinical features, and genotype (e.g., karyotype, presence of viral genomes) of each entity. In the following sections, we will focus on those that are most common and clinically important (summarized in Table 9.7). We also will touch on a few rare entities that nevertheless deserve brief mention because of unusual or pathogenically informative characteristics.

Chronic Lymphocytic Leukemia/Small Lymphocytic Lymphoma

Chronic lymphocytic leukemia (CLL) and small lymphocytic lymphoma (SLL) are identical, differing only in the extent of peripheral blood involvement; if the peripheral blood lymphocyte count exceeds 5000 cells/µL, the patient is diagnosed with CLL. Most cases fit the criteria for CLL, which is the most common leukemia of adults in the Western world. For unclear reasons, CLL/SLL is less common in Asia.

Pathogenesis. CLL/SLL is an indolent, slowly growing tumor in which increased tumor cell survival is more important than tumor cell proliferation per se. CLL/SLL cells express high levels of BCL2, a protein that inhibits apoptosis. Also of critical importance are signals generated by surface immunoglobulin (the B-cell receptor, or BCR). BCR signals flow through an intermediary called Bruton tyrosine kinase (BTK) and ultimately turn on the transcription factor NF-κB, which contributes to the expression of genes that promote the survival of CLL/SLL cells.

Through unclear mechanisms, the accumulation of CLL/SLL cells suppresses normal B-cell function, often resulting in hypogammaglobulinemia. Paradoxically, approximately 15% of patients develop autoantibodies against their own red cells or platelets. When present, the autoantibodies are made by nonmalignant bystander B cells, indicating that CLL/SLL cells impair immune tolerance.

Morphology. Involved lymph nodes are diffusely effaced by sheets of small lymphocytes and scattered ill-defined areas containing larger, actively dividing cells (Fig. 9.16A). The small lymphocytes have dark, round nuclei and scanty cytoplasm (see Fig. 9.16B). The foci of mitotically active cells are called *proliferation centers,* which are pathognomonic for CLL/SLL. The marrow, spleen, and liver are also involved in almost all cases. In patients with CLL, there is an absolute *lymphocytosis* of small, mature-looking lymphocytes. These circulating cells are fragile and frequently disrupted on histologic preparations; they are called *smudge cells.*

Clinical Features. The diagnosis is based on increased lymphocytes in the peripheral blood and confirmed by flow cytometry, which reveals a population of cells expressing B-cell markers such as CD20, CD5 (which is also expressed on normal T cells), and clonal surface immunoglobulin light chain (either kappa or lambda). In SLL, tissue biopsy of an enlarged lymph node is required for diagnosis.

The prognosis is generally good because CLL usually follows a very indolent course. If diagnosed when the patient is asymptomatic, the median survival is greater than 10 years, even without treatment. Symptomatic patients are treated with antibodies against CD20, inhibitors of

Table 9.7 Characteristics of Non-Hodgkin Lymphomas and Chronic Lymphoid Leukemias

Entity	Cell of Origin	Associated Characteristics
Small lymphocytic lymphoma/chronic lymphocytic leukemia	Mature B cell	Occurs in older adults; usually involves lymph nodes, marrow, spleen; and peripheral blood; indolent
Follicular lymphoma	Germinal center B cell	Translocations involving *BCL2;* presents with generalized lymphadenopathy; indolent
Mantle cell lymphoma	Naïve mature B cell	Translocations involving the cyclin D1 gene; presents with generalized lymphadenopathy; moderately aggressive
Extranodal marginal zone lymphoma	Mature B cell	Arises at sites of chronic inflammation; very indolent
Diffuse large B-cell lymphoma	Germinal center or post–germinal center B cell	Heterogeneous, may arise at extranodal sites; variably associated with translocations involving *BCL2, BCL6,* and *MYC;* aggressive
Burkitt lymphoma	Germinal center B cell	Usually arises at extranodal sites; translocations involving *MYC* in virtually all cases; subset of cases associated with EBV; aggressive
Hairy cell leukemia	Mature B cell	Spleen and marrow involvement; most cases have *BRAF* mutations; indolent
Adult T-cell leukemia/lymphoma	CD4-positive T cell	Usually presents with lymph node and blood involvement; uniformly associated with HTLV-1 infection; frequent hypercalcemia; aggressive
Peripheral T-cell lymphoma	Mature T cells	Heterogeneous; often associated with systemic symptoms stemming from cytokine release; aggressive

EBV, Epstein-Barr virus; HTLV-1, human T-cell lymphotropic virus 1.

B-cell receptor signaling, and BCL2 antagonists. The presence of *TP53* mutations portends a worse prognosis. Cure may only be achieved with hematopoietic stem cell transplantation, which is reserved for younger patients who fail conventional therapies. A small fraction of CLL/SLL cases transform to aggressive tumors resembling diffuse large B-cell lymphoma (Richter transformation); once transformation occurs, the median survival time is less than 1 year.

Follicular Lymphoma

Follicular lymphoma is strongly associated with a (14;18) translocation that increases the expression of the antiapoptotic *BCL2* gene.

Follicular lymphoma constitutes approximately 25% of cases of adult non-Hodgkin lymphoma in the United States, making it the most common "indolent" non-Hodgkin lymphoma. Like CLL/SLL, it occurs less frequently in Asian populations. The cell of origin is a germinal center B cell.

Pathogenesis. More than 85% of follicular lymphomas have a characteristic (14;18) translocation that fuses the *BCL2* gene on chromosome 18 to the *IGH* (immunoglobulin heavy chain) locus on chromosome 14, resulting in "overexpression" of BCL2 protein, an inhibitor of apoptosis (see Chapter 1). In about a third of cases, additional mutations in genes encoding histone-modifying proteins are seen.

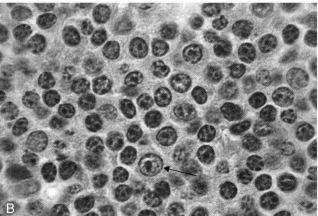

Fig. 9.16 Chronic lymphocytic leukemia/small lymphocytic lymphoma: lymph node. (A) Low-power view shows diffuse effacement of nodal architecture. (B) At high power, a majority of the tumor cells have the appearance of small, round lymphocytes. A "prolymphocyte," a larger cell with a centrally placed nucleolus, also is present in this field *(arrow).* (A, Courtesy of Dr. José Hernandez, Department of Pathology, University of Texas Southwestern Medical School, Dallas.)

Morphology. Lymph nodes are usually effaced by a distinctly *nodular proliferation* (Fig. 9.17A). Most commonly, the predominant neoplastic cells are so-called *centrocytes,* cells slightly larger than resting lymphocytes that have angular "cleaved" nuclei with indentations and linear infoldings, coarse condensed chromatin, and indistinct nucleoli (Fig. 9.17B). Centrocytes are mixed with variable numbers of *centroblasts,* larger cells with vesicular chromatin, several nucleoli, and modest amounts of cytoplasm. Uncommonly, centroblasts predominate, a feature that correlates with more aggressive clinical behavior. The tumor cells express the B-cell marker CD20, germinal center B-cell markers, surface immunoglobulin, and high levels of BCL2. Because BCL2 is not expressed in normal germinal center B cells, stains for BCL2 help distinguish follicular lymphoma from follicular hyperplasia.

Clinical Features. Follicular lymphoma affects adults older than 50 and usually manifests as painless generalized lymphadenopathy. The marrow is involved at diagnosis in approximately 80% of cases. Although the natural history is prolonged (overall median survival is approximately 10 years), the disease is not curable; therapy is reserved for patients with bulky, symptomatic disease. Treatment includes "gentle" chemotherapy, antibodies against CD20, and BCR signaling inhibitors. In 30% to 40% of patients, follicular lymphoma progresses to diffuse large B-cell lymphoma (DLBCL). DLBCL arising from follicular lymphoma has a worse prognosis than de novo diffuse DLBCL, described later.

Mantle Cell Lymphoma

Mantle cell lymphoma is strongly associated with an (11;14) translocation that increases expression of the *cyclin D1* gene.

Mantle cell lymphoma is derived from cells resembling the naïve B cells that are found in the mantle zones of normal lymphoid follicles. It constitutes approximately 6% of all non-Hodgkin lymphomas and occurs mainly in men older than 50 years.

Pathogenesis. Cyclin D1 stimulates growth by forming a complex with cyclin-dependent kinases and inactivating RB, promoting progression of cells from the G_1 phase to the S phase of the cell cycle (see Chapter 5). Overexpression of cyclin D1 overwhelms the braking effect of RB, driving lymphoma cell growth. Additional driver mutations have also been identified in genes encoding a variety of signaling molecules, transcription factors, and epigenetic regulators.

Morphology. Lymph nodes are effaced by tumor cells growing in diffuse or vaguely nodular patterns. The tumor cells usually are slightly larger than normal lymphocytes and have an irregular nucleus, inconspicuous nucleoli, and scant cytoplasm. The bone marrow is involved in most cases and the peripheral blood in about 20% of cases. The tumor cells express surface IgM and IgD, the B-cell antigen CD20, and CD5, and have high levels of cyclin D1 protein, a finding that is diagnostically helpful.

Clinical Features. Most patients present with fatigue and lymphadenopathy and are found to have generalized disease involving the bone marrow, spleen, liver, and (often) the gastrointestinal tract. These tumors are moderately aggressive and incurable. Treatment involves the use of low-dose chemotherapy, antibodies against CD20, and drugs that inhibit B-cell receptor signaling. The median survival is 4 to 6 years.

Extranodal Marginal Zone Lymphoma

Extranodal marginal zone lymphoma is an example of a cancer that arises within and is sustained by chronic inflammation.

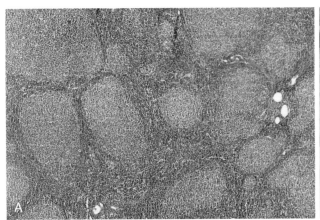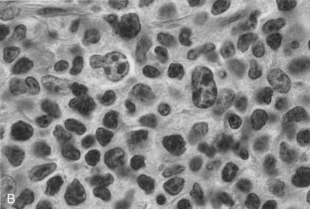

Fig. 9.17 Follicular lymphoma: lymph node. (A) Nodular aggregates of lymphoma cells are present throughout. (B) At high magnification, small lymphoid cells with condensed chromatin and irregular or cleaved nuclear outlines (centrocytes) are mixed with a population of larger cells with nucleoli (centroblasts). (A, Courtesy of Dr. Robert W. McKenna, Department of Pathology, University of Texas Southwestern Medical School, Dallas.)

Extranodal marginal zone lymphoma is an indolent tumor derived from antigen-stimulated B cells. It occurs most commonly in organs with epithelial linings, such as the gastrointestinal tract (so-called MALTomas [mucosa-associated lymphoid tumors]), salivary glands, lungs, orbit, and breast.

Pathogenesis. This lymphoma arises most often in tissues that are inflamed due to autoimmune disorders (e.g., Sjögren syndrome, Hashimoto thyroiditis) or chronic infection (e.g., *Helicobacter pylori* gastritis). Eradication of *H. pylori* with antibiotic therapy often leads to regression of the tumor cells, which depend on inflammatory cytokines secreted by *H. pylori*–specific T cells for their growth and survival. It is thought that the disease begins as a polyclonal immune reaction, and after subsequent, still-unknown driver mutations, a neoplastic clone emerges that remains dependent on antigen-stimulated T-helper cells for signals to drive growth and survival. Hence, withdrawal of the responsible antigen, such as *H. pylori* proteins, causes tumor involution.

Morphology. The clonal B cells infiltrate the epithelium of involved tissues and collect in small aggregates *(lymphoepithelial lesions).* The cytoplasm may be abundant and pale or exhibit plasma cell differentiation. The tumor cells express the B-cell antigen CD20 and surface immunoglobulin, usually IgM.

Clinical Features. Extranodal marginal zone lymphomas typically present as swellings of the salivary gland, thyroid, or orbit, or are discovered incidentally in the setting of *H. pylori*–induced gastritis. Unlike other non-Hodgkin lymphomas, when localized they are often cured by simple excision followed by radiotherapy, or (in the case of *H. pylori*-associated disease) may also completely regress in response to antibiotic therapy.

Diffuse Large B Cell Lymphoma

Diffuse large B-cell lymphoma is the most common type of lymphoma, accounting for approximately 35% of non-Hodgkin lymphomas in the United States.

Diffuse large B-cell lymphoma (DLBCL) occurs at all ages but is most common in adults older than 50 years. It is derived from antigen-stimulated B cells and encompasses a heterogeneous group of neoplasms that demonstrate substantial morphologic, immunophenotypic, and genotypic variation.

Pathogenesis. Among the most common driver mutations in DLBCL are chromosomal translocations that lead to the overexpression of several different oncogenes, including the following:

- *BCL6.* About one third of DLBCLs have rearrangements of *BCL6,* located on chromosome 3q27, and an even higher fraction have point mutations in the *BCL6* promoter. Both aberrations result in increased levels of BCL6 protein, an important transcriptional regulator of gene expression in germinal center B cells.
- *BCL2.* Approximately 30% of tumors have a (14;18) translocation involving the *BCL2* gene that results in overexpression of the antiapoptotic BCL2 protein. Some of these tumors may represent "transformed" follicular lymphomas, which virtually always have the t(14;18).
- *MYC.* Approximately 5% to 10% of DLBCLs have rearrangements involving *MYC,* a gene encoding a transcription factor that regulates many aspects of growth-promoting metabolism, such as the Warburg effect.

In addition to these translocations, numerous other driver mutations have been identified that affect various epigenetic regulators, signaling molecules, and transcription factors that have important functions in B cells.

Morphology. The neoplastic B cells are large, at least three to four times the size of resting lymphocytes; however, there is considerable histologic variation. Cells with oval nuclear contours, dispersed chromatin, several distinct nucleoli, and modest amounts of pale cytoplasm may predominate (Fig. 9.18), or the cells may have a round or multilobate vesicular nucleus, one or two prominent centrally placed nucleoli, and abundant pale or basophilic cytoplasm. Occasionally, the tumor cells are anaplastic and include tumor giant cells resembling Reed-Sternberg cells, the malignant cells of Hodgkin lymphoma (described later). The tumors express the B-cell antigen CD20, and many express surface IgM and/or IgG. Other protein markers such as BCL2, BCL6, and MYC are variably expressed.

Several distinctive clinicopathologic subtypes are included in the category of DLBCLs.
- *EBV-associated DLBCLs* arise in the setting of AIDS, iatrogenic immunosuppression (e.g., in transplant recipients), and in elderly persons. In the posttransplantation setting, these tumors often begin as EBV-driven polyclonal B-cell proliferations that may regress if immune function is restored.
- *Human herpesvirus type 8* (HHV8, also called Kaposi sarcoma herpesvirus [KSHV]) *is associated with rare primary effusion lymphomas,* which may arise within the pleural cavity, pericardium, or peritoneum. These tumors are latently infected with HHV8, which encodes proteins homologous to several known

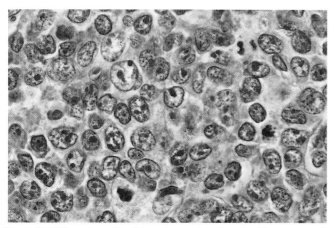

Fig. 9.18 Diffuse large B cell lymphoma: lymph node. The tumor cells have large nuclei with open chromatin and prominent nucleoli. (Courtesy of Dr. Robert W. McKenna, Department of Pathology, University of Texas Southwestern Medical School, Dallas.)

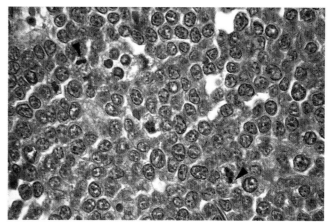

Fig. 9.19 Burkitt lymphoma: lymph node. The tumor cells and their nuclei are fairly uniform, giving a monotonous appearance. Note the high level of mitotic activity *(arrowheads)* and prominent nucleoli. The "starry sky" pattern produced by interspersed, lightly staining, normal macrophages is better appreciated at a lower magnification. (Courtesy of Dr. Robert W. McKenna, Department of Pathology, University of Texas Southwestern Medical School, Dallas.)

oncoproteins, including cyclin D1. Most affected patients are immunosuppressed.

- *Mediastinal large B-cell lymphoma* occurs most often in young women and appears to originate from an unusual population of thymic B cells. This tumor frequently has chromosomal amplifications that lead to the overexpression of the immune checkpoint proteins PD-L1 and PD-L2, suggesting that immune evasion plays an important role in its pathogenesis.
- *Double-hit lymphoma* refers to unusual tumors that have dual translocations involving *MYC* and another oncogene, most commonly *BCL2*. The combination of a potent progrowth oncogene *(MYC)* and a strong prosurvival oncogene *(BCL2)* yields tumors that exhibit very aggressive behavior with substantially worse outcomes than conventional DLBCL.

Clinical Features. Although most common in older adults, DLBCL can occur at any age; it constitutes about 15% of childhood lymphomas. Patients typically present with a rapidly enlarging, often symptomatic mass at one or several sites. Extranodal presentations are common; the gastrointestinal tract is the most common extranodal site, but DLBCL can arise in virtually any organ or tissue. Unlike the more indolent lymphomas (e.g., follicular lymphoma), involvement of the liver, spleen, and bone marrow is uncommon at diagnosis.

Without treatment, DLBCL is aggressive and rapidly fatal. With intensive combination chemotherapy and anti-CD20 immunotherapy, complete remissions are achieved in 60% to 80% of patients; of these, approximately 50% remain free of disease and appear to be cured. For others, other aggressive treatments (e.g., hematopoietic stem cell transplantation) offer hope.

Burkitt Lymphoma

Burkitt lymphoma is associated with translocations involving the *MYC* gene that result in overexpression of the MYC transcription factor.

Burkitt lymphoma is endemic in parts of Africa and occurs sporadically in other geographic areas, including the United States. Histologically, the African and nonendemic diseases are identical, although there are clinical and virologic differences. The cell of origin is a germinal center B cell.

Pathogenesis. MYC is a master regulator of Warburg metabolism (aerobic glycolysis), a cancer hallmark associated with rapid cell growth (see Chapter 5). Burkitt lymphoma may be the fastest-growing human tumor. Most translocations fuse the *MYC* gene on chromosome 8 with

the *IGH* gene on chromosome 14, which is transcriptionally active in B cells; variant translocations involving the Ig κ and λ light-chain loci on chromosomes 2 and 22, respectively, also are observed. The net result of each is the same: the dysregulation and overexpression of the MYC protein. In most endemic cases and about 20% of sporadic cases, the tumor cells are latently infected with EBV, but the precise role that EBV plays in the pathogenesis is uncertain.

Morphology. The tumor cells are intermediate in size and have round or oval nuclei and two to five distinct nucleoli (Fig. 9.19). There is a moderate amount of basophilic or amphophilic cytoplasm that often contains small, lipid-filled vacuoles. Very high rates of proliferation and apoptosis are characteristic, the latter associated with numerous tissue macrophages containing ingested nuclear debris that create a *"starry sky" pattern.* Tumor cells express surface IgM, the B-cell marker CD20, and germinal center B-cell markers.

Clinical Features. Both the endemic and nonendemic forms affect mainly children and young adults: Burkitt lymphoma accounts for approximately 30% of childhood non-Hodgkin lymphomas in the United States. The disease usually arises at extranodal sites. Endemic tumors often manifest as maxillary or mandibular masses, whereas in North America, tumors involving the bowel, retroperitoneum, and ovaries are more common. Burkitt lymphoma is highly aggressive; however, with very intensive chemotherapy regimens, a majority of patients can be cured.

Other Neoplasms of Mature Lymphoid Cells

Among the many other forms of lymphoid neoplasia in the World Health Organization classification, several with distinctive or clinically important features are worthy of a brief discussion.

- *Hairy cell leukemia* is an uncommon, indolent B-cell neoplasm with a distinctive morphology characterized by the presence of fine, hairlike cytoplasmic projections. Virtually all cases are associated with driver mutations in the serine/threonine kinase BRAF, which acts downstream of RAS. It occurs mainly in older males, and its manifestations result from infiltration of the bone marrow and spleen, which is usually enlarged. Pancytopenia is seen in more than half of cases. Scattered "hairy cells" can be identified in the peripheral blood smear in most cases. The disease is progressive if untreated but is extremely sensitive to certain chemotherapeutic agents and responds well to BRAF inhibitors. The overall prognosis is excellent.

- *Mycosis fungoides* and *Sézary syndrome* are tumors of neoplastic CD4+ T cells that are found in the skin, and are hence grouped under cutaneous T-cell lymphoma. Mycosis fungoides usually manifests as a rash that progresses over time to plaques and cutaneous tumors, followed by systemic dissemination. The neoplastic T cells have a cerebriform appearance produced by marked infolding of the nuclear membranes, and they infiltrate the upper dermis and epidermis. Sézary syndrome is characterized by a generalized exfoliative erythroderma and the presence of tumor cells (Sézary cells) in the peripheral blood. Patients diagnosed with early-phase mycosis fungoides often survive for many years, whereas patients with tumor-phase disease, disseminated disease, or Sézary syndrome survive on average for 1 to 3 years.

- *Adult T-cell leukemia/lymphoma* (ATL) is a neoplasm of CD4+ T cells caused by a retrovirus, human T-cell leukemia virus type 1 (HTLV-1). HTLV-1 infection is endemic in southern Japan, the Caribbean basin, and West Africa, and occurs sporadically elsewhere, including in the southeastern United States. The role of the virus in lymphogenesis is unclear but likely involves certain viral proteins and sustained proliferation of infected T cells. Adult T-cell leukemia/lymphoma is associated with skin lesions, lymphadenopathy, hepatosplenomegaly, hypercalcemia, and variable lymphocytosis. Most cases are very aggressive and respond poorly to treatment. The median survival time is only 8 months.

- *Peripheral T-cell lymphoma* encompasses a heterogeneous group of tumors that make up about 10% of non-Hodgkin lymphomas. In general, these are aggressive tumors that respond poorly to therapy. Moreover, because these are tumors of functional T cells, patients often suffer from symptoms related to tumor-derived inflammatory products, even when the tumor burden is relatively low.

Hodgkin Lymphoma

Hodgkin lymphomas are characterized by the presence of distinctive tumor giant cells known as Reed-Sternberg cells and variants.

Historically, Hodgkin lymphoma was considered apart from non-Hodgkin lymphomas because the diagnostic Reed-Sternberg cells have a distinctive appearance and comprise only a small fraction of the cells in the tumor. Although the Hodgkin lymphomas are now understood to be tumors of B-cell origin, they continue to be distinguished because of their unique biology and response to therapy.

Five subtypes of Hodgkin lymphoma are recognized: (1) nodular sclerosis, (2) mixed cellularity, (3) lymphocyte rich, (4) lymphocyte depletion, and (5) lymphocyte predominant. In the first four subtypes, the Reed-Sternberg cells share certain morphologic and immunophenotypic features (described later), and as a result these are lumped together under the rubric classic Hodgkin lymphoma.

Pathogenesis. All subtypes of Hodgkin lymphoma are caused by driver mutations in cancer genes; these are best characterized in classic Hodgkin lymphoma. NF-κB, a transcription factor that supports B-cell survival, is commonly upregulated by various mutations, and genes encoding PD-L1 and PD-L2, two immune checkpoint activators, are often amplified, which leads to their overexpression and helps Reed-Sternberg cells evade the host immune response. EBV is found in the Reed-Sternberg cells in as many as 70% of cases of the mixed-cellularity subtype and a smaller fraction of other "classic" forms of Hodgkin lymphoma.

Morphology. The sine qua non of classic Hodgkin lymphoma is the Reed-Sternberg cell (Fig. 9.20), a very large cell with an enormous multilobate nucleus, exceptionally prominent inclusion-like nucleoli, and abundant cytoplasm. Reed-Sternberg cells and their variants have a characteristic immunophenotype: They express CD15 and CD30 and do not express CD45 (leukocyte common antigen), B-cell antigens, or T-cell antigens. Differences in the appearance of the

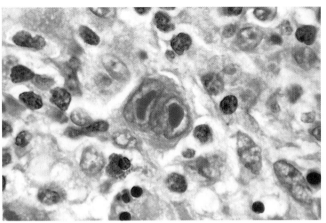

Fig. 9.20 Hodgkin lymphoma: lymph node. A binucleate Reed-Sternberg cell with large, inclusion-like nucleoli and abundant cytoplasm is surrounded by lymphocytes, macrophages, and an eosinophil. (Courtesy of Dr. Robert W. McKenna, Department of Pathology, University of Texas Southwestern Medical School, Dallas.)

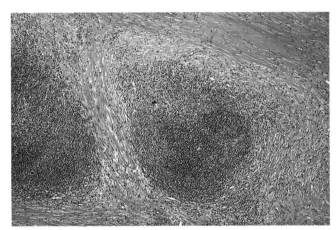

Fig. 9.21 Hodgkin lymphoma, nodular sclerosis type: lymph node. A low-power view shows well-defined bands of pink, acellular collagen that have subdivided the tumor cells into nodules. (Courtesy of Dr. Robert W. McKenna, Department of Pathology, University of Texas Southwestern Medical School, Dallas.)

Reed-Sternberg variants and the tissue response to these cells defines the most common subtypes of classical Hodgkin lymphoma:

- *Nodular sclerosis Hodgkin lymphoma* often involves the mediastinum of adolescents or young adults. It is defined by the presence of lacunar cells, Reed-Sternberg variants with a single multilobate nucleus, multiple small nucleoli and abundant, pale-staining cytoplasm, and collagen bands, which divide involved tissues into circumscribed nodules (Fig. 9.21). Also present are varying proportions of reactive lymphocytes, eosinophils, and macrophages, which are drawn in by cytokines produced by Reed-Sternberg cells and stromal cells in involved tissues.

- *Mixed-cellularity Hodgkin lymphoma* is most common in patients older than 50 years and comprises about 25% of cases overall. Classic Reed-Sternberg cells are plentiful within a heterogeneous inflammatory infiltrate containing small lymphocytes, eosinophils, plasma cells, and macrophages.

- The *lymphocyte-rich* and *lymphocyte-depleted* subtypes of classic Hodgkin lymphoma are both rare. As the names imply, they are characterized by the presence of unusually prominent or sparse infiltrates of reactive small lymphocytes, respectively. The

Reed-Sternberg cells and variants resemble those seen in the mixed cellularity subtype.

- Set apart from classical Hodgkin lymphoma is the *lympho-cyte-predominant subtype,* which accounts for about 5% of cases. It is defined by the presence of lymphohistiocytic (L&H) variant Reed-Sternberg cells with a delicate multilobed, puffy nucleus resembling popped corn (popcorn cell). L&H variants are found within large nodules containing mainly small B cells admixed with variable numbers of macrophages. Unlike the Reed-Sternberg variants in classic Hodgkin lymphoma, L&H variants express B-cell markers (e.g., CD20) and do not express CD15 and CD30.

Regardless of subtype, the diagnosis is based on the identification of Reed-Sternberg cells or variants in the appropriate background of reactive cells. Cells resembling Reed-Sternberg cells may be seen in other cancers and some reactive conditions; thus, immunophenotyping is often required for diagnosis.

Clinical Features. Hodgkin lymphoma usually manifests as painless lymphadenopathy or, with the nodular sclerosis subtype, symptoms related to the presence of a mediastinal mass. The systemic effects of cytokines cause anemia of chronic inflammation, leukocytosis, and so-called B symptoms (fever, weight loss, night sweats). Staging guides therapy and determines the prognosis. Younger patients with more favorable subtypes tend to present with low-stage disease and are free of so-called B symptoms, whereas patients with more extensive disease are more likely to have B symptoms and anemia. Initial treatment is with chemotherapy, sometimes with involved field radiotherapy for large tumor masses.

The overall outlook is excellent. The 5-year survival rate for patients with low-stage disease is over 90%. Even with widespread disease, the overall 5-year disease-free survival rate is around 50%. Immune checkpoint inhibitors have produced excellent responses in patients with relapsed, refractory disease and may soon be added to frontline therapeutic regimens.

Plasma Cell Neoplasms and Related Entities

These B-cell proliferations are composed entirely or in part of plasma cells and virtually always secrete a monoclonal immunoglobulin or immunoglobulin fragments.

Collectively, plasma cell neoplasms and related disorders account for about 15% of the deaths caused by lymphoid neoplasms. The most important of these neoplasms, multiple myeloma, is discussed next.

Multiple Myeloma

Multiple myeloma is one of the most common hematologic malignancies: Approximately 20,000 new cases are diagnosed in the United States each year. The median age at diagnosis is 70 years. It is more common in males and in people of African origin. It principally involves the marrow and usually is associated with lytic lesions throughout the skeletal system.

The most frequent immunoglobulin produced by myeloma cells is IgG (60%), followed by IgA (20% to 25%); in the remaining 15% to 20% of cases, the plasma cells produce only κ or λ immunoglobulin light chains. Only rarely are IgM, IgD, or IgE produced. Even in myelomas that produce complete immunoglobulins, immunoglobulin light chains are often synthesized in excess of immunoglobulin heavy chains, resulting in free, unpaired light chains. Once secreted, the small free light chains are excreted in the urine as *Bence-Jones proteins.* As described in the following, free light chains have important pathologic effects.

Morphology. Myeloma often has chromosomal translocations that fuse the *IGH* locus on chromosome 14 to proto-oncogenes such as the cyclin D1 gene. A wide variety of other driver mutations have been described. Proliferation of myeloma cells is supported by the cytokine interleukin 6 (IL-6).

The proliferating plasma cells have deleterious effects on the skeleton, the immune system, and the kidney, all of which contribute to morbidity and mortality:

- Several factors produced by myeloma cells cause bone resorption and lead to hypercalcemia and pathologic fractures, most frequently in the spine and femur.
- Myeloma causes defects in humoral immunity, increasing the risk for bacterial infections.
- Myeloma leads to renal failure owing to (1) obstructive proteinaceous casts comprised of precipitated Bence-Jones proteins; (2) light-chain deposition in the glomeruli or the interstitium, either as amyloid or linear deposits; (3) hypercalcemia, which leads to dehydration and renal stones; and (4) frequent bouts of bacterial pyelonephritis due to defective humoral immunity.

Morphology. Multiple myeloma usually manifests with multifocal destructive skeletal lesions that most commonly involve the vertebral column, ribs, skull, pelvis, femur, clavicle, and scapula. Radiologically, the bone lesions appear as punched-out defects 1 to 4 cm in diameter (Fig. 9.22A). The marrow contains increased numbers of plasma cells, typically more than 30% of the cellularity (see Fig. 9.22B). Renal involvement *(myeloma nephrosis)* is associated with proteinaceous casts that obstruct the distal convoluted tubules and the collecting ducts. Often, epithelial cells adjacent to the casts become necrotic or atrophic because Bence-Jones proteins are toxic. Other common pathologic processes involving the kidney include metastatic calcification, light-chain (AL) amyloidosis, and bacterial pyelonephritis.

Clinical Features. The diagnosis relies on the detection of a serum monoclonal immunoglobulin (a so-called M protein, for myeloma) and/or high levels of free immunoglobulin light chains in the serum or the urine; the identification of a large number of plasma cells in the marrow; and the characteristic radiologic findings. Hypercalcemia and renal failure also are common at the time of presentation. The prognosis is variable. Patients with multiple bony lesions, if untreated, rarely survive for more than 6 to 12 months, whereas patients with "smoldering myeloma" may be asymptomatic for many years.

Although cures have yet to be achieved, several recently developed therapies have improved outcomes. Misfolded immunoglobulin chains accumulate in myeloma cells and cause cell stress by activating the unfolded protein response (see Chapter 1). Inhibitors of the proteasome, a cellular organelle that disposes of misfolded proteins, induce apoptosis of myeloma cells and are effective therapies. The thalidomide-like compound lenalidomide also has activity against myeloma because of its ability to activate certain ubiquitin ligases, which tag proteins with ubiquitin, thereby marking them for proteasomal degradation. Bisphosphonates, drugs that inhibit bone resorption, reduce pathologic fractures and limit hypercalcemia. Hematopoietic stem cell transplantation prolongs life but has not yet proven to be curative. Trials of CAR-T cells that recognize plasma cell antigens are ongoing.

Other Plasma Cell Neoplasms and Related Entities

All these tumors are associated with the production of monoclonal immunoglobulins, marking them as clonal proliferations of antibody-producing B lymphocytes or plasma cells. Three tumors in this group merit discussion.

- *Monoclonal gammopathy of undetermined significance (MGUS)* is seen in patients without signs or symptoms who have monoclonal immunoglobulins in their blood. MGUS is very common in older adults, and about 1% of cases transform into a symptomatic neoplasm, most often multiple myeloma, each year.

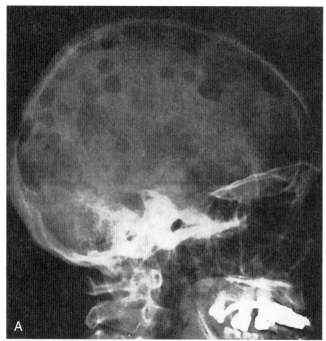

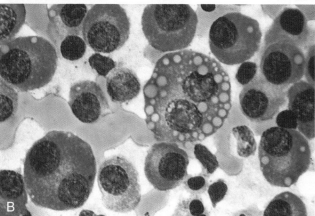

Fig. 9.22 Multiple myeloma. (A) Radiograph of the skull, lateral view. The sharply punched-out bone defects are most obvious in the calvaria. (B) Bone marrow aspirate. Normal marrow cells are largely replaced by plasma cells, including atypical forms with multiple nuclei, prominent nucleoli, and cytoplasmic droplets containing immunoglobulin.

- *Lymphoplasmacytic lymphoma* is a B-cell neoplasm of older adults that is composed of a mixture of small B cells and variable numbers of plasma cells. The plasma cell component secretes monoclonal IgM that often causes a hyperviscosity syndrome (*Waldenström macroglobulinemia*) marked by tinnitus, visual impairment, and neurologic dysfunction. Eventually, involvement of the marrow leads to cytopenias. Lymphoplasmacytic lymphoma is responsive to agents used for other indolent B-cell lymphomas (antibodies against CD20, inhibitors of B-cell receptor signaling). The overall survival time after diagnosis averages 4 to 5 years.
- *Primary or immunocyte-associated amyloidosis* results from a monoclonal proliferation of plasma cells producing immunoglobulin light chains that are deposited as amyloid (see Chapter 4). Some patients have overt multiple myeloma, but others have only a minor clonal population of plasma cells that nevertheless causes significant disease because of the synthesis of a pathogenic immunoglobulin.

Histiocytic Neoplasms

The term *histiocytosis* is an "umbrella" designation for a variety of proliferative disorders of dendritic cells or macrophages. Some, such

as very rare histiocytic sarcomas, are highly malignant neoplasms, whereas others are benign reactive hyperplasias. Between these two extremes lie a group of tumors comprised of Langerhans cells, the *Langerhans cell histiocytoses*, which merit a brief description.

Pathogenesis. All forms of Langerhans cell histiocytosis are associated with driver mutations that activate the serine/threonine kinase BRAF. BRAF is a component of the RAS signaling pathway that supports cellular proliferation and survival. Tumors without BRAF mutations often have mutations in a different serine/threonine kinase called MAP2K1 that acts downstream of BRAF, further implicating this pathway in the pathogenesis.

> *Morphology.* Proliferating Langerhans cells have abundant cytoplasm and vesicular nuclei, similar to that of tissue macrophages (also known as histiocytes); hence, the term *histiocytosis*. Numerous reactive eosinophils are often admixed. Langerhans cells express a unique protein called langerin and can be identified by staining for langerin and CD1a.

Clinical Features. Langerhans cell histiocytosis can be grouped into several clinicopathologic entities.
- The most common subtype is *unifocal unisystem disease,* in which the proliferation is confined to a single site in a single organ system, most commonly bone but also soft tissues such as the lung, skin, or gut. It may be asymptomatic or cause pain, tenderness, and pathologic fractures. It is indolent and is cured by local excision or irradiation.
- *Multifocal unisystem disease* usually affects children and typically manifests with multiple erosive bony masses. In about 50% of cases, involvement of the posterior pituitary stalk of the hypothalamus leads to diabetes insipidus. The combination of calvarial bone defects, diabetes insipidus, and exophthalmos is referred to as the *Hand-Schüller-Christian triad.* Some patients experience spontaneous regressions; others are treated effectively with chemotherapy.
- *Multisystem disease (Letterer-Siwe disease)* is an aggressive disorder that usually occurs in children younger than 2 years of age. It often manifests with cutaneous lesions that mimic seborrheic skin eruptions and frequently leads to hepatosplenomegaly, lymphadenopathy, pulmonary lesions, and destructive osteolytic bone lesions. Extensive marrow infiltration may lead to pancytopenia and predispose the patient to recurrent infections. The disease is rapidly fatal if untreated. With intensive chemotherapy, 50% of patients survive 5 years.

BLEEDING DISORDERS

Bleeding disorders may stem from abnormalities of vessels, platelets, or coagulation factors, alone or in combination (summarized in Table 9.8). As described in Chapter 3, normal clotting involves the vessel wall, platelets, and clotting factors. Laboratory tests that are relevant to hemostasis quantify and functionally characterize coagulation factors and platelets. The most important tests for investigation of suspected coagulopathies include:
- *Prothrombin time (PT).* This test assesses the extrinsic and common coagulation pathways. A prolonged PT can result from deficiencies of factors V, VII, and X; prothrombin; or fibrinogen.
- *Partial thromboplastin time (PTT).* This test assesses the intrinsic and common coagulation pathways. Prolongation of PTT can be caused by deficiencies of factors V, VIII, IX, X, XI, and XII; prothrombin; or fibrinogen.
- *Platelet count.* The normal reference range is 150,000 to 450,000/µL.
- *Tests of platelet function.* No single test provides an adequate assessment of platelet function. Aggregation tests that measure the response of platelets to certain agonists and qualitative and quantitative tests of von Willebrand factor (described later) are both used in clinical practice.

Table 9.8 Bleeding Disorders

Mechanism	Causes	Clinical Features
Vascular fragility	Vitamin C deficiency (scurvy) Systemic amyloidosis Chronic glucocorticoid use Inherited connective tissue disorders Vasculitis	Ecchymoses, skin and mucous membranes

Platelet dysfunction	Thrombocytopenia
	  Immune-mediated
	  Consumptive (DIC, HUS, TTP)
	  Marrow underproduction (tumors, other infiltrative disorders, aplastic anemia)
	Qualitative defects
	  Drugs (aspirin, other platelet inhibitors)
	  Myeloid neoplasms
	  Inherited defects (von Willebrand disease, Glanzmann thrombasthenia, Bernard-Soulier syndrome)
		Petechial bleeding, mucosae and skin
		Epistaxis
		Prolonged immediate bleeding from minor trauma
		Menorrhagia

Coagulation factor deficiencies	Inherited
	  Hemophilia A
	  Hemophilia B
	  Acquired
	Underproduction (vitamin K deficiency, liver disease)
	Factor inhibitors (antibodies, drugs)
	Consumptive (DIC)
		Hemorrhages in sites subject to mechanical trauma (e.g., joints)
		Delayed bleeding after surgery (e.g., circumcision)
		Bleeding in deep soft tissues (e.g., psoas muscle)

Additional more specialized tests are used to measure the levels of specific clotting factors and fibrin split products or to assess the presence of circulating anticoagulants.

Abnormalities of vessels that lead to bleeding include a range of miscellaneous, uncommon disorders, whereas disorders of platelets and coagulation factors are relatively common.

Thrombocytopenia

Thrombocytopenia is defined as a platelet count of less than 150,000/μL. Excessive posttraumatic bleeding is seen only when the platelet counts are reduced to 20,000 to 50,000/μL, and spontaneous bleeding is unlikely until counts fall below 5000/μL. Bleeding typically occurs from small, superficial blood vessels and produces petechiae or large ecchymoses in the skin, the mucous membranes of the gastrointestinal and urinary tracts, and other sites. The most feared complication of thrombocytopenia is hemorrhage into the central nervous system, which is uncommon but may be fatal.

Major causes of thrombocytopenia are listed in Table 9.9. Clinically important thrombocytopenia may be caused by reduced production or increased destruction of platelets. Splenomegaly depresses platelet counts because of the sequestration of platelets but in and of itself does not cause clinically significant thrombocytopenia. Reduced production is generally due to a problem with hematopoiesis that also affects red cell and granulocyte production. In contrast, increased destruction of platelets may be seen as an isolated abnormality in several disorders that merit a brief discussion.

Immune Thrombocytopenic Purpura

Immune thrombocytopenic purpura (ITP) is an autoimmune disease caused by antibodies that bind platelet surface proteins, leading to opsonization of the platelets and their removal from the circulation by macrophages.

The disease has two clinical subtypes. Acute ITP is a self-limited form seen mostly in children after viral infections. Chronic ITP is a relatively common disorder that most often affects women between

Table 9.9 Causes of Thrombocytopenia

Decreased Production of Platelets

Generalized Bone Marrow Dysfunction

Aplastic anemia: congenital and acquired
Marrow infiltration: leukemia, disseminated cancer

Selective Impairment of Platelet Production

Drug-induced: alcohol, thiazides, cytotoxic drugs
Infections: measles, HIV infection

Ineffective Megakaryocytopoiesis

Megaloblastic anemia

Decreased Platelet Survival

Immunologic Destruction

Autoimmune:
Primary: immune thrombocytopenic purpura
Secondary: B-cell tumors (e.g., chronic lymphocytic leukemia); autoimmune disorders (systemic lupus erythematosus); infections (infectious mononucleosis, HIV)
Isoimmune: posttransfusion and neonatal
Drug-associated: quinidine, heparin, sulfa compounds

Nonimmunologic Destruction

Disseminated intravascular coagulation
Hemolytic-uremic syndrome
Thrombotic thrombocytopenic purpura
Microangiopathic hemolytic anemia
Dengue fever

Sequestration

Hypersplenism

Dilutional

Multiple transfusions (e.g., for massive blood loss)

HIV, human immunodeficiency virus.

the ages of 20 and 40 years. The spleen is an important site of anti-platelet antibody production and the major site of destruction of the IgG-coated platelets, so splenectomy is beneficial. Chronic ITP is an isolated disorder that must be distinguished from secondary ITP due to other conditions (e.g., systemic lupus erythematosus, drug exposure, HIV infection, and B-cell malignancies).

The onset of chronic ITP is insidious. Common findings include petechiae, easy bruising, epistaxis, gum bleeding, and hemorrhages after minor trauma. Serious intracerebral or subarachnoid hemorrhages are rare, but occur. The diagnosis rests on the clinical features, the presence of thrombocytopenia, and the response to therapy. Most patients are first treated with glucocorticoids, which inhibit macrophage function and rapidly correct the platelet count and sometimes produce sustained responses, even after discontinuance. For others, splenectomy, anti–B-cell therapies (e.g., anti-CD20 antibodies), and thrombopoietin-like drugs are often effective at controlling the thrombocytopenia.

Heparin-Induced Thrombocytopenia

This special type of drug-induced thrombocytopenia merits a brief mention because of its clinical importance. Moderate to severe thrombocytopenia develops in 3% to 5% of patients after 1 to 2 weeks of treatment with heparin. It is caused by IgG antibodies that bind to platelet factor 4 on platelet membranes in a heparin-dependent fashion. Antibody binding activates platelets and induces their aggregation, thereby exacerbating thrombosis, the condition that heparin is used to treat. Both venous and arterial thromboses occur, even in the setting of marked thrombocytopenia, and may cause severe morbidity (e.g., loss of limbs) and death. Cessation of heparin therapy breaks the cycle of platelet activation and consumption.

Thrombotic Microangiopathies

The term *thrombotic microangiopathies* encompasses a spectrum of clinical syndromes that include thrombotic thrombocytopenic purpura (TTP) and hemolytic-uremic syndrome (HUS). Their causes are different, but all are characterized by abnormal platelet activation and deposition of platelet-rich thrombi in the microcirculation, leading to thrombocytopenia and anemia. In contrast to DIC, activation of coagulation factors is not a prominent feature of HUS or TTP; consequently, the PT and PTT are usually normal or only slightly deranged. Because both disorders prominently involve the kidney, they are discussed in Chapter 11.

Coagulation Disorders

Coagulation disorders result from either congenital or acquired deficiencies of protein factors that are required for clotting.
Acquired deficiencies are more common and are most often caused by:
- *Vitamin K deficiency.* This usually occurs in the setting of broad-spectrum antibiotic therapy, intestinal malabsorption, or impaired nutrition, and results in inadequate synthesis of prothrombin and clotting factors VII, IX, and X and a severe coagulation defect. Warfarin is an anticoagulant drug that acts by inhibiting the synthesis of vitamin K-dependent factors.
- *Liver disease.* The liver synthesizes several coagulation factors and also removes many activated coagulation factors from the circulation; thus, hepatic parenchymal diseases are common causes of complex coagulation disorders.
- *Disseminated intravascular coagulation* (DIC; discussed later) often leads to deficiencies of multiple factors.
- *Autoantibodies* against coagulation factors cause acquired deficiencies limited to a single factor.

Hereditary deficiencies of many coagulation factors also have been identified. Of these, only von Willebrand disease, hemophilia A, and hemophilia B are sufficiently common to warrant further consideration.

Von Willebrand Disease

Von Willebrand disease is a bleeding disorder caused by qualitative or quantitative defects in von Willebrand factor.

Von Willebrand disease is characterized by spontaneous bleeding from mucous membranes, excessive bleeding after dental procedures or surgery, and menorrhagia. It is more prevalent in persons of European descent and is believed to affect approximately 1% of people in the United States, making it the most common inherited bleeding disorder.

Von Willebrand factor (vWF) is mainly synthesized in endothelial cells and megakaryocytes and exists in the plasma as large multimers of up to 20 MDa in weight (Fig. 9.23). It also is found in the subendothelium, where it binds to collagen. vWF has two major functions:
- *vWF binds to platelet glycoproteins,* allowing vWF to serve as a molecular "glue" between subendothelial collagen and platelets following endothelial damage (see Fig. 9.23).
- *vWF binds factor VIII,* a cofactor for factor IX, increasing its half-life in the circulation and enhancing delivery of factor VIII to sites of primary hemostasis.

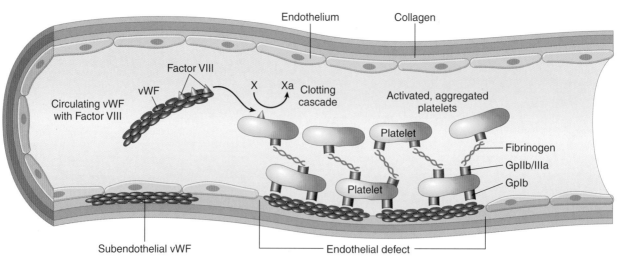

Fig. 9.23 Structure and function of factor VIII–von Willebrand factor *(vWF)* complex. Factor VIII and vWF circulate as a complex. vWF also is present in the subendothelial matrix of normal blood vessels. Factor VIII takes part in the coagulation cascade by activating factor X by means of factor IX *(not shown)*. vWF causes adhesion of platelets to subendothelial collagen, primarily through the glycoprotein Ib *(GpIb)* platelet receptor.

Von Willebrand disease is thus associated with defects in both platelet function and coagulation; only the platelet defect produces clinical findings, except in rare patients with homozygous von Willebrand disease who have severe factor VIII deficiency.

The classic and most common variant of von Willebrand disease is an autosomal dominant disorder with reduced circulating vWF and a measurable but clinically insignificant decrease in factor VIII levels that prolongs the PTT. Less common varieties of von Willebrand disease have mutations causing qualitative defects in vWF that lead to abnormally large or small vWF multimers, preventing normal primary hemostasis.

The diagnosis is reached by measuring the quantity, size, and function of vWF. vWF function is assessed using the *ristocetin platelet agglutination test.* Ristocetin "activates" the binding of vWF to platelet glycoproteins, creating interplatelet bridges that cause platelets to clump (agglutination), an easily quantified event that serves as a useful assay of vWF function.

Hemophilia A

Hemophilia A, the most common hereditary cause of serious bleeding, is an X-linked disorder caused by deficiency of factor VIII.

Almost all affected individuals are males. Approximately 30% of cases are caused by new mutations; in the remainder, there is a positive family history. Severe hemophilia A is observed in people with marked deficiencies of factor VIII (activity levels < 1% of normal). Milder deficiencies may only manifest after trauma or other hemostatic stresses. The varying degrees of factor VIII deficiency are due to the existence of many different causative mutations.

In symptomatic cases, there is a tendency toward easy bruising and massive hemorrhage after trauma or surgical procedures. In addition, "spontaneous" hemorrhages frequently are encountered in tissues that are subject to mechanical stress, particularly joints, where recurrent bleeds *(hemarthroses)* lead to progressive deformities that can be crippling. Bleeds into deep soft tissues (e.g., muscles) and the brain also may occur.

The diagnosis is suspected based on a characteristic bleeding history in an infant or young child and the identification of a prolonged PTT, and is confirmed with specific factor assays. Hemophilia A is usually treated with factor VIII infusions. In approximately 15% of those with severe hemophilia A, replacement therapy is complicated by the development of neutralizing antibodies against factor VIII, which is recognized

as a "foreign" antigen. These difficult-to-treat patients may benefit from therapy using a bispecific antibody that cross-links factor IX to factor X, greatly diminishing the physiologic requirement for factor VIII.

Hemophilia B–Factor IX Deficiency

Severe factor IX deficiency is an X-linked disorder that is clinically indistinguishable from hemophilia A but much less common. The diagnosis is made using specific assays of factor IX. It is treated by infusion of recombinant factor IX.

Disseminated Intravascular Coagulation

Disseminated intravascular coagulation is a condition in which excessive activation of clotting results in the formation of thrombi in many tissues and secondary deficiencies of platelets and coagulation factors.

Disseminated intravascular coagulation (DIC) occurs as a complication of a wide variety of disorders. DIC can give rise to either tissue hypoxia and microinfarcts caused by microthrombi or to a bleeding disorder related to depletion of the elements required for hemostasis (hence the term *consumptive coagulopathy*).

Pathogenesis. Clotting can be initiated by either the extrinsic pathway, which is activated by tissue factor; or the intrinsic pathway, which is activated when factor XII interacts with collagen or other negatively charged substances. Both pathways generate thrombin, which cleaves fibrinogen to form a fibrin clot. Clotting is normally limited to the site of injury by a number of factors (see Chapter 3).

DIC may be triggered by (1) excessive release of tissue factor or other thromboplastic substances into the circulation or (2) widespread endothelial cell damage (Fig. 9.24). Severe endothelial cell injury exposes subendothelial tissue factor and collagen. Even mild endothelial damage can unleash procoagulant activity by stimulating tissue factor expression while suppressing expression of anticoagulant factors (e.g., thrombomodulin). Endothelial injury has a central role in systemic inflammatory response syndrome (SIRS) triggered by sepsis and other systemic insults (see Chapter 3); DIC is a frequent complication of SIRS. Disorders associated with DIC are listed in Table 9.10. Of these, DIC is most often associated with sepsis,

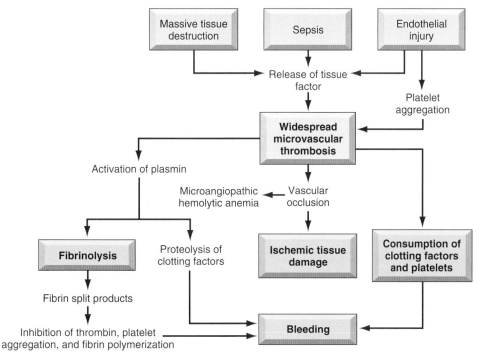

Fig. 9.24 Pathophysiology of disseminated intravascular coagulation.

Table 9.10 Major Disorders Associated with Disseminated Intravascular Coagulation

Obstetric Complications
Abruptio placentae
Retained dead fetus
Septic abortion
Amniotic fluid embolism
Toxemia

Infections
Sepsis (gram-negative and gram-positive)
Meningococcemia
Rocky Mountain spotted fever
Histoplasmosis
Aspergillosis

Neoplasms
Adenocarcinomas of pancreas, prostate, lung, and stomach
Acute promyelocytic leukemia

Massive Tissue Injury
Trauma
Burns
Extensive surgery

Miscellaneous
Acute intravascular hemolysis, snakebite, giant hemangioma, shock, heat stroke, vasculitis, aortic aneurysm, liver disease

Table 9.11 Causes of Splenomegaly

Massive Splenomegaly (weight >1000 g)
Myeloproliferative neoplasms (chronic myeloid leukemia, primary myelofibrosis)
Lymphoid leukemias (chronic lymphocytic leukemia and hairy cell leukemia)
Lymphoma
Infectious diseases (e.g., malaria)
Storage diseases (e.g., Gaucher disease)

Moderate splenomegaly (weight 500 to 1000 g)
Chronic congestive splenomegaly (portal hypertension or splenic vein obstruction)
Acute leukemias
Hemolytic anemias (hereditary spherocytosis, thalassemia, immunohemolytic anemia)
Amyloidosis
Niemann-Pick disease
Chronic infections (tuberculosis)
Sarcoidosis

Mild splenomegaly (weight < 500 g)
Infectious mononucleosis
Miscellaneous disorders (sepsis, systemic lupus erythematosus)

obstetric complications, malignancy, and major trauma (especially to the brain).

Once initiated, DIC has two consequences: (1) fibrin deposition in the circulation (thrombosis) and (2) depletion of platelets and clotting factors with secondary release of plasminogen activators, causing a bleeding disorder that is paradoxically superimposed on the excessive clotting. Plasmin cleaves not only fibrin (fibrinolysis) but also factors V and VIII, thereby reducing their concentration further. In addition, fibrinolysis creates fibrin degradation products that inhibit platelet aggregation, have antithrombin activity, and impair fibrin polymerization, all of which contribute to bleeding.

Clinical Features. Depending on the balance between clotting and bleeding tendencies, the range of clinical manifestations is enormous, from mere laboratory abnormalities to multiorgan failure, circulatory collapse, and massive, sometimes fatal, bleeding. In general, acute DIC (e.g., that associated with infection or obstetric complications) is dominated by bleeding, whereas chronic DIC (e.g., as occurs in those with cancer) more often causes thrombosis. Laboratory tests reveal thrombocytopenia, prolongation of the PT and PTT, increased fibrin split products, and decreased fibrinogen. The presence of thrombi in small vessels also creates shear stress that disrupts red cells, producing so-called microangiopathic hemolytic anemia. Red cell fragments called schistocytes are characteristically seen in the peripheral blood.

The prognosis is dictated by the underlying disorder and the severity of the DIC. Acute DIC is life threatening and is treated aggressively with anticoagulants if thrombosis dominates or by administration of clotting factors (fresh frozen plasma) and platelets if bleeding is the principal problem. In contrast, chronic DIC is sometimes identified unexpectedly by laboratory testing. In either circumstance, the only definitive intervention is treatment of the underlying cause.

DISORDERS OF SPLEEN AND THYMUS

SPLENOMEGALY

Primary disorders of the spleen are rare, but as an important component of the innate and adaptive immune system and a filter for the blood, the spleen is secondarily involved by many systemic disorders. In virtually all instances, the spleen responds by enlarging (splenomegaly), an alteration that produces a set of stereotypical signs and symptoms. Disorders may be grouped according to the degree of splenomegaly that they characteristically produce (Table 9.11).

When enlarged, the spleen and its resident macrophages often remove excessive numbers of formed blood elements, resulting in anemia, leukopenia, or thrombocytopenia; this is referred to as *hypersplenism*. Platelets are particularly susceptible to sequestration in the interstices of the red pulp; as a result, *thrombocytopenia* is more prevalent and severe in persons with splenomegaly than is anemia or neutropenia.

DISORDERS OF THE THYMUS

The thymus has a crucial role in T-cell maturation and is frequently involved by T-cell acute lymphoblastic leukemia (T-ALL). The focus here is on the two most frequent (albeit still uncommon) disorders of the thymus, thymic hyperplasia and thymoma, both of which may be associated with systemic autoimmune diseases.

Thymic Follicular Hyperplasia

The most frequent cause of thymic enlargement is formation of lymphoid follicles and hyperplasia of germinal center B cells, which are not normally present in the thymus. Thymic follicular hyperplasia is found in most patients with *myasthenia gravis* (see Chapter 18) and may occur in other autoimmune diseases, such as systemic lupus erythematosus and rheumatoid arthritis. Neither the cause of the thymic hyperplasia nor its contribution to the associated autoimmune disorders is understood, but removal of the hyperplastic thymus may lead to remittance of the myasthenia.

Thymoma

Thymomas are neoplasms derived from thymic epithelial cells. They may arise at any age, but most occur in middle-aged adults. They may be benign or malignant. Most include variable numbers of nonneoplastic immature T cells. In about 30% of cases, thymoma is associated with an autoimmune disorder (e.g., myasthenia gravis, systemic lupus erythematosus, pure red cell aplasia). Removal of the thymoma may lead to remittance of myasthenia gravis but is less effective in treating other associated disorders..

10

Lung and Upper Respiratory Tract

OUTLINE

Acute Respiratory Distress Syndrome, 163
Obstructive Lung Diseases, 164
    Chronic Obstructive Pulmonary Disease, 165
    Asthma, 166
    Bronchiectasis, 168
Restrictive Lung Diseases, 168
    Fibrosing Diseases, 168
    Pneumoconioses, 169
    Granulomatous Diseases, 170
Pulmonary Diseases of Vascular Origin, 171
    Pulmonary Embolism, Hemorrhage, and Infarction, 171
    Pulmonary Hypertension, 172
    Diffuse Alveolar Hemorrhage Syndromes, 172
Pulmonary Infections, 172
    Community-Acquired Bacterial Pneumonias, 173

Nosocomial Bacterial Pneumonias, 174
Aspiration Pneumonias, 174
Lung Abscess, 174
Tuberculosis, 175
Community-Acquired Viral Pneumonias, 177
Fungal Infections, 179
Opportunistic Infections, 180
Lung, Pleural, and Upper Airway Tumors, 181
    Lung Carcinoma, 181
    Carcinoid Tumors, 184
    Malignant Mesothelioma, 184
    Nasopharyngeal Carcinoma, 185
    Carcinoma of the Larynx, 185

The lung is anatomically designed to replenish oxygen and remove carbon dioxide from the blood. Gas exchange depends on a network of capillaries that lie closely apposed to sac-like terminal air spaces called alveoli that are separated from the blood by a thin layer comprised of epithelial cells, a small amount of extracellular matrix, and a layer of endothelial cells. A broad range of diseases involve the lung, including inflammatory, infectious, and neoplastic disorders, many of which present with signs and symptoms related to abnormalities of gas exchange. In this chapter, we focus on common disorders that affect the lung and the upper airways.

ACUTE RESPIRATORY DISTRESS SYNDROME

Acute respiratory distress syndrome is a disorder in which damage to alveoli throughout the lungs causes edema and leads to respiratory failure.

Acute respiratory distress syndrome affects approximately 190,000 patients per year in the United States and is also referred to clinically as acute lung injury. It is characterized by the rapid onset of life-threatening respiratory insufficiency, cyanosis, and severe arterial hypoxemia.

Pathogenesis. Acute respiratory distress syndrome may occur in association with primary pulmonary diseases or systemic inflammatory disorders. The most frequent triggers are pneumonia and sepsis, followed by aspiration, severe trauma, pancreatitis, and transfusion reactions. All of these disorders may cause widespread injury to alveolar endothelial and epithelial cells, leading to an accumulation of edema fluid in the alveolar interstitium and the air spaces and producing a characteristic "whiteout" of the lungs on imaging studies. Pulmonary macrophages respond to the injury by producing proinflammatory mediators (Fig. 10.1) that activate endothelial cells. Adhesion molecules that bind neutrophils are upregulated, leading to sequestration of the neutrophils in pulmonary capillaries. Locally produced cytokines also activate the neutrophils, which release a variety of products (e.g., reactive oxygen species, proteases) that may further damage the alveolar epithelium and endothelium.

Morphology. The histologic manifestation of acute respiratory distress syndrome is *diffuse alveolar damage*. In the acute phase, the lungs are dark red, firm, and heavy. Microscopic examination reveals congestion, necrosis of alveolar epithelial cells, interstitial and intraalveolar edema and hemorrhage, and (particularly with sepsis) collections of neutrophils in capillaries. The alveoli are often lined by *hyaline membranes* consisting of fibrin-rich edema fluid mixed with debris from necrotic epithelial cells (Fig. 10.2). In the *organizing stage,* alveolar epithelium proliferates to regenerate the alveolar lining. Healing may lead to resolution or to the development of fibrotic thickening of the alveolar walls.

Clinical Features. Acute respiratory distress syndrome usually develops within 72 hours of the initial insult. Most patients require intubation and mechanical ventilation, which improves oxygenation, but, nonetheless, approximately one third of patients die, usually because of the underlying disorder (e.g., sepsis) or multiorgan failure. Most patients who survive recover normal respiratory function within 6 to 12 months, but others have chronic respiratory insufficiency from residual alveolar fibrosis.

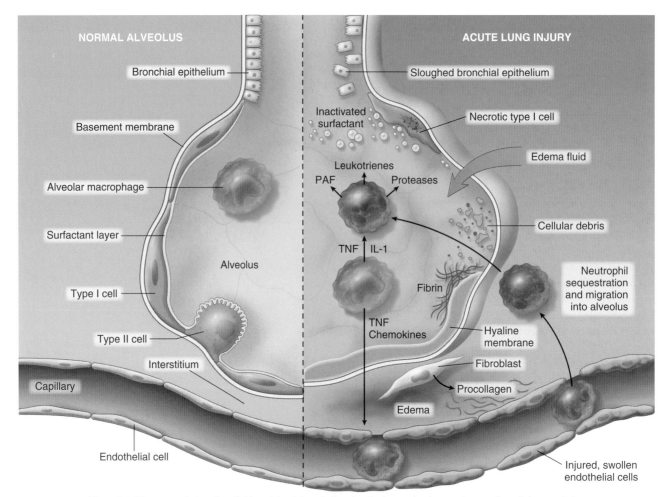

Fig. 10.1 The normal alveolus *(left)* and the injured alveolus in the early phase of acute lung injury and the acute respiratory distress syndrome. Under the influence of proinflammatory cytokines such as IL-8 and IL-1 and tumor necrosis factor (TNF) (released by macrophages), neutrophils are sequestered in the pulmonary microvasculature and then egress into the alveolar space, where they are activated. Activated neutrophils release factors (leukotrienes, reactive oxygen species, proteases, and platelet-activating factor [PAF]) that contribute to local tissue damage, accumulation of edema fluid, surfactant inactivation, and hyaline membrane formation. Subsequently, the release of macrophage-derived fibrogenic cytokines such as transforming growth factor-β (TGF-β) and platelet-derived growth factor (PGDF) stimulate fibroblast growth and collagen deposition associated with the healing phase of injury. (Modified from Ware LB: Pathophysiology of acute lung injury and the acute respiratory distress syndrome, *Semin Respir Crit Care Med* 27:337, 2006.)

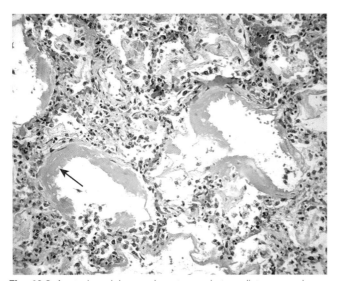

Fig. 10.2 Acute lung injury and acute respiratory distress syndrome. Diffuse alveolar damage. Some alveoli are collapsed, and others are distended; many are lined by pink hyaline membranes *(arrow)*.

OBSTRUCTIVE LUNG DISEASES

Chronic diseases that decrease pulmonary gas exchange are divided into (1) *obstructive (airway) disease,* characterized by an increase in resistance to air flow caused by partial or complete airway obstruction at any level, and (2) *restrictive disease,* characterized by reduced expansion of the lung parenchyma and decreased total lung capacity. In obstructive diseases, the forced vital capacity (FVC) is normal or slightly decreased, whereas the expiratory flow rate, usually measured as the forced expiratory volume at 1 second (FEV_1), is significantly decreased. Thus, the ratio of FEV to FVC is decreased. By contrast, in restrictive diseases (discussed later), the FVC is reduced and the expiratory flow rate is normal or reduced proportionately. Hence, the ratio of FEV to FVC is near normal.

The three major obstructive lung disorders—emphysema, chronic bronchitis, and asthma—have characteristic clinical and pathologic features in their prototypical forms (Table 10.1). Because emphysema and chronic bronchitis often coexist to varying degrees, we will discuss them together under the rubric of chronic obstructive pulmonary disease (COPD). We will finish by discussing asthma, a reversible form of obstructive airway disease, and bronchiectasis, an obstructive disorder with distinctive clinicopathologic features.

Chronic Obstructive Pulmonary Disease

Chronic obstructive pulmonary disease is characterized by obstructive airway and alveolar abnormalities caused by inhalation of noxious particles or gases, most often due to smoking tobacco.

Chronic obstructive pulmonary disease (COPD) affects more than 5% of the adults in the United States, where it is the third leading cause of death, exceeded only by cardiovascular disease and cancer. Airflow limitation is caused by a combination of mechanical obstruction of airways by mucous secretions and fibrosis (*chronic bronchitis*) and functional obstruction due to parenchymal destruction (*emphysema*), both in response to chronic inflammation. Chronic bronchitis is defined by the presence of a persistent productive cough for at least 3 consecutive months in at least 2 consecutive years. Emphysema is defined by the presence of enlarged air spaces distal to the terminal bronchioles and the destruction of alveolar walls.

Pathogenesis. Inhaled tobacco smoke and other noxious particles initiate several processes that result in parenchymal destruction (emphysema) and airway disease (bronchiolitis and chronic bronchitis). Factors that influence the development and severity of chronic bronchitis and emphysema include the following:

- *Inhalation of noxious particles.* Tobacco smoke contains numerous toxic substances and carcinogens that damage cells directly and induce deleterious reactive changes, such as hypertrophy of mucous glands in the trachea and bronchi and an increase in mucin-secreting goblet cells in the epithelial surfaces of smaller bronchi and bronchioles.
- *Inflammation.* Cell injury caused by toxic effects of inhaled agents induces the production of inflammatory mediators (including leukotrienes, interleukin-8 [IL-8], tumor necrosis factor [TNF], and others) that recruit leukocytes from the circulation, amplifying the inflammatory process. The resulting chronic inflammation produces fibrosis of the bronchiolar wall and narrowing of bronchial lumens. In some patients, inflammation also causes hyperresponsiveness of the bronchial smooth muscle, leading to bronchospasm.
- *Proteases* released from neutrophils are thought to have a central role in the emphysematous changes that accompany COPD. This idea is based in part on the predisposition of patients with a genetic deficiency of α1-antitrypsin to develop emphysema. α1-antitrypsin is an inhibitor of proteases (e.g., elastase, which digests elastic fibers) that are secreted by neutrophils. Most α1-antitrypsin–deficient individuals develop emphysema, which occurs at an earlier age and is of greater severity if the individual smokes. Small airways are normally held open by the elastic recoil of the lung parenchyma. The loss of elastic tissue in the walls of alveoli that surround respiratory bronchioles reduces radial traction, leading to collapse of the respiratory bronchioles during expiration and functional airflow obstruction.
- *Microbial infection* is often present but has a secondary role, chiefly by maintaining inflammation and exacerbating symptoms.

Morphology. Both emphysematous and bronchitic changes are seen in most cases. The classification of emphysematous change in COPD and other settings is based on the macroscopic appearance of the lung (Fig. 10.3). The most common pattern in smokers is *centriacinar emphysema*, which preferentially affects the terminal respiratory bronchiole. The lesions are more common and usually more severe in the upper lobes, particularly in the apical segments. Histologic examination reveals destruction of alveolar walls leading to air space enlargement, without overt fibrosis (Supplemental eFig. 10.1). Terminal and respiratory bronchioles also may be deformed because of the loss of septa that help tether these structures in the parenchyma. *Panacinar emphysema* is usually seen in the setting of α1-antitrypsin deficiency and results in greater expansion of lung volume than does centriacinar emphysema. Panacinar emphysema tends to occur more commonly in the lower zones and in the anterior margins of the lung; it is usually most severe at the bases.

The bronchitic component of COPD is marked by hyperemia of the bronchial and tracheal mucosa and excessive mucinous or mucopurulent secretions. The most characteristic microscopic feature is the enlargement of mucous-secreting glands (Supplemental eFig. 10.2). Variable numbers of inflammatory cells, including lymphocytes, macrophages, and neutrophils, are seen in the bronchial mucosa.

Clinical Features. Clinical features vary depending on the relative severity of the emphysematous and bronchitic changes. When emphysema is prominent, *dyspnea* is the first symptom. It begins insidiously and is steadily progressive. The classic presentation of emphysematous COPD is one in which the patient is barrel-chested and dyspneic, with obviously prolonged expiration, sitting forward in a hunched-over position. Hyperventilation maintains adequate gas exchange and blood gas values are relatively normal until late in the course. In patients in whom chronic bronchitis with or without bronchospasm dominates,

Table 10.1 Disorders Associated with Airflow Obstruction: The Spectrum of Chronic Obstructive Pulmonary Disease

Clinical Entity	Anatomic Site	Major Pathologic Changes	Etiology	Signs/Symptoms
Chronic bronchitis	Bronchus	Mucous gland hypertrophy and hyperplasia, hypersecretion	Tobacco smoke, air pollutants	Cough, sputum production
Emphysema	Acinus	Air space enlargement, wall destruction	Tobacco smoke	Dyspnea
Asthma	Bronchus	Smooth muscle hypertrophy and hyperplasia, excessive mucus, inflammation	Immunologic or undefined causes	Episodic wheezing, cough, dyspnea
Bronchiectasis	Bronchus	Airway dilation and scarring	Persistent or severe infections	Cough, purulent sputum, fever

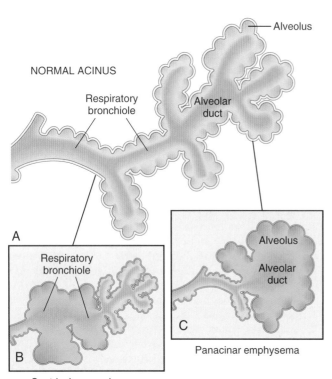

NORMAL ACINUS

— Alveolus

Respiratory
bronchiole

Alveolar
duct

A

Respiratory
bronchiole

Alveolus

Alveolar
duct

B

C

Centriacinar emphysema

Panacinar emphysema

Fig. 10.3 Major patterns of emphysema. (A) Diagram of normal structure of the acinus, the fundamental unit of the lung. (B) Centriacinar emphysema with dilation that initially affects the respiratory bronchioles. (C) Panacinar emphysema with initial distention of all the peripheral structures (i.e., the alveolus and alveolar duct); the disease later extends to affect the respiratory bronchioles.

cough and wheezing are common initial complaints. For unclear reasons, dyspnea is less prominent, and these patients tend to retain carbon dioxide, becoming hypoxic and often cyanotic. In most patients with COPD, symptoms fall between these two extremes. Pulmonary function tests reveal reduced FEV_1, a normal or near-normal FVC, and a reduced FEV_1-to-FVC ratio.

The therapeutic approach includes smoking cessation programs (to slow the decline in pulmonary function), vaccination against influenza and pneumococcus (to prevent acute exacerbations due to infection), bronchodilators (to counter inflammation-induced bronchospasm), and antiinflammatory agents such as corticosteroids. Hypoxia-induced pulmonary vascular spasm and loss of pulmonary capillary surface area from alveolar destruction cause the gradual development of secondary pulmonary hypertension, which in 20% to 30% of patients leads to right-sided congestive heart failure (cor pulmonale; see Chapter 8). Common causes of death in patients with COPD include heart failure, pneumonia, and pulmonary thromboembolism.

Asthma

Asthma is a chronic inflammatory disorder that causes episodic bronchospasm associated with airway obstruction.

Asthma is a common disorder that has increased in incidence in the Western world over the past 4 decades. One proposed explanation for this trend is the hygiene hypothesis, according to which a lack of exposure to environmental antigens, particularly microorganisms, in early childhood results in defects in immune tolerance and subsequent hyperreactivity to immune stimuli later in life.

Pathogenesis. Factors contributing to the development of asthma include a genetic predisposition to type I hypersensitivity (atopy), acute and chronic airway inflammation, and bronchial hyperresponsiveness to a variety of stimuli. Asthma may be subclassified as atopic (evidence of allergen sensitization) or nonatopic (no evidence of type I hypersensitivity). In both types, bronchospasm may be triggered by diverse exposures, including allergens, respiratory infections (especially viral infections), airborne irritants (e.g., smoke, fumes), cold air, stress, and exercise.

Atopic asthma is the most common type and is an example of an IgE-mediated type I hypersensitivity reaction (Fig. 10.4). It usually begins in childhood. Affected children develop type 2 helper T-cell (Th2) responses to various allergens present in dust, pollen, animal dander, or food. Cytokines produced by Th2 T cells account for most of the features: IL-4 and IL-13 stimulate IgE production, IL-5 activates eosinophils, and IL-13 also stimulates mucous production. IgE binds to submucosal mast cells, which on exposure to allergens release their granule contents and secrete cytokines and other mediators. Mast cell–derived mediators produce two waves of reaction:

- The *early-phase reaction* is dominated by bronchoconstriction, mucous production, and vasodilation. Bronchoconstriction is triggered by mediators released from mast cells (histamine, prostaglandins, and leukotrienes) and also by reflex neural pathways.
- The *late-phase reaction* is attributed to chemokines (including eotaxin, a potent chemoattractant and activator of eosinophils) released by cells such as epithelial cells that promote the recruitment of Th2 cells, eosinophils, and other leukocytes, amplifying an inflammatory reaction that is initiated by resident immune cells.

Nonatopic asthma is not associated with allergen sensitization; a positive family history of asthma is less common. Respiratory infections due to viruses (e.g., rhinovirus, parainfluenza virus) and inhaled air pollutants (e.g., sulfur dioxide, ozone, nitrogen dioxide) are common triggers, but exposures to cold air or exercise may also trigger an attack. Although the mechanisms of non-atopic asthma are not well understood, mast cell activation is common to both atopic and nonatopic variants.

Morphology. Bronchi and bronchioles are occluded by thick, tenacious mucus plugs containing whorls of shed epithelium (Curschmann spirals). Numerous eosinophils and Charcot-Leyden crystals (crystalloids made of galectin-10, a protein derived from eosinophils) also are present. Other characteristic morphologic changes, collectively called airway remodeling, include thickening of the airway wall, submucosal fibrosis, increased submucosal vascularity, an increase in the size of submucosal glands, goblet cell metaplasia, and hypertrophy of bronchial smooth muscle (Supplemental eFig. 10.3)

Clinical Features. An asthma attack leads to severe dyspnea and wheezing due to bronchoconstriction and mucous plugging, producing air-trapping in distal air spaces and progressive hyperinflation of the lungs. Attacks usually last from 1 hour to several hours and subside spontaneously or with therapy. Intervals between attacks are characteristically asymptomatic, but subtle persistent deficits can be detected by pulmonary function tests. The usual therapeutic approach involves avoidance of irritants and allergens and the use of antiinflammatory drugs (particularly corticosteroids) and bronchodilators. Newer therapies for atopic asthma include anti-IgE antibody and antibodies against Th2 cytokines or their receptors. In most cases, asthma is disabling but not lethal. However, occasionally a severe paroxysm occurs that does not respond to therapy and persists for days and even weeks (*status asthmaticus*), resulting in hypercapnia, acidosis, and severe hypoxia that may prove fatal.

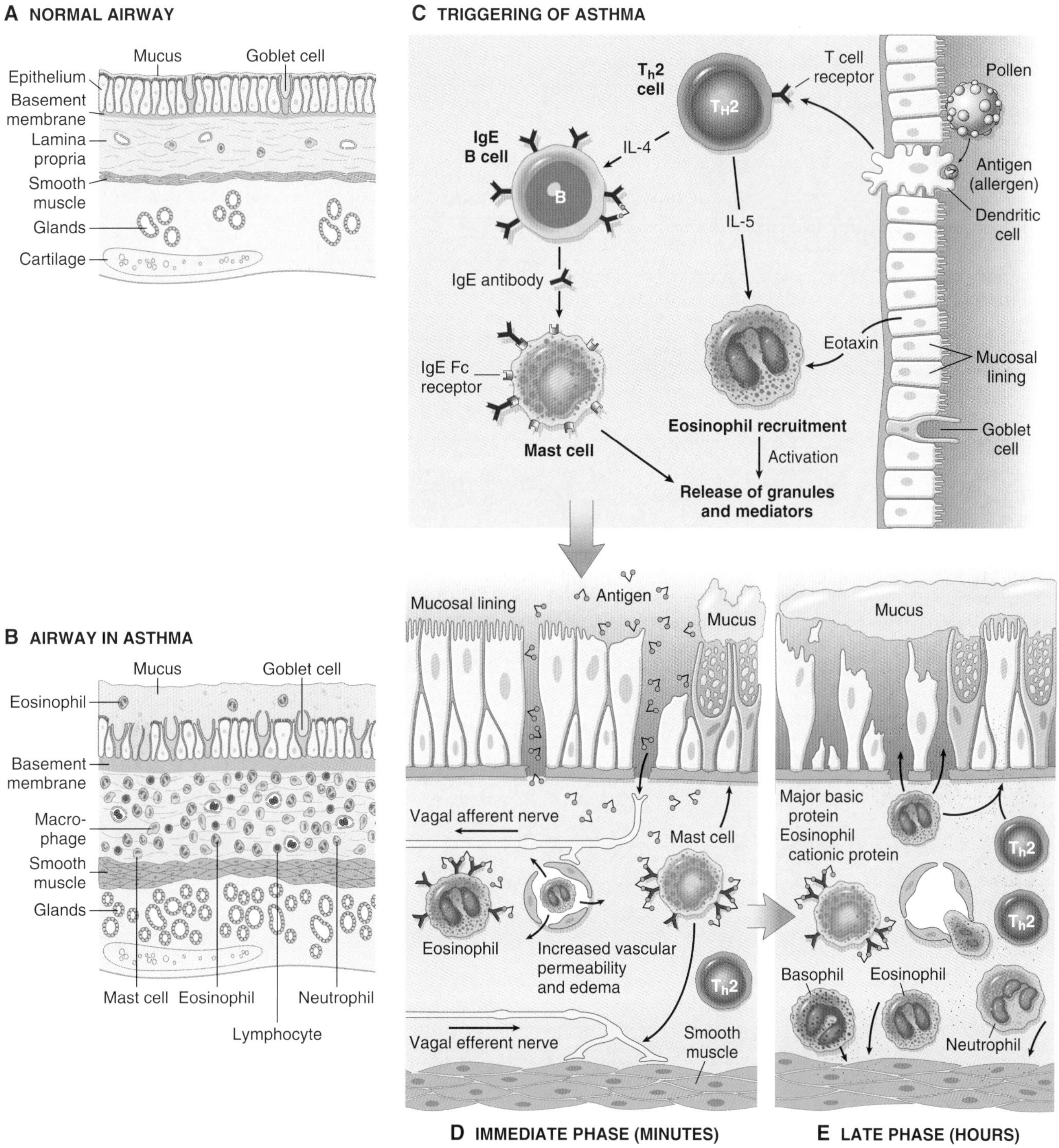

A NORMAL AIRWAY

Epithelium
Basement membrane
Lamina propria
Smooth muscle
Glands
Cartilage

Mucus
Goblet cell

C TRIGGERING OF ASTHMA

T$_H$2 cell
T cell receptor
Pollen
IgE B cell
IL-4
Antigen (allergen)
Dendritic cell
IgE antibody
IL-5
Eotaxin
IgE Fc receptor
Mucosal lining
Goblet cell
Eosinophil recruitment
Activation
Mast cell
Release of granules and mediators

B AIRWAY IN ASTHMA

Mucus
Goblet cell
Eosinophil
Basement membrane
Macrophage
Smooth muscle
Glands
Mast cell   Eosinophil   Neutrophil
Lymphocyte

Mucosal lining
Antigen
Mucus
Vagal afferent nerve
Mast cell
Eosinophil
Increased vascular permeability and edema
T$_h$2
Vagal efferent nerve
Smooth muscle

D IMMEDIATE PHASE (MINUTES)

Mucus
Major basic protein
Eosinophil cationic protein
T$_h$2
T$_h$2
Basophil   Eosinophil
Neutrophil

E LATE PHASE (HOURS)

Fig. 10.4 (A and B) Comparison of a normal airway and an airway involved by asthma. The asthmatic airway is marked by accumulation of mucus in the bronchial lumen secondary to an increase in the number of mucous-secreting goblet cells in the mucosa and hypertrophy of submucosal glands; chronic inflammation marked by the presence of eosinophils, macrophages, and other inflammatory cells; a thickened basement membrane; and hypertrophy and hyperplasia of smooth muscle cells. (C) In the atopic form, inhaled allergens elicit a Th2-dominated response favoring IgE production and eosinophil recruitment. (D) On reexposure to antigen, the binding of antigen to IgE on Fc receptors triggers mast cell activation. Mast cells release preformed mediators that directly and via neuronal reflexes induce bronchospasm and increase vascular permeability, mucous production, and recruitment of leukocytes. (E) Recruited leukocytes release additional mediators that initiate the late phase of an asthma "attack." Factor released from eosinophils also causes damage to the epithelium.

Bronchiectasis

Bronchiectasis is the permanent dilation of bronchi and bronchioles caused by destruction of smooth muscle and supporting elastic tissue; it typically results from or is associated with chronic necrotizing infections.

Pathogenesis. Either chronic obstruction or chronic infection may initiate the development of bronchiectasis. Obstruction, which may be due to tumors, foreign bodies, or mucous impaction (as in cystic fibrosis; see Chapter 6), impairs the clearance of secretions, providing a favorable environment for superimposed infection. The resultant inflammatory damage to the bronchial wall and the accumulating exudate further distend the airways, leading to irreversible dilation. Conversely, a persistent necrotizing bacterial infection in the bronchi or bronchioles may lead to poor clearance of secretions, obstruction, and inflammation with peribronchial fibrosis and traction on the bronchi, culminating again in bronchiectasis. Such infections are more common in those with immunodeficiency states or rare inherited disorders (primary ciliary dyskinesia, also called the immotile cilia syndrome) that impair ciliary function and mucociliary clearance of the airways.

Morphology. Bronchiectasis usually affects the lower lobes, particularly air passages that are vertically aligned. When caused by tumors or foreign bodies, it may be localized to a single lung segment. Affected airways are markedly dilated (Fig. 10.5) and show intense acute and chronic inflammation in the walls of the bronchi and bronchioles associated with desquamation of the lining epithelium and areas of ulceration. Many different bacterial species, including aerobes and anaerobes, may be involved. In some instances, the necrosis destroys the bronchial or bronchiolar walls, producing an abscess cavity.

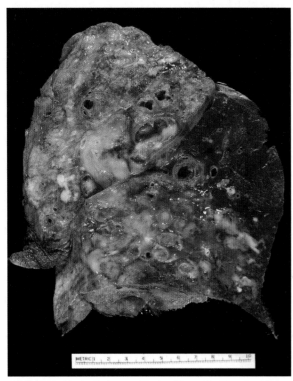

Fig. 10.5 Bronchiectasis in a patient with cystic fibrosis who underwent lung resection for transplantation. The cut surface of the lung shows markedly dilated bronchi filled with purulent mucus that extend to subpleural regions.

Clinical Features. Bronchiectasis is characterized by a severe cough and expectoration of mucopurulent sputum, sometimes associated with dyspnea and hemoptysis. Symptoms often are episodic and may be precipitated by upper respiratory tract infections or superinfection by new pathogenic agents. Severe disease may lead to obstructive ventilatory defects, hypoxemia, hypercapnia, pulmonary hypertension, and cor pulmonale. Treatment includes the use of antibiotics (to prevent and to treat disease flares), mucolytic agents (to help clear secretions), and surgery (for localized disease).

RESTRICTIVE LUNG DISEASES

Restrictive lung diseases are a heterogeneous group of disorders characterized by bilateral pulmonary fibrosis and varying degrees of inflammation. They are subclassified based on clinicopathologic features (Table 10.2), but there is considerable overlap among some of these conditions. The hallmark of these disorders is reduced compliance (stiff lungs), necessitating an increased effort to breathe (dyspnea), and damage to the alveolar epithelium and interstitial vasculature, leading to an abnormal ventilation–perfusion ratio and hypoxia. Forced vital capacity (FVC), which is a reflection of total lung volume, is decreased. Chest radiographs show small nodules, irregular lines, or "ground-glass shadows." With progression, patients may develop respiratory failure, pulmonary hypertension, and cor pulmonale (see Chapter 8). At advanced stages, the etiology of the underlying disease may be difficult to determine because of diffuse scarring and destruction of the lung (end-stage or "honeycomb" lung).

Fibrosing Diseases
Idiopathic Pulmonary Fibrosis

Idiopathic pulmonary fibrosis is a progressive disorder of unknown etiology characterized by patchy, progressive bilateral interstitial fibrosis that usually leads to "end-stage" lung and respiratory failure.

Pathogenesis. The interstitial fibrosis is believed to result from repeated injury and defective repair of alveolar epithelium (Fig. 10.6). The clearest etiologic clues come from genetic studies. Germline loss-of-function mutations in telomerase are associated with increased risk, suggesting that cellular senescence contributes to a profibrotic phenotype. Other affected individuals have a genetic variant that alters the production

Table 10.2 Categories of Chronic Interstitial Lung Disease

Fibrosing Diseases
Usual interstitial pneumonia (idiopathic pulmonary fibrosis)
Nonspecific interstitial pneumonia
Cryptogenic organizing pneumonia
Collagen vascular disease–associated
Pneumoconiosis
Therapy-associated (drugs, radiation)
Granulomatous Diseases
Sarcoidosis
Hypersensitivity pneumonia
Eosinophilic Diseases
Loeffler syndrome
Drug allergy–related
Idiopathic chronic eosinophilic pneumonia
Smoking-Related Diseases
Desquamative interstitial pneumonia
Respiratory bronchiolitis

of a particular mucin, MUC5B, or have a germline mutation in a surfactant gene. These affected genes are only expressed in lung epithelial cells, implicating epithelial abnormalities in the initiation of the disease in at least some patients.

Morphology. The pleural surface of the lung is "cobblestoned" due to the retraction of scars, and the cut surface shows firm, rubbery, white areas of fibrosis. Microscopically, there is patchy *interstitial fibrosis* that varies in intensity. The earliest lesions demonstrate exuberant fibroblast proliferation, but over time these areas become more collagenous and less cellular (Supplemental eFig. 10.4). Usually both early and late lesions are seen. The fibrosis causes collapse of alveolar walls and formation of cystic spaces lined by hyperplastic epithelium *(honeycomb fibrosis).* Secondary vascular changes due to superimposed pulmonary hypertension are often present. Similar morphologic features may be present in entities such as asbestosis and rheumatologic diseases; therefore, idiopathic pulmonary fibrosis is a diagnosis of exclusion.

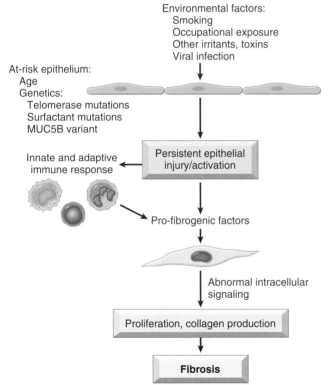

Fig. 10.6 Proposed pathogenic mechanisms in idiopathic pulmonary fibrosis.

Clinical Features. Idiopathic pulmonary fibrosis is more common in males and is a disease of aging, virtually never occurring before 50 years of age. It presents with a nonproductive cough and progressive dyspnea. On physical examination, characteristic "dry" or "Velcro-like" crackles are heard during inspiration. Cyanosis and cor pulmonale may develop in later stages of the disease. Antifibrotic therapies have produced positive outcomes in clinical trials and are approved for use, but the overall prognosis is poor. Survival is only 3 to 5 years after diagnosis and lung transplantation is the only definitive treatment. Other rare pulmonary diseases associated with fibrosis need to be considered in the differential diagnosis of idiopathic pulmonary fibrosis. Rheumatologic diseases, such as systemic sclerosis, rheumatoid arthritis, and systemic lupus erythematosus, may be complicated by pulmonary fibrosis and should be excluded clinically.

Pneumoconioses

Pneumoconiosis **is a term coined to describe lung disorders caused by inhalation of mineral dusts, most commonly coal dust, silica, and asbestos.**

Table 10.3 indicates the pathologic conditions associated with each of these mineral dusts and the major industries in which the dust exposure may occur.

Pathogenesis. The reaction of the lung to mineral dusts depends on the size, shape, solubility, and reactivity of the particles. Particles that are 1 to 5 μm in diameter are most dangerous because they tend to lodge at bifurcations in distal airways. Coal dust is relatively inert, and large amounts must be deposited before clinically detectable lung disease is produced. Silica, asbestos, and beryllium are more reactive than coal dust, resulting in fibrotic reactions at lower concentrations.

The pulmonary alveolar macrophage is central to the initiation and perpetuation of inflammation, lung injury, and fibrosis. Following phagocytosis by macrophages, the particles activate the inflammasome and induce production of cytokines such as IL-1, initiating an inflammatory response. In addition, particles may damage the membrane of phagolysosomes, leading to cell injury that amplifies the inflammatory reaction. Chronic inflammation leads to interstitial fibroblast proliferation and collagen deposition. Tobacco smoking exacerbates the deleterious effects of all inhaled mineral dusts, more so with asbestos than other particles.

Coal worker's pneumoconiosis has decreased in incidence as work in coal mines has declined, but silicosis and asbestosis remain important health problems and merit a brief mention.

Silicosis

Silicosis is currently the most prevalent chronic occupational disease in the world.

Pathogenesis. Silicosis is caused by the inhalation of crystalline silica, mostly in occupational settings (e.g., sandblasting and hard rock mining). After inhalation, silica particles are phagocytosed by macrophages; this induces the release of IL-1 and other inflammatory mediators.

Table 10.3 Mineral Dust–Induced Lung Disease

Agent	Disease	Exposure
Coal dust	Simple coal worker's pneumoconiosis: macules and nodules Complicated coal worker's pneumoconiosis	Coal mining
Silica	Silicosis	Sandblasting, quarrying, mining, stone cutting, foundry work, ceramics
Asbestos	Asbestosis, pleural effusions, pleural plaques, or diffuse fibrosis; mesothelioma; carcinoma of the lung and larynx	Mining, milling, and fabrication of ores and materials; installation and removal of insulation

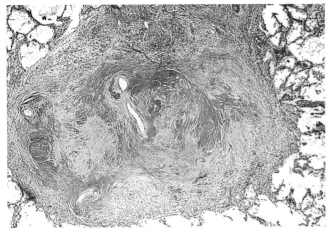

Fig. 10.7 Collagenous silicotic nodules. (Courtesy of Dr. John Godleski, Brigham and Women's Hospital, Boston.)

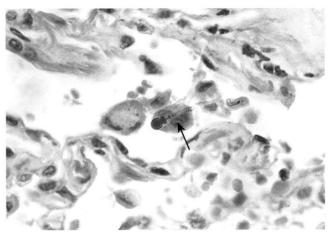

Fig. 10.8 High-power detail of an asbestos body, revealing the typical beading and knobbed ends *(arrow)*.

Morphology. Inflammation produced by silica results in silicotic nodules, composed of concentric whorls of collagen fibers surrounding an amorphous center (Fig. 10.7). Examination of the nodules by polarized microscopy reveals birefringent silica particles. As the disease progresses, individual nodules coalesce into hard, collagenous scars, and with further progression a honeycomb pattern of fibrosis may develop. Fibrotic lesions also may occur in hilar lymph nodes and the pleura.

Clinical Features. Silicosis usually is detected on routine chest radiographs, which show a fine nodularity in the upper lung zones. The disease is slowly progressive, ultimately impairing pulmonary function to such a degree that physical activity is limited. There is an increased susceptibility to tuberculosis, possibly because silica interferes with local host defenses, and there may be an increased risk of lung cancer.

Asbestosis

Asbestos exposure is associated with interstitial and pleural pulmonary fibrosis and an increased risk of cancers of the lung and the pleura.

Pathogenesis. Asbestos is a family of crystalline hydrated silicates with a fibrous geometry. Exposure comes through the workplace, but individuals living in the same household also may be exposed secondarily. As with silica crystals, once phagocytosed by macrophages, asbestos fibers activate the inflammasome and damage phagolysosomal membranes, stimulating the release of proinflammatory and fibrogenic mediators. The oncogenic effects of asbestos may be mediated by reactive free radicals generated by asbestos fibers, which preferentially localize in the distal lung close to the mesothelial layer. Carcinogens that are adsorbed onto the asbestos fibers also may contribute to the pathogenicity of the fibers. The adsorption of carcinogens in tobacco smoke onto asbestos fibers may explain the remarkable synergy between tobacco smoking and the development of lung carcinoma in asbestos workers.

Morphology. The pulmonary interstitial fibrosis is associated with *asbestos bodies:* golden brown, beaded rods with a translucent center consisting of asbestos fibers coated with iron-containing proteinaceous material (Fig. 10.8). Fibrosis also develops in the visceral pleura, causing adhesions between the lungs and the chest wall, often in the form of well-circumscribed plaques of dense collagen (Supplemental eFig. 10.5).

Clinical Features. The clinical findings are indistinguishable from those of other chronic interstitial lung diseases. Progressively worsening dyspnea appears 10 to 20 years after exposure, usually accompanied by a cough and sputum production. The interstitial lung disease may remain static or progress to congestive heart failure, cor pulmonale, and death. Pleural plaques are usually asymptomatic and are detected on radiographs as circumscribed densities. The risk for developing lung carcinoma is increased about 5-fold for asbestos workers, whereas the risk for mesothelioma, normally a very rare tumor, is more than 1000 times greater. Concomitant cigarette smoking greatly increases the risk for lung carcinoma but not for mesothelioma.

Granulomatous Diseases

Sarcoidosis

Sarcoidosis is a disease of unknown etiology characterized by noncaseating granulomatous inflammation in many tissues and organs.

Sarcoidosis is discussed here because it may present as a restrictive lung disease. Bilateral hilar lymphadenopathy associated with lung involvement is often seen at presentation. Eye and skin involvement also is common, and either may occasionally be the presenting feature.

Pathogenesis. Sarcoidosis occurs throughout the world, with a predilection for adults younger than 40 years of age. The incidence is relatively high in Danish and Swedish populations and in people of African descent. A higher prevalence also has been noted among nonsmokers. The cause is unknown but appears to involve some exposure that produces a sustained CD4+ Th1 T-cell response at sites of disease, leading to local production of interferon-γ, recruitment and activation of macrophages, and formation of noncaseating granulomas. There is a familial and racial clustering of cases, suggesting the involvement of genetic factors.

Morphology. The cardinal histopathologic feature is the *nonnecrotizing granuloma,* a discrete, compact collection of epithelioid macrophages admixed with multinucleated giant cells that are rimmed by a zone rich in CD4+ T cells (Supplemental eFig. 10.6). Newly formed granulomas are surrounded by a ring of fibroblasts; over time, these proliferate and lay down collagen that replaces the granuloma with a hyalinized scar. These granulomas are seen in the lung, hilar lymph nodes, skin, eye, lacrimal glands, and other sites of active disease.

Clinical Features. In many individuals, the disease is asymptomatic and is discovered incidentally on routine chest films. In others, peripheral lymphadenopathy, cutaneous lesions, eye involvement, splenomegaly, or hepatomegaly are the presenting manifestations. In about two thirds of symptomatic cases, there is a gradual appearance of respiratory symptoms or constitutional signs and symptoms (fever, fatigue, weight loss, anorexia, night sweats). A definitive diagnostic test does not exist, and establishing the diagnosis requires the presence of clinical and radiologic findings that are consistent with the disease, the exclusion of other disorders with similar presentations, and the identification of noncaseating granulomas in involved tissues. In particular, tuberculosis must be excluded. Sarcoidosis is unpredictable: It may be chronic and progressive or have periods of activity interspersed with remissions. Overall, 65% to 70% of affected individuals recover with minimal or no residual manifestations. Another 20% develop permanent lung dysfunction or visual impairment. In the remaining 10% to 15%, refractory disease may lead to fatal pulmonary fibrosis and cor pulmonale.

Hypersensitivity Pneumonitis

Hypersensitivity pneumonitis is an immunologically mediated inflammatory lung disease that primarily affects the alveoli and is therefore often called allergic alveolitis.

Hypersensitivity pneumonitis is usually an occupational disease resulting from heightened sensitivity to certain inhaled antigens (Table 10.4). It manifests predominantly as a restrictive lung disease. The responsible occupational and household exposures are diverse, but the associated syndromes are similar and probably have a common pathophysiologic basis. The host response to antigens usually involves both B cells and T cells, and "loose," poorly formed granulomas are found in the lungs of two thirds of affected patients (Supplemental eFig. 10.7). In chronic cases, bilateral upper-lobe–dominant interstitial fibrosis occurs.

Hypersensitivity pneumonitis may manifest as an acute reaction, with cough, dyspnea, and constitutional signs and symptoms appearing 4 to 8 hours after exposure, or as a chronic disease characterized by an insidious onset of cough, dyspnea, malaise, and weight loss. If antigenic exposure ceases after an acute attack, the pulmonary symptoms resolve within days. Failure to remove the inciting agent from the environment may result in chronic interstitial pulmonary disease.

PULMONARY DISEASES OF VASCULAR ORIGIN

Pulmonary Embolism, Hemorrhage, and Infarction

Pulmonary thromboembolism most often originates from thrombi in deep leg veins and usually complicates the course of other diseases.

It is estimated that pulmonary embolism causes about 50,000 deaths per year in the United States, but the true incidence is unknown: Even among hospitalized patients no more than one third are diagnosed before death. Autopsy data on the incidence vary from 1% in the general hospitalized population to 30% in individuals dying after burns, trauma, or fractures.

Pathogenesis. Blood clots that occlude large pulmonary arteries usually originate from thrombi involving the popliteal vein of the leg or the larger veins above it. As discussed in Chapter 3, the following risk factors are paramount: (1) prolonged bed rest (particularly with leg immobilization);

Table 10.4 Sources of Antigens Causing Hypersensitivity Pneumonitis

Source of Antigen	Types of Exposures
Bacteria	Dairy barns (farmer's lung)
Mycobacteria	Metal-working fluids, sauna, hot tub
Birds	Pigeons, dove feathers, ducks, parakeets
Chemicals	Isocyanates (auto painters), zinc, dyes
Fungi, yeasts	Contaminated wood, humidifiers, central hot air heating ducts, peat moss plants

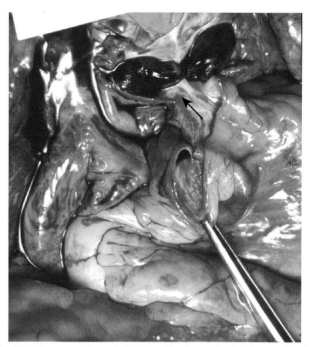

Fig. 10.9 Large saddle embolus from the femoral vein lying astride the main left and right pulmonary arteries. (Courtesy of Dr. Linda Margraf, Department of Pathology, University of Texas Southwestern Medical School, Dallas.)

(2) surgery (especially orthopedic surgery on the knee or hip); (3) severe trauma (including burns or multiple fractures); (4) congestive heart failure; (5) in women, the period around parturition or the use of oral contraceptive pills with high estrogen content; (6) disseminated cancer; and (7) primary disorders of hypercoagulability (e.g., factor V Leiden).

The consequences of pulmonary thromboembolism depend on the size of the occluded pulmonary artery and the cardiopulmonary status of the patient. Pulmonary arterial occlusion immediately increases the pulmonary artery pressure, partly from the blockage of flow and possibly also from vasospasm caused by neurogenic mechanisms, and induces ischemia of the downstream pulmonary parenchyma. Large, abrupt increases in pulmonary artery pressure may produce acute right-sided heart failure *(acute cor pulmonale)* and, sometimes, sudden death. Hypoxemia also develops as a result of multiple mechanisms, including ventilation–perfusion mismatch; widening of the difference in arterial-venous oxygen saturation, due to decreased cardiac output; and right-to-left shunting, which occurs in individuals with a patent foramen ovale.

Because the lungs are oxygenated by bronchial arteries and directly from air in the alveoli, ischemic necrosis (infarction) is the exception rather than the rule. It occurs only if there is cardiac dysfunction or the bronchial circulation is compromised, or if the lung at risk is underventilated due to underlying pulmonary disease.

Morphology. A large embolus may obstruct the main pulmonary artery or its major branches or lodge astride the bifurcation as a saddle embolus (Fig. 10.9). Death may follow so suddenly that morphologic alterations in the lung are absent. Smaller emboli lodge in medium-sized and small-sized pulmonary arteries. With adequate circulation and bronchial arterial flow, the involved lung remains viable, but alveolar hemorrhage may occur as a result of ischemic damage to endothelial cells. With a compromised cardiovascular status (e.g., congestive heart failure), infarction results, particularly if the occlusion occurs in the periphery of the lung. Characteristically, acute infarcts are raised, wedge-shaped, hemorrhagic, red-blue areas (Supplemental eFig. 10.8). With time, fibrous replacement eventually converts the infarct into a white-gray scar.

Clinical Features. Most emboli are small and clinically silent, though 5% of cases result in sudden death. In fatal cases, typically more than 60% of the total pulmonary vasculature is obstructed by a large embolus or multiple simultaneous smaller emboli. Patients with obstruction of small- to medium-sized pulmonary branches (10% to 15% of cases) may present with dyspnea, chest pain referred to the pleura, and hemoptysis. In a small subset of patients (<5% of cases), recurrent "showers" of emboli lead to pulmonary hypertension and chronic right-sided heart failure (cor pulmonale).

Emboli usually resolve after the initial event. However, a small, relatively innocuous embolus may presage a larger one, and patients who have experienced a pulmonary embolism have a 30% chance of having a second one. Prophylactic therapy in those at risk includes anticoagulation, early ambulation (postoperative and postpartum patients), isometric leg exercises, and intermittent pneumatic calf compression for bedridden patients. Those with recurrent or "uninduced" thromboembolism are treated with anticoagulants, usually for life.

Pulmonary Hypertension

Pulmonary hypertension may be caused by a decrease in the cross-sectional area of the pulmonary vascular bed or, less commonly, by increased pulmonary vascular blood flow.

Pathogenesis. Pulmonary hypertension falls into several groups:

- *Pulmonary arterial hypertension,* a collection of disorders that includes heritable causes. The best characterized of the hereditary causes are mutations that affect the bone morphogenetic protein (BMP) signaling pathway.
- *Pulmonary hypertension due to heart disease,* including congenital heart disease and acquired systolic and diastolic dysfunction and valvular disease, all of which can lead to volume overload on the right side of the heart.
- *Pulmonary hypertension due to lung diseases and/or hypoxia,* including COPD and obstructive sleep apnea, and interstitial lung disease from other causes, such as rheumatologic disorders.
- *Chronic thromboembolic pulmonary hypertension,* due to the decrease in the cross-sectional area of the functional pulmonary vascular bed, leading to an increase in pulmonary vascular resistance.

> *Morphology.* All forms of pulmonary hypertension are associated with hypertrophy of the pulmonary muscular and elastic arteries, arterial sclerosis, and right ventricular hypertrophy (Supplemental eFig. 10.9). The arterioles and small arteries are most prominently affected by medial hypertrophy and intimal fibrosis, sometimes narrowing the lumens to pinpoint channels.

Clinical Features. Pulmonary hypertension produces symptoms only when the disease is advanced. The presenting features are usually dyspnea and fatigue, but some patients have anginal chest pain. Over time, respiratory distress, cyanosis, and right ventricular hypertrophy appear, and death from decompensated cor pulmonale ensues within 2 to 5 years in 80% of patients. Treatment choices depend on the underlying cause. For those with secondary disease, therapy is directed at the trigger (e.g., thromboembolic disease or hypoxemia). Several vasodilators have been used with varying success. Lung transplantation is the definitive treatment for selected patients.

Diffuse Alveolar Hemorrhage Syndromes

Pulmonary hemorrhage is a dramatic complication of some interstitial lung disorders. Among these so-called pulmonary hemorrhage syndromes are Goodpasture syndrome and granulomatosis with polyangiitis.

Goodpasture Syndrome

Goodpasture syndrome is an uncommon autoimmune disease in which lung and kidney injury are caused by autoantibodies against the basement membranes of renal glomeruli and pulmonary alveoli.

Pathogenesis. The pathogenic autoantibodies bind to type IV collagen, a component of the basement membranes of pulmonary alveoli and renal glomeruli, giving rise to necrotizing hemorrhagic interstitial pneumonitis and rapidly progressive glomerulonephritis.

> *Morphology.* The lungs are heavy and have areas of red-brown consolidation resulting from diffuse alveolar hemorrhage. Microscopic examination shows focal necrosis of alveolar walls associated with intraalveolar hemorrhage and abundant hemosiderin due to earlier episodes of hemorrhage. The diagnosis is established by identifying the characteristic linear pattern of immunoglobulin deposition (usually IgG) in renal (see Chapter 11) or pulmonary biopsy specimens.

Clinical Features. Goodpasture syndrome usually occurs in patients in their teens or twenties and shows a male preponderance. Most patients are active smokers. Plasmapheresis and immunosuppressive therapy are used to decrease the levels of the pathogenic antibodies and have improved a once-dismal prognosis. With severe renal disease, renal transplantation is eventually required.

Granulomatosis and Polyangiitis

This form of vasculitis (formerly called Wegener granulomatosis) causes upper-respiratory or pulmonary manifestations in more than 80% of patients and is discussed in Chapter 7. The lung lesions are characterized by necrotizing vasculitis (angiitis) and granulomatous parenchymal inflammation. The signs and symptoms stem from involvement of the upper respiratory tract (chronic sinusitis, epistaxis, nasal perforation) and the lungs (cough, hemoptysis, chest pain). Antineutrophil cytoplasmic antibodies (PR3-ANCAs) are present in close to 95% of cases.

PULMONARY INFECTIONS

Pulmonary infections in the form of pneumonia are responsible for one sixth of all deaths in the United States.

Pneumonia is broadly defined as any infection in the lung. Normally, the lung parenchyma remains sterile because of highly effective immune and nonimmune defense mechanisms. The vulnerability of the lung to infection stems from the frequent inhalation of airborne microbes and aspiration of nasopharyngeal flora during sleep, and is exacerbated by lung diseases, which often lower local immune defenses. In addition, lifestyle choices interfere with host immune defenses and facilitate infections: Cigarette smoke compromises mucociliary clearance and pulmonary macrophage activity, and alcohol impairs neutrophil function and cough and epiglottic reflexes (increasing the risk for aspiration).

Bacterial pneumonias are classified according to the etiologic agent or, if no pathogen is isolated, by clinical setting. Seven distinct clinical settings are recognized, each associated with certain pathogens (Table 10.5). Thus, the clinical setting can be a helpful guide when antimicrobial therapy has to be given empirically.

With this brief introduction, we turn next to some of the more common forms of pneumonia, starting with bacterial pneumonia.

Community-Acquired Bacterial Pneumonias

***Streptococcus pneumoniae* (pneumococcal) pneumonia is the most common cause of community-acquired bacterial pneumonia.**

Pneumococcal pneumonia occurs with increased frequency in the setting of chronic diseases (e.g., heart failure, COPD, or diabetes) and congenital or acquired defects in immunoglobulin production. Splenic macrophages have an important role in the removal of pneumococci from the blood; individuals with decreased or absent splenic function are at high risk of developing sepsis. These patients benefit from pneumococcal vaccines. The presence of numerous neutrophils in sputum containing gram-positive, lancet-shaped diplococci supports the diagnosis, but false-positive results are common. Isolation of pneumococci from blood cultures is more specific but less sensitive.

Other important causes of community-acquired bacterial pneumonia include the following:

- *Haemophilus influenzae.* Both encapsulated and unencapsulated forms of *H. influenzae* may be responsible. Adults at risk for developing infections include those with chronic pulmonary diseases such as COPD, cystic fibrosis, and bronchiectasis. Encapsulated *H. influenzae* type B was formerly an important cause of epiglottitis and suppurative meningitis in children, but vaccination in infancy has significantly reduced the risk.
- *Moraxella catarrhalis* mainly infects older adults and is a common cause of acute exacerbation of COPD.
- *Staphylococcus aureus* frequently causes secondary bacterial pneumonia after viral respiratory illnesses and is associated with a high incidence of complications, such as lung abscess and empyema. Staphylococcal pneumonia occurring in association with right-sided staphylococcal endocarditis is a serious complication of intravenous drug use.
- *Klebsiella pneumoniae* is the most frequent cause of gram-negative bacterial pneumonia and primarily afflicts debilitated and malnourished individuals, particularly chronic alcoholics. Thick and gelatinous sputum is characteristic because the organism produces an abundant viscid capsular polysaccharide, which is not easily cleared by coughing.
- *Legionella pneumophila* is the agent of Legionnaire disease. *L. pneumophila* flourishes in artificial aquatic environments, such as water-cooling towers and within the tubing system of potable water supplies. Transmission occurs through inhalation of aerosolized organisms or aspiration of contaminated drinking water. *Legionella* pneumonia occurs more frequently in individuals with cardiac, renal, immunologic, or hematologic diseases. It frequently requires hospitalization and has a fatality rate of 30% to 50% in immunosuppressed individuals.
- *Mycoplasma pneumoniae* infections are particularly common among children and young adults. They occur sporadically or as local epidemics in closed communities (schools, military camps, prisons).

Morphology. **Bacterial pneumonia has two anatomic distributions: bronchopneumonia and lobar pneumonia.**

Patchy lung involvement is the dominant characteristic of bronchopneumonia (Supplemental eFig. 10.10), whereas involvement of a large portion of a lobe or of an entire lobe defines lobar

Table 10.5 The Pneumonia Syndromes and Implicated Pathogens

Community-Acquired Bacterial Pneumonias
Streptococcus pneumoniae
Haemophilus influenzae
Moraxella catarrhalis
Staphylococcus aureus
Legionella pneumophila
Enterobacteriaceae *(Klebsiella pneumoniae)* and *Pseudomonas* spp.
Mycoplasma pneumoniae
Chlamydia pneumoniae
Coxiella burnetii (Q fever)

Community-Acquired Viral Pneumonias
Respiratory syncytial virus, human metapneumovirus, parainfluenza virus (children); influenza A and B (adults); adenovirus (military recruits)

Nosocomial Pneumonias
Gram-negative rods belonging to Enterobacteriaceae (*Klebsiella* spp., *Serratia marcescens, Escherichia coli*) and *Pseudomonas* spp.
S. aureus (usually methicillin-resistant)

Aspiration Pneumonias
Anaerobic oral flora *(Bacteroides, Prevotella, Fusobacterium, Peptostreptococcus)*, admixed with aerobic bacteria *(S. pneumoniae, S. aureus, H. influenzae,* and *Pseudomonas aeruginosa)*

Chronic Pneumonias
Nocardia
Actinomyces
Granulomatous: *Mycobacterium tuberculosis* and atypical mycobacteria, *Histoplasma capsulatum, Coccidioides immitis, Blastomyces dermatitidis*

Necrotizing Pneumonias and Lung Abscess
Anaerobic bacteria (extremely common), with or without mixed aerobic infection
S. aureus, K. pneumoniae, Streptococcus pyogenes, and type 3 pneumococcus (uncommon)

Pneumonias in the Immunocompromised Host
Cytomegalovirus
Pneumocystis jiroveci
Mycobacterium avium complex
Invasive aspergillosis
Invasive candidiasis
"Usual" bacterial, viral, and fungal organisms

pneumonia (Supplemental eFig. 10.11). These patterns often overlap, however, and patchy disease may become confluent over time, producing complete lobar consolidation. Most important from the clinical standpoint are identification of the causative agent and determination of the extent of disease.

In lobar pneumonia, the inflammatory response can be divided into four successive stages: (1) congestion; (2) red hepatization, characterized by exuberant alveolar exudates containing neutrophils, red cells, and fibrin (Fig. 10.10A) that create a red, firm, airless, liver-like consistency; (3) gray hepatization, marked by progressive disintegration of red cells and the persistence of a fibrin- and neutrophil-rich exudate (Fig. 10.10B); and (4) resolution, marked by resorption of exudate and clearance of inflammatory cells, sometimes with fibrosis (referred to as organization) (Fig. 10.10C). A pleural fibrinous reaction (pleuritis) is often present in the early stages that may resolve or organize, leaving fibrous thickening or permanent adhesions. In contrast, bronchopneumonia is usually multilobar, frequently bilateral, and often basal because secretions gravitate to the lower lobes. Histologically, a neutrophil-rich exudate fills the bronchi, bronchioles, and adjacent alveolar spaces.

Complications of pneumonia include (1) abscess formation; (2) spread of infection to the pleural cavity, causing empyema; and (3) bacteremic dissemination leading to the infection of the heart valves, pericardium, brain, kidneys, spleen, or joints.

Clinical Features. Typical community-acquired acute bacterial pneumonia presents with the abrupt onset of high fever, shaking chills, and cough producing mucopurulent sputum; occasional patients have hemoptysis. When pleuritis is present, there is pleuritic pain and a pleural friction rub. The whole lobe is radiopaque in lobar pneumonia, whereas there are focal opacities in bronchopneumonia due to abundant alveolar exudates and fluid. The pneumonia improves rapidly following administration of effective antibiotics. Less than 10% of patients requiring hospitalization die, mostly from complications such as empyema, meningitis, endocarditis, or pericarditis or due to some predisposing factor, such as debility or chronic alcoholism.

Nosocomial Bacterial Pneumonias

Nosocomial (hospital-acquired) pneumonias are defined as pulmonary infections acquired in the course of a hospital stay. Nosocomial infections are common in individuals with severe underlying disease, the immunosuppressed, and those taking prolonged antibiotic regimens. Patients on mechanical ventilation are a particularly high-risk group. Gram-negative rods (members of *Enterobacteriaceae* and *Pseudomonas* spp.) and *S. aureus* are the most common culprits.

Aspiration Pneumonias

Aspiration pneumonia occurs in patients with abnormal gag and swallowing reflexes, such as patients who are severely debilitated or unconscious (e.g., after a stroke or following a drug overdose). The resultant pneumonia is partly chemical, due to the irritating effects of gastric acid, and partly bacterial. Typically, more than one organism is recovered on culture, aerobes being more common than anaerobes. Aspiration pneumonia is often necrotizing and complicated by abscess formation, and is a frequent cause of death in individuals predisposed to aspiration.

Lung Abscess

Lung abscess refers to a cavitary area of suppurative necrosis within the pulmonary parenchyma. The causative organisms may be introduced into the lung by several mechanisms:

- *Aspiration* of infective material from carious teeth or infected sinuses or tonsils, gastric contents, or oropharyngeal infectious organisms
- *As a complication of necrotizing bacterial pneumonias,* particularly those caused by *S. aureus, Streptococcus pyogenes, K. pneumoniae,* and *Pseudomonas* spp.
- *Secondary to bronchial obstruction* (e.g., by bronchogenic carcinoma or a foreign body)
- *Septic embolism,* from infective endocarditis of the right side of the heart
- *Hematogenous spread of bacteria* in disseminated pyogenic infection; this occurs most characteristically in staphylococcal bacteremia and often results in multiple lung abscesses

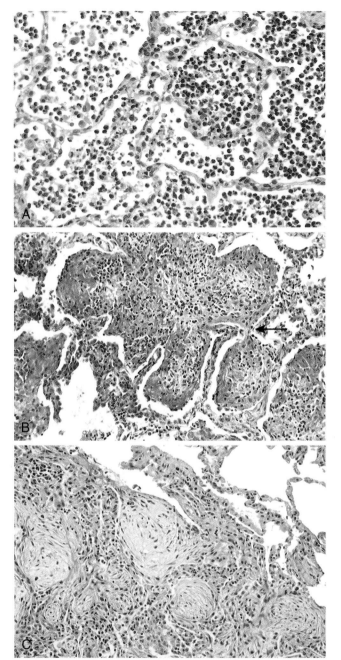

Fig. 10.10 (A) Acute pneumonia. The congested septal capillaries and extensive neutrophil exudation into alveoli correspond to early red hepatization. Fibrin nets have not yet formed. (B) Early organization of intraalveolar exudates, seen in areas to be streaming through the pores of Kohn *(arrow)*. (C) Advanced organizing pneumonia, featuring transformation of exudates to fibrous masses surrounded by infiltrates of macrophages and fibroblasts.

Morphology. Abscesses typically consist of a cavity filled with organisms and acute inflammatory exudate surrounded by variable amounts of fibrous scarring and mononuclear infiltration (lymphocytes, plasma cells, macrophages) (Supplemental eFig. 10.12). Abscesses resulting from aspiration are more common in the right lung (with its more vertical airways) and are most often single. Abscesses that develop in the course of pneumonia or bronchiectasis commonly are multiple, basal, and diffusely scattered. Septic emboli and abscesses arising from hematogenous seeding are commonly multiple and may affect any region. With enlargement, the abscess may rupture into airways or sometimes into the pleural cavity, producing a bronchopleural fistula, with associated pneumothorax or empyema.

Clinical Features. Lung abscess usually is associated with cough and copious amounts of foul-smelling, purulent, or sanguineous sputum; occasionally, hemoptysis occurs. Spiking fever and malaise are common. Abscesses occur in 10% to 15% of patients with bronchogenic carcinoma; thus, when a lung abscess is found in an older adult, underlying carcinoma must be considered. Treatment includes antibiotic therapy and, if needed, surgical drainage. The underlying condition such as obstruction also needs to be addressed. Overall, the mortality rate is in the range of 10%.

Tuberculosis

Tuberculous is a communicable infectious agent that causes disease in the setting of altered T-cell immunity.

Tuberculosis is caused by *Mycobacterium tuberculosis* and usually involves the lungs, but may affect any organ or tissue in the body. More than 2 billion individuals are infected worldwide (more than one third of the world's population), with approximately 10 million new cases and 1.5 million deaths per year. Tuberculosis flourishes under conditions of poverty, crowding, and chronic debilitating illness. In the United States, it is a disease of older adults, the urban poor, patients with AIDS, and members of minority communities. Disease states that impair local or systemic immunity also increase the risk; included among these are diabetes mellitus, Hodgkin lymphoma, silicosis, chronic renal failure, malnutrition, alcoholism, and immunosuppression. In some areas of the world, HIV infection is the dominant risk factor for the development of tuberculosis.

Etiology and Pathogenesis. Mycobacteria are slender rods that are acid-fast (i.e., they resist decolorization after staining with the Ziehl-Neelsen stain). *M. tuberculosis hominis* is responsible for most cases. The main reservoir of infection is individuals with active pulmonary disease, defined as disease with ongoing bacillary proliferation and tissue damage. Transmission is airborne; it usually occurs by inhalation of organisms in aerosols generated by cough and expectoration or by exposure to contaminated secretions of infected individuals.

Primary pulmonary tuberculosis is the form of disease that develops upon first exposure in a previously unsensitized patient. The usual sequence of events from inhalation of the infectious inoculum to containment of the primary focus is illustrated in Fig. 10.11 and can be outlined as follows:
- *Entry into macrophages.* Virulent strains of mycobacteria are taken up into macrophage endosomes, a process mediated by several receptors that recognize components of mycobacterial cell walls.
- *Replication in macrophages.* Once internalized, the organisms inhibit microbicidal responses by preventing the fusion of lysosomes with the phagocytic vacuole, allowing the mycobacterium to persist and proliferate. This early phase of primary tuberculosis in the nonsensitized patient lasts about 3 weeks and is characterized by bacillary proliferation within pulmonary alveolar macrophages and air spaces, eventually resulting in bacteremia and seeding of the organisms to multiple sites. Despite the bacteremia, most individuals are asymptomatic or have a mild flulike illness.
- *Development of cell-mediated immunity.* Mycobacterial antigens reach draining lymph nodes and are processed and presented to CD4+ T cells by dendritic cells and macrophages. The T cells develop into Th1 effector cells that secrete interferon-γ and TNF.
- *T cell–mediated macrophage activation and killing of bacteria.* Activated Th1 cells return to sites of infection and release interferon-γ and TNF. These cytokines recruit monocytes, activate macrophages, and direct the formation of granulomas, collections of activated macrophages with an enhanced capacity to kill mycobacteria. The importance of TNF is underscored by the fact that patients who are treated with TNF antagonists are at increased risk for active tuberculosis.

- *Granulomatous inflammation and tissue damage.* In addition to stimulating macrophages to kill mycobacteria, the enhanced immune response triggered by Th1 cells also produces tissue damage and caseous necrosis. In many individuals, this response halts the infection before clinically significant tissue destruction or illness occur, but if there are immune deficits due to aging or immunosuppression, the infection progresses and the ongoing immune response results in substantial tissue damage.

In the large majority of otherwise healthy individuals with an effective T cell immune response, the only consequence of primary tuberculosis are small foci of scarring within the lungs and lymph nodes. These foci often harbor viable bacilli and may serve as a nidus for disease reactivation at a later time if host defenses wane. Uncommonly, in patients who have inherited or acquired defects in T-cell immunity, the initial infection leads to *progressive primary tuberculosis.* The incidence of progressive primary tuberculosis is particularly high in HIV-positive patients with significant immunosuppression (i.e., CD4+ T-cell counts below 200 cells/μL). Because of an inadequate CD4+ T-cell response, infected tissues in such individuals often lack caseating granulomas and contain unusually large numbers of acid-fast bacilli *(nonreactive tuberculosis).*

Secondary tuberculosis (reactivation tuberculosis) is the pattern of disease that arises in a previously sensitized individual when host defenses are weakened by aging or other acquired factors, often many decades after the initial infection. It also may result from reinfection, either because the protection afforded by the primary infection has waned or because of exposure to a large inoculum of virulent bacilli. Whatever the source of the organism, only a few patients (<5%) with primary disease subsequently develop secondary tuberculosis.

Secondary pulmonary tuberculosis is usually localized to the apex of one or both upper lobes, possibly because high oxygen tension in the apices somehow favors growth of the bacilli. Because of preexistent hypersensitivity, the bacilli usually excite a prompt, exuberant tissue response in the form of granuloma formation and caseous necrosis (Chapter 2). Due to necrosis, cavitary lesions often appear that erode into and disseminate along airways. Once this occurs, bacilli appear in the sputum and the patient poses an infectious risk for others. This pattern of secondary tuberculosis also is typical of HIV-positive patients with modest immune deficiency (CD4+ T-cell counts over 300 cells/μL). However, with more severe immune deficiency (e.g., HIV-positive patients with CD4+ T-cell counts less than 200 cells/μL), the picture resembles progressive primary tuberculosis, with lower and middle lobe consolidation, hilar lymphadenopathy, and noncavitary disease. The extent of immune deficiency also determines the frequency of extrapulmonary involvement, rising from 10% to 15% in mild immune deficiency patients to greater than 50% in those with severe immune deficiency. Loss of hypersensitivity in a *M. tuberculosis*–infected patient (indicated by tuberculin negativity) is an ominous sign of fading resistance to the organism and often is a harbinger of disease reactivation and spread.

The central role of T-cell immunity is highlighted by the observation that individuals with inherited mutations in any component of the Th1 pathway or with acquired T-cell immunodeficiency are very susceptible to infections with mycobacteria, even low-virulence ("atypical") mycobacteria. These rare inherited disorders are collectively called *Mendelian susceptibility to mycobacterial disease (MSMD).*

Morphology. Patterns of spread of tuberculosis are depicted in Fig. 10.12.
- *Primary tuberculosis* typically begins in the lungs. With immune sensitization, small foci of inflammation with granulomatous reaction and caseous necrosis appear, typically in subpleural

A PRIMARY TUBERCULOSIS: INFECTION BEFORE ACTIVATION OF CELL-MEDIATED IMMUNITY

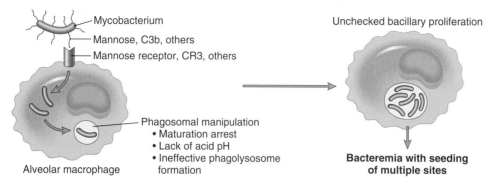

B SECONDARY (REACTIVATION) TUBERCULOSIS: INITIATION AND CONSEQUENCES OF CELL-MEDIATED IMMUNITY

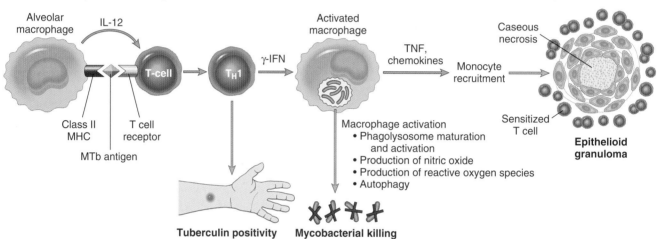

Fig. 10.11 Sequence of events in the natural history of primary pulmonary tuberculosis. This sequence commences with inhalation of virulent strains of *Mycobacterium* and culminates in the development of immunity and delayed hypersensitivity to the organism. (A) Events occurring in the first 3 weeks after exposure. (B) Events thereafter. The development of resistance to the organism is accompanied by conversion to a positive result on tuberculin skin testing. Cells and bacteria are not drawn to scale. IFN-γ, interferon-γ; MHC, major histocompatibility complex; MTb, *Mycobacterium tuberculosis;* TNF, tumor necrosis factor.

location. The bacilli travel through lymphatic vessels to regional lymph nodes, where they also incite a host response (Fig. 10.13A to C). The combination of parenchymal and nodal lesions is called the Ghon complex (Supplemental eFig. 10.13). Lymphatic and hematogenous dissemination also occurs during the first few weeks. Development of cell-mediated immunity controls the infection in approximately 95% of cases, and the Ghon complex undergoes progressive fibrosis and sometimes calcification. Despite seeding of other organs, no lesions develop.

- *Secondary pulmonary tuberculosis* usually begins as a small focus of inflammation near the apical pleura. Such foci are sharply circumscribed and have a variable amount of central caseous necrosis and peripheral fibrosis. Histologically, active lesions show characteristic coalescent granulomas with central caseation, within which tubercle bacilli can be identified. In some instances, the parenchymal focus undergoes fibrosis and leaves only a fibrocalcific scar. Localized apical secondary pulmonary tuberculosis may heal or may progress along several different pathways (Supplemental eFig. 10.14).
- In *progressive pulmonary tuberculosis,* the area of caseation expands and erodes into adjacent structures. Erosion into a

bronchus evacuates the caseous center, creating a ragged, irregular cavity, and penetration of blood vessels results in hemoptysis. If the treatment is inadequate or host defenses are impaired, the infection may disseminate widely through the airways, lymphatic channels, and the vascular system.

- *Miliary tuberculosis* occurs when organisms reach the bloodstream and then recirculate to the lung via the pulmonary arteries. The lesions appear as small (2-mm) yellow-white foci throughout the lungs (the term *miliary* is derived from the resemblance of these foci to millet seeds). The pleural cavity also is invariably involved, leading to pleural effusions, tuberculous empyema, or obliterative fibrous pleuritis. Vascular dissemination may give rise to miliary disease in many other organs (e.g., liver, spleen, kidneys, meninges) (Supplemental eFig. 10.15). Involvement of lymph nodes is the most frequent form of extrapulmonary tuberculosis, usually occurring in the cervical region (scrofula), but virtually any tissue may be involved.

Clinical Features. Most cases of primary tuberculosis are asymptomatic or self-limited. The development of delayed hypersensitivity after a primary infection can be detected by several different tests, each

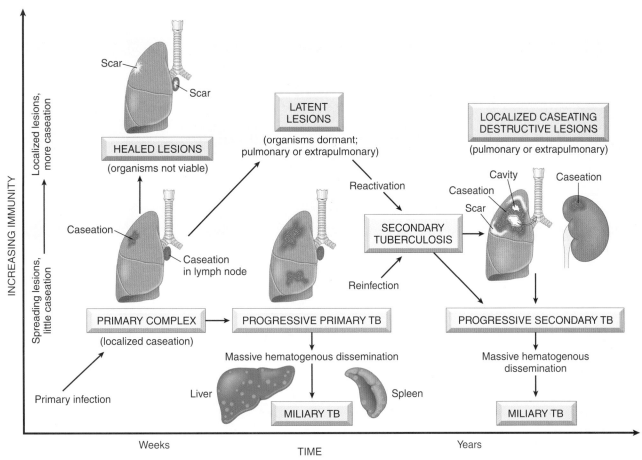

Fig. 10.12 The natural history and spectrum of tuberculosis. (Adapted from a sketch provided by Dr. R.K. Kumar, The University of New South Wales, School of Pathology, Sydney, Australia.)

with certain advantages. The tuberculin (Mantoux) test, involves the injection of purified protein derivative (PPD) under the skin, while the interferon-γ release assay, is performed by mixing patient blood cells with tubercle bacillus antigens and measuring interferon-γ production. Positive results for either test signify exposure to mycobacterial antigens, but neither differentiates between past infection and active disease. Another limitation is that altered host immunity may produce a false-negative reaction (anergy), particularly in those with active tuberculosis and T-cell immunodeficiency. Because the rate of development of active tuberculosis in normal healthy individuals with latent tuberculosis is only 0.1% per year, testing is restricted to those with a high risk of exposure (e.g., healthcare workers) or those at increased risk for development of active disease due to underlying health conditions, in whom prophylactic treatment may be beneficial.

Active tuberculosis leads to systemic manifestations, probably related to the release of cytokines by activated macrophages (e.g., TNF and IL-1). These systemic signs and symptoms often appear early in the course and include malaise, anorexia, weight loss, fever, and night sweats. With progressive pulmonary involvement, increasing amounts of sputum, at first mucoid and later purulent, are produced. When cavitation is present, the sputum contains tubercle bacilli and hemoptysis frequently occurs. Extrapulmonary manifestations of tuberculosis are legion and depend on the organ system involved.

The diagnosis may be suspected based on the history and the detection of lung consolidation or cavitation and is established by identification of tubercle bacilli. The most common method for diagnosing tuberculosis is demonstration of organisms in sputum by acid-fast staining or by staining with fluorescent dyes. The Mantoux test and interferon-γ release assay support the diagnosis in suspected cases. Various culture techniques are used to determine drug sensitivity, and nucleic acid assays are used to identify the mycobacterium and, in some instances, detect mutations that lead to drug resistance.

The prognosis depends on the extent of the infection, the immune status of the host, and the antibiotic sensitivity of the organism. Multidrug resistance (resistance to two or more of the primary tuberculosis drugs) is becoming more common. The prognosis is guarded in those with multidrug-resistant tuberculosis.

Community-Acquired Viral Pneumonias

The most common causes of community-acquired viral pneumonias are influenza types A and B, respiratory syncytial virus, human metapneumovirus, adenovirus, rhinoviruses, rubeola virus, and varicella virus (Table 10.5). Nearly all of these agents also cause upper-respiratory tract infections (common cold).

Pathogenesis. These viruses share a propensity to infect and damage the respiratory epithelium, producing an inflammatory response. When the process extends to the alveoli, there is usually interstitial inflammation, but some outpouring of fluid into alveolar spaces may also occur, which can mimic bacterial pneumonia radiologically. Moreover, respiratory epithelial necrosis limits mucociliary clearance and predisposes to secondary bacterial infections. Serious complications of viral infections are more likely in infants, older adults, malnourished patients, alcoholics, and immunosuppressed individuals.

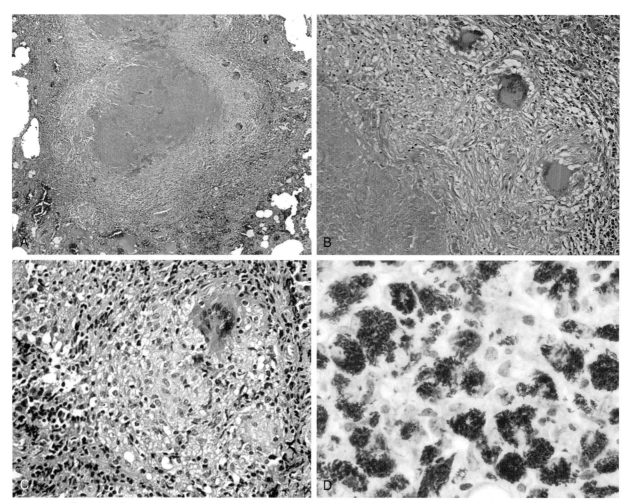

Fig. 10.13 The morphologic spectrum of tuberculosis. A characteristic tubercle at low magnification (A) and at higher power (B) shows central granular caseation surrounded by epithelioid and multinucleate giant cells. This is the usual response in individuals who develop cell-mediated immunity to the organism. (C) Occasionally, even in immunocompetent patients, tubercular granulomas may not show central caseation; hence, irrespective of the presence or absence of caseous necrosis, use of special stains for acid-fast organisms is indicated when granulomas are present. (D) In this specimen from an immunosuppressed patient, sheets of macrophages packed with mycobacteria are seen (acid-fast stain).

Morphology. Viral pneumonia may be patchy, or may involve whole lobes bilaterally or unilaterally. Affected areas are congested, and the inflammatory reaction (mostly lymphocytes and monocytes) is largely confined to the walls of the alveoli. Alveolar spaces are usually clear, but in severe infections, diffuse alveolar damage with hyaline membranes may develop (Supplemental eFig. 10.16). Generally, disease is followed by reconstitution of the normal architecture. Superimposed bacterial infection manifests with the typical appearance of bronchopneumonia.

Clinical Features. The clinical course of viral pneumonia is varied: It may present as a severe upper respiratory tract infection or "chest cold" that goes undiagnosed, or manifest as a fulminant, life-threatening infection in immunocompromised patients. Symptoms include the acute onset of fever, headache, muscle aches, and malaise and, later, cough, with minimal sputum. Inflammatory exudate in the alveolar walls decreases the oxygenation of blood flowing through the affected lung, leading to ventilation–perfusion mismatch and a degree of respiratory distress that is often out of proportion to the radiographic findings. Identifying the causative agent can be difficult. Treatment is largely supportive, and most patients recover spontaneously without any sequelae.

Influenza

Influenza virus is an unusual RNA virus that frequently mutates or recombines its genome, leading to the periodic emergence of pathogenic strains to which human populations have little or no immunity.

The threat of an influenza epidemic remains a grave concern for public health: The great 1918 influenza pandemic killed 20 million to 40 million people.

Pathogenesis. Influenza virus has a single-stranded RNA genome bound by a nucleoprotein that determines the virus type—A, B, or C. Infections with types A and B are much more common than with type C. The surface of the virus is composed of a lipid bilayer containing viral hemagglutinin (H) and neuraminidase (N), which determine the virus subtype (e.g., H1N1, H3N2). Host antibodies to hemagglutinin and neuraminidase prevent and ameliorate, respectively, infection with the influenza virus. Type A viruses infect humans, pigs, horses, and birds and are the major cause of pandemic and epidemic influenza infections. Epidemics of influenza occur when mutations of the hemagglutinin and neuraminidase antigens allow the virus to escape most host antibodies (*antigenic drift*). Pandemics, which last longer and are

Morphology. In uncomplicated cases, the infected lung shows changes similar to other viral pneumonias, with mononuclear inflammatory infiltrates and edema of the alveolar wall. Severe infections can lead to diffuse alveolar damage and acute respiratory distress syndrome, or may be complicated by superimposed bacterial pneumonia by organisms such as *S. aureus.*

more widespread than epidemics, occur when both the hemagglutinin and neuraminidase are replaced through recombination of RNA segments with those of animal viruses (such as bird or pig viruses), making all members of a species susceptible to the new influenza virus *(antigenic shift).* The first flu pandemic of this century, in 2009, resulted from an antigenic shift involving a virus of swine origin (as did the influenza virus from the 1918 epidemic).

Clinical Features. Comorbidities such as diabetes, heart disease, lung disease, and immunosuppression are associated with a higher risk for severe infection. Treatment involves supportive care and (if diagnosed early) neuraminidase inhibitors, which are active against both influenza A and B and can shorten the duration of symptomatic disease. Influenza vaccines provide reasonable protection against the disease, especially in vulnerable infants and older adults.

Fungal Infections
Histoplasmosis, Coccidioidomycosis, and Blastomycosis

Infections caused by the dimorphic fungi *Histoplasma capsulatum, Coccidioides immitis,* and *Blastomyces dermatitidis* range from isolated pulmonary involvement in immunocompetent individuals to disseminated disease in immunocompromised patients.

In the United States, dimorphic fungi have characteristic geographic distributions:

- *H. capsulatum* is endemic in the Ohio and central Mississippi River valleys and along the Appalachian Mountains in the Southeast. Warm, moist soil containing droppings from bats and birds provides a medium for the growth of the mycelial form, which produces infectious spores.
- *C. immitis* is endemic in the southwestern and western regions of the United States, particularly in California's San Joaquin Valley, where coccidial infection is known as "valley fever."
- *B. dermatitidis* has a distribution in the United States that overlaps with that of histoplasmosis.

Morphology. The yeast forms are distinctive, which helps in their identification in tissue sections:

- *H. capsulatum:* round to oval, small yeast forms measuring 2 to 5 μm in diameter (Fig. 10.14A)
- *C. immitis:* thick-walled, nonbudding spherules, 20 to 60 μm in diameter, often filled with small endospores (see Fig. 10.14B)
- *B. dermatitidis:* round to oval, large yeast forms (5 to 25 μm in diameter) that reproduce by characteristic broad-based budding (see Fig. 10.14C and D).

Primary pulmonary disease mimics tuberculosis and consists of aggregates of macrophages filled with organisms, which evolve into small granulomas complete with giant cells and central necrosis, followed by fibrosis and calcification. Similar lesions may be seen in draining lymph nodes. Differentiation from tuberculosis requires identification of the yeast forms (best seen with silver stains). If T-cell

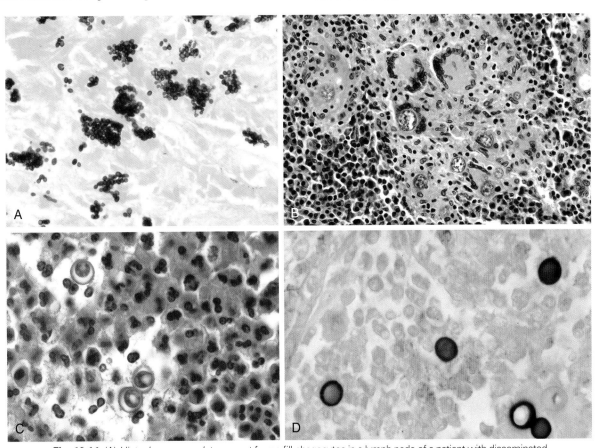

Fig. 10.14 (A) *Histoplasma capsulatum* yeast forms fill phagocytes in a lymph node of a patient with disseminated histoplasmosis (silver stain). (B) Coccidioidomycosis with intact spherules within multinucleated giant cells. (C) Blastomycosis, with rounded budding yeasts, larger than neutrophils. Note the characteristic thick wall and nuclei (not seen in other fungi). (D) Silver stain highlights the broad-based budding seen in *Blastomyces dermatitidis* organisms.

function is suppressed, well-formed granulomas are absent and the infection often disseminates. In such cases, focal collections of macrophages containing yeast forms are seen in multiple organs.

Clinical Features. Clinical manifestations may take the form of acute (primary) pulmonary infection, chronic (granulomatous) pulmonary disease, or disseminated miliary disease. Symptoms and signs in most primary infections resemble those of a "flu-like" syndrome and are usually self-limited. In the vulnerable host, chronic cavitary pulmonary disease develops, with a predilection for the upper lobe, resembling the secondary form of tuberculosis. Infections also may to give rise to perihilar mass lesions that resemble bronchogenic carcinoma radiologically. Symptoms may include cough, hemoptysis, dyspnea, and chest pain. In infants or immunocompromised adults, particularly those with HIV infection, disseminated disease may develop, characterized by a febrile illness marked by hepatosplenomegaly, anemia, leukopenia, and thrombocytopenia. Disseminated disease is difficult to treat and may prove fatal.

Opportunistic Infections

Opportunistic microbes do not cause disease in healthy individuals but may cause serious infections in individuals whose immune systems are suppressed by disease or therapy.

Opportunistic pulmonary pathogens include cytomegalovirus and certain fungi, which are discussed further in the following.

Cytomegalovirus Infection

Infection by cytomegalovirus (CMV), a member of the herpesvirus family, manifests in various forms depending on the age and the immune status of the host.

Most people are exposed to CMV at some point during life. Infection of the fetus transplacentally can lead to serious congenital abnormalities. Transmission occurs more commonly in children or adults exposed to infected saliva, secretions, or semen. Transmission may also occur through organ transplantation and blood transfusion. In healthy children and adults, CMV infection is usually asymptomatic, but there may be a self-limited infectious mononucleosis–like illness. Following infection, the virus remains latent within leukocytes, the major reservoirs of the virus throughout life.

When T-cell immunity is suppressed, as in recipients of organ or hematopoietic stem cell transplants and in patients with AIDS, latent CMV infection may be reactivated or, less commonly, primary CMV infection can occur. The disease mainly affects the lungs (pneumonitis), gastrointestinal tract (colitis), and retina (retinitis). Infected cells are markedly enlarged, and contain prominent intranuclear basophilic inclusions set off from the nuclear membrane by a clear halo (Fig. 10.15). Within the cytoplasm of these cells, smaller basophilic inclusions also may be seen.

Diagnosis of CMV infection is made by demonstration of characteristic viral inclusions in tissue sections, viral culture, rising antiviral antibody titer, and PCR assay–based detection of CMV DNA. The latter has revolutionized the approach to monitoring patients after transplantation.

Pneumocystis Infection

Pneumocystis jiroveci is an opportunistic fungus that causes clinical disease almost exclusively in immunocompromised individuals. Patients with AIDS are extremely susceptible to infection with *P. jiroveci* (although it is seen much less often since the advent of effective antiviral therapy), and it also may cause disease in severely malnourished infants and individuals who are immunosuppressed following organ transplantation or treatment with cytotoxic chemotherapy or corticosteroids.

Pneumocystis infection is largely confined to the lung, where it produces an interstitial pneumonitis. Involved areas contain a

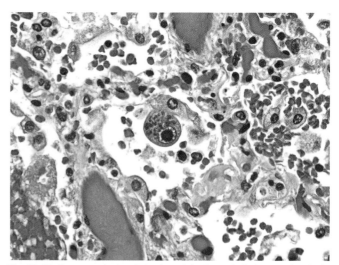

Fig. 10.15 Cytomegalovirus infection of the lung. A distinct nuclear inclusion and multiple cytoplasmic inclusions are seen in an enlarged cell.

characteristic intraalveolar, foamy exudate that appears pink with a hematoxylin-eosin (H&E) stain (cotton candy exudate) (Fig. 10.16A). Silver staining of tissue sections reveals round or cup-shaped cysts (4 to 10 μm in diameter) within the alveolar exudates (Fig. 10.16B).

The diagnosis should be considered in any immunocompromised patient with respiratory symptoms and abnormal findings on chest radiograph. Fever, dry cough, and dyspnea occur in 90% to 95% of patients. The most sensitive and effective method of diagnosis is to identify the organism in sputum or bronchoalveolar lavage fluid using immunofluorescence. If treatment is initiated before widespread involvement, the outlook for recovery is good; however, because residual organisms are likely to persist, particularly in patients with AIDS, relapses are common unless the underlying immunodeficiency is corrected or prophylactic therapy is given.

Candidiasis

Candida albicans is the most common cause of fungal disease. It is a normal inhabitant of the oral cavity, gastrointestinal tract, and vagina. Candidiasis can involve the mucous membranes, skin, and deep organs such as the lungs (invasive candidiasis). Of these varied presentations, several merit a brief mention:

- *Superficial infection on mucosal surfaces of the oral cavity (thrush)* is the most common presentation. Thrush is seen in newborns and debilitated patients, in individuals receiving oral corticosteroids or broad-spectrum antibiotics (which destroy competing normal bacterial flora), and in HIV-positive patients. Proliferation of the fungi creates gray-white pseudomembranes composed of matted organisms, inflammatory cells, and tissue debris.
- *Vaginitis* is extremely common in women, especially those who are diabetic or pregnant or are taking oral contraceptive pills.
- *Esophagitis* is common in patients with AIDS and in those with hematolymphoid malignancies. These patients present with dysphagia (painful swallowing) and retrosternal pain; endoscopy demonstrates white plaques and pseudomembranes.
- *Skin infection* can manifest in many different forms, including infection of the nail, nail folds, hair follicles, penile skin, and moist, intertriginous skin such as armpits or webs of the fingers and toes. Diaper rash is a cutaneous candidal infection seen in the perineum of infants, in the region of contact with wet diapers.
- *Invasive candidiasis* implies blood-borne dissemination of organisms to various tissues or organs. Patients with acute leukemias who are profoundly neutropenic after chemotherapy are particularly prone to the development of invasive disease.

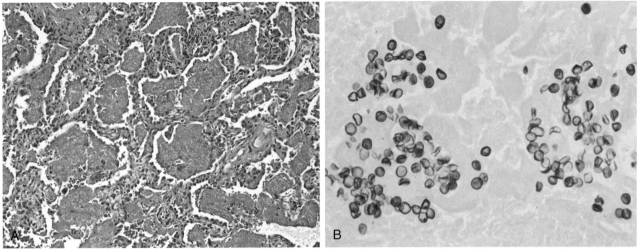

Fig. 10.16 *Pneumocystis* pneumonia. (A) The alveoli are filled with a characteristic foamy acellular exudate. (B) Silver stain demonstrates cup-shaped and round cysts within the exudate.

- In tissue sections, *C. albicans* demonstrates yeast-like forms (blastoconidia), pseudohyphae, and true hyphae (Fig. 10.17A). Pseudohyphae are an important diagnostic clue and represent budding yeast cells joined end to end at constrictions, thus simulating true fungal hyphae. The organisms are visible with routine H&E stains but are better highlighted with a variety of special "fungal" stains (Gomori methenamine–silver, periodic acid–Schiff).

Cryptococcosis

Two species of *Cryptococcus* cause disease. *Cryptococcus neoformans* almost exclusively infects immunocompromised hosts, particularly patients with AIDS or hematolymphoid malignancies. *Cryptococcus gatti* is an emerging pathogen that causes disease in immunocompetent individuals. Both fungi appear as 5- to 10-μm yeasts, have thick, gelatinous capsules, and reproduce by budding (Fig. 10.17D). Periodic acid–Schiff staining effectively highlights the yeast forms. The capsular polysaccharide antigen is the substrate for the cryptococcal latex agglutination assay, which is positive in more than 95% of patients infected with either species.

Both cryptococcal species are acquired by inhalation of aerosolized contaminated soil or bird droppings. The fungus initially localizes in the lungs and then disseminates to other sites, particularly the meninges. The immune response may be minimal (in immunodeficient hosts) or granulomatous (in a more reactive host). In the central nervous system, these fungi grow in gelatinous masses within the meninges or expand the perivascular Virchow-Robin spaces, producing so-called *soap-bubble lesions*.

Opportunistic Molds

Mucormycosis and invasive aspergillosis are uncommon infections that occur mainly in immunocompromised hosts, particularly those with profound neutropenia. Poorly controlled diabetics also are at high risk. Mucormycosis is caused by fungi of the *Zygomycetes* class. Both zygomycetes and *Aspergillus* have a predilection for invading blood vessel walls, causing hemorrhage, vascular necrosis, and infarction (Fig. 10.17B).

In rhinocerebral and pulmonary mucormycosis, zygomycetes colonize the nasal cavity or sinuses and then spread directly into the brain, orbit, and other local structures. Patients with diabetic ketoacidosis are most likely to develop a fulminant invasive form of rhinocerebral mucormycosis. Invasive aspergillosis preferentially localizes to the lungs, and infection most often manifests as a necrotizing pneumonia (Fig. 10.17C). Systemic dissemination, especially to the brain, is a complication that is often fatal.

LUNG, PLEURAL, AND UPPER AIRWAY TUMORS

Lung Carcinoma

Lung carcinoma is most frequently caused by exposure to carcinogens in tobacco smoke.

The American Cancer Society estimated that there would be approximately 228,820 new cases of lung cancer in 2019 and 135,720 deaths. The incidence is gradually decreasing, largely attributable to changes in smoking habits in the population. The peak incidence is in adults past 50 years of age. At diagnosis, more than 50% of patients have distant metastases, and an additional one fourth have disease in the regional lymph nodes. The prognosis remains dismal: The 5-year survival rate for all stages of lung cancer combined is about 24%.

Carcinomas of the lung are classified based on histologic features into four major types: adenocarcinoma, squamous cell carcinoma, large cell carcinoma, and small cell carcinoma (a subtype of neuroendocrine carcinoma). Adenocarcinoma, squamous cell carcinoma, and large cell carcinoma are often grouped together for clinical purposes under the term "non–small cell carcinoma" in recognition of the differences in behavior and treatment of these tumors as compared to small cell carcinoma. Squamous cell and small cell carcinomas have the strongest association with smoking, but an association with adenocarcinoma also exists. Adenocarcinoma is the most common type and occurs at a higher frequency than other types in women, never-smokers, and individuals under 45 years of age.

Pathogenesis. Most carcinomas of the lung arise by a stepwise accumulation of driver mutations induced by carcinogens in tobacco smoke. Certain genetic changes associated with lung cancer are found in the benign-appearing bronchial epithelium of smokers (field effect). The mutations found in smoking-related cancers show a "signature" that is specific for the mutagenic effects of carcinogens in tobacco smoke. About 90% of lung cancers occur in active smokers or those who stopped recently, and there is a nearly linear correlation between the frequency of lung cancer and pack-years of cigarette smoking. Cessation of smoking decreases the risk for developing lung cancer over time, but never to baseline levels. Passive smoking (proximity to cigarette smokers) also increases the risk for developing lung cancer, as does smoking of pipes and cigars, albeit only modestly.

Other carcinogenic influences act in concert with smoking or may independently cause lung cancer. Examples of occupational

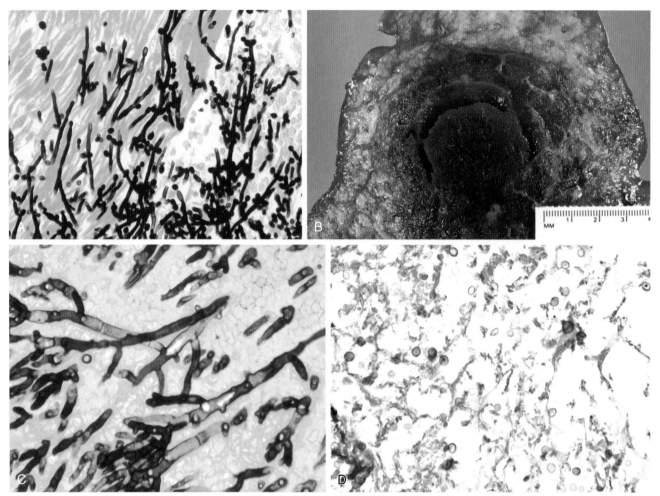

Fig. 10.17 The morphology of fungal infections. (A) *Candida* organism has pseudohyphae and budding yeasts (silver stain). (B) Invasive aspergillosis (gross appearance) of the lung in a hematopoietic stem cell transplant recipient. (C) Gomori methenamine–silver (GMS) stain shows septate hyphae with acute-angle branching, consistent with *Aspergillus*. (D) Cryptococcosis of the lung in a patient with AIDS. The organisms are somewhat variable in size. (B, Courtesy of Dr. Dominick Cavuoti, Department of Pathology, University of Texas Southwestern Medical School, Dallas.)

carcinogens include exposure to radiation (in uranium miners), exposure to asbestos, and inhalation of dusts containing arsenic, chromium, nickel, or vinyl chloride. The risk associated with exposure to asbestos and tobacco smoking is multiplicative: Nonsmokers exposed to asbestos have a 5-fold risk of developing lung cancer, whereas in heavy smokers exposed to asbestos, the risk is elevated approximately 55-fold.

Not all individuals exposed to tobacco smoke develop cancer (~11% of heavy smokers do), and it is likely that the mutagenic effect of carcinogens is modified by hereditary (genetic) factors. Individuals with certain polymorphisms involving the P-450 genes have an increased capacity to activate procarcinogens found in cigarette smoke, and are thus exposed to larger doses of carcinogens and incur a greater risk of developing lung cancer. Similarly, individuals whose peripheral blood lymphocytes undergo chromosomal breakage after exposure to carcinogens in tobacco smoke (mutagen-sensitive genotype) have a greater than 10-fold increased risk for developing lung cancer over control subjects.

Some of the mutations that drive lung cancer growth activate tyrosine kinases, which are excellent drug targets. Tyrosine kinase mutations are most common in adenocarcinomas, particularly those arising in nonsmoking women, and affect several different kinases, such as the epidermal growth factor receptor (EGFR), ALK, ROS1, HER2, and c-MET. Each of these kinases is optimally targeted by a different drug, which has spurred a new era of "personalized" lung cancer treatment, in which the genetics of the tumor guide therapy.

Morphology. Adenocarcinomas are usually peripherally located and may display a variety of growth patterns, including acinar (gland-forming) (Fig. 10.18A and B), papillary, mucinous, and solid types. These tumors often have spread by the time of diagnosis, possibly because they produce few symptoms early in their course due to peripheral location.

Squamous cell carcinomas tend to arise centrally in major bronchi and eventually spread to hilar nodes. Large lesions may undergo central necrosis, giving rise to cavitation. These tumors often become symptomatic when the tumor obstructs a bronchus, leading to distal collapse of alveoli (atelectasis) and superimposed infection (Fig. 10.19A). On histologic examination, these tumors show a wide range of differentiation (Fig. 10.19B).

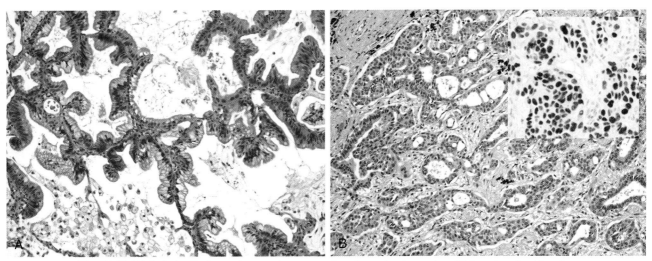

Fig. 10.18 (A) Early in situ lung adenocarcinoma growing along alveolar septae. (B) Invasive gland-forming lung adenocarcinoma; *inset* shows thyroid transcription factor 1 (TTF-1) positivity, which is seen in a majority of cases.

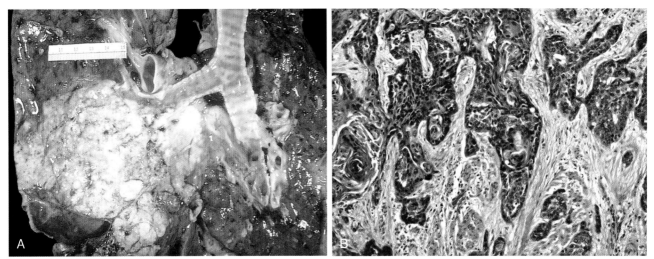

Fig. 10.19 Squamous cell carcinoma. (A) Squamous cell carcinoma appearing as a central (hilar) mass that is invading contiguous parenchyma. (B) Well-differentiated squamous cell carcinoma, showing keratinization and pearls.

Large cell carcinomas are undifferentiated malignant epithelial tumors that lack the cytologic features of neuroendocrine carcinoma and show no evidence of glandular or squamous differentiation.

Small cell lung carcinomas generally appear as pale gray, centrally located masses that extend into the lung parenchyma. These cancers are composed of relatively small tumor cells with a round to fusiform shape, scant cytoplasm, and finely granular chromatin. Numerous mitotic figures are present (Fig. 10.20). These tumors may secrete a host of polypeptide hormones that result in paraneoplastic syndromes. By the time of diagnosis, most tumors will have metastasized to the hilar and mediastinal lymph nodes. In the 2015 World Health Organization classification, small cell lung carcinoma is grouped together with large cell neuroendocrine carcinoma, another very aggressive tumor that exhibits neuroendocrine morphology and expresses neuroendocrine markers.

Each of these lung cancer subtypes tends to spread to lymph nodes and, sooner or later, to distant sites. Involvement of the left supraclavicular node *(Virchow node)* is characteristic and sometimes calls attention to an occult primary tumor. When advanced, these cancers often extend into the pleural or pericardial space, leading to inflammation and malignant effusions. They may compress or infiltrate the superior vena cava to cause vena cava syndrome. Apical neoplasms may invade the brachial or cervical sympathetic plexus, causing severe pain in the distribution of the ulnar nerve or Horner syndrome (ipsilateral enophthalmos, ptosis, miosis, and anhidrosis).

Clinical Features.   Carcinomas of the lung are insidious and often have spread beyond the lung before symptoms appear. Uncommonly, squamous cell carcinomas or adenocarcinomas are detected before metastasis or local spread, making a surgical cure possible. Unresectable adenocarcinomas associated with targetable mutations in tyrosine kinases such as EGFR often respond to specific inhibitors. A few patients with these types of lesions have long-term remissions on the order

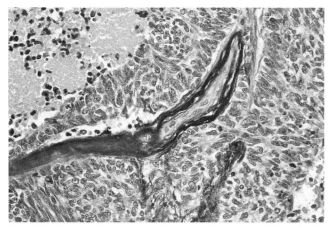

Fig. 10.20 Small cell carcinoma with small deeply basophilic cells and areas of necrosis *(top left)*. Note basophilic staining of vascular walls due to encrustation by DNA from necrotic tumor cells (Azzopardi effect).

of years, but relapse within several months to a year is more typical. Inevitably, resistant tumors have new mutations that either alter the drug target (e.g., an additional mutation in *EGFR* that prevents drug binding) or that circumvent the tumor's dependence on the drug target. Immune checkpoint inhibitors produce responses in some tumors, particularly those that are smoking related (likely because the high burden of carcinogen-induced mutations creates more tumor neoantigens).

By contrast, the picture for small cell lung cancers has changed little. These tumors invariably spread before diagnosis, and surgical resection is not an option. Small cell lung cancers are very sensitive to chemotherapy but rapidly recur, and targeted therapies have yet to be developed. The median survival with treatment is 1 year, and only 5% of patients are alive at 10 years.

Up to 10% of patients with lung cancer develop *paraneoplastic syndromes* related to hormones secreted by the tumor cells. These syndromes include (1) hypercalcemia (from secretion of a parathyroid hormone–related peptide [PTHrP]); (2) Cushing syndrome (from increased production of adrenocorticotropic hormone [ACTH]); (3) the syndrome of inappropriate secretion of antidiuretic hormone (ADH); (4) neuromuscular syndromes, including a myasthenic disorder, peripheral neuropathy, and polymyositis; (5) clubbing of the fingers and hypertrophic pulmonary osteoarthropathy; and (6) coagulation abnormalities, including migratory thrombophlebitis and disseminated intravascular coagulation. Hypercalcemia is most often encountered

with squamous cell neoplasms, the hematologic syndromes with adenocarcinomas, and the neurologic syndromes with small cell neoplasms.

Carcinoid Tumors

Carcinoid tumors are malignant neuroendocrine tumors that contain dense-core neurosecretory granules in their cytoplasm and sometimes secrete biologically active polypeptide hormones.

Carcinoid tumors mainly arise in the lung and in the gastrointestinal tract. Bronchial carcinoids occur in young adults (mean 40 years) and represent about 5% of all pulmonary neoplasms.

Morphology. Most carcinoids originate in the main bronchi, either as an obstructing polypoid, spherical, intraluminal mass (Fig. 10.21A) or a mucosal plaque that penetrates the bronchial wall and fans out in the peribronchial tissue (collar-button lesion). The lesions are well demarcated. Although 5% to 15% of carcinoids have metastasized to the hilar nodes at presentation, distant metastases are rare. The tumor consists of nests of uniform cells that have regular round nuclei with "salt-and-pepper" chromatin, absent or rare mitoses, and little pleomorphism (see Fig. 10.21B).

Clinical Features. Most pulmonary carcinoid tumors manifest with signs and symptoms related to their intraluminal growth, including cough, hemoptysis, and bronchial and pulmonary infections. Peripheral tumors are often asymptomatic and are discovered incidentally. Only rarely do pulmonary carcinoids cause the *carcinoid syndrome*, characterized by intermittent attacks of diarrhea, flushing, and cyanosis; these symptoms are much more commonly produced by carcinoids arising in the gastrointestinal tract. The reported 5- and 10-year survival rates for carcinoid tumors are above 85%.

Malignant Mesothelioma

Malignant mesothelioma is strongly associated with exposure to airborne asbestos.

This rare cancer of mesothelial cells usually arises in the parietal or visceral pleura or, much less commonly, in the peritoneum and pericardium. Approximately 80% to 90% of individuals with mesothelioma have a history of exposure to asbestos. Those who work directly with asbestos (shipyard workers, miners, insulators) are at greatest risk, but mesothelioma has occurred in individuals whose only exposure was living in proximity to an asbestos factory or being a relative of an asbestos worker. The latent period after the initial exposure is long, often 25 to 40 years. Smoking does not increase the incidence of mesothelioma, in contrast to lung carcinoma.

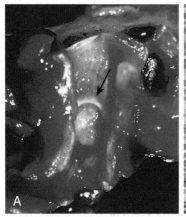
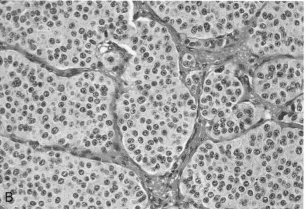

Fig. 10.21 Bronchial carcinoid. (A) Carcinoid growing as a spherical, pale mass *(arrow)* protruding into the lumen of the bronchus. (B) Histologic appearance demonstrating small, rounded, uniform nuclei and moderate cytoplasm. (Courtesy Dr. Thomas Krausz, Department of Pathology, University of Chicago Pritzker School of Medicine, Chicago.)

Pathogenesis. Once inhaled, asbestos fibers remain in the body for life, and the lifetime risk after exposure does not diminish over time. Asbestos occurs in two distinct geometric forms, *serpentine* and *amphibole* (needlelike). Amphiboles are more pathogenic than serpentine forms, perhaps because the straight fibers align with the airstream and are delivered more deeply into the lungs. It is hypothesized that asbestos fibers preferentially accumulate in alveoli at the periphery, near the mesothelial cell layer, where they induce the production of reactive oxygen species that cause DNA damage and mutations. Sequencing of mesothelioma genomes has revealed multiple driver mutations, many of which cluster in pathways involved in DNA repair, cell cycle control, and growth factor signaling. One of the most commonly mutated genes in sporadic mesothelioma, *BAP1*, encodes a tumor suppressor involved in DNA repair that also is affected by germline mutations in families with a high incidence of mesothelioma.

Morphology. Malignant mesotheliomas are often preceded by pleural fibrosis and *plaque formation,* both readily seen on imaging. Once established, the tumor spreads along the pleura widely, either by contiguous growth or by the diffuse seeding of pleural surfaces. At autopsy, the affected lung typically is encased in a layer of yellow-white, firm tumor that obliterates the pleural space (Fig. 10.22). The neoplasm may be locally invasive, but distant metastases are uncommon. Normal mesothelial cells are biphasic, giving rise to pleural lining cells, as well as the underlying fibrous tissue. In line with this potential, mesotheliomas conform to one of three morphologic appearances: (1) epithelial; (2) sarcomatous, in which spindled, occasionally fibroblastic-appearing cells grow in sheets; and (3) biphasic, having both sarcomatous and epithelial areas.

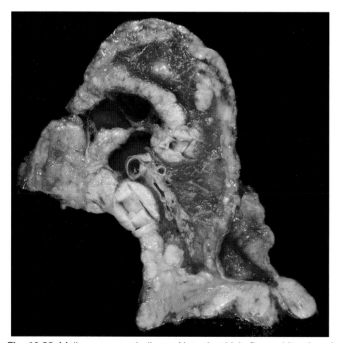

Fig. 10.22 Malignant mesothelioma. Note the thick, firm, white pleural tumor that encases this bisected lung.

Clinical Features. Malignant mesothelioma is a lethal tumor. The median survival is less than 1 year in untreated patients and only slightly greater in treated patients. Because the tumor encases the lung, surgical resection requires removal of the entire lung and pleura (extrapleural pneumonectomy). Combination chemotherapy extends life, but only by a matter of months.

Nasopharyngeal Carcinoma

Nasopharyngeal carcinoma is a rare neoplasm that merits a brief comment because of its strong association with Epstein-Barr virus (EBV) and its high frequency among the Chinese, raising the possibility of viral oncogenesis on a background of genetic susceptibility. The EBV genome is found in virtually all nasopharyngeal carcinomas, including those that occur outside the endemic areas in Asia. It is thought that EBV infects the host by first replicating in the nasopharyngeal epithelium, and in some individuals, this may lead to transformation of the epithelial cells. The tumor typically is composed of large epithelial cells with indistinct cell borders and prominent nucleoli (Supplemental eFig. 10.17). There often is a striking influx of intratumoral T cells, which are believed to be responding to viral antigens.

Nasopharyngeal carcinomas invade locally, spread to cervical lymph nodes, and then metastasize to distant sites. They tend to be radiosensitive, and 5-year survival rates of 50% are reported even for patients with cancers that have spread locally. They also are highly responsive to immune checkpoint inhibitors, providing a new therapeutic strategy for tumors that do not respond to conventional therapy.

Carcinoma of the Larynx

Nearly all cases of laryngeal carcinoma occur in smokers.

Carcinoma of the larynx represents only 2% of all cancers. It most commonly occurs after 40 years of age and is more common in men than in women. In addition to smoking, alcohol consumption and asbestos exposure are associated with increased risk. Human papillomavirus (HPV) genomes are present in about 15% of tumors, and these tumors have a better prognosis than those that are HPV-negative. Most laryngeal cancers are typical squamous cell carcinomas.

Carcinoma of the larynx manifests clinically with persistent hoarseness. The location of the tumor within the larynx has a significant bearing on the prognosis. Glottic tumors are often symptomatic early in their course due to effects on speech, and spread beyond the larynx is uncommon. In contrast, the supraglottic larynx is rich in lymphatic spaces, and nearly one third of these tumors metastasize to regional (cervical) lymph nodes, and subglottic tumors tend to produce symptoms only after they have spread. With surgery, radiation therapy, or combination treatment, many patients can be cured, but about one third die of the disease. The usual cause of death is widespread metastases and cachexia, sometimes complicated by pulmonary infection.

11

Kidney

OUTLINE

Overview of Renal Diseases, 186
Diseases of Glomeruli, 187
  Mechanisms of Glomerular Injury, 187
  Minimal Change Disease, 187
  Membranous Nephropathy, 187
  Focal Segmental Glomerulosclerosis, 189
  Membranoproliferative Glomerulonephritis, 191
  C3 Glomerulopathies, 191
  Diabetic Nephropathy, 191
  Acute Poststreptococcal Glomerulonephritis, 192
  Lupus Nephritis, 193
  Rapidly Progressive Glomerulonephritis, 193
  IgA Nephropathy, 194
  Hereditary Nephritis, 194

Diseases of Tubules and Interstitium, 195
  Acute Pyelonephritis, 195
  Chronic Pyelonephritis, 196
  Drug-Induced Tubulointerstitial Nephritis, 197
  Acute Tubular Injury, 197
  Cystic Diseases, 198
Diseases of Blood Vessels, 199
  Nephrosclerosis, 199
  Malignant Hypertension, 199
  Thrombotic Microangiopathies, 199
Renal Stones (Urolithiasis), 201
  Hydronephrosis, 202
Tumors of the Kidney, 202
  Renal Cell Carcinoma, 202
  Wilms Tumor, 203

OVERVIEW OF RENAL DISEASES

The major diseases of the kidney initially involve one of the four main structural renal components, but in all diseases, all other components of the kidney may be affected secondarily.

The four main structural components of the kidney are:

- *Glomeruli,* functional units that filter the blood, retaining macromolecules and cells and excreting soluble materials and fluid (Supplemental eFig. 11.1)
- *Tubules,* which control the amount of fluid, ions, and small molecules that are excreted by regulating the reabsorption of these substances
- The *interstitium,* which provides the supporting scaffold
- *Blood vessels,* which deliver arterial blood to be filtered and return venous blood to the circulation

Renal injury caused by different mechanisms tends to preferentially affect particular structures; for example, glomerular diseases are often immunologically mediated, whereas tubular and interstitial disorders are more likely to be caused by toxic or infectious agents. We will therefore discuss individual diseases by focusing on the primary site of renal injury, recognizing that because the components of the kidney are functionally linked, as disease advances all parts of the kidney may be affected. It is also important to appreciate that the kidney has a large functional reserve; thus, early signs of kidney disease are often missed, and substantial damage may occur before renal dysfunction becomes clinically apparent.

Renal diseases manifest with different clinical syndromes (Table 11-1).

The nature of the syndrome often provides valuable clues about the underlying diagnosis and, therefore, the most effective therapy. The major renal syndromes fall into several broad categories.

Table 11.1 Glomerular Syndromes

Syndrome	Manifestations
Nephritic syndrome	Hematuria, azotemia, variable proteinuria, oliguria, edema, and hypertension
Rapidly progressive glomerulonephritis	Acute nephritis, proteinuria, and acute renal failure
Nephrotic syndrome	>3.5 gm/day proteinuria, hypoalbuminemia, hyperlipidemia, lipiduria
Chronic renal failure	Azotemia → uremia progressing for months to years
Isolated urinary abnormalities	Glomerular hematuria and/or subnephrotic proteinuria

Acute kidney injury (not listed) is most often the result of diseases affecting tubules.

- *Renal failure* is the loss of renal function. *Acute renal failure* is the clinical state that results from rapidly developing renal injury. It may present with reduced or no urine output (*oliguria* or *anuria,* respectively), hypertension, and other signs of renal dysfunction. Laboratory tests reveal an increase in blood urea nitrogen (BUN) and serum creatinine, collectively termed *azotemia.* These changes are caused by a reduced glomerular filtration rate (GFR), which may result from intrinsic diseases of the kidney (e.g., glomerular or tubular diseases) or extrarenal causes (e.g., severe hypertension or hemolytic-uremic syndrome). The causative abnormalities outside the kidney may be prerenal (reduced fluid volume and, therefore, reduced glomerular perfusion) or postrenal (obstruction to the outflow tract). When the azotemia is severe enough to cause clinical signs and symptoms, the term *uremia* is used.

- *Acute kidney injury* refers to abrupt onset of azotemia with oliguria or anuria. It is most often caused by severe tubular injury (previously called *acute tubular necrosis*, or ATN), but also may result from acute, usually severe, injury to glomeruli, vessels, or the interstitium.
  - *Rapidly progressive glomerulonephritis (RPGN)* is a distinct entity that also can cause acute renal failure.
- *Nephrotic syndrome* has diverse causes that share a common pathophysiology: a derangement in the capillary walls of the glomeruli that results in increased permeability to plasma proteins and proteinuria (urinary protein loss >3.5g/24 hours). The protein loss leads to hypoalbuminemia, which reduces the plasma colloid osmotic pressure, and the resulting transudation of fluid across small blood vessels produces generalized edema. Hyperlipidemia is also often seen. There is frequently retention of salt and water, which exacerbates the edema.
- *Nephritic syndrome* is caused by inflammatory lesions of the glomerulus (hence the term *nephritis*), characterized by hematuria, azotemia, and hypertension. It is seen in diseases in which glomerular inflammation is prominent. Proteinuria, if present, is modest.
- *Chronic kidney disease* is caused by progressive scarring of the kidneys and loss of renal parenchyma, eventually resulting in electrolyte and metabolic abnormalities. It is often asymptomatic for a long time, until uremia develops, but can be preceded by one of several clinical syndromes mentioned above. It culminates in *end-stage renal disease,* which can be treated only by dialysis or transplantation.
- *Other clinical manifestations* of kidney disease include asymptomatic hematuria.

DISEASES OF GLOMERULI

Salient features of the most common primary glomerular diseases are summarized in Table 11.2. Here we discuss first the general mechanisms of glomerular injury and then diseases that are frequently encountered clinically or that illustrate important principles of pathogenesis. As we shall see in this discussion, pathologic analysis of renal biopsies is often the mainstay of diagnosis.

Mechanisms of Glomerular Injury

Most glomerular diseases are immunological in origin, caused by deposition of immune complexes or antibodies in the glomerular capillary wall (Fig. 11.1).

- *Immune complex deposition.* Complexes of antigen and antibody are usually formed in the circulation and are prone to deposit in glomeruli because of the high vascular pressure that drives the filtration of plasma to form urine, as well as the negative charge and permeability characteristics of the glomerular basement membrane (GBM), which promote the stable attachment of antibodies. Two nonexclusive mechanisms of antibody deposition in the glomerulus have been established: (1) deposition of circulating antigen–antibody complexes in the glomerular capillary wall or mesangium (e.g., in systemic lupus erythematosus [SLE]), and (2) antibodies reacting in situ within the glomerulus, either with fixed (intrinsic) glomerular antigens or with extrinsic molecules that are planted in the glomerulus. When antibody binding is patchy (resembling deposition of circulating complexes) it is called *in situ immune complex* formation. Immune complex deposits are seen as granular areas containing immunoglobulin or complement products by immunofluorescent staining or as electron-dense "lumpy bumpy" deposits on the GBM by electron microscopy. Once immune complexes are formed in the glomerulus, they may activate the complement system and recruit leukocytes via complement products, as well as by Fc receptor binding (see Chapter 4), resulting in local inflammation (glomerulonephritis with nephritic syndrome). In

other instances, depending on the makeup and anatomic location of the deposits, they may instead disrupt the glomerular permeability barrier without causing inflammation (nephrotic syndrome).
- *Deposition of anti-GBM antibody.* Less frequently, antibodies bind to antigens that are evenly distributed along the GBM, resulting in a linear pattern of immunofluorescent staining (e.g., Goodpasture syndrome). The subsequent injury is caused by inflammation triggered by complement and Fc receptor–dependent mechanisms, as in immune complex diseases.
- *Other mechanisms of glomerular injury.* Some diseases are caused by defective regulation of complement activation, resulting in uncontrolled deposition of proinflammatory complement products in the glomerulus. In other cases, epithelial cells (podocytes) that line the glomerular capillary wall may be injured (e.g., by toxins or unknown causes), or abnormal glomerular permeability may be the result of mutations in genes encoding proteins of the slit diaphragm (the filtration membrane of the foot processes of the podocytes). Podocytes are intimately involved in maintaining the barrier function of the GBM, and podocyte abnormalities are a virtually universal feature of diseases associated with nephrotic syndrome.

Minimal Change Disease

Minimal change disease is the most common cause of nephrotic syndrome in children; its unique feature is the absence of glomerular pathology by light microscopic evaluation.

Pathogenesis. There are no deposits of antibodies or immune complexes in the glomerulus, and no inflammation. Because of the leakiness of the GBM to albumin, a permeability-inducing circulating factor is suspected, but attempts to identify this elusive culprit have failed, and the pathogenesis of the disease remains unknown.

> *Morphology.* The glomeruli appear normal by light microscopy. Electron microscopic evaluation reveals diffuse effacement of podocyte foot processes (Fig. 11.2); it is not known if this is the cause or consequence of proteinuria.

Clinical Features. The disease typically presents with nephrotic syndrome in a previously healthy child, most commonly between the ages of 1 and 7 years. Classically, the protein loss is selective, primarily of low-molecular-weight proteins such as albumin. The majority of patients respond well to corticosteroid therapy, but proteinuria recurs in 60% of initial responders, many of whom become steroid dependent. In adults the response to steroids is slower and relapses are more common.

Membranous Nephropathy

Membranous nephropathy is caused by immune complex deposition in the glomerular capillary wall, resulting in the nephrotic syndrome.

Pathogenesis. In the majority of cases, immune complexes are formed *in situ* by autoantibodies binding to endogenous podocyte antigens (e.g., phospholipase A2 receptor) or planted antigens. Thus, membranous nephropathy is an autoimmune disease, and, like most diseases in this group, its etiology is unknown. In up to 80% of cases, membranous nephropathy is primary with no associated disease; less commonly, it is seen in association with other well-defined autoimmune diseases, such as SLE. It may also be secondary to infections (e.g., malaria, syphilis, and hepatitis B) or tumors (e.g., melanoma and carcinomas of the lung and colon), or may occur in patients taking therapeutic drugs (e.g., penicillamine, captopril, nonsteroidal antiinflammatory agents); all of these conditions may elicit antibodies that may bind to antigens that are planted in the GBM. The formation of subepithelial immune deposits leads to complement activation on the surface of podocytes and generates the membrane attack complex (C5 to C9). This in turn causes podocyte and GBM injury and proteinuria.

Table 11.2 Summary of Major Primary Glomerular Diseases

Disease	Most Frequent Clinical Presentation	Pathogenesis	Glomerular Pathology		
			Light Microscopy	Fluorescence Microscopy	Electron Microscopy
Minimal change disease	Nephrotic syndrome	Unknown; permeability-inducing factor?	Normal	Negative	Loss of foot processes; no deposits
Membranous nephropathy	Nephrotic syndrome	Deposition of immune complexes; in most cases of primary disease the antigen is unknown	Diffuse GBM thickening	Granular deposits of IgG and C3; diffuse	Subepithelial deposits with interspersed spikes of GBM material; loss of foot processes
Diabetic nephropathy	Nephrotic syndrome	Unclear; may include increased synthesis of GBM material stimulated by growth factors; glomerular hyperfiltration because of microvascular disease	GBM thickening, mesangial sclerosis, nodular deposits of matrix material	Nonspecific	GBM thickening
Focal segmental glomerulosclerosis (FSGS)	Nephrotic syndrome, sometimes with microscopic hematuria and hypertension	Unknown; podocyte injury, glomerular hyperfiltration?	Focal and segmental sclerosis and accumulation of matrix material ("hyaline")	Focal IgM + C3 in some cases, reflecting nonspecific trapping	Effacement of podocyte foot processes
Membranoproliferative glomerulonephritis (MPGN type I)	Nephrotic/nephritic syndrome	Immune complex deposition	Proliferation of mesangial and epithelial cells; GBM thickening; splitting	Granular deposits of IgG and C3	Subendothelial deposits
Dense deposit disease	Nephrotic/nephritic syndrome	Unregulated activation of alternative pathway of complement because of autoantibody that binds to and stabilizes C3 convertase	Mesangial proliferative or membranoproliferative patterns of proliferation; GBM thickening; splitting	C3; no IgG or C1q	Ribbon-like electron-dense deposits in GBM
C3 glomerulonephritis	Nephrotic/nephrotic syndrome	Same as dense deposit disease	Mesangial proliferative or membranoproliferative patterns of proliferation	C3; no IgG or C1q	Mesangial and subendothelial electron-dense "waxy" deposits
Acute poststreptococcal glomerulonephritis	Nephritic syndrome	Immune-complex mediated; circulating or planted antigen	Diffuse proliferation of endothelial and other glomerular cells; leukocytic infiltration	Granular deposits of IgG and C3 in GBM and mesangium	Primarily subepithelial humps; subendothelial deposits in early disease stages
Lupus nephritis	Nephrotic or nephritic syndrome	Immune-complex mediated, circulating self-antigens (mainly nuclear antigens)	Variable; diffuse proliferative GN or primarily membranous pattern	Granular deposits of IgG and C3 in GBM and mesangium	Subendothelial, subepithelial, or mesangial deposits
Rapidly progressive glomerulonephritis (RPGN)	Nephritic syndrome, renal failure	Anti-GBM antibodies (Goodpasture syndrome), immune complexes, (in association with other disease such as SLE) or "pauci-immune" (sometimes with ANCA vasculitis)	Extracapillary proliferation with crescents; necrosis	Linear IgG and C3, immune complexes, or negative in different forms; fibrin in crescents	Typically no deposits; GBM disruptions; fibrin
IgA nephropathy	Recurrent hematuria or proteinuria	Unknown	Focal mesangial proliferative glomerulonephritis; mesangial widening	IgA ± IgG, IgM, and C3 in mesangium	Mesangial and paramesangial dense deposits
Hereditary nephritis	Proteinuria, hematuria	Mutation of the genes encoding the α3, α4, or α5 chain of type IV collagen (Alport syndrome)	Glomerulosclerosis	No deposits	Thinning and lamination of the basement membrane

Diabetic nephropathy is discussed in Chapter 16. FSGS and membranous nephropathy are the most common causes of idiopathic nephrotic syndrome in adults. Their relative incidence varies in different population groups. *ANCA,* Antineutrophil cytoplasmic antibodies; *GN,* glomerulonephritis; *GBM,* glomerular basement membrane.

A

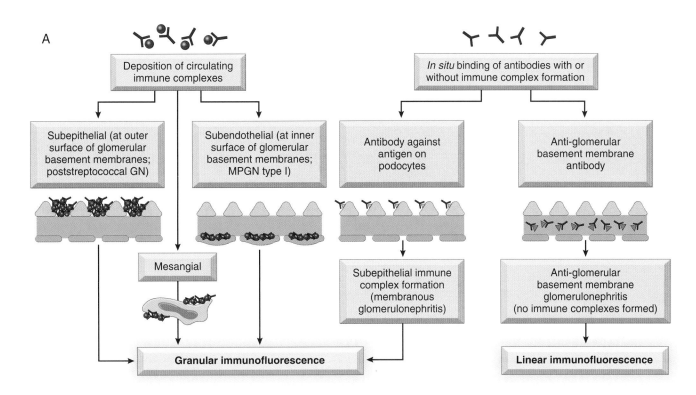

B

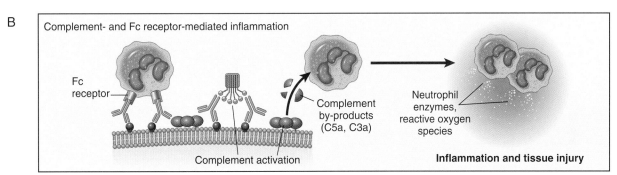

Fig. 11.1 Antibody-mediated glomerular injury. (A) Injury can result either from the deposition of circulating immune complexes or from antibody binding to glomerular components followed by formation of complexes in situ. Deposition of circulating immune complexes gives a granular immunofluorescence pattern. Anti–glomerular basement membrane (anti-GBM) antibody glomerulonephritis is characterized by a linear immunofluorescence pattern; there is no immune deposit formation in this disease. (B) The antibodies in these deposits activate complement, leading to recruitment of leukocytes and inflammatory damage. Growth factors produced during this reaction may also stimulate proliferation of glomerular cells.

Morphology. The main histologic finding is diffuse thickening of the GBM, caused by deposition of immune complexes and the formation of "spikes" of basement membrane material around the deposits (Fig. 11.3). Podocyte foot processes are diffusely effaced, as in other diseases with proteinuria. There is typically no inflammation.

Clinical Features. Membranous nephropathy usually presents in adults between the ages of 30 and 60 years and follows an indolent and slowly progressive course. The onset is sudden and is characterized by nephrotic syndrome, usually without antecedent illness. Unlike in minimal change disease, the proteinuria is "nonselective," meaning that large proteins also leak into the urine. The disease does not respond well to corticosteroid therapy, and other immunosuppressive drugs such as cyclophosphamide and cyclosporin are used. Patients who go into remission following treatment or spontaneously tend to do well, but about 20% have a remitting and relapsing course and about 10% develop renal failure.

Focal Segmental Glomerulosclerosis

Focal segmental glomerulosclerosis (FSGS) is a common cause of nephrotic syndrome; it is characterized by sclerosis of a subset and portions of glomeruli and may occur as a primary disease or secondary to other disorders.

Pathogenesis. Injury to podocytes is thought to represent the initiating event of primary FSGS, though the mechanism of injury is usually unknown. As in minimal change disease, circulating factors that may damage podocytes have been suggested but not identified. In most cases, FSGS is primary, but it may develop secondary to HIV infection, heroin abuse, other forms of glomerular disease (e.g., immunoglobulin A [IgA] nephropathy), or inherited defects in cytoskeletal or podocyte proteins. FSGS may also be seen in the context of reduced renal mass (e.g., due to ablation or disease) in which increased blood flow to the remaining kidney causes hemodynamic injury to the glomeruli.

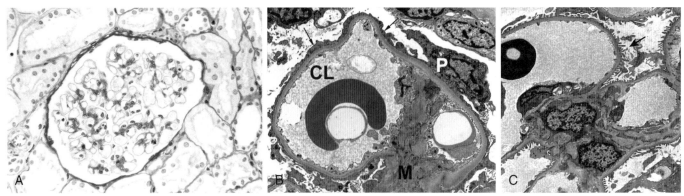

Fig. 11.2 Minimal change disease. (A) Glomerulus showing normal basement membranes and absence of proliferation (PAS stain). (B) Ultrastructural characteristics of minimal change disease include effacement of foot processes *(arrows)* and absence of deposits; compare with the podocyte foot processes *(arrow)* in the normal glomerulus (C). CL, Capillary lumen; M, mesangium; P, podocyte. (C, Courtesy Dr. Vighnesh Wala-valkar, Department of Pathology, University of California San Francisco.)

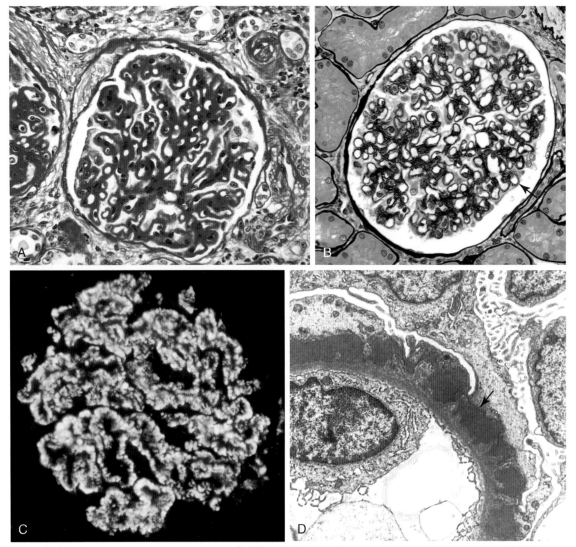

Fig. 11.3 Membranous nephropathy. **(**A and B) Diffuse thickening of the glomerular basement membrane (GBM) without proliferation of cells or inflammation (A, periodic acid–Schiff stain; B, silver stain). In (B), the arrow points to "spikes" of matrix material projecting from the GBM. (C) Granular deposits of IgG by immunofluorescence along the GBM. (D) Subepithelial deposits on the basement membrane (B) with effacement of foot processes overlying the deposits *(arrow)*. (B, Courtesy Dr. Charles Lassman, UCLA School of Medicine, Los Angeles.)

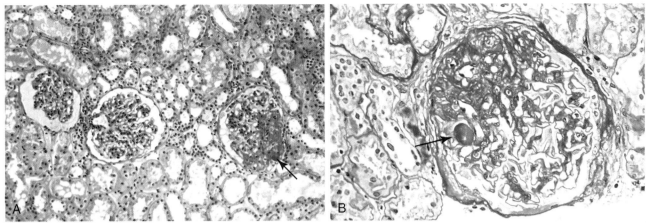

Fig. 11.4 Focal segmental glomerulosclerosis (FSGS). (A) Low-power view showing segmental sclerosis in one of three glomeruli *(arrow)*. (B) Involvement of a segment of a glomerulus, with sclerosis and hyaline deposit *(arrow)*.

Morphology. FSGS is characterized by sclerosis of some but not all glomeruli (hence focal), and in each affected glomerulus, only a portion of the glomerulus and not the entire structure is affected (hence segmental). In affected glomeruli, there is increased matrix protein in the mesangium that obliterates glomerular capillaries and also the deposition of matrix material (which appears pink in hematoxylin-and-eosin [H&E] stains and is called *hyaline*) throughout the abnormal segment (Fig. 11.4). Immunofluorescence microscopy shows nonspecific trapping of antibodies but no immune complexes. Electron microscopy reveals diffuse foot process effacement. In patients with HIV, the disease can be very severe and is associated with collapse of the entire glomerular tuft and epithelial cell hyperplasia, both manifestations of severe glomerular injury.

Clinical Features. The classic presentation is the nephrotic syndrome, sometimes associated with microscopic hematuria and hypertension. The proteinuria is nonselective and the response to immunosuppressive drugs is poor; about half the patients develop end-stage renal disease within 10 years.

Membranoproliferative Glomerulonephritis

Membranoproliferative glomerulonephritis is characterized by alterations in the glomerular basement membrane as well as proliferation of glomerular cells.

Pathogenesis. Membranoproliferative glomerulonephritis (MPGN) is caused by immune complex deposition, but the inciting antigen is not known in most cases. Less commonly, MPGN is secondary to other diseases, such as SLE, viral hepatitis, and other chronic infections. In these cases, the immune complexes may be composed of antibodies bound to self nucleoproteins (in SLE) or to microbial antigens (in the setting of infection).

Morphology. Glomeruli are enlarged due to the proliferation of mesangial and endothelial cells and infiltration of leukocytes, and the lobular architecture of the glomerular tuft appears exaggerated (Fig. 11.5). Parts of these cells and the mesangial matrix extend into the capillary wall, and together with the immune complex deposits, they create the appearance of a split GBM (like a tram track) visible with special stains. Immunofluorescence and electron microscopy reveal granular deposits of antibodies and complement proteins.

Clinical Features. The most common presentation is the nephrotic syndrome, but some patients show a nephritic clinical pattern. The prognosis is poor: Most patients have variable degrees of renal insufficiency, and many progress to end-stage renal disease.

C3 Glomerulopathies

C3 glomerulopathies are rare diseases caused by excessive activation of the alternative complement pathway.

The two diseases in this group, *dense deposit disease* (formerly called MPGN type II) and *C3 glomerulonephritis* (C3 GN), have a similar pathogenesis but distinct morphologic features.

Pathogenesis. Complement activation in dense deposit disease and C3 GN is most often caused by an autoantibody, called C3 nephritic factor, which binds and stabilizes the C3 convertase enzyme (see Chapter 4 for a discussion of complement activation). Less commonly, inherited mutations that disable complement regulatory proteins have the same biological consequence. Although uncontrolled complement activity can injure any cell, for unknown reasons the kidney is the major target of complement-mediated inflammation in these diseases, and nonrenal systemic lesions are uncommon.

Morphology. The histologic appearance is similar to that of MPGN. The diagnostic hallmark is bright immunofluorescent staining for C3 in the mesangium and glomerular capillary walls in the absence of deposition of antibodies or early components of the classical complement pathway (such as C4). In dense deposit disease, the deposits of complement proteins are much larger and the GBM is converted to a ribbon-like structure (Fig. 11.6).

Clinical Features. The usual presentation is the nephrotic syndrome or a mixed nephrotic-nephritic pattern. Most patients progress to renal failure, and the disease frequently recurs following renal transplantation because unregulated complement activation continues.

Diabetic Nephropathy

Diabetes is a systemic metabolic disease caused by deficiency of the glucose-regulating hormone insulin, resulting in elevated blood glucose. The kidney is frequently involved, and because of the great increase in the incidence of diabetes, diabetic nephropathy is now the commonest

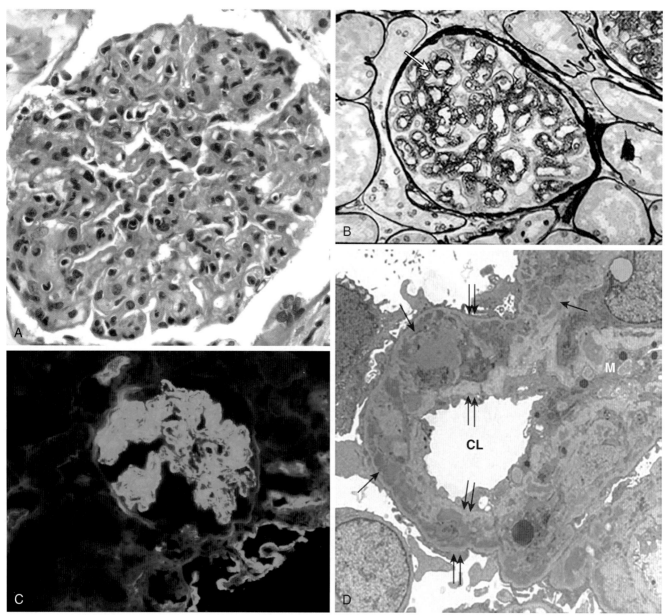

Fig. 11.5 Membranoproliferative glomerulonephritis (MPGN). (A) Mesangial cell proliferation, basement membrane thickening, leukocyte infiltration, and accentuation of lobular architecture. (B) Splitting of the GBM *(arrow)* seen with a silver stain. (C) Granular deposits of IgG in the GBM and mesangium. (D) Electron-dense deposits *(arrows)* in the glomerular capillary wall between duplicated (split) basement membranes *(double arrows)* and in mesangial regions *(M)*. CL, capillary lumen.

cause of chronic kidney disease in the United States. It is discussed in Chapter 16, in the context of diabetes.

Acute Poststreptococcal Glomerulonephritis

This uncommon sequela of streptococcal infections is caused by the glomerular deposition of immune complexes of streptococcal antigen and a specific antibody.

Pathogenesis. Acute poststreptococcal glomerulonephritis (GN) is a classic organ-specific immune complex disease caused by glomerular deposition of immune complexes resulting in proliferation of and damage to glomerular cells and infiltration of leukocytes, especially neutrophils. In less than 1% of cases of throat or skin infection by group A β-hemolytic streptococci, renal lesions develop 1 to 4 weeks after symptoms from the initial infection abate. In affected patients, for unknown reasons, streptococcal protein antigens persist and induce the formation of IgG antibodies, and immune complexes are formed in the circulation. These complexes are

deposited in the glomeruli, activate complement by the classical pathway, and induce acute inflammation that damages the glomeruli. Prevention of this complication is an important reason for rapid antibiotic treatment of the infection. Such treatment is readily available in higher-income countries, so this disease occurs primarily in lower-income countries. A similar disease may occur after infections with organisms other than streptococci, so the generic name *acute postinfectious GN* is sometimes preferred.

Morphology. Glomeruli show a diffuse increase in cellularity owing to the influx of inflammatory cells, mostly neutrophils, as well as the proliferation of glomerular cells (Fig. 11.7). Immunofluorescence shows a granular staining pattern for IgG and C3. Electron microscopy reveals large "humps" of deposited immune complexes, most often in the subepithelial region of the GBM, but sometimes in the subendothelial and intramembranous regions and in the mesangium, as well.

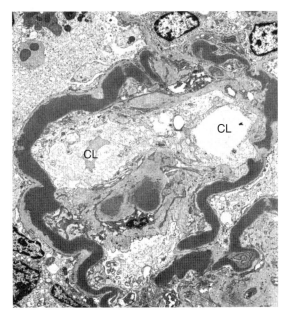

Fig. 11.6 Dense deposit disease. Dense homogeneous deposits in the GBM. CL, capillary lumen.

Clinical Features. Patients present with the acute nephritic syndrome, marked by hematuria, variable, typically mild proteinuria, azotemia, edema, and hypertension. Serum complement levels decrease during the acute phase. Most children with the disease recover, although rarely the disease may evolve into rapidly progressive GN (RPGN, described later). The prognosis in adults is significantly worse; about a third develop end-stage renal disease over 10 to 20 years.

Lupus Nephritis
Renal involvement is common in lupus and usually dominated by immune complex–mediated glomerulonephritis.

Systemic lupus erythematosus (SLE) is an autoimmune disease in which antinuclear autoantibodies are produced that form immune complexes with self nuclear antigens (see Chapter 4). Disease manifestations are mainly due to deposition of these complexes in vessels in different tissues. The kidney is a major site of immune complex deposition, and renal failure is one of the most serious complications of the disease. Autoantibodies against nonnuclear antigens also contribute to the disease, including those that bind to and deplete red cells or platelets (see Chapter 9) and others that affect coagulation, called antiphospholipid antibodies (see Chapter 3). Here we discuss the renal involvement; other aspects of SLE are discussed in Chapter 4.

Pathogenesis. The glomerular lesions are caused by the deposition of immune complexes, activation of complement, and subsequent recruitment and activation of leukocytes via complement products and by the deposited antibodies binding to leukocyte Fc receptors. This is the typical sequence of events in all immune complex diseases (see Chapter 4). Less commonly, there is evidence of tubulointerstitial nephritis and vasculitis, also caused mainly by immune complexes.

Morphology. The glomerular disease caused by the deposition of immune complexes is divided into six classes that have distinct pathologies (Fig. 11.8), clinical features, and prognostic implications. The glomerular lesions are classified on the basis of the site of deposition of the immune complexes (mesangial, subendothelial, subepithelial), the resulting proliferative reaction of the glomeruli (mesangial, focal or diffuse), and the extent of sclerosis of the glomerular tufts.

Of the six classes, *diffuse lupus nephritis* (called class IV) is the most common and severe form. The typical morphologic picture is proliferative GN affecting most glomeruli. The involved glomeruli show proliferation of endothelial, mesangial, and epithelial cells, sometimes with crescent formation (described later). Extensive subendothelial immune complex deposition may lead to GBM thickening, creating the appearance of "wire loops."

Other common renal lesions in SLE are tubulointerstitial inflammation, with or without immune complex deposition along the tubular basement membrane, and vasculitis with immune complex deposition and, sometimes, thrombosis. The prognosis worsens with increased severity of both of these lesions.

Clinical Features. Clinical manifestations range from mild hematuria and proteinuria to massive proteinuria with nephrotic syndrome (as in idiopathic membranous nephropathy) and progressive renal failure.

Rapidly Progressive Glomerulonephritis
This group of diseases shares clinical and morphologic features (especially the formation of crescents in glomeruli) but may have diverse etiologies.

Because crescents are the *sine qua non* of RPGN, it is also called *crescentic GN.*

Pathogenesis. RPGN may be caused by different immune mechanisms.
- Anti-GBM autoantibodies, often reactive with antigens in the noncollagenous component of the GBM, are deposited along the GBM, activate complement, and induce destructive inflammation. In some patients, the antibodies also bind to basement membranes of pulmonary alveolar capillaries, causing lung hemorrhages; the combination of renal and pulmonary involvement is called *Goodpasture syndrome.*
- RPGN may be a manifestation of a known immune complex disease, such as acute postinfectious GN or lupus. In some cases of RPGN, immune complexes are detected in the absence of another underlying disease.
- Pauci-immune crescentic GN is defined by the presence of the characteristic glomerular lesion in the absence of detectable antibodies or immune complexes. Anti–neutrophil cytoplasmic antibodies (PR3-ANCAs) are typically present in the serum, with or without associated systemic vasculitis (see Chapter 7). Thus, pauci-immune crescentic GN may be a manifestation of a systemic vasculitis or idiopathic (limited to the kidney).

Morphology. The morphologic changes in RPGN are reflections of severe glomerular injury. This is manifested in some cases with segmental capillary necrosis, breaks in the GBM (visible by electron microscopy), and the deposition of fibrin in the Bowman space. The glomeruli show proliferation outside the capillary loops, giving rise to distinctive proliferative lesions called *crescents* that obliterate the Bowman space (Fig. 11.9). Crescents consist of proliferating epithelial cells lining the Bowman capsule and infiltrating monocytes and other leukocytes. In addition to extracapillary proliferation, cellular proliferation may also be seen in the capillary loops and mesangium, similar to what is seen in other forms of immune complex–mediated injury. Immunofluorescence microscopy reveals linear or granular staining for IgG and C3 along the GBM (except in the pauci-immune type). Electron microscopy may show ruptures in the GBM, with or without immune deposits.

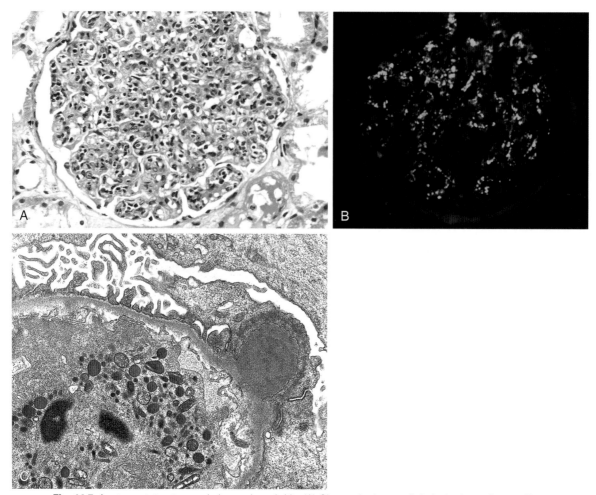

Fig. 11.7 Acute poststreptococcal glomerulonephritis. (A) Glomerular hypercellularity is due to intracapillary leukocytes and proliferation of intrinsic glomerular cells. (B) Immunofluorescent stain demonstrates discrete, coarsely granular deposits of IgG (and C3), corresponding to deposit seen in (C). (C) Typical electron-dense subepithelial deposit and a neutrophil in the lumen. (A to C, Courtesy Dr. H. Rennke, Brigham and Women's Hospital, Boston. B, Courtesy D. J. Kowaleska, Cedars-Sinai Medical Center, Los Angeles.)

Clinical Features. RPGN, regardless of the underlying cause, presents with a rapidly developing severe nephritic syndrome, typically with hematuria, moderate proteinuria, oliguria, and azotemia. The prognosis depends on the proportion of glomeruli involved; more than 80% portends a poor outcome. Removal of anti-GBM antibodies by plasma exchange can benefit patients with such antibodies.

IgA Nephropathy

IgA nephropathy is a frequent cause of recurrent hematuria in children and young adults. It often follows an upper respiratory infection. Deposits of IgA are detected in the mesangium by immunofluorescent staining (Supplemental eFig. 11.2). The suspected pathogenesis is unusual: It is postulated that the respiratory infection induces increased mucosal IgA production as part of the host's immune response and that some of this IgA is abnormally glycosylated. This abnormal IgA appears to the immune system as a foreign protein, and itself elicits an antibody response. The complexes of IgA and anti-IgA are deposited in the kidney and may activate complement, causing glomerular injury. Histologically, glomeruli may be normal or show subtle inflammatory changes, along with the characteristic IgA deposits. Patients present with hematuria following a respiratory or other infection, which usually resolves spontaneously and recurs often. Most patients maintain renal function for decades, but a minority slowly progress to end-stage renal disease.

Hereditary Nephritis

Hereditary nephritis refers to a group of rare diseases caused by inherited mutations in genes encoding GBM proteins. In the most severe form, *Alport syndrome,* there is accompanying sensorineural deafness and ocular abnormalities. *Thin basement membrane disease* is the cause of most cases of so-called benign familial hematuria. Both forms of hereditary nephritis are caused by mutations affecting type IV (basement membrane) collagen. Most Alport syndrome cases are caused by mutations in the α5 collagen gene, which is located on the X chromosome, so males are affected more frequently and more severely than females. Rare autosomal recessive and dominant cases are linked to other genes. Patients with the Alport syndrome present in childhood or the teenage years with hematuria, sometimes accompanied by proteinuria, and may progress to renal failure in 2 to 3 decades.

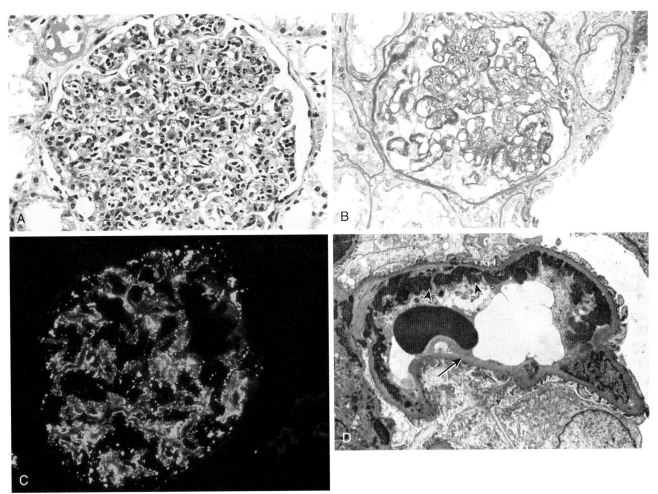

Fig. 11.8 Lupus nephritis. (A) Diffuse proliferative glomerulonephritis. Note the marked increase in cellularity throughout the glomerulus (H&E stain). (B) Membranous pattern of nephritis showing a glomerulus with several "wire loop" lesions representing extensive deposits of immune complexes (periodic acid–Schiff stain). (C) Deposition of IgG antibody in a granular pattern, detected by immunofluorescence. (D) Electron micrograph showing subendothelial deposits *(arrowheads)* in the GBM. The *arrow* indicates the basement membrane. (A and B, Courtesy Dr. Helmut Rennke, Department of Pathology, Brigham and Women's Hospital, Boston. C, Courtesy Dr. Jean Olson, Department of Pathology, University of California San Francisco. D, Courtesy Dr. Edwin Eigenbrodt, Department of Pathology, University of Texas, Southwestern Medical School, Dallas.)

DISEASES OF TUBULES AND INTERSTITIUM

The most frequent causes of disorders of these structures are inflammatory and result in a group of conditions collectively called *tubulointerstitial nephritis;* and toxic or ischemic damage to the tubular epithelium, called *acute tubular injury.* When the inflammation is the result of an infection, it usually involves the renal pelvis (part of the collecting system in the urine outflow tract) and is therefore called *pyelonephritis;* it may be acute or chronic. *Cystic diseases* of the kidney are generally considered separately from diseases of the tubules and interstitium, but we will discuss them at the end of this section because the cysts arise from tubular epithelium.

Acute Pyelonephritis

This inflammation of the renal pelvis and kidney is caused by bacteria that usually ascend from the lower urinary tract.

Pathogenesis. The causative organisms are predominantly gram-negative bacilli, most often *Escherichia coli,* which spread from the gastrointestinal tract. The organisms first infect the nearby urethral urothelium and then ascend through the bladder and the ureter to the kidney. Because of the shorter length of the urethra, females are more susceptible than males. Normally, antimicrobial properties of the bladder wall and periodic emptying of the bladder keep the urine sterile. Outflow obstruction, such as that caused by an enlarged prostate or uterine prolapse, causes stasis of urine and predisposition to lower urinary tract infection and therefore pyelonephritis. Vesicoureteral reflux, sometimes due to a congenital defect in the ureterovesicular valve, is another predisposing factor because contaminated urine from the bladder can leak back into the ureters. Instrumentation of the urinary tract can also allow upward movement of bacteria. Much less commonly, acute pyelonephritis results from hematogenous spread from distant infection, particularly in individuals with some immune abnormality, as in the setting of multiple myeloma (see Chapter 9).

Morphology. One or both kidneys show parenchymal abscesses that may coalesce to form large areas of liquefaction and purulent inflammation (Fig. 11.10). Collections of neutrophils fill the tubules and can extend to involve the interstitial space. Glomeruli are typically spared. Diabetic patients with pyelonephritis are prone to develop necrosis of the tips of papillae (papillary necrosis), likely because of the underlying microvascular disease and resulting ischemia (Supplemental eFig. 11.3).

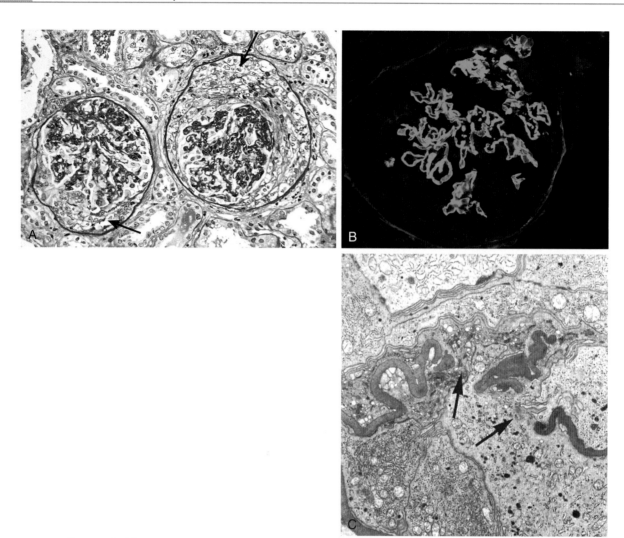

Fig. 11.9 Rapidly progressive (crescentic) glomerulonephritis. (A) Note the collapsed glomerular tufts and the crescent-shaped mass of proliferating parietal epithelial cells and leukocytes inside the Bowman capsule *(arrows)* (PAS stain). (B) Immunofluorescence showing linear deposit of anti-GBM antibody characteristic of Goodpasture syndrome, one form of RPGN. (C) Electron micrograph showing characteristic wrinkling of GBM with focal disruptions *(arrows)*. (A, Courtesy Dr. M. A. Venkatachalam, University of Texas Health Sciences Center, San Antonio, Texas.)

Clinical Features. The disease typically presents with sudden onset of pain in the costovertebral angle overlying one of the kidneys and systemic signs of infection. It is usually unilateral (unlike glomerular disorders). The urine contains neutrophils, sometimes attached to proteinaceous material (forming white cell casts); bacteria can be cultured from urine samples. Antibiotic treatment typically leads to resolution, but it may recur in patients with predisposing factors, and the prognosis is poorer in individuals who develop papillary necrosis.

Chronic Pyelonephritis

Chronic infection and the resultant scarring of the kidney may develop in patients with urinary reflux or obstruction.

Pathogenesis. As discussed previously, reflux of urine from the bladder to the ureters due to congenital vesicoureteral reflux or acquired obstruction to the flow of urine (caused, for instance, by renal calculi) can lead to repeated bacterial infection. The result is chronic inflammation, tissue loss, and fibrosis. Often, the acute phase is subtle and may not even be noticed by affected individuals, who present with the insidious development of chronic renal failure.

Morphology. One or both kidneys show uneven scarring involving the pelvis and calyces, which may be markedly deformed (Fig. 11.11). In contrast, in chronic diseases of the glomerulus or blood vessels, both kidneys are diffusely and almost equally affected. In chronic pyelonephritis, the scars may extend through the cortex to the kidney surface. The histologic picture is typical of chronic inflammation, with interstitial fibrosis and infiltrates of mononuclear cells (lymphocytes, plasma cells, and macrophages). Tubules may be dilated or shrunken, and often contain casts of protein from which the fluid has been resorbed (called colloid casts, referring to the homogeneous protein-rich material, similar to the colloid seen in the thyroid gland). The scarring may lead to narrowing or obliteration of blood vessels, diminished renal perfusion, activation of the renin–angiotensin system, and systemic hypertension.

Clinical Features. Chronic pyelonephritis is an important cause of chronic kidney disease. Patients come to medical attention because of the gradual onset of renal failure (azotemia) or hypertension, or because kidney disease is found upon laboratory testing, either routine or for other suspected conditions. Imaging studies are usually diagnostic; by the time symptoms appear, bacteria are rarely detected in the urine.

Drug-Induced Tubulointerstitial Nephritis

Renal injury can be caused by diverse therapeutic agents, most commonly by immune mechanisms.

Pathogenesis. The long list of drugs linked to kidney injury includes antibiotics, diuretics, and nonsteroidal antiinflammatory drugs, among others. Drugs may bind to and modify self proteins, creating "neoantigens" that elicit an IgE response (type I hypersensitivity) or a T-cell response (type IV hypersensitivity) (see Chapter 4). The renal pathology is not dose dependent, it occurs after a lag following drug exposure, and it recurs upon exposure to the same drug or chemically related drugs; all of these features are consistent with an underlying immune mechanism.

> *Morphology.* The interstitium is edematous and contains an infiltrate of mononuclear cells (lymphocytes and macrophages), sometimes with abundant eosinophils and neutrophils (Fig. 11.12). Drugs that evoke a T-cell response may elicit the formation of noncaseating granulomas.

Clinical Features. Rash, fever, and eosinophilia, usually within two weeks after drug exposure, are early systemic manifestations of a drug reaction. Renal manifestations include hematuria and, in some cases, eosinophils in the urine. Acute kidney injury with oliguria and elevation of the serum creatinine occurs in about 50% of cases. Clinical recognition of drug-induced kidney injury is imperative, because withdrawal of the offending drug is followed by recovery, although it may take several months for renal function to return to normal.

Acute Tubular Injury

Severe injury to tubular epithelial cells is caused by ischemia or exposure to toxins and results in an acute decline in renal function.

Clinicians often use the term *acute tubular necrosis (ATN)*, but frank necrosis is rare; therefore, acute tubular injury (ATI) is preferred. The resultant clinical syndrome is also called *acute kidney injury (AKI)*, previously referred to as acute renal failure.

Pathogenesis. Ischemic ATI results from reduced blood flow, usually due to hypotensive shock caused by blood loss, sepsis, or the systemic inflammatory response syndrome (SIRS), which is initiated by severe tissue injuries (see Chapter 3). Acute hemolysis, as in a transfusion reaction, can also lead to ATI. Diverse toxins, such as heavy metals (e.g., mercury) and solvents (e.g., carbon tetrachloride), drugs such as gentamicin, and radiographic contrast agents can cause a nephrotoxic form of ATI. Because of their high metabolic demand, tubular epithelial cells are particularly vulnerable to ischemia and toxins (Supplemental eFig. 11.4). In addition, because tubules absorb water, the concentration of toxins increases in the lumen. Necrotic epithelial cells may be shed into the lumen, causing outflow obstruction. Both of these

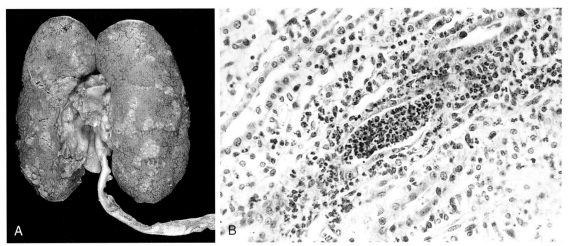

Fig. 11.10 Acute pyelonephritis. (A) Cortical surface shows pale areas of inflammation and abscess formation. (B) Neutrophilic infiltrates in the tubules and interstitium.

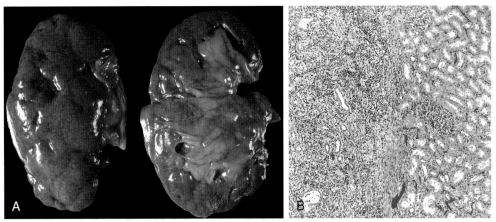

Fig. 11.11 Chronic pyelonephritis. (A) Shrunken kidney with irregular, coarse scars. (B) Tubular atrophy and interstitial fibrosis with foci of chronic inflammation. (Courtesy ExpertPath, copyright Elsevier.)

alterations contribute to a decrease in the GFR, which exacerbates the tubular ischemia, setting up an inexorable cycle of injury.

Morphology. Tubular epithelial cells show the hallmarks of cell injury (see Chapter 1), including the loss of brush borders, vacuolization, detachment, coagulative necrosis, and sloughing (Fig. 11.13). These are often accompanied by ruptures in the tubular basement membrane (tubulorrhexis). The interstitium is edematous. During recovery, the epithelial cells may show signs of regeneration, including a low cuboidal morphology and mitoses.

Clinical Features. ATI presents with the abrupt onset of oliguria and azotemia, which may rapidly progress to uremia. Recovery is possible with treatment of the underlying condition and appropriate supportive care (dialysis, careful management of fluids and electrolytes).

Cystic Diseases

Renal cystic diseases range from focal incidental findings of no clinical significance to bilateral lesions that destroy both kidneys.

Simple cysts are the most common form of cystic disease and are detected at postmortem examination or during radiologic studies; they have no clinical significance. In contrast, *autosomal dominant polycystic kidney disease,* which accounts for almost 10% of chronic kidney diseases, causes substantial morbidity.

Autosomal Dominant Polycystic Kidney Disease

As the name implies, this disease is inherited in an autosomal dominant fashion; however, in as many as 25% of patients there is no family history, either because other affected members of the family have died or have a mild form of the disease that is asymptomatic, or because the disease is caused by a new mutation.

Pathogenesis. The mutated gene is *PKD1* in 85% to 95% of patients and *PKD2* in the remainder. The encoded proteins, polycystin-1 and polycystin-2, respectively, heterodimerize and co-localize in tubular epithelial cells to nonmotile primary cilia, which sense fluid flow and regulate numerous cellular functions. Abnormalities of polycystin-1 or polycystin-2 are believed to lead to defective ciliary function and increased secretion of fluid from epithelial cells, eventually resulting in cyst formation. Thus, this disease is an example of a *ciliopathy.* Although germline mutations of the *PKD* genes are present in all renal tubular cells of affected individuals, cysts develop in only some tubules, most likely owing to a sporadic somatic mutation in the second normal *PKD* allele.

Morphology. The kidneys are progressively replaced by fluid-filled cysts and may attain enormous sizes (Fig. 11.14). The intervening renal parenchyma undergoes ischemic atrophy because of the pressure of the expanding cysts. Evidence of superimposed hypertension or infection is common. Asymptomatic liver cysts are present in about a third of patients, and cerebral aneurysms in the circle of Willis are found in 10% to 30%.

Clinical Features. Clinical manifestations related to kidney disease typically appear around the fourth decade of life. These include local pain, hematuria, hypertension, and a heavy, dragging sensation in the abdomen. Intermittent gross hematuria commonly occurs. The most important complications, because of their deleterious effect on already marginal renal function, are hypertension, due to activation of the renin-angiotensin system in the setting of diminished blood flow, and urinary infection. Progression is slow; ultimately, end-stage renal disease occurs, but the time course is highly variable. Patients are also at high risk of subarachnoid hemorrhage because of the association with cerebral aneurysms.

Autosomal Recessive Polycystic Kidney Disease

The rare autosomal recessive polycystic disease occurs in childhood. It is caused by mutations in the *PKHD1* gene, which encodes a putative membrane receptor protein called fibrocystin. Like polycystin, fibrocystin is found in cilia in tubular epithelial cells, but its function remains unknown. Grossly, numerous small cysts in the cortex and medulla give the kidney a sponge-like appearance. The disease is invariably bilateral. In almost all cases, multiple epithelium-lined liver cysts and a proliferation of portal bile ducts also are present.

Other Cystic Kidney Diseases

Numerous other familial and sporadic cystic diseases are known. *Familial juvenile nephronophthisis,* which is characterized by a variable number of medullary cysts, is an autosomal recessive disease that is the most common genetic cause of end-stage renal disease in children and young adults. As with other types of polycystic disease, the majority of the genes implicated in nephronophthisis encode components of epithelial cilia. Grossly, the kidneys are small, have contracted granular

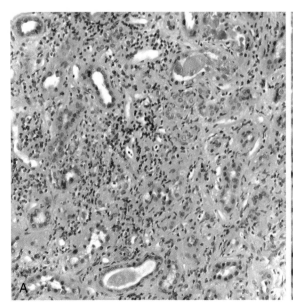
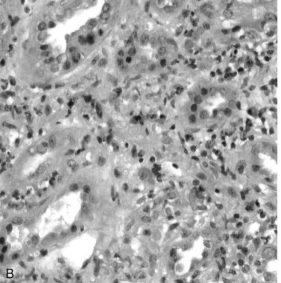

Fig. 11.12 Drug-induced tubulointerstitial nephritis. (A) Chronic inflammatory infiltrate in the interstitium with tubular injury. (B) Prominent eosinophilic infiltrate. (Courtesy ExpertPath, copyright Elsevier.)

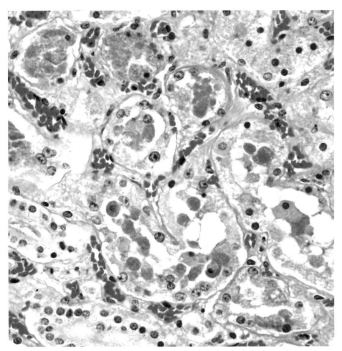

Fig. 11.13 Acute tubular injury. Necrotic tubular epithelial cells and cellular debris in tubular lumens. Congestion of peritubular capillaries is prominent. (Courtesy ExpertPath, copyright Elsevier.)

surfaces, and show cysts in the medulla, most prominently at the corticomedullary junction. Microscopically, there is widespread cortical atrophy and interstitial fibrosis.

Renal cystic disease may also arise in the setting of prolonged dialysis. Numerous medullary and cortical cysts are seen. There is an almost 30-fold increased risk of renal cell carcinoma, which develops in 7% of dialyzed patients observed for 10 years.

DISEASES OF BLOOD VESSELS

Although all diseases of the kidney may secondarily affect the renal vasculature, there are several vascular diseases in which the renal blood vessels are major targets.

Nephrosclerosis

Hypertension causes progressive narrowing of the small renal arteries, resulting in chronic ischemia and damage to the renal parenchyma.

Pathogenesis. The pathogenesis of hypertension is discussed in Chapter 7. In the kidney, the common (benign) form of hypertension causes endothelial dysfunction and hemodynamic stress, resulting in fibrous intimal and medial thickening of walls, primarily in small arteries. In arterioles, plasma proteins leak into the vessel wall and, together with increased synthesis of the basement membrane, produce pink hyaline material. The intima and media are thickened with increased collagen-like fibrous material. These vascular lesions are called *hyaline arteriolosclerosis,* sclerosis referring to the scar-like thickening of the vessel walls. The resulting narrowing of the small vessels causes ischemia, which not only damages renal tissues but also activates the renin–angiotensin system, thereby increasing the blood pressure. Thus, the cycle of hypertension and vascular narrowing becomes mutually reinforcing. These lesions are less severe and differ from those in malignant hypertension (described later), so this hypertension-related kidney disease is also commonly known as *benign nephrosclerosis.*

Morphology. The kidneys are atrophic and the surface is finely granular, due to tissue loss (mostly tubular atrophy) and interstitial fibrosis. The hyaline thickening of arterioles leads to narrowing of their lumen (Fig. 11.15).

Clinical Features. Patients may develop mild azotemia or proteinuria, but the lesions rarely produce renal failure.

Malignant Hypertension

This rare form of severe hypertension causes destructive lesions in renal arterioles and small arteries.

Malignant hypertension, defined as a rapid increase in blood pressure to greater than 200/120 mm Hg, occurs in less than 5% of individuals with hypertension, but often causes acute renal failure.

Pathogenesis. Small arteries and arterioles in the kidney suffer the major consequences of malignant hypertension. Endothelial injury and leakage of plasma proteins into the vessel wall produce fibrinoid necrosis, so named because it has the appearance of fibrin. Platelets are activated and aggregate in the injured vessels, releasing growth factors that stimulate the proliferation of cells in the adjacent intima, leading to luminal narrowing. Vessel damage may be severe enough to produce small hemorrhages.

It should be noted that there is considerable clinical and morphologic overlap between malignant hypertension and thrombotic microangiopathies. About 30% of cases of malignant hypertension have microangiopathic hemolytic anemia (discussed below) and conversely, severe hypertension can occur in primary forms of hemolytic uremic syndrome. Endothelial injury is a common pathogenic factor in these disorders.

Morphology. There may be small petechial hemorrhages on the surface of the cortex, caused by the rupture of small blood vessels, giving a "flea-bitten" appearance. Arterioles show fibrinoid necrosis, and larger vessels show proliferation of intimal cells, producing an "onion-skin" appearance (Fig. 11.16). Arterioles and small arteries are severely narrowed.

Clinical Features. The clinical features of malignant hypertension include papilledema (caused by fluid leakage from injured retinal vessels), encephalopathy (resulting from increased intracranial pressure), cardiovascular abnormalities (secondary to the massive increase in blood pressure), and renal failure. Headache, nausea, vomiting, and visual disturbances are early symptoms. The renal manifestations, which develop soon thereafter, start with hematuria and rapidly progress to azotemia. The syndrome is a medical emergency, requiring urgent treatment with antihypertensive agents. About 50% of patients survive at least 5 years; 90% of deaths are caused by uremia, and the other 10% are caused by cerebral hemorrhage or cardiac failure.

Thrombotic Microangiopathies

These diverse diseases are characterized by microvascular thrombi, microangiopathic hemolytic anemia, platelet consumption, and, occasionally, renal failure.

Several forms of these diseases are primary and are discussed here (Table 11.3). Secondary forms of thrombotic microangiopathies (TMAs) are those associated with severe hypertension, systemic sclerosis, and other conditions. Two forms of primary TMA that involve the kidney are called *hemolytic-uremic syndrome (HUS)* and *thrombotic thrombocytopenia purpura (TTP).*

Pathogenesis. The various forms of TMA have different pathogenic mechanisms.

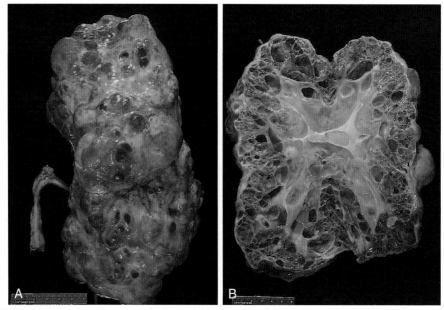

Fig. 11.14 Autosomal dominant adult polycystic kidney, viewed from the external surface (A) and bisected (B). The kidney is markedly enlarged, with numerous dilated cysts.

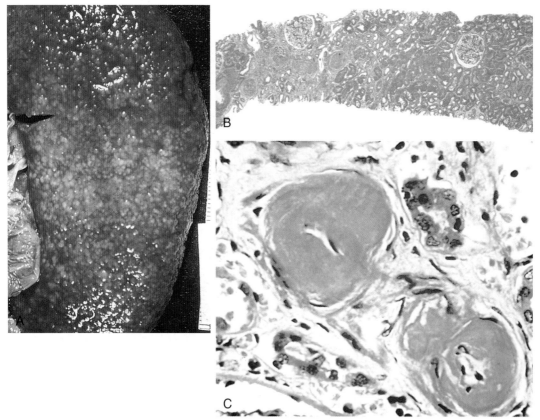

Fig. 11.15 Benign nephrosclerosis. (A) The external surface is finely granular because of scarring, and the cut surface shows cortical atrophy. (B) Tubular atrophy resulting from vascular narrowing, and interstitial fibrosis. The biopsy is stained with the trichrome stain, which stains collagen blue. (C) Two arterioles with hyaline deposition, marked thickening of the walls, and a narrowed lumen. (B, Courtesy Dr. Vighnesh Walavalkar, Department of Pathology, University of California San Francisco; C, Courtesy Dr. M. A. Venkatachalam, Department of Pathology, University of Texas Health Sciences Center, San Antonio, Texas.)

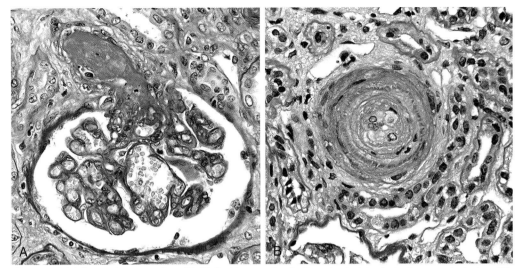

Fig. 11.16 Malignant hypertension. (A) Fibrinoid necrosis of afferent arteriole, typically an acute lesion. (B) Hyperplastic arteriolosclerosis (onion-skin lesion, more often seen in cases with long-standing hypertension. PAS stain. (Courtesy ExpertPath, copyright Elsevier.)

- *Shiga toxin–associated HUS* is caused by infections by bacteria *(E. coli, Shigella)* that produce a toxin that damages endothelial cells, especially in renal glomeruli, resulting in thrombosis.
- *Atypical* (or *complement-mediated) HUS* is caused by inherited or acquired abnormalities leading to excessive complement activation. Precisely why this leads to microvascular thrombosis is not known. It is notable that the lesions are different from those in C3 glomerulopathies, discussed earlier, implying that the pathogenic abnormalities are also distinct.
- *Thrombotic thrombocytopenic purpura (TTP),* another form of systemic TMA, is caused by deficiency of a protease called ADAMTS13 that cleaves and thereby limits the size of multimers of von Willebrand factor. The abnormally large multimers resulting from ADAMTS13 deficiency cause platelet activation and aggregation and the deposition of thrombi in multiple organs, including the kidneys. ADAMTS13 deficiency may result from mutations in the gene (inherited form) or autoantibodies against the protein (acquired). In both HUS and TTP, the thrombi are "platelet-rich" and there is a deficiency of circulating platelets (thrombocytopenia) due to their consumption, sometimes associated with hemorrhages (purpura).

Morphology. All forms of TMA show thrombi mostly in glomerular capillaries and arterioles (Supplemental eFig. 11.5). In severe cases, this may produce ischemic necrosis of the renal cortex. The narrowing caused by thrombi in small vessels creates sheer forces that shred red cells, leading to hemolysis and the appearance of red cell fragments *(schistocytes)* in peripheral blood smears (see Chapter 9).

Clinical Features. Patients usually present with the sudden onset of oliguria, hematuria, bleeding problems, and microangiopathic hemolytic anemia. Shiga toxin–associated HUS is a major cause of acute renal failure in children. If the acute kidney injury is managed with dialysis, most patients recover within weeks; the long-term prognosis (over 15 to 25 years), however, is not uniformly favorable, as about 25% of affected children eventually develop renal insufficiency. Atypical HUS has a poorer prognosis; only 60% to 70% of patients recover renal function, and about 20% die. In TTP, the dominant symptoms more often are related to involvement of organs other than the kidney, such as the brain. Without therapy, TTP typically follows a rapidly fatal course, with survival rates of approximately 10%. Fortunately, timely treatment greatly lowers the risk of death and includes replacing the missing ADAMTS13 enzyme and/or removing the pathogenic autoantibody, typically by plasma exchange.

RENAL STONES (UROLITHIASIS)

Renal stones (calculi) can produce local symptoms and obstruct urine outflow.

Pathogenesis. Stones form in the renal calyces and pelvis when the concentration of the stone's constituents in the urine exceeds their solubility, leading to supersaturation and precipitation of the chemical. The most common stones (~80%) consist of *calcium oxalate,* with or without admixed calcium phosphate. Most patients with this type of stone excrete high levels of calcium in the urine, which may be secondary to unexplained, excessive absorption of calcium from the gut. Only a minority of patients with calcium stones has elevated blood calcium. Less common than calcium stones are *magnesium-containing stones* that typically arise in the setting of alkaline urine, most often secondary to bacterial infections of the urinary tract by organisms such as *Proteus vulgaris,* which increase

Table 11.3 Primary Thrombotic Microangiopathies

	Forms	Etiology and Pathogenesis
Shiga toxin–mediated HUS	Acquired	Shiga toxin–producing *E. coli* *Shigella dysenteriae* serotype 1
Complement-mediated HUS	Inherited	Complement dysregulation due to genetic abnormalities (relatively common)
	Acquired	Acquired complement dysregulation due to autoantibodies (rare)
TTP	Inherited	Genetic ADAMTS13 deficiency (rare)
	Acquired	ADAMTS13 deficiency due to autoantibodies (relatively common)

ADAMTS13, von Willebrand factor cleaving protease; HUS, hemolytic-uremic syndrome; TTP, thrombotic thrombocytopenic purpura.

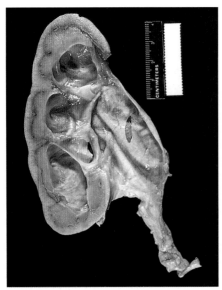

Fig. 11.17 Hydronephrosis, showing marked dilation of the pelvis and calyces and thinning of renal parenchyma.

the urine pH by splitting urea. Gout and other conditions in which blood uric acid levels are elevated are associated with *uric acid stones*. About 50% of individuals with uric acid stones, however, have neither hyperuricemia nor increased urine urate, but instead demonstrate an unexplained tendency to excrete a persistently acidic urine (pH < 5.5). *Cystine stones* are almost invariably associated with a genetic defect in renal transport of certain amino acids, including cystine.

> *Morphology.* Stones are usually unilateral and small (2 to 3 mm); they are most commonly present in the renal pelvis and calyces and the bladder (Supplemental eFig. 11.6). Large stones lodged in the renal pelvis may cause significant renal damage.

Clinical Features. Small stones that pass through the ureter can cause severe paroxysms of flank pain radiating toward the groin *(renal colic)*, often associated with gross hematuria. Because they obstruct the flow of urine, stones of all types predispose to bacterial infections. In most cases, the diagnosis is readily made radiologically.

Hydronephrosis

Urinary outflow obstruction causes dilation of the renal pelvis and calyces, called hydronephrosis.

Pathogenesis. Outflow obstructions leading to hydronephrosis may be the result of congenital structural anomalies or acquired calculi, benign prostatic hyperplasia, tumors that compress the ureters, pregnancy, or paralysis of the bladder (e.g., after spinal cord injury). Retroperitoneal fibrosis, which is a manifestation of IgG4 related disease, causes bilateral hydronephrosis. Filtration continues, causing dilation of the affected calyces and pelvis. Unusually high pressure generated in the renal pelvis and transmitted back through the collecting ducts results in compression of the renal vasculature, leading to arterial insufficiency and venous stasis. The initial functional disturbances are largely tubular, manifested primarily by an impaired concentrating ability. Dilation of the renal pelvis and calyces is readily detectable by radiologic imaging, and if unilateral, kidney function is usually maintained until late in the course. With complete bilateral obstruction, irreversible renal injury occurs in as little as 3 weeks.

> *Morphology.* The pelvis and calyces are dilated, and the kidney parenchyma is compressed and becomes atrophic (Fig. 11.17). The earliest microscopic lesions are tubular dilation, followed by atrophy and interstitial fibrosis; glomeruli become atrophic if the obstruction is severe and prolonged.

Clinical Features. Anuria results if the obstruction is bilateral and complete, but this is rarely the case. Paradoxically, incomplete bilateral obstruction causes polyuria rather than oliguria as a result of defects in tubular concentrating mechanisms, and this may obscure the true nature of the lesion. Hydronephrosis is typically diagnosed by imaging, either incidentally or as part of the evaluation of the underlying cause of the obstruction.

TUMORS OF THE KIDNEY

The most important and common tumor of the kidney is renal cell carcinoma, representing 2% to 3% of cancers in adults and 80% to 85% of primary renal tumors. Wilms tumor is the commonest renal tumor of children.

Renal Cell Carcinoma

This malignant tumor of the tubular epithelium is strongly associated with acquired mutations that mimic adaptive responses to hypoxia and has a striking propensity to metastasize through blood vessels.

Pathogenesis. The most common histologic form of the tumor is *clear cell carcinoma*. This tumor is usually sporadic, but there is also a rare familial form that occurs at high frequency in association with *von Hippel-Lindau (VHL) disease*. This association has led to the discovery that the most frequent driver mutation in both the familial and sporadic forms is loss or inactivation of the *VHL* gene. As discussed in Chapter 5, VHL regulates adaptive responses to hypoxia, and in its absence there is overexpression of vascular endothelial growth factor (VEGF), a key regulator of angiogenesis. The uncommon *papillary* type of renal cell carcinoma is associated with activating mutations in the oncogene *MET* (also mutated in papillary thyroid cancer), which encodes a receptor tyrosine kinase that stimulates pathways leading to increased cell growth and survival.

> *Morphology.* Grossly, the clear cell type of renal cell carcinoma is usually solitary, has areas of necrosis and hemorrhage, and exhibits a propensity to invade into renal veins. Microscopically, the cells contain abundant lipid and glycogen, accounting for the clear appearance of the cells after tissue processing (Fig. 11.18). Because of their origin from tubules, they can arise anywhere in the cortex. Papillary tumors, as the name implies, have papillae with fibrovascular cores. They tend to be bilateral and multiple (Supplemental eFig. 11.7).

Clinical Features. Carcinomas of the kidney are most common from the sixth to seventh decades, and men are affected about twice as often as women. The risk is higher in smokers, hypertensive and obese patients, and those who have had occupational exposure to cadmium. The risk for developing renal cell cancer is increased 30-fold in individuals with acquired polycystic disease as a complication of chronic dialysis. In more than 50% of cases, these tumors present with hematuria. In other cases, they present as palpable masses causing flank pain, or are detected incidentally during imaging for other conditions. Uncommon manifestations include fever, polycythemia (related to erythropoietin production by the tumor cells), and various paraneoplastic syndromes (hypercalcemia, hypertension, Cushing syndrome, or feminization or masculinization) because of aberrant hormone production. Metastases, especially to the lungs and bones, are frequent.

Wilms Tumor

Wilms tumor is often caused by inherited or acquired mutations in genes that regulate renal and gonadal development.

Wilms tumor accounts for about 5% of pediatric cancers.

Pathogenesis. Although Wilms tumor is usually a sporadic disease, about 10% of cases are associated with rare congenital syndromes: WAGR (*W*ilms tumor, *a*niridia, *g*enital abnormalities, and intellectual disability) syndrome, Denys-Drash syndrome (Wilms tumor, gonadal dysgenesis, and early-onset nephropathy), and Beckwith-Wiedemann syndrome (Wilms tumor and enlargement of individual body organs or entire body segments). The genetic basis of these disorders

has provided important insights into the pathogenesis of the tumor. Approximately one third of patients with WAGR syndrome and almost 90% of patients with Denys-Drash syndrome develop this tumor. The gene that is mutated in WAGR and Denys-Drash syndrome is *WT1*, which encodes a nuclear protein that regulates the expression of genes that are required for renal and gonadal development. It is postulated that the failure of normal development of the kidney results in compensatory overproliferation of primordial cells (the renal blastema, or nephrogenic rests), and the tumors arise from these rests. Numerous other genes associated with both sporadic and congenital Wilms tumors have been identified, but how, or even if, they interfere with normal renal development is not known.

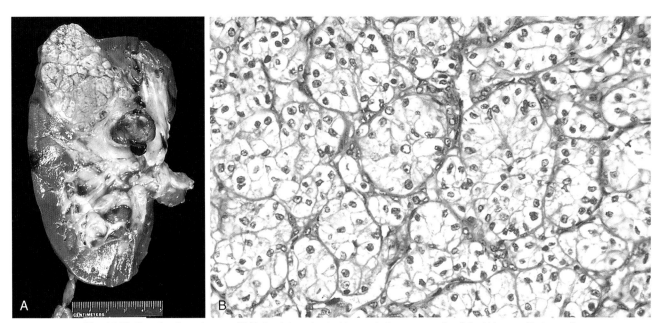

Fig. 11.18 Renal cell carcinoma. (A) Yellowish, spherical tumor in the upper pole of the kidney, with tumor in the dilated, thrombosed renal vein. (B) The clear cell microscopic pattern of renal cell carcinoma.

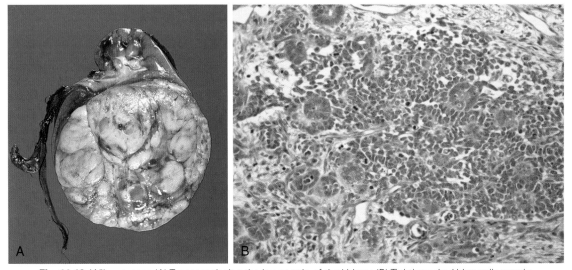

Fig. 11.19 Wilms tumor. (A) Tumor replacing the lower pole of the kidney. (B) Tightly packed blue cells consistent with the blastemal component, and interspersed primitive tubules representing the epithelial component.

Morphology. Wilms tumor typically is a large, solitary, well-circumscribed mass, although 10% are either bilateral or multicentric (Fig. 11.19). Microscopically, the tumor cells recapitulate different stages of nephrogenesis, with admixtures of blastemal, stromal, and epithelial cell types. The blastemal component consists of small, blue, primitive-looking, undifferentiated cells; the epithelial part usually takes the form of abortive tubules or glomeruli; and the stromal cells are immature spindle cells, sometimes showing skeletal muscle or cartilage differentiation. Approximately 5% of tumors contain foci of anaplastic cells with large, hyperchromatic, pleomorphic nuclei and abnormal mitoses; these tumors are often associated with *TP53* mutations and are relatively resistant to chemotherapy. Nephrogenic rests are present in about 35% of solitary Wilms tumors and almost all bilateral tumors (but are found in only about 1% of normal kidneys because they regress in childhood).

Clinical Features. Patients are typically younger than 10 years old and present with a palpable abdominal mass. Less often, the presenting features are fever and abdominal pain, hematuria or, occasionally, intestinal obstruction as a result of pressure from the tumor. The treatment generally consists of nephrectomy and chemotherapy, sometimes supplemented with radiation therapy. The overall prognosis is very good.

12

Gastrointestinal System

OUTLINE

Congenital Anomalies of the Gastrointestinal Tract, 205
Disorders of the Esophagus, 205
   Esophageal Obstruction, 205
   Esophageal Varices, 205
   Esophagitis, 205
   Esophageal Tumors, 207
Disorders of the Stomach, 207
   Gastritis and Peptic Ulcer Disease, 207
   Tumors of the Stomach, 209
Disorders of the Small and Large Intestines, 211
   Diarrheal Diseases, 211

Inflammatory Bowel Disease, 213
Other Inflammatory Diseases, 215
Tumors and Related Conditions of the
   Intestines, 216
Obstructive and Vascular Diseases, 219
Disorders of the Oral Cavity
  and Salivary Glands, 220
   Inflammatory Disorders of the Oral Cavity, 220
   Tumors and Tumor-like Lesions of the Oral
    Cavity, 220
   Diseases of the Salivary Glands, 220

The gastrointestinal (GI) tract is a hollow tube consisting of the esophagus, stomach, small intestine, colon, rectum, and anus. Each region has unique but complementary functions that serve to regulate the intake, processing, and absorption of ingested nutrients and the disposal of waste products. The intestines also are the principal site where the immune system interfaces with a diverse array of antigens present in food and gut microbes. In this chapter, we discuss mainly the inflammatory and neoplastic diseases of the GI system. We conclude with a brief consideration of disorders affecting the oral cavity and salivary glands.

CONGENITAL ANOMALIES OF THE GASTROINTESTINAL TRACT

A variety of developmental anomalies can affect the GI tract and are usually either asymptomatic or cause obstruction.

Atresia, fistulae, and duplications may occur in any part of the GI tract. When present within the esophagus they are discovered shortly after birth, usually due to regurgitation during feeding. A true diverticulum is a blind outpouching of the alimentary tract that communicates with the lumen and includes all three layers of the bowel wall. The most common true diverticulum is the *Meckel diverticulum*, which occurs in the ileum. Meckel diverticulum occurs as a result of failed involution of the vitelline duct, which connects the lumen of the developing gut to the yolk sac. This solitary diverticulum extends from the antimesenteric side of the bowel (Supplemental eFig. 12.1). The "rule of 2s" helps to remember the characteristics of Meckel diverticula, which are:
- Occur in approximately 2% of the population
- Generally present within 2 feet (60 cm) of the ileocecal valve
- Approximately 2 inches (5 cm) long
- Twice as common in males

- Most often symptomatic by age 2 (only approximately 4% are ever symptomatic). In the rare symptomatic cases, common presentations are gastrointestinal bleeding and acute abdominal complaints.

DISORDERS OF THE ESOPHAGUS

Esophageal Obstruction

Obstruction may be mechanical or functional. Mechanical obstruction results from strictures following esophageal injury, developmental defects, and tumors. Stenosis-associated dysphagia usually is progressive; difficulty eating solid foods typically occurs long before problems with liquids. Functional obstruction, called achalasia, results from defects in the tone of the lower esophageal sphincter (LES). Achalasia is characterized by the triad of incomplete LES relaxation, increased LES tone, and esophageal aperistalsis. Achalasia results from loss of distal esophageal inhibitory neurons. In idiopathic cases, there is inflammatory degeneration of the neurons. Secondary loss may occur in Chagas disease caused by infection with *Trypanosoma cruzi*.

Esophageal Varices

Portal hypertension can lead to the development of esophageal varices, an important cause of upper GI bleeding.

Portal hypertension (e.g., due to cirrhosis) induces development of collateral channels to shunt blood from the portal circulation to the caval circulation, creating dilated veins (varices) (see Chapter 13) (Supplemental eFig. 12.2). Esophageal varices appear as tortuous dilated veins within the submucosa of the distal esophagus and proximal stomach. Varices often are asymptomatic but are prone to rupture, which can lead to massive hematemesis and death.

Esophagitis

Inflammation of the lining of the esophagus may be caused by gastric acid, ingested chemicals, immune reactions, and infectious agents.

Esophagitis is one of the most common GI disorders of adults in the United States; its major forms are discussed next.

Reflux Esophagitis (Gastroesophageal Reflux Disease)

Gastroesophageal reflux disease (GERD) is the most common GI ailment with which patients present in the outpatient setting, and drugs for its usual symptom, heartburn, are among the most frequently used medicines.

Pathogenesis. When the esophageal mucosa is exposed to gastric acid, injury and inflammation occur. Conditions that decrease LES tone or increase abdominal pressure contribute to GERD and include alcohol and tobacco use, obesity, central nervous system depressants, pregnancy, hiatal hernia, delayed gastric emptying, and increased gastric volume.

> *Morphology.* The esophageal mucosa is infiltrated with varying numbers of eosinophils (Supplemental eFig. 12.3). Neutrophils may also be present, especially in severe cases and those with ulceration or accompanying infection.

Clinical Features. Symptoms include heartburn, dysphagia, and regurgitation of sour gastric contents. In more severe cases, there may be attacks of chest pain that are mistaken for heart disease.

Barrett Esophagus

This complication of chronic GERD is characterized by metaplastic conversion of the normal squamous esophageal epithelium to columnar epithelium, typically with goblet cells (Fig. 12.1A,B). Endoscopically, areas of Barrett esophagus appear as tongues or patches of velvety red mucosa extending upward from the gastroesophageal junction. Dysplasia develops in 0.2% to 1% of individuals with Barrett esophagus each year and is a precursor of adenocarcinoma, a cardinal example of the well-recognized relationship between chronic inflammation, tissue injury, and neoplasia. Although most individuals with Barrett esophagus do not develop dysplasia or esophageal cancer, the vast majority of esophageal adenocarcinomas are associated with Barrett esophagus. Therefore, periodic surveillance endoscopy with biopsy to screen for dysplasia is recommended.

Eosinophilic Esophagitis

This inflammatory condition of the esophagus usually develops in response to a reaction to allergens in foods such as cow milk and soy products. It is associated with other manifestations of atopy, such as atopic dermatitis, allergic rhinitis, and asthma. Eosinophils are present in the esophageal mucosa, typically in far greater numbers than in GERD (see Fig. 12.1C), and disease may involve the mid or upper esophagus. Symptoms include dysphagia and intolerance of food containing the responsible allergen. Unlike in GERD, proton pump inhibitors are of limited efficacy in eosinophilic esophagitis, but the disease often responds to the exclusion of offending agents from the diet and treatment with systemic steroids.

Chemical and Infectious Esophagitis

The mucosa of the esophagus may be damaged directly by a variety of irritants, including alcohol, acids and alkalis, hot fluids, and drugs in pill form that adhere to the esophageal lining. The injury and associated inflammation cause pain but are usually self-limited. Infectious esophagitis is most frequent in immunodeficient individuals. The common agents include herpes simplex virus, cytomegalovirus (Supplemental eFig. 12.4A-C), and *Candida.*

Esophageal Lacerations

The most common esophageal lacerations are *Mallory-Weiss tears,* which are often induced by severe retching or vomiting. The roughly linear lacerations of Mallory-Weiss syndrome are longitudinally oriented and usually cross the gastroesophageal junction. These superficial tears generally heal quickly and do not need surgical intervention. By contrast, severe, transmural esophageal tears *(Boerhaave syndrome)* result in mediastinitis, are catastrophic, and require prompt surgical intervention.

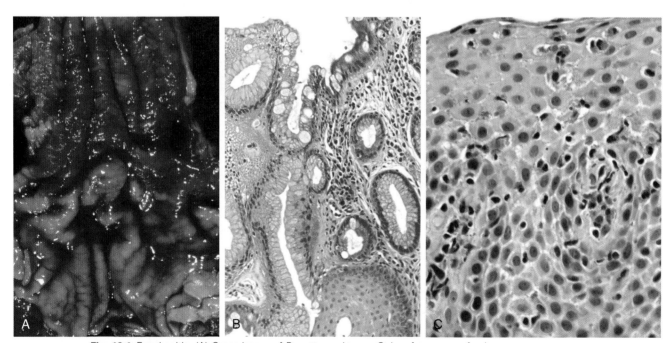

Fig. 12.1 Esophagitis. (A) Gross image of Barrett esophagus. Only a few areas of pale squamous mucosa remain within the predominantly metaplastic, reddish mucosa of the distal esophagus. (B) Histologic appearance of the gastroesophageal junction in Barrett esophagus. Note the transition between esophageal squamous mucosa *(lower right)* and metaplastic mucosa containing goblet cells *(upper).* (C) Eosinophilic esophagitis with numerous intraepithelial eosinophils.

Esophageal Tumors

The two major types of esophageal cancer are adenocarcinoma and squamous cell carcinoma. Squamous cell carcinoma is more common in Asia. Its incidence in the United States is decreasing, but the incidence of adenocarcinoma is going up.

- *Adenocarcinoma* usually arises in regions of Barrett esophagus in patients with long-standing GERD. Progression from the dysplasia of Barrett esophagus to carcinoma involves sequential acquisition of genetic and epigenetic changes. *TP53* mutations and chromosomal copy number changes are often seen. The tumors are most often located in the distal esophagus; early lesions appear as flat or raised patches in otherwise intact mucosa, whereas later tumors may form large exophytic masses associated with dysphagia (Supplemental eFig. 12.5). On microscopic examination, tumors typically produce mucin and form glands. Patients present with pain, difficulty in swallowing, vomiting, and weight loss. By the time signs and symptoms appear, the tumor usually has invaded the submucosal lymphatic vessels; due to the advanced stage at diagnosis, the overall 5-year survival rate is less than 25%.
- *Squamous cell carcinoma* is associated primarily with alcohol and tobacco use (which synergize to increase risk), as well as caustic esophageal injury, achalasia, Plummer-Vinson syndrome (iron deficiency anemia, dysphagia, and esophageal webs), frequent consumption of very hot beverages, and previous radiation therapy to the mediastinum. It is more common in people of African descent than in Caucasians, a difference not accounted for by known risk factors. Unlike adenocarcinoma, these tumors are located in the upper or middle third of the esophagus and initially appear as small, gray-white, plaque-like thickenings that can evolve into polypoid tumor masses that protrude into and obstruct the lumen, or into ulcerated, diffusely infiltrative lesions (see Supplemental eFig. 12.6). Histologically, most are well to moderately differentiated.

The overall 5-year survival rate is 9%, which increases to 75% in patients with superficial carcinomas.

DISORDERS OF THE STOMACH

Gastritis and Peptic Ulcer Disease

Gastritis is inflammation of the gastric mucosa resulting from exposure to acid and other injurious agents, and is usually due to an imbalance between damaging factors and mechanisms that protect the stomach lining from these agents.

Gastritis may be acute or chronic.

Acute Gastritis

Acute gastritis may be asymptomatic or it may cause epigastric pain, nausea, and vomiting. In more severe cases, there may be ulceration and hemorrhage, resulting in hematemesis (vomiting of blood) and blood loss.

Pathogenesis. The gastric lumen is strongly acidic, with a pH close to 1—more than 1 million times more acidic than the blood. It also contains proteases and other enzymes. This harsh environment contributes to digestion of food but also has the potential to damage the mucosa. Multiple mechanisms have evolved to protect the gastric mucosa (Fig. 12.2). Mucin secreted by surface epithelial cells forms a thin layer of mucus that shields the mucosa; it has a neutral pH as a result of secretion of bicarbonate ions by epithelial cells. The rich blood supply of the gastric mucosa efficiently buffers and removes protons that diffuse back into the lamina propria. Gastritis can occur after disruption of any of these protective mechanisms or augmentation of injurious exposures. The main causes of chemical gastritis include the following:

- *Nonsteroidal antiinflammatory drugs (NSAIDs)* inhibit production of prostaglandins, which normally stimulate mucin and bicarbonate

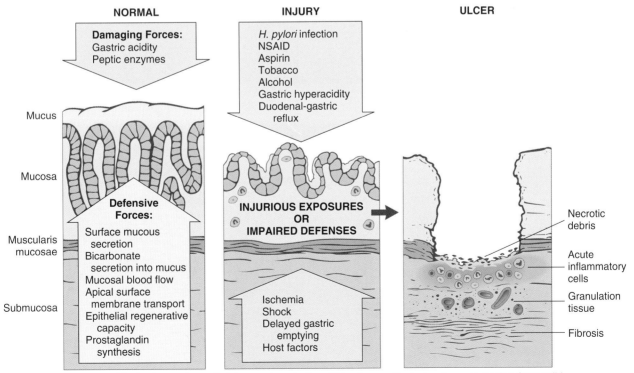

Fig. 12.2 Mechanisms of gastric injury and protection. This diagram illustrates the progression from mild forms of injury to ulceration that may occur with acute or chronic gastritis. Ulcers include layers of necrotic debris, inflammation, and granulation tissue; scarring, which develops over time, is present only in chronic lesions. NSAID, nonsteroidal antiinflammatory drug.

secretion and mucosal blood flow. Ingestion of these drugs is a frequent cause of gastric mucosal injury.
- *Uremia and infection by Helicobacter pylori* (discussed later) may inhibit gastric bicarbonate transporters.
- *Chemical exposures,* especially to acids and alkalis, alcohol, and chemotherapeutic drugs, may directly injure the gastric mucosa.

Acute gastritis is characterized by the presence of neutrophils within the epithelial layer; in severe cases, there is erosion of the mucosa leading to hemorrhage, which may be life threatening.

Stress-Related Gastritis

Patients with severe trauma, burns, extensive surgery, and critical illnesses are prone to developing acute gastritis in the form of stress ulcers:
- *Curling ulcers* occur in the proximal duodenum and are associated with severe burns or trauma.
- *Cushing ulcers* arise in the stomach, duodenum, or esophagus of those with intracranial disease and have a high incidence of perforation.

Pathogenesis. Stress-related mucosal injury may stem from local ischemia due to systemic hypotension or reduced blood flow caused by vasoconstriction (triggered by sympathetic nervous or other neural impulses), as well as increased acid production secondary to stimulation of the vagus nerve. Systemic acidosis may exacerbate the damage by lowering the intracellular pH of mucosal cells.

Morphology. The mucosa shows shallow erosions or acute ulcers, often multiple. Unlike chronic peptic ulcers, there is no scarring of the ulcer bed or thickening of the blood vessel wall.

Clinical Features. Most critically ill patients admitted to intensive care units show some evidence of gastritis, which may lead to severe bleeding and even perforations. Treatment of the underlying condition usually results in resolution of the inflammation and repair of the epithelium.

Helicobacter pylori *Gastritis*

Infection with the *H. pylori* bacillus causes chronic gastritis and duodenal and gastric ulcers.

Pathogenesis. H. pylori is a spiral-shaped bacillus detectable in gastric mucosal biopsies from the majority of patients with duodenal ulcer and chronic gastritis, although the incidence is decreasing in higher-income countries. Infection rates are inversely correlated with patient age, and the infection is often acquired during childhood, especially in areas with crowded living conditions and poor sanitation. The bacteria invade the gastric mucosa and, without therapy, generally persist for life. As a result of improved sanitation, the incidence of H. pylori infection in children has fallen.

The bacteria are thought to cause gastric epithelial injury by several mechanisms, including the following:
- Release of *bacterial enzymes* and other toxic products that directly damage epithelial cells
- Increased production of *gastric acid,* in part by stimulating gastrin secretion and in part by reducing the production of physiologic inhibitors of acid secretion
- Production of *proteases* that degrade normally protective glycoproteins in the mucous layer, exposing epithelial cells to the harsh gastric contents
- Stimulation of acute and chronic *inflammation* and cytokine release

H. pylori infection is also associated with an increased risk of gastric carcinoma and lymphoma (discussed later).

Morphology. Bacteria are present in the mucus overlying epithelial cells (Fig. 12.3), particularly foveolar cells in the antrum; increased acid production and gastritis typically occur in the antral region. Intestinal metaplasia, characterized by the presence of goblet cells and columnar absorptive cells, may be present. Variable numbers of neutrophils are seen in the lamina propria, epithelium, and gastric pits. The lamina propria also contains lymphocytes and macrophages, as is typical of chronic inflammation, and sheets of plasma cells. The mucosa may contain lymphoid follicles with germinal centers.

Clinical Features. Patients present with typical signs of gastritis, such as epigastric pain, nausea, and vomiting. The bacteria may be identified in gastric biopsies using immunohistochemical stains and by culture. Ureases produced by the bacteria break down urea into ammonia, which can be detected by breath tests. A stool test for the presence of H. pylori antigen is used for the diagnosis of active disease. Antibiotics can eradicate H. pylori and allow resolution of gastritis. In untreated cases, the prolonged immune response in the mucosa-associated lymphoid tissue (MALT) can result in the development of low-grade extranodal marginal zone lymphomas (also called MALTomas). Intestinal metaplasia is a risk factor for the development of gastric carcinoma.

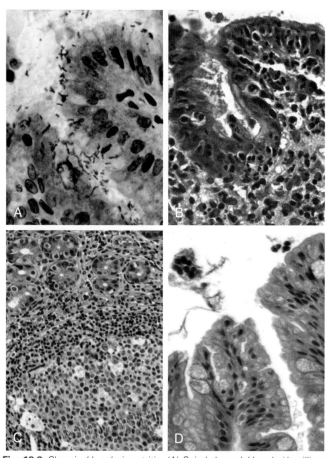

Fig. 12.3 Chronic *H. pylori* gastritis. (A) Spiral-shaped *H. pylori* bacilli are highlighted in this Warthin-Starry silver stain. Organisms are abundant within surface mucus. (B) Intraepithelial and lamina propria neutrophils are prominent. (C) Lymphoid aggregates with germinal centers and abundant subepithelial plasma cells within the superficial lamina propria are characteristic of *H. pylori* gastritis. (D) Intestinal metaplasia, recognizable as the presence of goblet cells admixed with gastric foveolar epithelium, can develop and is a risk factor for development of gastric adenocarcinoma.

Autoimmune Gastritis

Autoimmune gastritis has diverse consequences, including an increased risk of gastric cancer and development of vitamin B_{12} deficiency.

***Pathogenesis.* This form of gastritis is caused by an autoimmune attack on gastric parietal cells.**

Both autoreactive T cells and autoantibodies against parietal epithelial cells and intrinsic factor have been implicated in the pathogenesis; which is more important in causing parietal cell damage is uncertain, but detection of the antibodies is diagnostically helpful. Parietal cell loss leads to decreased production of gastric acid (achlorhydria) and intrinsic factor. Achlorhydria can allow bacterial overgrowth and secondary hyperplasia of gastrin-producing enteroendocrine cells. Loss of intrinsic factor reduces absorption of vitamin B_{12} and can lead to pernicious anemia, which is reversible (see Chapter 9). More ominous is irreversible neurologic damage.

Morphology. The acid-producing cells in the body and fundus of the stomach are lost, the mucosa in this region is thinned, and rugal folds are attenuated. The antrum is relatively spared (unlike in *H. pylori* gastritis). Intestinal metaplasia is common, and there is an increased risk of gastric cancer. The inflammatory infiltrate consists mainly of lymphocytes, macrophages, and plasma cells (Supplemental eFig. 12.7). Because of the atrophy of the glands, the disease is also called *atrophic gastritis,* or autoimmune metaplastic atrophic gastritis when metaplasia is present.

Clinical Features. Patients present with symptoms of chronic gastritis, but only a minority develop clinically apparent anemia. Serum antibodies reactive with parietal cells and intrinsic factor are present in most patients early in the disease. Often, there are other concomitant autoimmune diseases, such as autoimmune thyroid disease and diabetes.

Peptic Ulcer Disease

This common condition results from excess gastric acid and an impaired mucosal defense, most often the consequence of *H. pylori* infection and chronic NSAID use.

Pathogenesis. As mentioned earlier, NSAIDs inhibit prostaglandin production and thus impair a major pathway of mucosal protection, and *H. pylori* damages the gastric epithelium by the mechanisms detailed previously.

Morphology. Peptic ulcers are more frequent in the duodenum than in the stomach. They are commonly located within a few centimeters of the pyloric valve in the duodenum or near the interface of the antrum and the body in the stomach. In both sites, they are usually solitary, sharply punched-out defects (see Fig 2.7, Chapter 2). The base of benign ulcers is composed of granulation tissue and necrotic cell debris and inflammatory cells resting on a fibrous scar.

Clinical Features. The disease is most often seen in middle-aged or older adults. Patients usually present with epigastric burning or pain after meals, although a significant fraction present with GI bleeding, iron deficiency anemia due to chronic blood loss, or perforation, which is a medical emergency.

Tumors of the Stomach

Masses arising from the gastric mucosa include polyps, benign tumors called adenomas, and malignant tumors, of which the most common are adenocarcinomas.

Gastric Polyps and Adenomas

Gastric polyps may be inflammatory or neoplastic, whereas adenomas are neoplasms that may serve as precursors for cancers.

- *Polyps* are nodules or masses projecting from the mucosa. They are frequent incidental findings in endoscopies. The majority are inflammatory or hyperplastic, arising in areas of reactive hyperplasia caused by chronic gastritis (Supplemental eFig. 12.8A,B). In the gastric body and fundus, polyps are often multiple but usually of little consequence. Proton pump inhibitors used for the treatment of gastric acidity may give rise to fundic gland polyps because reduced acidity increases gastrin secretion, which in turn causes glandular hyperplasia. In Western countries, because the prevalence of *H. pylori* infection is low and the use of proton pump inhibitors is common, fundic gland polyps are the most frequent type of polyp.
- *Adenomas* represent about 10% of gastric polyps; the incidence increases with age, and most patients are between 50 and 60 years of age. Males are affected three times more often than females. Adenomas almost always occur on a background of chronic gastritis with atrophy and intestinal metaplasia. They exhibit varying degrees of epithelial dysplasia, and about a third become malignant, especially those larger than 2 cm in diameter (see Supplemental eFig. 12.8C).

Gastric Adenocarcinoma

Adenocarcinoma is the most common malignancy of the stomach. Its incidence is up to 20 times higher in Japan and many other countries outside of North America and northern Europe. In the United States, gastric cancer rates have dropped by more than 85% during the 20th century, presumably because of reduced exposure to one or more unknown carcinogens. There are two types of gastric adenocarcinomas: intestinal and diffuse. The intestinal type is more common and is associated with chronic gastritis, intestinal metaplasia, and dysplasia, which may be precancerous lesions. The diffuse type has no defined precursor lesion and is characterized by loss of the tumor suppressor E-cadherin.

Pathogenesis. The development of gastric adenocarcinoma is associated with particular mutations and infections; however, so far no clear sequence of events in its development has been established.

- Mutations in the gene encoding *E-cadherin,* an epithelial intercellular adhesion molecule, are found in gastric carcinomas of the diffuse type, both the rare familial cases and the more common sporadic ones. Many sporadic tumors in which the gene is not mutated have reduced expression owing to methylation of the E-cadherin promoter. These observations suggest that loss of E-cadherin is a key step in the development of diffuse gastric carcinoma.
- Patients with the familial adenomatous polyposis syndrome have mutations in the *adenomatous polyposis coli (APC)* gene, which is discussed later in the context of colon cancer. These patients also are at increased risk for intestinal-type gastric and duodenal cancer. Other mutations that have been identified include gain-of-function mutations in the gene for β-catenin, a transcription factor that is negatively regulated by E-cadherin and APC, and loss-of-function mutations in *TP53*.
- *H. pylori*–induced and autoimmune chronic gastritis are associated with intestinal-type gastric cancer, another example of the link between chronic inflammation and cancer (see Chapter 5).
- About 5% to 10% of gastric adenocarcinomas have evidence of Epstein-Barr virus (EBV) infection. The virus is clonal in such cases, meaning that the tumor originated from an EBV-infected cell, but precisely how EBV contributes to oncogenesis in gastric cancer is unknown.

Morphology. Intestinal-type tumors are bulky and composed of glands with mucin-producing cells that resemble those in colonic adenocarcinoma. Grossly, they can appear as an exophytic mass or an ulcerated lesion with heaped-up margins, unlike the "punched-out" appearance of peptic ulcers. Intestinal-type gastric cancer predominates in high-risk areas such as Japan (Fig. 12.4). Diffuse tumors have an infiltrative growth pattern, often without a discernible mass, and the cells lack intercellular adherens junctions. The tumor cells often contain large mucin vacuoles that push the nucleus to one side, producing a "signet-ring" appearance. These infiltrative tumors may elicit a strong fibrotic reaction that converts the wall of the stomach to a leathery consistency, called *linitis plastica*.

Clinical Features. The most common symptoms at the time of initial presentation are abdominal pain, dysphagia, and weight loss. Occult bleeding is frequent and may cause iron deficiency anemia. Gastric cancers spread locally to involve the duodenum, pancreas, and retroperitoneum. Metastases occur in regional lymph nodes and in distant organs, and when present indicate a poor prognosis.

Gastric Lymphoma

The stomach is a common site for extranodal lymphomas, which account for nearly 5% of gastric malignancies. Gastric lymphomas are of B-cell origin and mainly occur in two forms: indolent marginal zone lymphomas that remain localized to the stomach for long periods and are strongly associated with *H. pylori* infection, and aggressive, diffuse large B-cell lymphomas (Supplemental eFig. 12.9). Both are discussed further in Chapter 9.

Neuroendocrine Tumors (Carcinoid Tumors)

Most of these tumors are found in the GI tract, especially the small intestine. They grow more slowly than neuroendocrine carcinomas (hence the name *carcinoid*) and may come to medical attention because they secrete vasoactive and other hormone-like substances that cause flushing, sweating, bronchospasm, abdominal pain, diarrhea, and cardiac valve abnormalities, collectively known as the *carcinoid syndrome*. When the tumor is intestinal, the vasoactive mediators are metabolized in the liver; therefore, the presence of symptoms usually reflects metastatic disease. Foregut neuroendocrine tumors (in the stomach, duodenum, and esophagus) rarely spread. Gastrin-producing neuroendocrine tumors, called gastrinomas, are associated with increased gastric acid production, causing ulcers (*Zollinger-Ellison syndrome*). Midgut carcinoid tumors (small intestine) are often multiple and aggressive. Hindgut carcinoid tumors (appendix and colon) are usually incidental and benign. Histologically, all of these tumors contain uniform-appearing cells with abundant granular cytoplasm (Supplemental eFig. 12.10).

Gastrointestinal Stromal Tumor

Gastrointestinal stromal tumor (GIST) is the most common mesenchymal tumor of the abdomen, and over half occur in the wall of the stomach. It arises from the gastric pacemaker cells known as interstitial cells of Cajal. Of these tumors, 75% to 85% contain activating mutations in the gene encoding the tyrosine kinase KIT, which functions as the receptor for stem cell factor. Another 8% of tumors have activating mutations in the related platelet-derived growth factor (PDGF) receptor, also a tyrosine kinase; these two mutations are mutually exclusive, because they both activate the same signal transduction pathway. The constitutive kinase signaling stimulates unregulated cell proliferation. In GISTs without *KIT* or *PDGFRA* mutations, genes encoding components of the mitochondrial

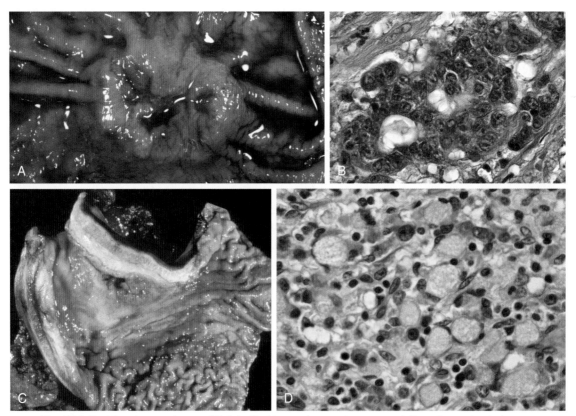

Fig. 12.4 Gastric adenocarcinoma. (A) Intestinal-type adenocarcinoma consisting of an elevated mass with heaped-up borders and central ulceration. (B) Intestinal-type adenocarcinoma composed of columnar, gland-forming cells infiltrating through desmoplastic stroma (C) Linitis plastica. The gastric wall is markedly thickened and rugal folds are partially lost. (D) Signet-ring cells can be recognized by their large cytoplasmic mucin vacuoles and peripherally displaced, crescent-shaped nuclei.

succinate dehydrogenase complex are often affected, a poorly understood example of an oncogenic effect stemming from altered metabolism. Histologically, the tumor consists of spindle-shaped or epithelioid cells (Supplemental eFig. 12.11). The peak incidence of gastric GIST is around 60 years of age. Large tumors come to attention because of mass effects or mucosal ulceration and its consequences. Primary treatment is by surgical resection; unresectable or recurrent tumors with *KIT* or *PDGFR* mutations are treated with tyrosine kinase inhibitors. The prognosis correlates with the tumor's size, mitotic index, and location, with gastric GISTs being somewhat less aggressive than those arising in the small intestine.

DISORDERS OF THE SMALL AND LARGE INTESTINES

Diarrheal Diseases

Diarrhea is defined as an increase in the mass, frequency, or fluidity of stool. Chronic diarrhea results in malabsorption, and the inadequate absorption of nutrients often has serious systemic consequences. Diarrhea can be classified into four major categories:

- *Secretory diarrhea* is characterized by isotonic stool and persists during fasting.
- *Osmotic diarrhea,* such as that occurring with lactase deficiency, is due to osmotic forces exerted by unabsorbed luminal solutes. The diarrheal fluid is at least 50 mOsm more concentrated than plasma, and the condition abates with fasting.
- *Malabsorptive diarrhea* caused by inadequate nutrient absorption is associated with steatorrhea and is relieved by fasting.
- *Exudative diarrhea* is due to inflammatory disease and characterized by purulent, bloody stools that continue during fasting.

Malabsorptive and Osmotic Diarrhea

Malabsorption manifests most commonly as chronic diarrhea and is characterized by the defective absorption of fats, fat- and water-soluble vitamins, proteins, carbohydrates, electrolytes, minerals, and water.

The chronic malabsorptive disorders most commonly encountered in Western countries are pancreatic insufficiency (secondary to cystic fibrosis), celiac disease, and Crohn disease (discussed later).

Lactase (disaccharidase) deficiency is another cause of malabsorptive diarrhea. It gives rise to osmotic diarrhea because without the enzyme, osmotically active lactose remains in the lumen. There are two types of lactase deficiency: a congenital form that is an autosomal recessive disorder and an acquired form caused by downregulation of lactase gene expression. The latter form is particularly common among Native Americans, Chinese populations, and people of African descent.

Infectious Diarrhea

Infectious enterocolitis is responsible for over 1 million deaths per year worldwide.

Infections are caused by diverse bacteria, viruses, and parasites (Table 12.1); are usually acquired from contaminated food or water; and typically present with diarrhea. *Campylobacter, Shigella, Salmonella,* and many other bacterial infections, including *Yersinia* and *Escherichia coli,* all induce a similar microscopic picture and give rise to *acute self-limited colitis.* The specific diagnosis is primarily by stool culture.

Here we summarize the features of some representative and common infections.

- *Cholera,* caused by *Vibrio cholerae,* is endemic in parts of India and Bangladesh. The infection is spread mainly by contaminated drinking water, and epidemics break out when natural disasters such as hurricanes and floods disrupt the water supply. The bacteria attach to the epithelium of the small intestine and secrete a toxin that activates a G-protein, leading to a sustained increase in intracellular cyclic AMP. This opens an ion channel that releases chloride ions into the lumen, creating an osmotic gradient that draws water into the lumen, producing secretory diarrhea. Most exposed individuals are asymptomatic or suffer only mild diarrhea; in severe disease, the volume of diarrhea may reach 1 L per hour, leading to dehydration, electrolyte imbalances, shock, and death. Although the mortality rate for severe cholera is 50% to 70% without treatment, fluid replacement can save more than 99% of patients.

- *E.coli diarrhea.* Various subspecies of *E. coli* cause "traveler's diarrhea" and other intestinal infections. The infection typically results in an acute, self-limited colitis, with neutrophil infiltrates and crypt abscesses, though some subtypes have other associations. Both enteroinvasive *E. coli* and enterohemorrhagic *E. coli* can cause dysentery (bloody diarrhea); the latter can also result in hemolytic-uremic syndrome.

- *Campylobacter jejuni* also causes traveler's diarrhea and can result in reactive arthritis, a triad of sterile arthritis, urethritis, and conjunctivitis that preferentially affects HLA-B27–positive men between 20 and 40 years of age. Other extraintestinal complications include erythema nodosum and Guillain-Barré syndrome.

- *Typhoid,* caused by *Salmonella typhi* and *Salmonella paratyphi,* affects almost 30 million people worldwide annually and is endemic in many developing countries. The bacteria are taken up by M (microfold) epithelial cells in the small intestine and engulfed by macrophages in the underlying Peyer patches. The infection and associated host reaction may produce large mucosal elevations and longitudinal ulcers in the ileum. Organisms can disseminate via lymphatics and blood vessels, often to the lymph nodes and spleen, causing reactive hyperplasia. Foci of parenchymal necrosis with macrophage aggregates, called typhoid nodules, may be found in the lymph nodes, liver, and bone marrow. Acute infection is associated with anorexia, vomiting, and bloody diarrhea. It is usually followed by an asymptomatic phase that gives way to bacteremia with systemic manifestations of inflammation (high fever), abdominal pain, skin rash, and a host of extraintestinal complications involving multiple organs.

- Unlike *S.typhi,* other species of *Salmonella* cause an acute self limited colitis, without systemic spread.

- *Shigella,* the most common cause of bloody diarrhea, secretes powerful exotoxins that cause ulceration of the colonic mucosa. These ulcers can mimic those in Crohn disease and, in severe cases, the mucosa may become hemorrhagic and pseudomembranes (overlying layers of necrotic debris and inflammatory cells) may form. Like typhoid, organisms are taken up by M cells, usually in the left colon but also the ileum. Complications are uncommon and include reactive arthritis (as with *Campylobacter* infection) and hemolytic-uremic syndrome.

- *Pseudomembranous colitis* is caused by overgrowth of *Clostridium difficile* in the setting of reduced numbers of normal colonic commensal bacteria (the "microbiome") due to broad-spectrum antibiotic therapy. *C. difficile* injures the colonic mucosal epithelium, and, in severe cases, pseudomembranes form on the epithelium. The surface epithelium is denuded, and damaged crypts are distended by a mucopurulent exudate that "erupts" to the surface in a fashion reminiscent of a volcano (Supplemental eFig. 12.12). Patients present with watery diarrhea, abdominal cramps, and systemic signs of inflammation. The diagnosis depends on the detection of *C. difficile* toxin in stool. Metronidazole or vancomycin is generally effective, but antibiotic-resistant and hypervirulent *C. difficile* strains are increasingly common. Fecal microbial transplantation to restore the normal microbiome has proven effective in patients with recurrent *C. difficile* infection.

- *Whipple disease* is a rare, multivisceral chronic disease caused by a gram-positive actinomycete named *Tropheryma whippelii.* Patients present with malabsorptive diarrhea, lymphadenopathy, and arthritis of undefined origin. Histologically, there is a dense accumulation of distended, foamy macrophages full of organisms in the lamina propria of the small intestine, the mesenteric lymph nodes, the

Table 12.1 Bacterial Infections of the Small and Large Intestines

Infection Type	Geographic Area of World	Reservoir	Transmission	Epidemiology	Affected GI Sites	Symptoms	Complications
Cholera	India, Africa	Shellfish	Fecal-oral, water	Sporadic, endemic, epidemic	Small intestine	Severe watery diarrhea	Dehydration, electrolyte imbalances
Campylobacter spp.	Developed countries	Chickens, sheep, pigs, cattle	Poultry, milk, other foods	Sporadic; children, travelers	Colon	Watery or bloody diarrhea	Arthritis, Guillain-Barré syndrome
Shigellosis	Worldwide; endemic in developing countries	Humans	Fecal-oral, food, water	Children, migrant workers, travelers, nursing home residents	Left colon, ileum	Bloody diarrhea	Reactive arthritis, urethritis, conjunctivitis, hemolytic-uremic syndrome
Salmonellosis	Worldwide	Poultry, farm animals, reptiles	Meat, poultry, eggs, milk	Children, older adults	Colon, small intestine	Watery or bloody diarrhea	Sepsis, abscess
Enteric (typhoid) fever	India, Mexico, Philippines	Humans	Fecal-oral, water	Children, adolescents, travelers	Small intestine	Bloody diarrhea, fever	Chronic infection, carrier state, encephalopathy, myocarditis, intestinal perforation
Yersinia spp.	Northern and central Europe	Pigs, cows, puppies, cats	Pork, milk, water	Clustered cases	Ileum, appendix, right colon	Abdominal pain, fever, diarrhea	Reactive arthritis, erythema nodosum
Escherichia coli							
Enterotoxigenic (ETEC)	Developing countries	Unknown	Food or fecal-oral	Infants, adolescents, travelers	Small intestine	Severe watery diarrhea	Dehydration, electrolyte imbalances
Enteropathogenic (EPEC)	Worldwide	Humans	Fecal-oral	Infants	Small intestine	Watery diarrhea	Dehydration, electrolyte imbalances
Enterohemorrhagic (EHEC)	Worldwide	Widespread, includes cattle	Beef, milk, produce	Sporadic and epidemic	Colon	Bloody diarrhea	Hemolytic-uremic syndrome
Enteroinvasive (EIEC)	Developing countries	Unknown	Cheese, other foods, water	Young children	Colon	Bloody diarrhea	Unknown
Enteroaggregative (EAEC)	Worldwide	Unknown	Unknown	Children, adults, travelers	Colon	Nonbloody diarrhea, afebrile	Poorly defined
Pseudomembranous colitis (*C. difficile*)	Worldwide	Humans, hospital patients	Antibiotics allow emergence	Immunosuppressed, antibiotic-treated	Colon	Watery diarrhea, fever	Relapse, toxic megacolon
Whipple disease	Rural more than urban	Unknown	Unknown	Rare	Small intestine	Malabsorption	Arthritis, CNS disease
Mycobacterial infection	Worldwide	Unknown	Unknown	Immunosuppressed, endemic	Small intestine	Malabsorption	Pneumonia, infection at other sites

CNS, Central nervous system; GI, gastrointestinal.

synovial membranes of affected joints, and the cardiac valves, brain, and other sites (Supplemental eFig. 12.13A and B).

- *Norovirus* infection is responsible for almost half the outbreaks of gastroenteritis worldwide and is a frequent cause of sporadic gastroenteritis in higher-income countries. The infection is usually self-limited. Local outbreaks are usually related to contaminated food or water, but person-to-person transmission underlies most sporadic cases.
- *Rotavirus* is the most common cause of severe childhood diarrhea worldwide. It selectively infects and destroys mature (absorptive) enterocytes in the small intestine, and the villus surface is repopulated by immature secretory cells, resulting in loss of absorptive function and net secretion of water and electrolytes, compounded by an osmotic diarrhea from incompletely absorbed nutrients. Children between 6 and 24 months of age are most vulnerable. Vaccines are now available, and their use is beginning to decrease the occurrence of rotavirus infection.
- *Parasitic infections* of the intestines affect more than half the world's population at some time in their lives. Although the small intestine can

harbor as many as 20 different parasites, only a few cause significant disease.

- *Ascaris lumbricoides* is a nematode that infects individuals by fecal-oral transmission of the parasite's eggs. In the intestine, the eggs hatch to release larvae, which penetrate the wall and enter the circulation to reach the lungs, from where they are coughed up and swallowed. Upon return to the small intestines, they mature into adult worms that induce an inflammatory reaction rich in eosinophils. Clinical manifestations may include lung inflammation caused by the migrating larvae, or intestinal and hepatobiliary symptoms during the late phase of the infection. The diagnosis is based on the detection of eggs in the stools.
- *Strongyloides stercoralis* larvae live in fecally contaminated soil and can penetrate the skin. From here, they migrate to the lungs, are coughed up and swallowed after reaching the oropharynx, and mature into adult worms in the intestine. Reproducing worms lay eggs that hatch in the intestine and release larvae that continue a cycle of autoinfection.

Table 12.2 Features of Crohn Disease and Ulcerative Colitis

Feature	Crohn Disease	Ulcerative Colitis
Macroscopic Features		
Bowel region affected	Ileum ± colon	Colon only
Rectal involvement	Sometimes	Always
Distribution	Skip lesions	Diffuse
Stricture	Yes	Rare
Bowel wall appearance	Thick	Thin
Inflammation	Transmural	Limited to mucosa and submucosa
Pseudopolyps	Moderate	Marked
Ulcers	Deep, knifelike	Superficial, broad-based
Lymphoid reaction	Marked	Moderate
Fibrosis	Marked	Mild to none
Serositis	Marked	No
Granulomas	Yes (~35%)	No
Fistulas/sinuses	Yes	No
Clinical Features		
Perianal fistula	Yes (in colonic disease)	No
Fat/vitamin malabsorption	Yes	No
Malignant potential	With colonic involvement	Yes
Recurrence after surgery	Common	No
Toxic megacolon	No	Yes

NOTE: Not all features may be present in a single case.

The usual clinical presentation is intermittent GI, pulmonary, or cutaneous symptoms that may continue for many years.

- *Necator americanus and Ancylostoma duodenale* are hookworms that also initiate infection by larval penetration through the skin. They develop in the lungs, and are swallowed and complete their maturation in the duodenum. Here the adult worms attach to the mucosa, suck blood, and reproduce. Because of the chronic blood loss, hookworm infections are a leading cause of iron deficiency anemia in lower-income countries.
- *Giardia lamblia,* a flagellated protozoan, is the most common pathogenic parasite in humans. Infection is acquired by ingestion of cysts in contaminated food or water. Trophozoites are released in the acidic environment of the stomach and damage intestinal microvilli, causing apoptosis of epithelial cells. The infection may lead to acute or chronic malabsorptive diarrhea.
- *Entamoeba histolytica* is a protozoan that also spreads by fecal-oral transmission. It infects as many as 500 million people worldwide and causes 40 million cases of dysentery and liver abscess annually. While amebiasis affects most commonly the cecum and ascending colon, any part of the large intestine can be involved. In about 40% of those with intestinal amebiasis, the parasites enter the splanchnic circulation and lodge in the liver to produce an abscess, which may persist after the intestinal infection has passed. Liver abscesses can extend into the lung and sometimes the heart. Individuals with amebiasis may present with abdominal pain, bloody diarrhea, or weight loss. Occasionally, acute necrotizing colitis and megacolon occur, both associated with significant rates of mortality.

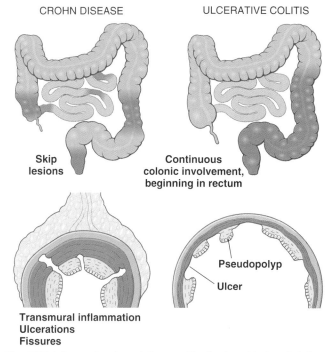

Fig. 12.5 Inflammatory bowel disease. Distribution of lesions in inflammatory bowel disease. The distinction between Crohn disease and ulcerative colitis is based primarily on morphology.

Inflammatory Bowel Disease

Inflammatory bowel disease refers to chronic inflammation of the intestines caused by dysregulated immune responses to commensal bacteria.

Inflammatory bowel disease (IBD) encompasses two entities: *Crohn disease* and *ulcerative colitis*. They share some clinical features and are treated with similar drugs, but there are also significant differences in these disorders (Table 12.2 and Fig. 12.5). Both Crohn disease and ulcerative colitis frequently present during adolescence or in young adults; some studies suggest a second, smaller peak in the incidence of both diseases after the fifth decade. In Western nations, IBD is most common among Caucasians and, in the United States, it occurs three to five times more often among eastern European (Ashkenazi) Jews than other ethnic groups.

Pathogenesis. The etiology of IBD is unknown, but the available evidence indicates that the disorder is caused mainly by aberrant immune responses to commensal bacteria. Crohn disease is likely the result of excessive CD4+ Th1 and Th17 responses to gut bacteria. The activated T cells elicit chronic inflammation in the wall of the intestine. The nature of the injurious immune response in ulcerative colitis is not defined. The triggers that cause these pathogenic immune responses are also unknown, but gene association studies implicate defects in innate immune defense, immune regulation, and epithelial integrity.

- Inadequate wound repair and epithelial barrier function may allow luminal bacteria and their products to enter the lamina propria, where immune cells are located. Polymorphisms in the gene encoding NOD2 are associated with Crohn disease in some populations. NOD2 is an innate immune receptor that recognizes cytoplasmic bacterial products and activates cellular defense mechanisms. The disease-associated variants may be less able to recognize and respond to bacteria, thus allowing bacteria to traverse the epithelium and trigger excessive immune activation.
- Inadequate regulation of T-cell responses is likely a fundamental basis of the disease. This defect may be in the activation and function of regulatory T cells or in cytokines that suppress inflammation, notably

interleukin-10. Both mechanisms are known to prevent proinflammatory immune responses to commensal microbes. Rare Mendelian diseases in which regulatory T cells are deficient or the interleukin-10 receptor or interleukin-10 genes are mutated manifest with severe colitis early in childhood, supporting the idea that abnormalities in these mechanisms may result in aberrant mucosal immune responses.

- Changes in the gut microbiome may contribute to the inflammation. The nature of these microbial changes has proved challenging to define, and it remains difficult to differentiate between microbial shifts as causes or results of disease. Some success with ingestion of probiotics (so-called good bacteria) and fecal transplants from healthy donors suggests that restoring the "healthy microbiome" may be beneficial.
- Defective autophagy may contribute to the dysregulated immune response. Autophagy is a host cellular response at times of nutrient deficiency, and is also involved in the clearance of microbes from the cytosol (see Chapter 1). Polymorphisms in an autophagy-associated gene, *ATG16L*, are associated with Crohn disease, perhaps by increasing the burden of intracellular microbes.

One model that unifies the roles of intestinal microbiota, epithelial function, and mucosal immunity suggests a cycle in which transepithelial flux of luminal bacterial components activates innate and adaptive immune responses. In a genetically susceptible host, the subsequent release of tumor necrosis factor and other immune signals impair the permeability of the intestinal epithelial barrier, which further increases the flux of luminal material. These events may establish a self-amplifying cycle in which a stimulus at any site may be sufficient to initiate IBD.

Long-standing IBD with severe inflammation increases the risk of colon cancer.

This risk is greater for ulcerative colitis than for Crohn disease mainly because colonic involvement is more extensive in ulcerative colitis. Other risk factors include the duration of disease and the frequency and persistence of active inflammation. Thus, IBD is another example of the link between inflammation and cancer. Dysplasia of the epithelium is often seen in areas of long-standing inflammation, and may be a precursor to adenocarcinoma.

Crohn Disease
Crohn disease is a chronic inflammatory disease of the terminal ileum and proximal colon that is associated with transmural inflammation and skip lesions.

> *Morphology.* Crohn disease, also known as *regional enteritis*, may occur in any area of the GI tract, but the most common sites at presentation are the terminal ileum, ileocecal valve, and cecum. The presence of multiple, sharply delineated areas of disease separated by uninvolved gut (skip lesions) is characteristic of Crohn disease. The intestinal wall is thickened as a consequence of transmural edema, inflammation, submucosal fibrosis, and hypertrophy of the muscularis propria, all of which contribute to stricture formation; ulcers, fissures, and fistulas are also seen. In cases with extensive transmural disease, mesenteric fat frequently wraps around the serosal surface (creeping fat). Microscopically, the entire wall of the intestine is involved. It may contain an infiltrate of neutrophils, often forming crypt abscesses (Fig. 12.6). Repeated cycles of crypt destruction and regeneration lead to distortion of the mucosal architecture; the normally straight and parallel crypts take on bizarre branching shapes and unusual orientations to one another. Submucosal noncaseating granulomas are seen in a third of the cases.

Clinical Features. Although the clinical manifestations are quite varied, most patients present with diarrhea, abdominal pain, and signs of systemic

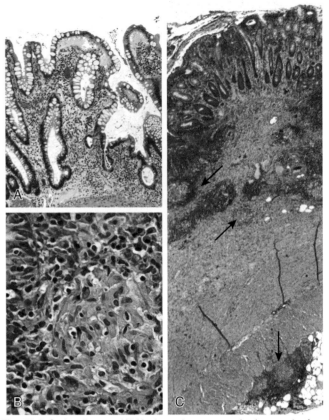

Fig. 12.6 Crohn disease. (A) Haphazard crypt organization results from repeated injury and regeneration. (B) Noncaseating granuloma. (C) Transmural Crohn disease with submucosal and serosal granulomas *(arrows)*.

inflammation, such as fever. Periods of disease activity typically are interrupted by asymptomatic intervals that last for weeks to many months. Disease reactivation can be associated with a variety of external triggers, including physical or emotional stress, dietary changes, NSAID use, and cigarette smoking. Fibrosing strictures and fistulas may develop, requiring surgical treatment. There may be inflammatory disorders outside the intestines, including uveitis, primary sclerosing cholangitis, and arthritis. The risk for the development of colonic adenocarcinoma is increased in long-standing colonic disease.

Ulcerative Colitis
Ulcerative colitis is a chronic inflammatory disease diffusely involving the mucosa of the colon and rectum.

> *Morphology.* The lesions always involve the rectum and spread contiguously for varying distances. The small intestine is not affected, although mild mucosal inflammation of the distal ileum (backwash ileitis) may be present in severe cases of pancolitis. The mucosal surface appears granular and may show multiple broad-based ulcerations, transitioning abruptly from normal mucosa (Fig. 12.7). Islands of regenerating epithelium often bulge into the lumen, creating small elevations called pseudopolyps. Unlike in Crohn disease, transmuralural thickening is absent, the serosal surface is normal, and strictures do not occur. Microscopically, the inflammation is continuous (without skip lesions) and limited to the mucosa and submucosa. There may be neutrophil infiltrates and crypt abscesses, but granulomas are not seen.

Clinical Features. Patients present with episodes of bloody diarrhea, abdominal pain, and cramps. Periods of remission followed by relapse are common. Colectomy cures intestinal disease, but extraintestinal

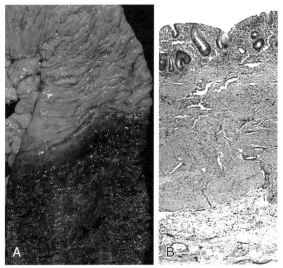

Fig. 12.7 Ulcerative colitis. (A) Sharp demarcation between active ulcerative colitis *(bottom)* and normal *(top)*. (B) This full-thickness histologic section shows that disease is limited to the mucosa.

manifestations such as primary sclerosing cholangitis (more common in ulcerative colitis than in Crohn disease) may persist.

Other Inflammatory Diseases

In addition to the entities grouped under IBD, the intestines are affected by several other inflammatory diseases caused by aberrant immune responses or infections. Some of the more common of these diseases are described next.

Celiac Disease (Gluten Enteropathy)

Celiac disease is an inflammatory disorder of the small intestine caused by an immune reaction to gluten.

Pathogenesis. Gluten, the major storage protein of wheat and related grains, is digested by enzymes in the gut to generate amino acids and peptides, including a peptide called gliadin that is resistant to further enzymatic digestion. It is deaminated by tissue transglutaminase and is then presented by antigen-presenting cells to CD4+ T cells. Virtually everyone ingests gluten, but only some individuals make T-cell responses to its antigenic components. This implies a genetic predisposition, and is consistent with a strong association with particular class II HLA alleles, specifically HLA-DQ2 and -DQ8. These class II MHC molecules are capable of binding gliadin and other gluten-derived peptides and presenting these antigens to CD4+ T cells. In susceptible individuals, gliadin may also stimulate cytokine secretion from epithelial cells, and these cytokines promote T-cell responses. The T cells, in turn, produce cytokines that damage the epithelium. CD8+ T cells and natural killer cells have been implicated in epithelial injury. Patients also make antibody responses to transglutaminase and gliadin, which are markers of disease activity but of uncertain pathogenic significance.

> *Morphology.* The characteristic findings are increased numbers of intraepithelial T lymphocytes, villus atrophy, hyperplasia of crypts, and increased numbers of plasma cells, mast cells, and eosinophils in the lamina propria (Fig. 12.8). Villus atrophy results in a decreased surface area of the mucosal brush border, accounting for the malabsorption.

Clinical Features. Pediatric celiac disease may manifest with classic symptoms (irritability, abdominal distention, anorexia, diarrhea, failure to thrive, weight loss, or muscle wasting). Cases with nonclassic symptoms tend to present at older ages and are often marked by abdominal pain,

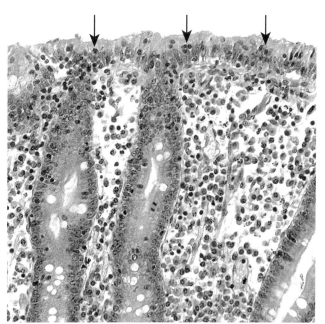

Fig. 12.8 Celiac disease. Advanced cases of celiac disease show complete loss of villi, or total villous atrophy. Note the dense plasma cell infiltrates in the lamina propria and intraepithelial lymphocytes *(arrows)*. (Courtesy ExpertPath, copyright Elsevier.)

nausea, vomiting, bloating, or constipation. Children with the disease may develop consequences of malabsorption, such as anemia, vitamin deficiencies, and growth retardation. In adults, celiac disease manifests most commonly between 30 and 60 years of age with bulky, foul-smelling stool (because of steatorrhea) and abdominal bloating, but other, more subtle presentations, such as iron deficiency anemia, also are seen. The diagnosis depends on the detection of antibodies to tissue transglutaminase and gliadin. Biopsy may be needed in some cases. The symptoms abate when gluten is excluded from the diet. Various autoimmune disorders are frequently associated with celiac disease, including dermatitis herpetiformis (an autoimmune blistering disease of the skin), type 1 diabetes, and other endocrine diseases. In long-standing disease, there is also an increased incidence of enteropathy-associated T-cell lymphoma, an aggressive tumor of intraepithelial T lymphocytes, and small-intestinal adenocarcinoma.

Sigmoid Diverticulitis

Diverticula are outpouchings of the mucosa and submucosa of the wall of the intestine caused by increased intraluminal pressure (Supplemental eFig. 12.14). The presence of multiple diverticula is known as *diverticulosis*. Diverticula are most often seen in the colon, especially the sigmoid colon because of discontinuities where nerves and blood vessels penetrate the outer muscle coat and weaken the wall. They develop in the sigmoid when the diet is low in fiber and the stool is relatively thick and viscous, resulting in increased peristaltic contractions. Obstruction of diverticula and stasis of luminal contents can lead to inflammation, called *diverticulitis*. Its great danger is perforation, because diverticular walls are thin, bulge outside the muscularis propria, and are easily damaged by inflammation. Perforation can result in localized abscess or diffuse peritonitis. Diverticular disease without inflammation, that is, diverticulosis, is usually asymptomatic, but may cause intermittent cramping, constipation, and diarrhea.

Appendicitis

The appendix is a true diverticulum of the cecum. Similar to other diverticula, it is prone to inflammation. Acute appendicitis is the result

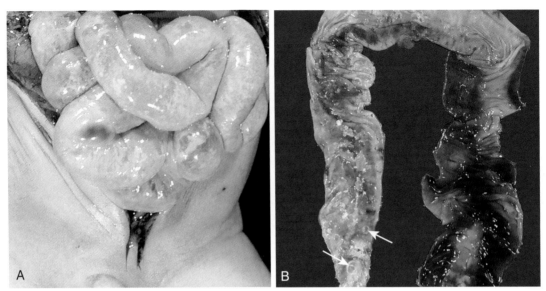

Fig. 12.9 Necrotizing enterocolitis. (A) At postmortem examination in a severe case, the entire small bowel was markedly distended and perilously thin (usually this appearance implies impending perforation). (B) The congested portion of the ileum corresponds to areas of hemorrhagic infarction and transmural necrosis. Submucosal gas bubbles (pneumatosis intestinalis) can be seen in several areas *(arrows)*.

of increased intraluminal pressure causing venous obstruction, usually superimposed on luminal obstruction by a small stone-like mass of stool *(fecalith)*. Ischemic injury and stasis favor bacterial proliferation, causing inflammation. Neutrophils are usually present in the wall, and abscesses may form. In severe cases, the inflamed appendix may rupture, leading to peritonitis and even sepsis. Patients usually present with acute abdominal pain, nausea, vomiting, and systemic signs of acute inflammation. Surgical removal of the inflamed appendix is definitive treatment.

Necrotizing Enterocolitis

Necrotizing enterocolitis (NEC) is a perinatal GI emergency that most commonly occurs in premature infants. It may be seen in as many as 10% of very-low-birth-weight infants (<1500 g), and its incidence is inversely proportional to gestational age. It is associated with enteral feeding and usually involves the terminal ileum, cecum, and ascending colon, but any part of the intestines may be affected. Involved areas show mucosal or transmural necrosis (Fig. 12.9), mucosal ulcers, bacterial contamination, and submucosal gas bubbles, presumably resulting from infection with gas-forming enteric bacteria, which are detectable radiologically. In severe cases, there is intestinal perforation and peritonitis. Babies present with bloody diarrhea, abdominal distention, and circulatory collapse in the most severe cases. The perinatal mortality rate is high, and almost half of the cases require resection of necrotic segments of bowel.

Tumors and Related Conditions of the Intestines

Polyps and tumors are more common in the colon than in the small intestine. Their clinical significance varies greatly, from incidental findings to fatal cancers.

Polyps

A polyp is any protruberance into the lumen from the normally flat mucosa. It may be nonneoplastic or neoplastic.

The neoplastic lesions, adenomas, are described later. The nonneoplastic polyps are of several types.

- *Hamartomatous polyps* are masses of normal tissue elements growing in a disordered and unorganized manner. The most common types are juvenile polyps, which consist of dilated cystic glands and have a tendency to bleed. *Peutz-Jeghers syndrome* is an autosomal dominant disorder characterized by multiple intestinal hamartomatous polyps (Supplemental eFig. 12.15) and mucocutaneous hyperpigmentation. About half the cases are associated with loss-of-function mutations affecting LKB1, a serine/threonine kinase that regulates cellular metabolism. Patients are prone to developing cancers of the GI tract and other tissues.
- *Hyperplastic polyps* are common epithelial proliferations, typically discovered in the sixth and seventh decades of life, often during routine colonoscopy. They are usually less than 5 mm in diameter and multiple but may be solitary. These polyps do not have malignant potential but must be distinguished from sessile serrated adenomas, which are precancerous lesions (described later).
- *Adenomatous polyps* are discussed in the following section.

Adenomas

Adenomas are benign colonic epithelial neoplasms that have the potential for malignant transformation.

Colorectal adenomas are present in almost 50% of adults over the age of 50 years living in Western countries. Although most do not become cancerous, the risk exists and is the reason for screening colonoscopy, which can be used to detect these tumors and remove them before they become malignant.

Morphology. Adenomas may be pedunculated (Fig. 12.10) or sessile. The histologic hallmark of adenomas is *epithelial dysplasia*, characterized by nuclear hyperchromasia, elongation, and stratification. The glandular architecture is used to classify adenomas into tubular, villous, or tubulovillous types, a distinction of no clinical significance by itself. However, size is an important risk factor for malignancy and is correlated with architecture: In general, tubular adenomas tend to be smaller than the other two types. Sessile serrated adenomas are a distinct type that lack epithelial dysplasia but have the same malignant potential as other adenomas; histologically, they are characterized by a serrated architecture that extends the full length of the glands, including the crypt base.

Clinical Features. Adenomas are typically asymptomatic, but occasionally bleed. They are usually removed by colonoscopy. The risk of cancer

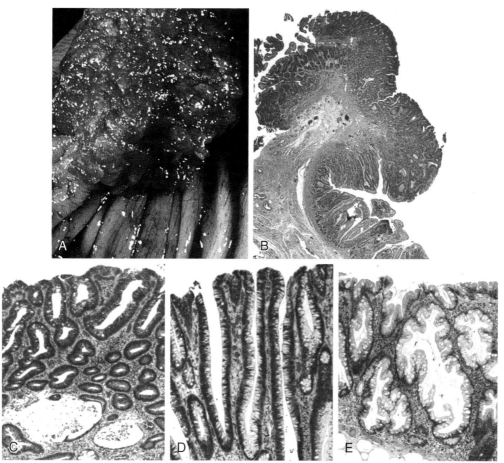

Fig. 12.10 Colonic adenoma. (A) Adenoma with a velvety surface. (B) Low-magnification photomicrograph of a pedunculated tubular adenoma. (C) Tubular adenoma with a smooth surface and rounded glands. In this case, crypt dilation and rupture, with associated reactive inflammation, can be seen at the bottom of the field. (D) Villous adenoma with long, slender projections that are reminiscent of small-intestinal villi. (E) Sessile serrated adenoma lined by goblet cells without typical cytologic features of dysplasia. This lesion is distinguished from a hyperplastic polyp by involvement of the crypts.

increases with increasing size of adenomas (>1 cm in diameter), an increasing number of lesions, and the presence of high-grade dysplasia.

Familial adenomatous polyposis is an autosomal dominant disorder in which more than 100 colorectal adenomas develop by the teenage years (Fig. 12.11). It is caused most often by mutations in the *APC* gene, discussed later in the context of colonic adenocarcinoma. All patients with this syndrome, if untreated, will develop colon cancer; therefore, the standard treatment is prophylactic colectomy. Some patients with polyposis do not have mutations in the *APC* gene but instead have mutations in genes involved in the repair of DNA mismatches (discussed next).

Adenocarcinoma

Adenocarcinoma of the colon accounts for almost 15% of all cancer-related deaths in the United States, and its study has provided important insights into the molecular mechanisms of carcinogenesis. Dietary factors, such as a low intake of unabsorbable vegetable fiber and a high intake of refined carbohydrates and fat, are associated with increased colorectal cancer rates. Several epidemiologic studies suggest that aspirin or other NSAIDs have a protective effect against recurrence of colon cancer and progression of adenomas to carcinoma. It is suspected that this effect is mediated by inhibition of the enzyme cyclooxygenase-2 (COX-2). This enzyme is highly expressed in 90% of colorectal carcinomas and 40% to 90% of adenomas and is known to promote epithelial proliferation, particularly in response to injury.

Pathogenesis. **The development of colonic adenocarcinoma occurs along three distinct pathways, one initiated by *APC* gene mutations and chromosomal instability, a second by mutations in mismatch repair genes, and a third by global genome hypermethylation, and all of these progress by stepwise accumulation of additional genetic abnormalities.**

- *The chromosomal instability pathway* is involved in 80% of colon cancers. Most of these tumors start with mutations in the *APC* gene (Fig. 12.12). Both copies of the gene have to be inactive; one may be absent in the germline and the other may be mutated or inactivated by epigenetic mechanisms in intestinal epithelial cells. The APC protein normally promotes degradation of the transcription factor β-catenin, a component of the Wnt signaling pathway. When APC function is lost, β-catenin accumulates, enters the nucleus, and activates transcription of several genes involved in cell survival and proliferation, including the oncogene *MYC*. Proliferating cells acquire additional mutations, the most common being in *KRAS*, which stimulates more cell growth. The development of full-blown cancer is usually associated with further mutations in tumor suppressor genes and copy number changes in many genes due to chromosomal instability.
- *The mismatch repair pathway.* Mismatch repair is the process that detects, excises, and repairs errors that may occur during DNA replication. Several proteins are involved in this process. The role of this

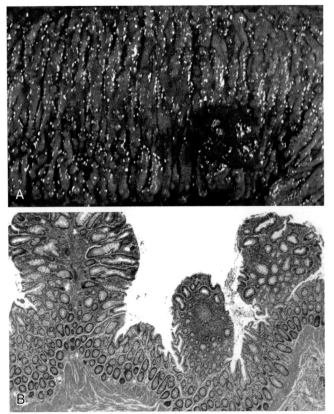

Fig. 12.11 Familial adenomatous polyposis. (A) Hundreds of small colonic polyps are present, along with a dominant polyp *(right)*. (B) Three tubular adenomas are present in this single microscopic field.

pathway was discovered when mutations in mismatch repair genes, most often genes called *MSH2* and *MLH1*, were discovered as the cause of the *hereditary nonpolyposis colorectal cancer syndrome*, also known as Lynch syndrome. Defects in the repair process result in high rates of mutation, mostly in regions containing short DNA repeats called *microsatellites*; therefore, the genetic abnormality is also called *microsatellite instability (MSI)*. Some of these microsatellite sequences lie within proto-oncogenes or tumor suppressor genes, and their mutation results in excessive, sustained growth (Fig. 12.13).

- *The hypermethylation, or CpG island methylator phenotype (CIMP), pathway* is characterized by downregulation of tumor suppressor genes due to DNA hypermethylation. These genes include *MLH1*, which results in a microsatellite-unstable (MSI+) tumor. CIMP pathway tumors without microsatellite instability (MSI–) are often associated with mutations in *BRAF*, a component of the RAS signaling pathway.

Morphology. Tumors in the proximal colon often grow as polypoid, exophytic masses that extend along one wall of the large-caliber cecum and ascending colon; these tumors rarely cause obstruction. By contrast, carcinomas in the distal colon tend to be annular lesions that cause constrictions and luminal narrowing, sometimes to the point of obstruction. The tumors consist of dysplastic epithelial cells, typically arrayed in glands that invade the submucosa and sometimes penetrate the wall of the colon (Fig. 12.14). The invasive tumor evokes a strong desmoplastic response, giving rise to a firm consistency. Some poorly differentiated tumors form few glands; others produce abundant mucin that accumulates within the intestinal wall, a feature associated with a poor prognosis. Tumors also may be composed of signet-ring cells similar to those in gastric cancer.

Clinical Features. Cecal and right-sided colon cancers are most often detected because of iron deficiency anemia caused by chronic bleeding

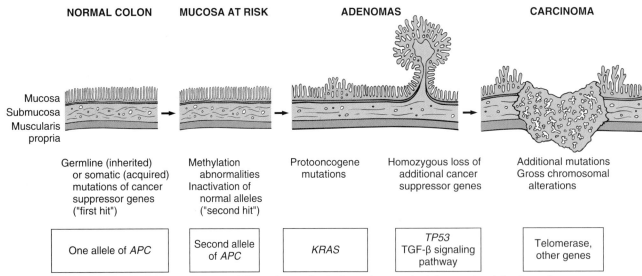

Fig. 12.12 The chromosomal instability pathway of colonic carcinogenesis. It is postulated that loss of one normal copy of the tumor suppressor gene *APC* occurs early. Individuals may be born with one mutant allele, making them extremely prone to the development of colon cancer, or inactivation of *APC* may occur later in life. This is the "first hit" according to Knudson's hypothesis (see Chapter 5). The loss of the intact copy of *APC* follows ("second hit") and sets the stage for adenoma formation. Other mutations involving *KRAS*, *SMAD2, and SMAD4* and the tumor suppressor gene *TP53* lead to the emergence of carcinoma, in which still more mutations occur. Although there may be a preferred temporal sequence for these changes, it is the aggregate effect of the mutations, rather than their order of occurrence, that appears most critical.

from the tumor; hence, iron deficiency anemia in older males and post-menopausal females must be assumed to be from an occult colon cancer until proven otherwise. Left-sided tumors cause narrowing of the lumen and thus produce changes in bowel habits and cramping. Metastases occur most commonly in regional lymph nodes and the liver. The main prognostic factors are the depth of local invasion and the presence of lymph node metastases.

Obstructive and Vascular Diseases

We conclude this section with a brief discussion of other conditions that affect the intestines.

Intestinal Obstruction

Mechanical obstruction occurs most often in the small intestine and is caused by diverse anatomic lesions (Fig. 12.15).

- *Adhesions* between loops of intestine may occur due to inflammation or scarring following abdominal surgery and are the most common cause of obstruction.
- *Tumors*

- *Herniation* of a segment of intestine through the umbilical or inguinal openings
- *Volvulus,* or twisting of the intestine, occurs most often in the sigmoid colon and cecum.
- *Intussusception* is telescoping of the bowel through a distal portion, sometimes caused by a tumor but usually without an identifiable cause.

The usual clinical presentation of acute small bowel obstruction is the sudden onset of vomiting, abdominal pain, and distention. The bowel is distended proximal to the block. If prolonged, the obstruction can compromise the blood supply to the intestinal wall.

Hirschsprung disease is a congenital disorder that causes intestinal obstruction from birth. It results from defective innervation of the colon due to the failure of migration of neural crest cells. Patients lack the ganglion cells of the Meissner and Auerbach enteric neural plexuses, so the distal colon has no peristaltic contractions, creating a functional block. In familial cases, the most common mutation is in the *RET* gene, which encodes a receptor tyrosine kinase. Hirschsprung disease always affects the rectum, but the length of the additional involved segments varies. The diagnosis is made by determining that ganglion cells are absent in a rectal biopsy.

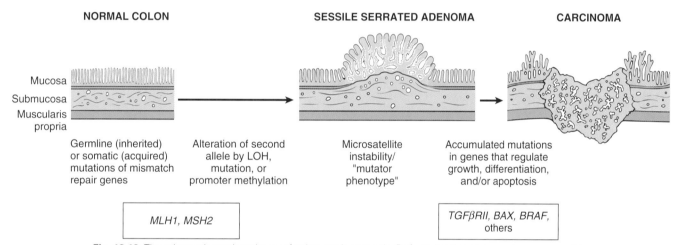

NORMAL COLON | SESSILE SERRATED ADENOMA | CARCINOMA

Mucosa
Submucosa
Muscularis propria

Germline (inherited) or somatic (acquired) mutations of mismatch repair genes

Alteration of second allele by LOH, mutation, or promoter methylation

Microsatellite instability/ "mutator phenotype"

Accumulated mutations in genes that regulate growth, differentiation, and/or apoptosis

MLH1, MSH2

TGFβRII, BAX, BRAF, others

Fig. 12.13 The mismatch repair pathway of colon carcinogenesis. Defects in mismatch repair genes result in microsatellite instability and permit accumulation of mutations in numerous genes. If these mutations affect genes involved in cell survival and proliferation, cancer may develop. LOH, Loss of heterozygosity.

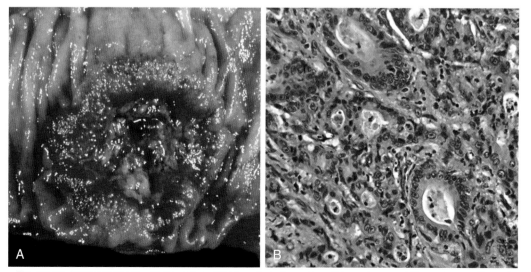

Fig. 12.14 Adenocarcinoma of the colon. (A) Ulcerated circumferential carcinoma of the rectum, with anal mucosa at the bottom. (B) Poorly differentiated adenocarcinoma forms a few glands but is largely composed of infiltrating nests of tumor cells. (Courtesy ExpertPath, copyright Elsevier.)

Herniation   **Adhesions**

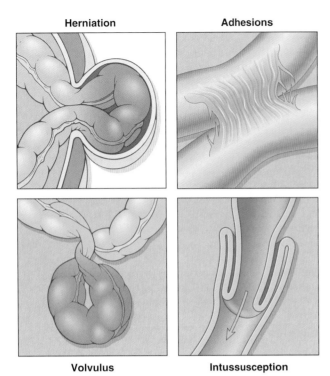

Volvulus   **Intussusception**

Fig. 12.15 Intestinal obstruction. The four major mechanical causes of intestinal obstruction are (1) herniation of a segment in the umbilical or inguinal regions, (2) adhesion between loops of intestine, (3) volvulus, and (4) intussusception.

Vascular Diseases

The most serious vascular disorder is *ischemic bowel disease*. Acute arterial obstruction, which may be caused by atherosclerosis, an aortic aneurysm, a thrombus, or an embolism, can lead to transmural infarction of segments of the bowel that are supplied by the obstructed vessels (Supplemental eFig. 12.16). Hypoperfusion secondary to cardiac failure, dehydration, or gradual arterial compromise typically causes sub-total mucosal or mural infarction; lesions frequently involve watershed zones that include the splenic flexure, where the superior and inferior mesenteric arterial circulations terminate, and, to a lesser extent, the sigmoid colon and rectum, where inferior mesenteric, pudendal, and iliac arterial circulations end. Patients typically present with abdominal pain. If not treated, the ischemic bowel can perforate, which is a surgical emergency.

DISORDERS OF THE ORAL CAVITY AND SALIVARY GLANDS

The oral cavity and salivary glands are frequent sites of inflammatory diseases and some tumors. The diseases are conceptually simple and are described only briefly.

Inflammatory Disorders of the Oral Cavity

A variety of infectious and noninfectious inflammatory disorders frequently involve the oral cavity. Among the most common are the following:

- *Aphthous ulcers* are painful superficial mucosal ulcerations (Supplemental eFig. 12.17) that affect as much as 40% of the population at some time, and tend to resolve spontaneously but recur. Their cause is not known.
- *Herpes simplex virus infection* presents with vesicles and ulcerations, commonly called *cold sores*. Most orofacial herpetic infections are

caused by herpes simplex virus type 1 (HSV-1), with the remainder being caused by HSV-2 (genital herpes). Primary infection occurs usually in childhood, and the virus establishes a latent infection that may persist for life. The infection may be reactivated by virtually any stress, including trauma, exposure to ultraviolet light and temperature extremes, pregnancy, other infections, and immune suppression. The lesions are similar to those in genital herpes (see Chapter 14).

- *Candida infection* occurs when this normal fungal inhabitant of the oral cavity grows excessively, which may occur in immunosuppressed individuals or when the normal microbiota are altered by antibiotic treatment. Some strains of *C. albicans* are more pathogenic than others. The most common type of infection is called *thrush*. Characteristically, a pseudomembrane consisting of fungal hyphae and inflammatory cells trapped within a protein-rich exudate covers the site of infection.
- *Pyogenic granuloma* is a vascular lesion of unknown etiology found on the gums of children, young adults, and pregnant women (Supplemental eFig. 12.18). The lesions consist of proliferating small blood vessels, similar to those in granulation tissue, which may create an alarming red appearance. The lesions may regress or become fibrotic.

Tumors and Tumor-like Lesions of the Oral Cavity

The most important proliferations involving the oral cavity are squamous cell carcinoma and its precursors.

- *Leukoplakia* is defined clinically as a white plaque in the oral cavity with no underlying cause (such as an infection) (Supplemental eFig. 12.19). Microscopically, it is an area of squamous cell hyperplasia. Lesions with dysplastic features may progress to squamous cell carcinoma. Surgical excision is therefore the accepted treatment. A related but less common entity, *erythroplakia,* is a red, velvety, sometimes eroded lesion that is flat or slightly depressed relative to the surrounding mucosa (Supplemental eFig. 12.20). Erythroplakia is associated with a greater risk for malignant transformation than leukoplakia.
- *Squamous cell carcinoma* is the most common malignant tumor of the oropharynx. Two mechanisms are implicated in tumor development: exposure to carcinogens (most commonly in tobacco) and infection with high-risk types of human papillomavirus (HPV) (up to 70% of cases, particularly those of the tonsils, base of tongue, and pharynx). The tumors associated with chemical carcinogens frequently harbor mutations in tumor suppressor genes such as *TP53* and oncogenes such as *RAS*. The prognosis of HPV-associated tumors is better than those that are not associated with HPV. The mechanisms by which HPV causes cancer are discussed in Chapter 5.

This tumor may appear as raised plaques or mucosal thickenings, and may ulcerate as it grows (Fig. 12.16). Histologically, it varies from well-differentiated and keratinizing to poorly differentiated and anaplastic. The most frequent sites of metastases are cervical lymph nodes.

Diseases of the Salivary Glands

The salivary glands are prone to a number of inflammatory and neoplastic disorders.

- *Sialadenitis* (inflammation of the salivary glands) may be caused by bacterial or viral infections (e.g., mumps), autoimmune diseases (e.g., Sjögren syndrome), obstruction by ductal stones, or physical agents (e.g., radiotherapy). A common manifestation of salivary gland damage is *xerostomia,* or dry mouth, caused by a reduced production of saliva. The most common inflammatory lesion of the salivary glands is *mucocele,* a cyst usually in the lower lip that is caused by blockage or rupture of a salivary duct with leakage of saliva into the connective tissue. The cyst is filled with fluid and inflammatory cells and lined by granulation or fibrous tissue.

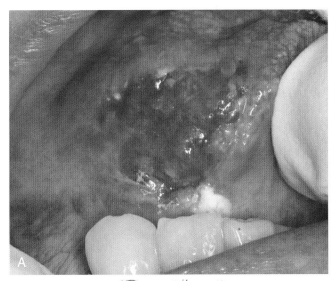

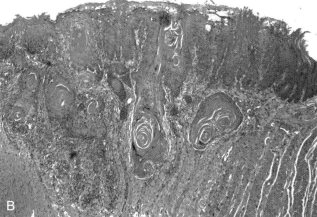

Fig. 12.16 Oral squamous cell carcinoma. (A) Gross appearance demonstrating ulceration and induration of the oral mucosa. (B) Histologic appearance demonstrating numerous nests and islands of malignant keratinocytes invading the underlying connective tissue stroma.

- *Tumors* of the salivary glands are relatively uncommon, representing less than 2% of all human tumors. Approximately 65% to 80% arise within the parotid, 10% in the submandibular gland, and the remainder in the minor salivary glands, including the sublingual glands. Only a minority (15% to 30%) of tumors in the parotid glands are malignant, whereas approximately 40% of submandibular, 50% of minor salivary gland, and 70% to 90% of sublingual tumors are cancerous. Thus, the likelihood that a salivary gland tumor is malignant is inversely proportional, roughly, to the size of the gland. The most common tumors are the following:
  - *Pleomorphic adenoma* is a benign tumor composed of a mixture of ductal epithelial and myoepithelial cells dispersed within loose myxoid or chondroid stroma (Supplemental eFig. 12.21). Because they have both epithelial and mesenchymal components, they are often called mixed tumors. However, all elements are clonal progeny of a common progenitor cell. The vast majority arise in the parotid gland. They frequently recur after excision and may undergo malignant transformation with time. The transformed tumors are among the most aggressive malignant salivary gland neoplasms, with mortality rates of 30% to 50% at 5 years.
  - *Warthin tumor* is a benign neoplasm that is the second most common salivary gland tumor. It arises almost exclusively in the parotid gland. It occurs more commonly in males than in females and there is an eight-fold increased risk in smokers compared with nonsmokers. The tumors are encapsulated and are composed of cystic spaces lined by a double layer of neoplastic epithelial cells resting on a dense lymphoid stroma sometimes bearing germinal centers (Supplemental eFig. 12.22).
  - *Mucoepidermoid carcinoma* is the most common malignant tumor of the salivary glands. It is composed of a mixture of squamous, mucous-secreting, and intermediate cells (Supplemental eFig. 12.23). The latter is a hybrid cell type with both squamous features and mucous-filled vacuoles, which are most easily detected with mucin stains. The tumors lack well-defined capsules and may be locally infiltrative. The prognosis depends on the grade: Low-grade tumors have a 5-year survival rate of more than 90%, whereas high-grade tumors have a 5-year survival rate of only 50%.

13

Liver, Biliary System, and Pancreas

OUTLINE

Disorders of the Liver, 222
    Clinical Consequences of Liver Disease, 222
    Viral Hepatitis, 223
    Other Infections of the Liver, 228
    Alcoholic Liver Disease, 228
    Nonalcoholic Fatty Liver Disease, 228
    Other Forms of Hepatitis, 229
    Inherited Diseases of the Liver, 230
    Circulatory Disorders of the Liver, 231

Nodules and Tumors of the Liver, 231
Disorders of the Biliary System, 233
    Cholangitis, 234
    Congenital Disorders Causing Jaundice, 235
    Cholelithiasis and Cholecystitis, 235
    Tumors of the Biliary System, 236
Disorders of the Pancreas, 236
    Pancreatitis, 236
    Tumors of the Pancreas, 237

This chapter focuses on the liver. Also discussed briefly are the biliary system and gallbladder, which are intimately linked to the liver anatomically and functionally, and the exocrine pancreas (composed of secretory glands) because the pancreas drains with the bile duct into the small intestine and is thus often included in the larger "pancreaticobiliary" system. The endocrine pancreas is discussed in Chapter 16.

DISORDERS OF THE LIVER

The liver is strategically located between the gastrointestinal (GI) tract and the systemic circulation, allowing it to process materials absorbed in the intestines before they are disseminated throughout the body. It has numerous critical functions, including the following.

- *Secretion of bile,* which contains chemicals that are required to digest fat and absorb certain factors, such as water-insoluble vitamins, in the intestines.
- *Metabolism* of sugar, fatty acids, and amino acids absorbed from the intestine via the portal vein and conversion of these nutrients into forms that are stored, used to produce energy, or used to synthesize proteins and other substances.
- *Detoxification* of the blood, removing potentially harmful compounds such as alcohol, drugs, and both exogenous and endogenous (such as ammonia) toxins.
- *Storage* of carbohydrates, lipids, and proteins, as well as vitamins and minerals.
- *Synthesis and secretion of many essential proteins,* including albumin, certain coagulation factors, growth factors, soluble transporters, and factors that regulate iron metabolism.

The cells of the liver, called *hepatocytes,* have tremendous regenerative capacity such that isolated injuries can usually be repaired. In addition, the liver has a significant functional reserve, so pathophysiologic and clinical derangements become apparent only after a large fraction of the liver is damaged. Other cells that play diverse roles in normal hepatic physiology and diseases include Kupffer cells (the resident phagocytes of the liver), endothelial cells that line vascular sinusoids, perisinusoidal cells that store vitamin A, and epithelial cells that line bile ducts.

Clinical Consequences of Liver Disease

The manifestations of liver disease depend on the nature, severity, and acuity of the insult.

- *Acute liver failure* is defined as liver disease that produces encephalopathy within 6 months of the initial diagnosis; if encephalopathy develops more rapidly, within 2 weeks, it is called *fulminant liver failure.* The most frequent morphologic correlate of acute liver failure is massive *hepatic necrosis,* usually accompanied by liver shrinkage due to loss of parenchyma (Supplemental eFig. 13.1). In the United States, acetaminophen overdose accounts for almost 50% of cases of acute liver failure; autoimmune hepatitis, other drugs and toxins, and acute hepatitis A and B infections account for most of the rest.

    Clinical manifestations of acute liver failure include the following.
- *Hepatic encephalopathy,* with symptoms ranging from subtle behavioral abnormalities, to confusion and stupor, to coma and death. The liver normally detoxifies ammonia, which is produced from breakdown of amino acids, from two sources: most of it comes from gut bacteria and is converted into glutamine and does not enter the systemic circulation, and some of it is produced by breakdown of amino acids and converted into urea, a relatively nontoxic substance that is readily excreted in urine. In liver failure, detoxification is impaired because of loss of hepatocyte function, and ammonia from the gut enters the systemic circulation through porta-systemic shunts. The accumulated ammonia enters the CNS, where it impairs neuronal function, and causes cerebral edema. Typical among the neurologic signs is *asterixis,* a nonrhythmic, rapid, extension-flexion movement of the head and extremities, best seen as "flapping" of the hands when the arms are held in extension with dorsiflexed wrists.
- *Jaundice* and *icterus* (yellow discoloration of the skin and sclera, respectively) are due to the retention of bilirubin. They stem from a failure to eliminate bilirubin and other solutes in the bile, which build up in the blood. Accumulation of bile in the liver is called *cholestasis.*
- *Coagulopathy* is secondary to the reduced synthesis of coagulation factors and results in bleeding, which may manifest as easy bruising or hemorrhage. Ironically, this bleeding tendency may be

Table 13.1 Laboratory Evaluation of Liver Disease

Test Category	Blood Measurement[a]
Hepatocyte structural integrity	Cytosolic hepatocellular enzymes[b] *Serum aspartate aminotransferase (AST)* *Serum alanine aminotransferase (ALT)* Serum lactate dehydrogenase (LDH)

Biliary excretory function	Substances normally secreted in bile[b]
	Serum bilirubin
	   Total: unconjugated plus conjugated
	   Direct: conjugated only
	Urine bilirubin
	Serum bile acids
	Plasma membrane enzymes (from damage to bile canaliculus)[b]
	Serum alkaline phosphatase
	Serum γ-glutamyl transpeptidase (GGT)

Hepatocyte function	Proteins secreted into the blood *Serum albumin*[c] *Prothrombin time (PT)*[b] *Partial thromboplastin time (PTT)*[b] Hepatocyte metabolism Serum ammonia[b] Aminopyrine breath test (hepatic demethylation)[c]

[a]The most commonly used tests are in italics.
[b]An elevation suggests liver disease.
[c]A decrease suggests liver disease.

exacerbated by the development of disseminated intravascular coagulation, uncontrolled clotting caused by the failure of the damaged liver to remove activated coagulation factors from the circulation.

- *Hepatorenal syndrome* is defined as kidney failure in the setting of acute or chronic liver disease in the absence of primary renal disease. Its mechanism is not well defined.

- *Chronic liver failure* is the result of prolonged liver injury, most often caused by alcoholic hepatitis, nonalcoholic fatty liver disease, and chronic viral hepatitis B and C. *Cirrhosis* is the morphologic change most often associated with chronic liver disease; it is marked by diffuse distortion of the liver architecture resulting from replacement by regenerative parenchymal nodules surrounded by fibrous bands. The fibrosis obstructs blood flow through the liver and results in impaired drainage of the portal vein, causing *portal hypertension.* This may lead to congestive splenomegaly (due to back pressure in the splenic vein), ascites (transudate in the peritoneal cavity), and esophageal varices (dilated veins prone to rupture and bleeding). An impaired ability to catabolize estrogens may cause symptoms of estrogen excess such as hypogonadism and gynecomastia in males and spider angiomata in both sexes. Most of the clinical manifestations of acute liver failure may also be seen in chronic liver failure.

Laboratory evaluation plays an important role in the diagnosis of liver disease (Table 13.1).

Viral Hepatitis

There are five types of hepatitis viruses, all of which cause destructive inflammation of the liver but differ in disease course and outcome.

The five viruses are named hepatitis A, B, C, D, and E and belong to different families. They all cause injury of the liver with inflammation, but some produce self-limited infection and others produce chronic infections (Table 13.2). Acute infection by each of the hepatotropic viruses may be symptomatic or asymptomatic. Hepatitis A virus (HAV) and hepatitis E virus (HEV) do not cause chronic

hepatitis, and only 5%–10% of adults who become infected with hepatitis B virus (HBV) develop chronic hepatitis. By contrast, hepatitis C virus (HCV) is notorious for producing chronic hepatitis, a risk factor for hepatocellular carcinoma. Fulminant hepatitis is unusual and is seen primarily with HAV, HBV, or hepatitis D virus (HDV) infections. Although HCV and HBV are responsible for most cases of chronic hepatitis, there are many other nonviral causes, including autoimmune hepatitis and drug- and toxin-induced hepatitis (discussed later).

Pathogenesis. **Hepatic injury in acute viral hepatitis is caused mostly by the host immune response.**

Hepatitis viruses are not strongly cytopathic, that is, they do not directly injure or kill infected cells. Rather, the presence of the virus is detected by the host's immune system, and natural killer cells and viral antigen-specific CD8+ cytotoxic T lymphocytes kill infected hepatocytes in an attempt to clear the infection. Chronic liver injury may result from persistent acute injury and the process of repair that follows. However, chronic hepatitis frequently develops without evidence of prior acute infection.

Hepatitis A Virus

Hepatitis A is an acute, self-limited infection.

Hepatitis A virus (HAV) usually causes a benign, self-limited infection, but in rare instances (in ~0.1% of cases) it produces fulminant hepatitis. The virus is acquired through contaminated food and water, and is endemic in many lower-income countries. Sporadic infections in higher-income countries may occur by eating shellfish from water contaminated with human sewage. HAV has an incubation period of 3 to 6 weeks and is shed in the stool for 2 to 3 weeks before and 1 week after the onset of jaundice. Viremia is transient; therefore, blood-borne transmission is rare. IgM anti-HAV antibody is detectable in the serum by the time symptoms appear and is a reliable marker of acute infection. It is gradually replaced by IgG anti-HAV antibody over several months. The clinical manifestations of acute infection are fever, jaundice, hepatomegaly, and abdominal pain. Because the immune response efficiently clears the virus and IgG antibody is produced for years, providing lifelong protection, patients recover in a few months and cannot be reinfected.

Hepatitis B Virus

Hepatitis B may cause a wide range of diseases, from self-limited acute hepatitis to fulminant hepatic necrosis to chronic infection with cirrhosis.

Hepatitis B virus (HBV) is acquired perinatally during childbirth in endemic countries, mostly in Asia, but elsewhere, it is acquired primarily though intravenous drug use (with contaminated needles) and by sexual transmission. The disease course is extremely variable (Fig. 13.1). HBV has a prolonged incubation period (2 to 26 weeks). Unlike HAV, HBV remains in the blood during active episodes of acute and chronic hepatitis. Approximately 70% of adults with newly acquired HBV have mild or no symptoms and do not develop jaundice. The remaining 30% have nonspecific constitutional symptoms. In most cases, the infection is self-limited and resolves without treatment; chronic disease develops in up to 10% of patients. The host immune response determines the outcome: Innate immune mechanisms protect the host during the initial infection, and a strong response by virus-specific CD4+ and CD8+ interferon γ–producing cells correlates with resolution of acute infection. It is unclear why chronic hepatitis develops in a minority of patients. In general, the younger an individual's age at the time of HBV

Table 13.2 The Hepatitis Viruses

Virus	Hepatitis A (HAV)	Hepatitis B (HBV)	Hepatitis C (HCV)	Hepatitis D (HDV)	Hepatitis E (HEV)
Viral genome	ssRNA	Partially dsDNA	ssRNA	Circular defective ssRNA	ssRNA
Viral family	Hepatovirus; related to picornavirus	Hepadnavirus	*Flaviviridae*	Subviral particle in Deltaviridae family	Calicivirus
Route of transmission	Fecal-oral (contaminated food or water)	Parenteral, sexual contact, perinatal	Parenteral; intranasal cocaine use is a risk factor	Parenteral	Fecal-oral
Incubation period	2-6 weeks	2-26 weeks (mean 8 weeks)	4-26 weeks (mean 9 weeks)	Same as HBV	4-5 weeks
Frequency of chronic liver disease	Never	5% to 10%	>80%	10% (coinfection); 90% to 100% for superinfection	In immunocompromised hosts only
Diagnosis	Detection of serum IgM antibodies	Detection of HBsAg or antibody to HBcAg; PCR for HBV DNA	ELISA for antibody detection; PCR for HCV RNA	Detection of IgM and IgG antibodies, HDV RNA in serum, or HDAg in liver biopsy	Detection of serum IgM and IgG antibodies; PCR for HEV RNA

dsDNA, Double-stranded DNA; HBcAg, hepatitis B core antigen; HBsAg, hepatitis B surface antigen; HDAg, hepatitis D antigen; ELISA, enzyme-linked immunosorbent assay; ssRNA, single-stranded RNA.
From Washington K: Inflammatory and infectious diseases of the liver. In Iacobuzio-Donahue CA, Montgomery EA, editors: *Gastrointestinal and liver pathology*, Philadelphia, 2005, Churchill Livingstone.

infection, the higher the risk of chronic infection. The risk for hepatocellular carcinoma is increased in chronic hepatitis, likely as a consequence of oncogenic mutations acquired during the prolonged period of inflammation and regeneration of surviving hepatocytes.

The HBV genome encodes several proteins that have pathogenic and clinical significance:

- *Nucleocapsid core protein* (HBcAg, hepatitis B core antigen) and a longer polypeptide with a precore and core region, designated HBeAg (hepatitis Be antigen)
- *Envelope glycoproteins* (HBsAg, hepatitis B surface antigen)
- A *polymerase (Pol)* with both DNA polymerase activity and reverse transcriptase activity
- *HBx protein,* which is required for virus replication and has been implicated in the pathogenesis of HBV-associated liver cancer

The course of the disease is followed clinically by monitoring certain serum markers (Fig. 13.2). Small amounts of HBV DNA can be detected using new PCR-based tests. HBsAg appears before the onset of symptoms and peaks during symptomatic disease. In resolving infections, HBsAg typically declines to undetectable levels by 12 weeks post-infection. Anti-HBs antibody is detected soon after HBsAg disappears from the blood and persists for life, providing protection against reinfection. IgM specific for HBc becomes detectable shortly before the onset of symptoms, concurrent with the elevation of serum aminotransferases (indicative of hepatocyte injury). Over the next few months, IgM anti-HBc is replaced by IgG anti-HBc antibody. In chronic infection, HBsAg persists in the serum for more than 6 months, together with HBV DNA and IgG anti-HBc antibody. Thus, the presence of HBsAg and IgM anti-HBc is diagnostic of acute infection, whereas the

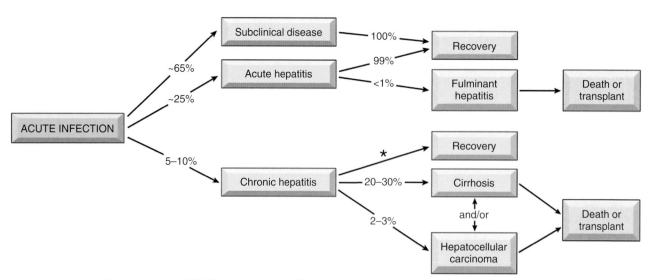

Fig. 13.1 Outcomes of HBV infection in adults. The potential outcomes with their approximate frequencies in the United States are shown. *Spontaneous HBsAg clearance occurs during chronic HBV infection at an estimated annual rate of 1% to 2% in Western countries.

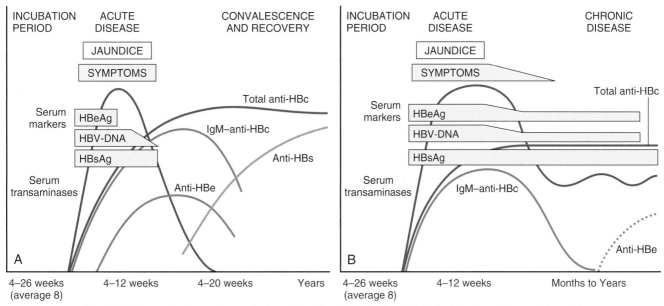

Fig. 13.2 Temporal changes in serologic markers for HBV infection. (A) Acute infection with resolution. (B) Progression to chronic infection. Note in some cases of chronic HBV infection, serum transaminases may become normal.

presence of HBsAg, HBV DNA, and IgG anti-HBc indicates chronic infection.

HBV vaccination is strongly protective, and adoption of the vaccine worldwide promises to greatly reduce or even abolish hepatitis B.

Hepatitis C Virus

Untreated hepatitis C typically causes chronic infection resulting in cirrhosis, liver failure, and a high risk of hepatocellular carcinoma.

Hepatitis C virus (HCV), like HBV, causes infection in children mainly following perinatal transmission, and in adults mainly through intravenous drug use and sexual transmission. Working in the medical or dental field is another risk factor: The risk for acquiring HCV by needle stick is about six times higher than that for HIV (1.8% vs. 0.3%).

The acute infection is asymptomatic in about 85% of patients; in symptomatic patients, anti-HCV antibodies are detected in only 50% to 70% of patients. In contrast to HBV, chronic disease occurs in the majority of HCV-infected individuals (50% to 80%), and cirrhosis eventually occurs in as many as one third of these individuals (Fig. 13.3). Patients with cirrhosis can develop the usual complications such as rupture of esophageal varices and hepatocellular carcinoma. Others with compensated cirrhosis may remain asymptomatic for years. The best predictor of progression to cirrhosis is the amount of chronic inflammation and fibrosis seen in liver biopsy (described later). Hepatocellular carcinoma is a late complication, seen not only with chronic HCV infection but also in other disorders associated with chronic inflammation, fibrosis, and long-standing hepatocellular damage and regeneration (e.g., chronic hepatitis from any cause and hemochromatosis).

Serologic assays are used to diagnose and follow HCV infection. HCV RNA is detectable for 1 to 3 weeks after infection, coincident with increases in serum aminotransferases. Anti-HCV antibodies are detected at this time or later in the disease but do not clear the virus. In chronic HCV infection, circulating HCV RNA persists in 90% of patients despite the presence of neutralizing antibodies and serves as a diagnostic marker of chronic infection. Episodic elevations in serum aminotransferases separated by periods of normal or near-normal enzyme levels can be seen.

The advent of new antiviral drugs promises to reduce the incidence of chronic HCV hepatitis. These drugs inhibit several viral proteins and RNA polymerase and, when used in combination, effectively suppress viral replication, leading to eradication of the infection. Currently, over 95% of HCV infections are curable, and this can be expected to improve further as new antiviral drugs become available. The major downside of this therapy is the very high cost.

Hepatitis D Virus

Also called the *delta agent,* hepatitis D virus (HDV) is a unique RNA virus that is dependent for its life cycle on coinfection with HBV because HBsAg is necessary for the production of complete HDV virions. Due to this dependency, HDV infection is prevented by vaccination against HBV. Coinfection with HDV occurs in two different ways:

- *Simultaneous coinfection by HDV and HBV.* This is associated with high rates of severe acute hepatitis and fulminant liver failure, particularly in intravenous drug users, and high rates of progression to chronic infection, often complicated by hepatocellular carcinoma.
- *Superinfection of a chronic HBV carrier by HDV.* Superinfection presents 30 to 50 days later as severe acute hepatitis in a previously unrecognized HBV carrier or as an exacerbation of preexisting chronic hepatitis B. It results in chronic HDV infection in 80% to 90% of cases. Superinfection may have two phases: an acute phase with active HDV replication and suppression of HBV with high serum transaminase levels, followed by a chronic phase in which HDV replication decreases, HBV replication increases, serum transaminase levels fluctuate, and the disease progresses to cirrhosis and hepatocellular cancer.

Hepatitis E Virus

Hepatitis E virus (HEV) is thought to be a common, underdiagnosed cause of acute hepatitis. It is prevalent in India, Asia, sub-Saharan Africa, and Mexico, where epidemics have been reported, but it is responsible for sporadic cases in Western countries. HEV is a zoonotic disease, with animal reservoirs that include monkeys, cats, pigs, and dogs. The virus is acquired through contaminated food and water and typically infects young to middle-aged adults. Similar to hepatitis A, the infection may be asymptomatic, cause self-limited acute hepatitis,

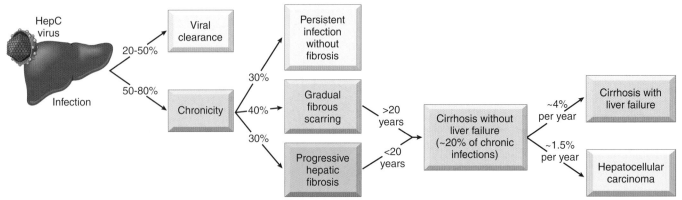

Fig. 13.3 Natural history of HCV infection. The possible outcomes of HCV infection and their approximate frequencies are shown.

or progress to fulminant hepatitis in a minority of cases. In most cases, HEV is not associated with chronic liver disease or persistent viremia. For unclear reasons, severe disease with a mortality rate of almost 20% is common in pregnant women.

Morphology of Infectious Hepatitis. The general morphologic features of acute and chronic viral hepatitis are depicted schematically in Fig. 13.4. The morphologic changes in acute and chronic viral hepatitis are shared among the hepatotropic viruses and can be mimicked by drug reactions or autoimmune hepatitis.

- **Acute viral hepatitis.** Hepatocytes may undergo necrosis or apoptosis. In the former, the cytoplasm appears empty, with scattered wisps of cytoplasmic remnants. Mononuclear cells predominate in all phases of viral hepatitis. In severe acute hepatitis, confluent hepatocyte necrosis surrounds central veins. With increasing severity, there is central-portal bridging necrosis, followed by parenchymal collapse. In acute HBV disease, there may be extensive hepatocyte destruction, often with little portal inflammation (Fig. 13.5). Bile stasis may be prominent. If the injury begins to resolve,

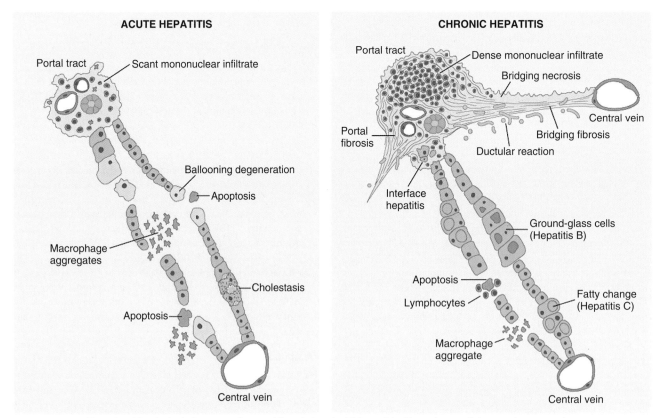

Fig. 13.4 Morphologic features of acute (A) and chronic (B) hepatitis. There is very little portal mononuclear infiltration in acute hepatitis (or sometimes none at all), but in chronic hepatitis, portal infiltrates are dense and prominent; in fact, they are the defining feature of chronic hepatitis. Bridging necrosis and fibrosis are shown only for chronic hepatitis, but bridging necrosis may also occur in more severe acute hepatitis. Ductular reactions in chronic hepatitis are minimal in early stages of scarring, but become extensive in late-stage disease.

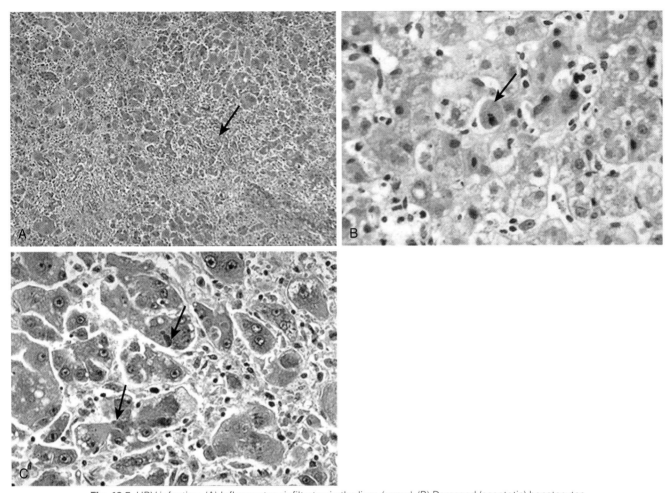

Fig. 13.5 HBV infection. (A) Inflammatory infiltrates in the liver *(arrow)*. (B) Damaged (apoptotic) hepatocytes *(arrow)*. (C) Intracanalicular bile stasis *(arrows)*. (Courtesy Drs. Ryan Gill and Sanjay Kakar, Department of Pathology, University of California San Francisco.)

there are regenerating hepatocytes with large nuclei and prominent nucleoli, often with mitoses. Apoptotic hepatocytes may stain deeply eosinophilic, forming so-called Councilman bodies.

- **Chronic viral hepatitis.** The defining histologic feature of chronic viral hepatitis is variable mononuclear cell infiltration around portal tracts (Fig. 13.6). Progression is marked by scarring, beginning with portal fibrosis and followed by extension of fibrous septa between portal tracts. Continued scarring and nodule formation lead to the development of cirrhosis (Supplemental eFig. 13.2). Certain histologic features suggest the viral etiology: In chronic hepatitis B, "ground-glass" hepatocytes (cells with endoplasmic reticulum swollen by HBsAg) are seen (Supplemental eFig 13.3), whereas chronic hepatitis C is characterized by large lymphoid aggregates and bile duct injury. Fatty change may also be seen.

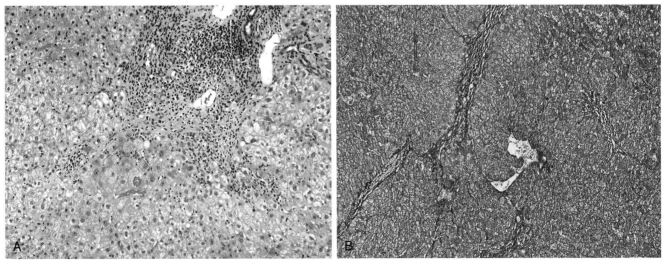

Fig. 13.6 Chronic HCV infection. Chronic hepatitis due to HCV, showing characteristic portal tract expansion by a dense lymphoid infiltrate (A) and bridging fibrosis (stained blue) connecting portal tracts (B).

Other Infections of the Liver

Infectious pathogens may reach the liver from the intestines via the portal vein; from distant sites via the hepatic artery (hematogenous spread); or from adjacent tissue, such as an infected gallbladder. Pyogenic bacteria typically cause mild inflammation with cholestasis, but in rare cases may lead to abscess formation. Several parasitic infections of the liver are major causes of morbidity and mortality in certain parts of the world:

- *Schistosomiasis,* most commonly found in Asia, Africa, and South America, is characterized by a granulomatous reaction associated with marked fibrosis that leads to noncirrhotic portal hypertension.
- *Entamoeba histolytica,* an important cause of dysentery, particularly in Africa, Mexico, parts of South America, and India, can ascend to the liver and produce large areas of necrosis (amebic liver abscesses).
- *Liver fluke infection (Fasciola hepatica, Opisthorchis* species, and *Clonorchis sinensis)* is most common in Southeast Asia and is associated with a high rate of cholangiocarcinoma.
- *Echinococcal infections* are most common in Asia, Australia, and parts of South America and Africa and may produce intrahepatic hydatid cysts.

Alcoholic Liver Disease

Prolonged alcohol ingestion causes fat deposition in the liver, which may progress to chronic inflammation and cirrhosis.

Alcoholic liver disease is a major health problem. The disease progresses in stages, starting with the deposition of fat in hepatocytes *(fatty liver,* or *steatosis),* seen in the majority of drinkers; progressing to inflammation *(steatohepatitis)* in about a third; and culminating in *cirrhosis* in 10% to 20%. These may develop sequentially or independently and do not represent a continuum.

Pathogenesis. Alcoholic liver disease manifests as various patterns of injury, but the mechanisms underlying progression from fatty liver to hepatitis and cirrhosis are not well defined.

- *Fatty liver.* Alcohol causes fat deposition by inhibiting the oxidation of hepatic fatty acids, shunting metabolic pathways away from catabolism toward lipid biosynthesis (lipogenesis), and inhibiting the formation of lipoproteins, which bind lipids and transport them out of the liver.
- *Steatohepatitis.* Influx of neutrophils, the hallmark of early alcoholic steatohepatitis, occurs due to an increased production of cytokines and chemokines from Kupffer cells or hepatocytes. Reactive oxygen species (ROS) generated in hepatocytes during oxidation of alcohol damage the cells and induce inflammation. The gut microbiome may contribute, if luminal bacteria gain access to tissues through damaged intestinal epithelium and produce substances that trigger inflammation. Acetaldehyde, a major metabolite of ethanol, causes lipid peroxidation of cell membranes.
- *Cirrhosis.* Sustained and progressive cell death gives rise to fibrosis, which is driven by cytokines and growth factors produced by Kupffer cells and other cells.
- *Hepatocellular carcinoma.* As in chronic liver diseases from other causes, there is an increased incidence of hepatocellular carcinoma.

Morphology. Fatty livers are enlarged, soft, yellow, and greasy to touch. Fat deposition begins in centrilobular hepatocytes as small (microvesicular) lipid droplets that coalesce to form large (macrovesicular) droplets that replace the cytoplasm and displace the nucleus (Fig. 13.7A). Lipid accumulation may spread to involve the entire lobule. *Steatohepatitis* is characterized by focal hepatocyte necrosis, eosinophilic cytoplasmic inclusions of tangled intermediate filaments *(Mallory bodies)* in the injured cells, and inflammatory infiltrates, predominantly neutrophils, which are most prominent around the degenerating hepatocytes (Fig. 13.7B). Fibrosis appears first in the centrilobular region and spreads outward, encircling clusters of surviving and regenerating hepatocytes and linking portal

triads. These areas of fibrosis become nodular, and their continuing division by more scarring leads to the classic morphologic appearance of *micronodular cirrhosis* (Fig. 13.7C).

Clinical Features. Alcoholic fatty liver is usually asymptomatic, but may give rise to hepatomegaly and mild elevations of serum bilirubin and the liver enzymes alkaline phosphatase and gamma-glutamyl transpeptidase (GGT) (reflecting intrahepatic cholestasis). The onset of alcoholic hepatitis is typically acute and follows a bout of heavy drinking. Patients present with fever, anorexia, and hepatomegaly, and laboratory tests reveal increased serum alkaline phosphatase and neutrophilic leukocytosis. Injury to hepatocytes causes elevation of serum transaminases, although to a lesser degree than seen in viral hepatitis (usually <500 U/mL). The serum aspartate aminotransferase (AST) level is usually higher than the serum alanine aminotransferase (ALT) level in a ratio of 2:1 or more. Acute alcoholic hepatitis is fatal in 10% to 20% of cases. Ten percent to 15% of patients develop cirrhosis, which presents with portal hypertension and its manifestations (e.g., splenomegaly, esophageal varices, and effects of elevated estrogens) and may progress to hepatic failure. In patients with alcoholic cirrhosis, about 1% of patients develop hepatocellular carcinoma annually.

Nonalcoholic Fatty Liver Disease

Nonalcoholic fatty liver disease (NAFLD) is associated with type 2 diabetes and obesity and is characterized by fatty liver, which may progress to hepatitis (nonalcoholic steatohepatitis, NASH) and cirrhosis.

The morphology resembles that seen in alcoholic liver disease but occurs in patients who consume little or no alcohol. NAFLD is closely linked to the metabolic syndrome, characterized by obesity, abnormal lipid profiles (increased triglycerides and low-density lipoproteins), and insulin resistance causing type 2 diabetes (Chapter 19). It is becoming an increasingly common cause of chronic liver disease worldwide in parallel with the alarming obesity epidemic.

Pathogenesis. The pathogenesis of NAFLD is not established, but several contributory factors have been proposed.

- *Obesity* leads to increased free fatty acids, which are mobilized from adipose tissue, taken up by the liver, and deposited in hepatocytes. The accumulation may be increased by diminished export of triglycerides out of the liver.
- *Insulin resistance* seems to play a key role in the progression of the disease, perhaps by altering lipid metabolism to favor accumulation of free fatty acids in hepatocytes.
- *Inflammation.* Free fatty acids activate the inflammasome, a cytosolic sensor of abnormal substances and products of damaged cells. This leads to the secretion of the cytokine interleukin-1, which induces inflammation (see Chapter 2).
- Free fatty acids may also increase the *generation of ROS* or disrupt mitochondrial function, injuring hepatocytes.
- *Other factors* that have been proposed include increased hepatic iron, hormones secreted by adipose tissue cells, and intestinal microbes.

Morphology. The disease progresses from fatty liver to inflammation (NASH) to cirrhosis (Fig. 13.8). The morphologic features are similar to those of alcoholic liver disease.

Clinical Features. Most patients are asymptomatic and NAFLD is discovered incidentally due to elevation of serum transaminases. Only a minority progresses to NASH and cirrhosis. Some patients with NASH may present with signs of early hepatitis; cirrhosis usually manifests with

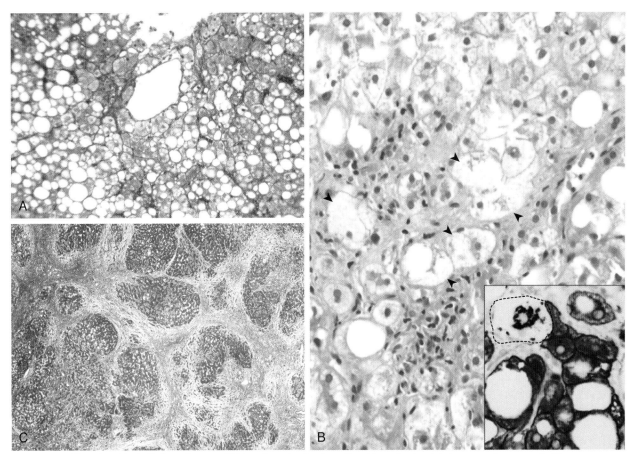

Fig. 13.7 Alcoholic liver disease. (A) Fatty liver. A mix of small and large fat droplets (seen as clear vacuoles) is most prominent around the central vein and extends outward to the portal tracts. Some fibrosis *(blue)* is present in a characteristic perisinusoidal "chicken wire fence" pattern. (B) "Ballooned" hepatocytes *(arrowheads)* associated with clusters of inflammatory cells. The *inset* stained for keratins 8 and 18 *(brown)* shows a ballooned cell *(dotted line)* in which keratins have been ubiquitinlated and have collapsed into an immunoreactive "Mallory-Denk" body, leaving the cytoplasm "empty." (C) Cirrhosis with nodules of regenerating hepatocytes *(red)* separated by bands of fibrosis *(blue)*. (C, Courtesy Dr. Elizabeth Brunt, Washington University, St. Louis.)

signs of chronic liver disease. NAFLD increases the risk of hepatocellular carcinoma, which may arise in the absence of significant scarring.

Other Forms of Hepatitis

Two other forms of hepatic injury and inflammation are sufficiently common to merit discussion, autoimmune hepatitis and drug- and toxin-induced hepatitis.

Autoimmune Hepatitis

Autoimmune hepatitis is a chronic autoimmune disease of the liver associated with the presence of multiple autoantibodies and often with other autoimmune diseases.

Pathogenesis. As in other autoimmune diseases, the etiology is unknown and likely involves a genetic predisposition (including an association with particular HLA alleles) and undefined environmental triggers. Multiple serum autoantibodies are present, including antibodies against nuclear antigens and various liver proteins. Hepatocyte injury is likely caused by autoreactive CD4+ and CD8+ T cells.

Morphology. The hallmark of the disease is early and extensive parenchymal destruction followed quite rapidly by fibrosis (typically more rapid than in viral hepatitis). There may be foci of confluent

necrotic hepatocytes or parenchymal collapse. Plasma cells are abundant in the inflammatory infiltrate (Supplemental eFig. 13.4).

Clinical Features. There is a female predominance (approximately 4:1). About 40% of patients present with acute illness. The mortality rate in patients with severe untreated autoimmune hepatitis is approximately 40% within 6 months of diagnosis, and cirrhosis develops in at least 40% of survivors. In general, the prognosis is better in adults than in children. Immunosuppressive therapy is effective and results in a long-term survival rate of around 80%; however, even with treatment, approximately 10% of patients eventually die of liver disease, typically after development of cirrhosis.

Drug- and Toxin-Induced Hepatitis

The liver is the body's major drug metabolizing and detoxifying organ, and is therefore exposed to many potentially injurious therapeutic and environmental chemicals.

Exposure to a toxin or therapeutic agent should always be included in the differential diagnosis of any form of liver disease.

Pathogenesis. Drug reactions are of two types.
* *Predictable reactions,* in which a chemical metabolized in hepatocytes, usually by the cytochrome P-450 system, generates toxic products that directly injure hepatocytes. The liver cell injury is dose

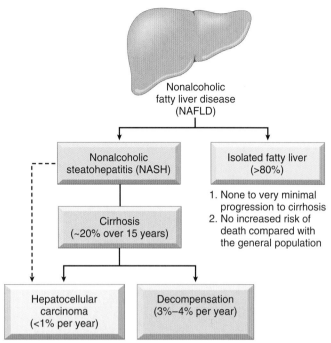

Nonalcoholic
fatty liver disease
(NAFLD)

Nonalcoholic
steatohepatitis (NASH)

Isolated fatty liver
(>80%)

1. None to very minimal
progression to cirrhosis
2. No increased risk of
death compared with
the general population

Cirrhosis
(~20% over 15 years)

Hepatocellular
carcinoma
(<1% per year)

Decompensation
(3%–4% per year)

Fig. 13.8 Natural history of nonalcoholic fatty liver disease. Isolated fatty liver disease shows a minimal risk for progression to cirrhosis or increased mortality rates, and nonalcoholic steatohepatitis shows an increased overall mortality rate, as well as an increased risk for cirrhosis and hepatocellular carcinoma.

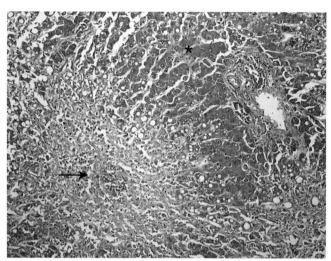

Fig. 13.9 Acetaminophen toxicity. Hepatocellular necrosis caused by acetaminophen overdose. Confluent necrosis is seen in the perivenular region (*arrow*). There is little inflammation. Residual normal tissue is indicated by the *asterisk*. (Courtesy of Dr. Matthew Yeh, University of Washington, Seattle.)

related and affects all people exposed to the drug. The classic example is acetaminophen. Hepatocyte injury usually starts in the centrilobular region, where the drugs are initially concentrated, and in severe cases spreads to involve entire lobules. Genetic differences among individuals, such as polymorphisms in cytochrome P-450 genes, may contribute to abnormal metabolism of the drug and direct liver injury.

- *Idiosyncratic reactions,* which are responsible for most cases of drug-induced liver injury. These reactions are unpredictable, occurring in only a subset of patients at doses that are usually nontoxic. The drug or its metabolite may modify self proteins to produce neoantigens that elicit immune reactions. Drugs that produce idiosyncratic liver injury include chlorpromazine, which causes cholestasis in patients who metabolize it slowly, several antibiotics, notably amoxicillin, and hundreds of others.

Morphology. The parenchymal injury is similar to that in other types of acute hepatitis, and includes focal or confluent hepatocyte necrosis (Fig. 13.9), steatosis, cholestasis, and inflammation. Occasionally, there may be noncaseating granulomas.

Clinical Features. Both classes of injury may be immediate or take weeks to months to develop. The clinical features are similar to those of other forms of acute liver disease. Progression to chronic hepatitis is unusual.

Inherited Diseases of the Liver

Several inherited diseases interfere with the metabolism of iron or copper, or lead to protein misfolding, thereby causing liver pathology.

Hemochromatosis

Hemochromatosis is caused by the increased intestinal absorption of iron, which is deposited in multiple parenchymal organs, the liver being a prominent site.

Pathogenesis. The increased absorption of iron is most often due to an autosomal recessive disorder called *hereditary hemochromatosis*

(primary hemochromatosis). Numerous mutations have been described in patients, most of which lower hepcidin production by the liver or interfere with hepcidin function. As discussed in Chapter 9, hepcidin is a critical negative regulator of iron absorption in the duodenum, and hepcidin defects therefore result in increased iron uptake. Inactivating mutations of *HFE* (for *Hereditary Fe* [iron]), which reduce hepcidin production, are seen in 70% of patients. Disease expression is variable and less severe in females due to iron losses associated with menstruation and increased iron requirements during pregnancy. Less commonly, hereditary hemochromatosis is caused by mutations in genes encoding proteins that are directly involved in iron trafficking, such as the receptor for transferrin (the plasma transport molecule for iron) or ferroportin (a transmembrane iron transporter). An acquired form of hemochromatosis (*secondary hemochromatosis*) may develop in patients who receive multiple blood transfusions or have chronic ineffective hematopoiesis, as occurs in β-thalassemia and certain myeloid neoplasms. When red cell production is inefficient due to premature death of red cell progenitors in the bone marrow, there is a compensatory increase in iron uptake from the gut due to suppression of hepatic hepcidin production by a hormone released from marrow progenitors called erythroferrone.

The excess iron, in the form of hemosiderin, is deposited in the liver, pancreas, heart, and other organs. It may increase the generation of ROS, which damage many cellular constituents, including lipids and DNA (see Chapter 1) and activate hepatic stellate cells to produce collagen.

Morphology. Iron is seen in the cytoplasm of hepatocytes as a brown pigment; its identity can be confirmed with special stains (Fig. 13.10). Increased fibrosis results in cirrhosis. The endocrine pancreas and the heart also show brown discoloration and evidence of parenchymal injury and fibrosis.

Clinical Features. Men are affected more commonly than women (5 to 7:1) and become symptomatic earlier in life (generally in the fourth to fifth decades). The principal manifestations include hepatomegaly, abdominal pain, increased skin pigmentation (particularly in sun-exposed areas), deranged glucose homeostasis or frank diabetes due to destruction of pancreatic islets (bronze diabetes), and cardiac dysfunction (arrhythmias, cardiomyopathy). The risk for hepatocellular carcinoma is increased 200-fold, presumably because of ongoing liver

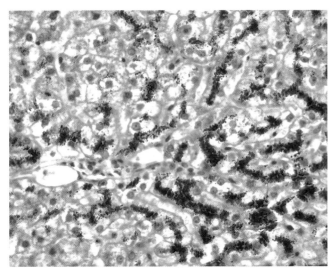

Fig. 13.10 Hereditary hemochromatosis. In this Prussian blue–stained section, hepatocellular iron appears blue. The parenchymal architecture is normal at this stage of disease, even with such abundant iron.

damage and the DNA-damaging effects of free radicals. Death may result from cirrhosis, hepatocellular carcinoma, or cardiac disease.

Wilson Disease

Wilson disease is an inherited disorder in which toxic levels of copper accumulate in the liver and other organs.

Pathogenesis. Wilson disease is an autosomal recessive disorder caused by loss-of-function mutations in the *ATP7B* gene, which encodes an ATPase that is expressed on the hepatocyte plasma membrane. This transmembrane protein mediates the ATP-dependent excretion of copper into bile and the incorporation of copper into apoceruloplasmin, which then is secreted into blood as ceruloplasmin. When ATP7B is defective, copper cannot be transported out of hepatocytes and it accumulates in the cytoplasm and in lysosomes, causing increased production of ROS, which damage the hepatocytes. Serum levels of ceruloplasmin, the copper transport protein, are reduced because in the absence of bound copper the protein has a decreased half-life.

> *Morphology.* The liver changes are variable, ranging from mild steatosis to hepatocyte necrosis (sometimes severe), to chronic hepatitis and cirrhosis.

Clinical Features. Common clinical presentations are acute or chronic liver disease and neuropsychiatric manifestations caused by copper deposition in the basal ganglia. A classical finding on physical examination in about half of patients are *Kayser-Fleischer rings,* discoloration of the cornea caused by copper deposition. Diagnostic laboratory findings include decreased serum ceruloplasmin and increased urinary excretion of copper.

α1-Antitrypsin Deficiency

This autosomal recessive disease is caused by mutations in the α1-antitrypsin gene that result in misfolding and reduced production of the α1-antitrypsin protein. α1-antitrypsin is an inhibitor of a number of proteases, and its deficiency results in excessive neutrophil-derived protease activity, often leading to emphysema (see Chapter 10). In hepatocytes, which produce large amounts of the protein, the misfolded protein triggers the unfolded protein response, culminating in apoptotic death of the cells. The histologic hallmark is the presence of periodic acid–Schiff (PAS)–positive globular cytoplasmic inclusions composed of aggregates of the mutant protein (Supplemental eFig. 13.5). About 10% to 20% of affected newborns with the mutations develop neonatal hepatitis with cholestatic jaundice, which may resolve or progress to cirrhosis.

Circulatory Disorders of the Liver

The liver is less susceptible to ischemic necrosis than many other organs because it has a dual blood supply (via the hepatic artery and portal vein). Some circulatory disorders are unique to the liver (Fig. 13.11) and are discussed here.

- *Portal vein obstruction* is often idiopathic. *Extrahepatic obstruction* may be caused by portal vein thrombosis, which may occur in the setting of cirrhosis, tumors, hypercoagulable states, local inflammation (such as pancreatitis or peritonitis), or surgical or other trauma to the vein. It results in portal hypertension. *Intrahepatic obstruction* of portal vein branches may be seen in schistosomiasis, but more often the cause is unknown. It may result in noncirrhotic portal hypertension or hepatocyte atrophy but usually does not cause infarction.

- *Hepatic vein thrombosis.* Thrombosis of the small intrahepatic branches of the hepatic vein, called *sinusoidal obstruction syndrome,* is seen most often after hematopoietic stem cell transplantation and cancer chemotherapy. Local endothelial injury leads to inflammation, congestion, and obstruction of hepatic venules. Thrombosis of two or more major hepatic veins, called the *Budd-Chiari syndrome,* results in centrilobular congestion and hepatocyte necrosis (Supplemental eFig. 13.6). About half of cases are caused by hypercoagulability due to the presence of a myeloproliferative neoplasm, such as polycythemia vera (see Chapter 9). The remainder has diverse causes, including hepatocellular carcinoma.

- *Passive congestion* is the result of cardiac failure and is a common finding in patients who die of heart disease. The liver may be enlarged, tense, and cyanotic. The centrilobular sinusoids are congested. The combination of decreased perfusion and congestion causes centrilobular necrosis, with a variegated appearance often referred to as a "nutmeg liver".

Nodules and Tumors of the Liver

Metastases to the liver from cancers of the GI tract and other organs are far more frequent than primary liver neoplasms in the Western world. By contrast, primary liver neoplasms are among the most common tumors in Asia and parts of Africa, particularly in regions where hepatitis B infection is highly prevalent. Here we discuss the more common proliferative and neoplastic lesions arising in the liver.

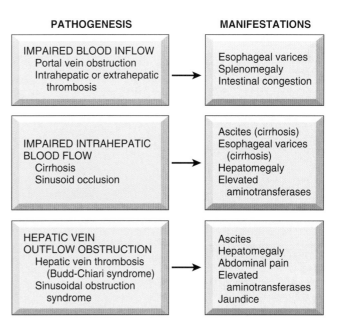

PATHOGENESIS	MANIFESTATIONS
IMPAIRED BLOOD INFLOW Portal vein obstruction Intrahepatic or extrahepatic thrombosis	Esophageal varices Splenomegaly Intestinal congestion
IMPAIRED INTRAHEPATIC BLOOD FLOW Cirrhosis Sinusoid occlusion	Ascites (cirrhosis) Esophageal varices (cirrhosis) Hepatomegaly Elevated aminotransferases
HEPATIC VEIN OUTFLOW OBSTRUCTION Hepatic vein thrombosis (Budd-Chiari syndrome) Sinusoidal obstruction syndrome	Ascites Hepatomegaly Abdominal pain Elevated aminotransferases Jaundice

Fig. 13.11 Hepatic circulatory disorders. Forms and clinical manifestations of compromised hepatic blood flow.

Focal Nodular Hyperplasia

Focal nodular hyperplasia (FNH) is a benign lesion that is believed to be nonneoplastic in origin. Its principal importance is that it produces a mass lesion that must be distinguished from true neoplasms, such as hepatocellular carcinoma.

Pathogenesis. FNH is thought to result from abnormally low vascular perfusion of a part of the liver, causing scarring and compensatory hyperperfusion, giving rise to hyperplasia of surviving hepatocytes. The blood vessels in the center of the nodules are anomalous and the likely basis of the hypoperfusion. It is possible that FNH is the result of a primary congenital vascular anomaly; supporting this idea, it is frequently associated with two congenital disorders of blood vessels, hereditary hemorrhagic telangiectasia and hepatic hemangioma.

> *Morphology.* The typical macroscopic finding is a single nodule with a central depressed scar (Fig. 13.12) in an otherwise normal liver. Microscopically, the central scar shows a large artery with branches radiating to the periphery, dividing the lesion into cords or small segments. The radiating septa show abnormal proliferating bile ductules. In between the septa are hyperplastic liver cells.

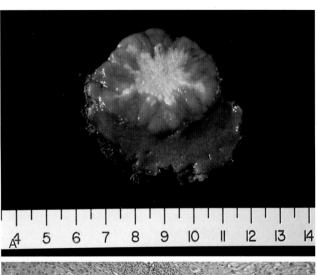

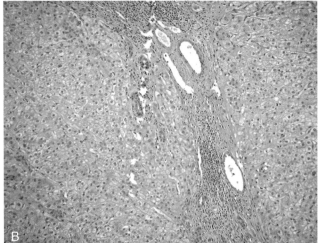

Fig. 13.12 Focal nodular hyperplasia. (A) Resected specimen showing lobulated contours and a central stellate scar. (B) Low-power photomicrograph showing a broad fibrous scar with mixed hepatic arterial and bile duct elements and chronic inflammation within hepatic parenchyma that lacks normal architecture because of hepatocyte regeneration.

Clinical Features. FNH is asymptomatic and is usually an incidental mass lesion found in young and middle-aged adults.

Hepatic Adenoma

Hepatic adenoma is a benign tumor that usually arises in a noncirrhotic liver in reproductive-age women. In the past, hepatic adenoma was commonly associated with oral contraceptive use, but this etiology has decreased with reduced estrogen doses; the major association now is with obesity and metabolic syndrome. Estrogens may stimulate the growth of established tumors. Driver mutations in several cancer genes have been described, including gain-of-function mutations in β-catenin. The morphology ranges from sheets of normal-appearing hepatocytes (Supplemental eFig. 13.7) to tumors with significant cytologic atypia. They are usually asymptomatic, but may cause local pain and, when large, rupture, resulting in intraabdominal bleeding. With accumulation of mutations, adenomas may undergo malignant transformation, particularly those with mutations of β-catenin.

Hepatocellular Carcinoma

This malignant tumor of hepatocytes is strongly associated with chronic liver disease, most often caused by hepatitis B and C viral infections.

More than 85% of cases of hepatocellular carcinoma (HCC) occur in regions with high rates of chronic HBV infection, such as parts of Asia and sub-Saharan Africa; significant exposure to the carcinogen aflatoxin (produced by fungi contaminating foods such as rice) is also common in these parts of the world. The incidence of HCC is rising in Western countries due to increasing prevalence of chronic liver disease related to HCV and NAFLD.

Pathogenesis. The major risk factors for HCC are chronic hepatitis caused by HBV and HCV, but increasingly alcoholic hepatitis, NAFLD, and other causes of chronic liver injury underlie HCC. Although it is often seen against a background of cirrhosis, cirrhosis *per se* is not a premalignant lesion. Rather, progression to cirrhosis and liver carcinogenesis are driven by chronic liver injury and take place in parallel. Viruses and other inducers of chronic hepatocyte injury and inflammation are not themselves oncogenic. It is believed that inflammation, with its attendant growth factors and cytokines, promotes the proliferation of normal and transformed cells and predisposes to oncogenic mutations. Aflatoxin is not only carcinogenic but also synergizes with HBV to increase the risk. Driver mutations include gain-of-function mutations in β-catenin, which are usually found in HBV-negative tumors, and loss-of-function mutations in *TP53*, which are strongly associated with aflatoxin exposure. The key oncogenic drivers in most cases are not known.

> *Morphology.* HCC may present as a solitary mass (Fig. 13.13), multiple nodules, or a diffuse infiltrate without defined borders, usually in a background of cirrhosis. Intrahepatic metastases occur and are seen as small satellite nodules surrounding a larger primary mass. The morphologic appearance of tumor cells varies from well differentiated to highly anaplastic. The cells in well-differentiated tumors resemble normal hepatocytes, but certain features of normal liver (e.g., bile ducts and hepatic triads) are absent.

Clinical Features. In Western populations, HCC rarely manifests before 60 years of age, and in almost 90% of cases, the malignancy emerges from a background of cirrhosis, most often caused by chronic HCV infection. In Asia and Africa, where HCC is associated with HBV infection, patients present at significantly younger ages, in part because those who acquire HBV in the neonatal period through maternal transmission have the highest incidence of chronic HBV infection. Throughout the world, HCC shows a pronounced male predominance.

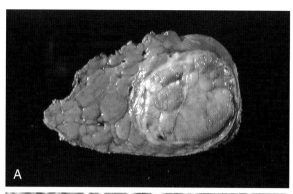

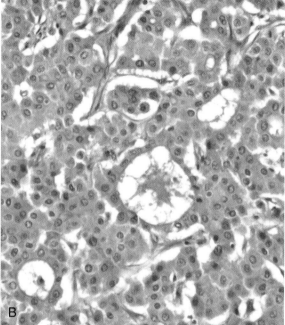

Fig. 13.13 Hepatocellular carcinoma. (A) Liver removed at autopsy showing a massive unifocal neoplasm replacing most of the right hepatic lobe in a noncirrhotic liver. (B) Malignant hepatocytes growing in distorted versions of normal architecture: large pseudoacinar spaces; malformed, dilated bile canaliculi; and thickened hepatocyte trabeculae.

Most patients present with vague symptoms such as abdominal pain, fatigue, or weight loss, while others present with jaundice or upper GI bleeding. Almost 50% of patients have elevated serum levels of α-fetoprotein, a protein made in hepatocytes, but measurement of α-fetoprotein has insufficient sensitivity and specificity to be a useful screening test. The tumor tends to invade blood vessels and metastasize hematogenously, particularly to the lungs. The 5-year survival rate for patients with large tumors is dismal, and the majority die within 2 years of diagnosis. Death usually occurs from (1) cachexia, (2) GI or esophageal variceal bleeding, or (3) liver failure with hepatic coma. Rarely, rupture of the tumor leads to fatal hemorrhage. Ultimately, the best hope for stemming the toll taken by HCC is prevention, which can be accomplished through HBV vaccination and treatment of HCV infection with antiviral drugs.

Cholangiocarcinoma

Malignant tumors of intrahepatic bile ducts, called cholangiocarcinoma, are described later in the section on diseases of the biliary system.

DISORDERS OF THE BILIARY SYSTEM

The biliary system consists of intrahepatic and extrahepatic bile ducts and the gallbladder. Grooves in the plasma membranes of hepatocytes

Table 13.3   Major Causes of Jaundice

Predominantly Unconjugated Hyperbilirubinemia
Excess Production of Bilirubin
Hemolytic anemia
Resorption of blood from internal hemorrhage (e.g., alimentary tract bleeding, hematomas)
Ineffective erythropoiesis (e.g., pernicious anemia, thalassemia)
Reduced Hepatic Uptake
Drug interference with membrane carrier systems
Impaired Bilirubin Conjugation
Physiologic jaundice of the newborn
Diffuse hepatocellular disease (e.g., viral or drug-induced hepatitis, cirrhosis)
Predominantly Conjugated Hyperbilirubinemia
Decreased Hepatocellular Excretion
Drug-induced canalicular membrane dysfunction (e.g., oral contraceptives, cyclosporine)
Hepatocellular damage or toxicity (e.g., viral or drug-induced hepatitis, total parenteral nutrition, systemic infection)
Impaired Intrahepatic or Extrahepatic Bile Flow
Inflammatory destruction of intrahepatic bile ducts (e.g., primary biliary cirrhosis, primary sclerosing cholangitis, graft-versus-host disease, liver transplantation)
Gallstones
External compression (e.g., carcinoma of the pancreas)

form *bile canaliculi*, into which bile is secreted. The canaliculi converge to form ducts of increasing size. Bile contains *bilirubin*, a waste product created by degradation of heme from senescent red cells that are destroyed by macrophages in the spleen, liver, and bone marrow. Bilirubin released from macrophages is bound by plasma albumin and transported to the liver, where it is conjugated with glucuronic acid which makes it water soluble and facilitates excretion in bile and urine.

Diseases that result in the obstruction of intrahepatic or extrahepatic bile ducts and accumulation of bile in the liver, a condition called *cholestasis* (Supplemental eFig 13.8), produce increases in conjugated bilirubin (measured as *direct bilirubin*). Unconjugated bilirubin (measured as *indirect bilirubin*) may be increased by overproduction (e.g., red cell hemolysis, when production overwhelms the capacity of the conjugation system), displacement from albumin (e.g., certain drugs), or underconjugation (e.g., acquired hepatocellular disease or inherited disorders that interfere with bilirubin conjugation [described later]). If unconjugated bilirubin levels rise, it may diffuse into tissues, particularly the brain in infants, and produce toxic injury *(kernicterus)*.

Different diseases are preferentially associated with elevation of conjugated or unconjugated bilirubin in the blood, which can help with the differential diagnosis (Table 13.3). Other diagnostic clues may come from measurement of the levels of alkaline phosphatase and gamma-glutamyl transferase (GGT) in the blood. GGT is a sensitive marker of hepatobiliary disease, whereas elevation of alkaline phosphatase out of proportion to GGT levels is strongly associated with biliary obstruction. Clinically, jaundice appears when bilirubin levels are at least twice normal and is most easily appreciated as yellow discoloration of the conjunctiva of the eye (inaccurately referred to as scleral icterus). Patients also may develop pruritus, skin xanthomas (focal accumulation of cholesterol), malabsorption of fat-soluble vitamins as well as other nutrients, and dark urine. Chronic biliary obstruction may result in injury to hepatocytes and ultimately cirrhosis.

Disorders affecting the intrahepatic and extrahepatic components of the biliary tract are discussed together because many diseases of the biliary system involve both and they share many clinical features.

Cholangitis

Inflammation of the bile ducts may be caused by infection or immune reactions. *Ascending cholangitis* is an infection of the biliary tract by enteric bacteria that usually occurs as a complication of extrahepatic duct obstruction, most commonly by gallstones. If undetected or not treated, it may lead to sepsis. The two major autoimmune cholangiopathies, primary biliary cholangitis and primary sclerosing cholangitis, differ in significant ways (Table 13.4) and are described next.

Primary Biliary Cholangitis

Primary biliary cholangitis (PBC) is an autoimmune disease that leads to inflammation and destruction of small- and medium-sized intrahepatic bile ducts.

Pathogenesis. The triggers that initiate PBC are unknown. Serum antimitochondrial antibodies are the most characteristic finding, but their role in initiating or sustaining bile duct damage is unknown. The disease is associated with other autoimmune disorders, such as Sjögren syndrome, suggesting that it arises in the context of a genetic predisposition to autoimmune disorders.

> *Morphology.* In active disease, the intralobular bile ducts contain infiltrates of T lymphocytes and plasma cells, sometimes with granuloma formation, and many ducts are destroyed (Fig. 13.14). The proliferation of surviving bile ducts (*ductular reaction*) is often seen (Supplemental eFig. 13.9).

Clinical Features. PBC (previously called *primary biliary cirrhosis*) is primarily a disease of middle-age women, with a female-to-male ratio of 6:1. Its peak incidence is between 40 and 50 years of age. Most patients are diagnosed while asymptomatic following a workup triggered by the identification of an elevated serum alkaline phosphatase level or severe itching. Hypercholesterolemia is common. Early treatment with oral ursodeoxycholic acid has dramatically improved outcomes by slowing the disease progression through unknown mechanisms. With time, even with treatment, secondary features may emerge, including skin hyperpigmentation, xanthelasmas, steatorrhea, and osteomalacia and/or osteoporosis due to malabsorption of vitamin D. Liver transplantation is the favored treatment for individuals with advanced liver disease.

Primary Sclerosing Cholangitis

Primary sclerosing cholangitis is a presumed autoimmune disease characterized by inflammation and obliterative fibrosis (sclerosis) of intrahepatic and extrahepatic bile ducts.

Pathogenesis. The pathogenesis is unclear, but an immunologic basis is suspected. Up to 80% cases are associated with serum antineutrophil cytoplasmic antibodies (ANCAs), which are found in various forms of vasculitis (see Chapter 3), and almost two thirds of patients also have ulcerative colitis. First-degree relatives of patients with PSC are at an increased risk for developing the disease, suggesting that genetic factors contribute.

> *Morphology.* Strictures causing "beading" of the biliary tract are a classic feature that can be detected by MRI. Inflammation is prominent in larger ducts, whereas small bile ducts often show circumferential "onion-skin" fibrosis around a narrowed lumen with little or no inflammation (Supplemental eFig. 13.10).

Clinical Features. PSC tends to occur in the third through fifth decades of life and has a 2:1 male predominance. Chronic pancreatitis and chronic cholecystitis due to involvement of the pancreatic ducts and gallbladder are also seen. In some patients, sclerosing cholangitis is associated with autoimmune pancreatitis. PSC follows a protracted course of 5 years to decades, and severely afflicted patients have symptoms typical of chronic cholestatic liver disease, including steatorrhea. Unlike PBC, there is no satisfactory medical therapy. Liver transplantation is the only definitive treatment for individuals with end-stage liver disease. Cholangiocarcinoma develops in up to 7% of patients, usually with a fatal outcome.

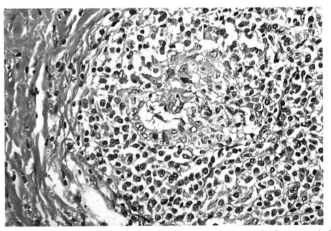

Fig. 13.14 Primary biliary cholangitis. A portal tract is markedly expanded by an infiltrate of lymphocytes and plasma cells. Note the granulomatous reaction to the injured bile duct (called a florid duct lesion).

Table 13.4 Main Features of Primary Biliary Cholangitis and Primary Sclerosing Cholangitis

Parameter	Primary Biliary Cholangitis	Primary Sclerosing Cholangitis
Age	Median age 50 years	Median age 30 years
Gender	90% female	70% male
Clinical course	Progressive	Unpredictable, but usually progressive
Associated conditions	Sjögren syndrome (70%)	Inflammatory bowel disease (70%)
	Scleroderma (5%)	Pancreatitis (≤25%)
	Thyroid disease (20%)	
Serology	95% AMA-positive	0% to 5% AMA-positive (low titer)
	20% ANA-positive	6% ANA-positive
	40% ANCA-positive	65% ANCA-positive
Radiology	Normal	Strictures and beading of large bile ducts; pruning of smaller ducts
Duct lesion	Florid duct lesions and loss of small ducts only	Inflammatory destruction of extrahepatic and large intrahepatic ducts; fibrotic obliteration of medium and small intrahepatic ducts

AMA, Antimitochondrial antibody; ANA, antinuclear antibody; ANCA, antineutrophil cytoplasmic antibody.

Congenital Disorders Causing Jaundice

Because glucuronosyltransferase, the hepatic enzyme that conjugates bilirubin and thus promotes its excretion, is not fully expressed until about 2 weeks of age, almost every newborn develops transient and mild unconjugated hyperbilirubinemia, termed *neonatal jaundice* or *physiologic jaundice of the newborn.* Sustained jaundice may result from inherited defects, obstruction, or cholestasis of uncertain origin.

- *Inherited defects.* Mutation of the *UGT1A1* gene, which encodes glucuronosyltransferase, results in defective conjugation of bilirubin and unconjugated hyperbilirubinemia. The common mild form is called *Gilbert syndrome,* and the more severe form is a rare fatal disorder called *Crigler-Najjar syndrome. Dubin-Johnson syndrome* is an autosomal recessive disease caused by defects in the transport protein responsible for the secretion of conjugated bilirubin from hepatocytes into bile canaliculi. This defect leads to the accumulation of a dark, melanin-like pigment in the liver, but patients are otherwise normal.
- *Biliary atresia* is obstruction of the extrahepatic biliary tract occurring within the first 3 months of life. Infants with biliary atresia present with neonatal cholestasis, but exhibit a normal birth weight and postnatal weight gain. There is a slight female predominance. Initially stools are normal, but they become acholic as the disease progresses. In the fetal form, bile ducts do not develop normally; it is associated with developmental anomalies of other organs. In the more common perinatal form, the biliary system develops normally but is injured after birth. Its etiology is unknown but may involve viral infection or toxin exposure. The hepatic or common bile ducts show inflammation and strictures caused by fibrosis.
- *Neonatal hepatitis* is a poorly defined entity in which infants present with cholestasis and jaundice. There is usually no liver inflammation (hence the name "hepatitis" is a misnomer). The majority of cases are likely due to various toxic, metabolic, or infectious causes.

Cholelithiasis and Cholecystitis

The most common disorders of the gallbladder are caused by the formation of stones, which frequently lead to the obstruction of the extrahepatic bile duct and acute inflammation of the gallbladder and biliary tree (cholecystitis and cholangitis).

Cholelithiasis

The formation of gallstones, called cholelithiasis, is a common clinical problem, especially in Western countries and Latin America, and the removal of stone-laden gallbladders is among the most common surgical procedures.

Pathogenesis. There are two major types of stones, and the mechanisms that underlie their formation are different.

- *Cholesterol stones,* which contain crystallized cholesterol monohydrate, constitute about 80% of gallstones in Western countries. Excess cholesterol, in the form of free cholesterol or bile salts, can only be eliminated from the body in bile. Cholesterol is rendered water-soluble by forming micelles with bile salts and lecithins. When cholesterol concentrations exceed the solubilizing capacity of bile (supersaturation), cholesterol can no longer remain dispersed and crystallizes out of solution, leading to stone formation.
- *Pigment stones,* made of bilirubin calcium salts, form when the bile contains a high concentration of unconjugated bilirubin, as may occur in patients with chronic red cell hemolysis (e.g., sickle cell anemia and hereditary spherocytosis).

The incidence of gallstones increases with age. Ethnicity and heredity clearly are risk factors, but how they contribute to stone formation is unknown. Obesity and estrogens also increase gallstone formation; the latter likely contributes to the higher incidence in women as compared with men.

Morphology. Cholesterol stones arise in the gallbladder. They are yellowish and usually multiple (Supplemental eFig. 13.11). Pigment stones are brown or black and may arise anywhere in the biliary tract (Supplemental eFig. 13.12).

Clinical Features. Although the majority of individuals with gallstones are asymptomatic for life, gallstones present a risk of biliary obstruction, which may have a range of consequences depending on the position of the obstruction. The most dangerous complication is obstruction of the common bile duct causing blockage of the pancreatic duct and acute pancreatitis, described later. Other serious complications include empyema of the gallbladder, perforation, and formation of fistulas with adjacent bowel loops. Gallstones also increase the risk of carcinoma of the gallbladder, probably because of the associated chronic inflammation and epithelial repair.

Cholecystitis

Inflammation of the gallbladder almost always occurs in association with gallstones.

Acute Cholecystitis. Acute cholecystitis is precipitated in more than 90% of cases by obstruction of the neck of the gallbladder or the cystic duct by gallstones, and is the most common significant complication of gallstones. Obstruction of bile outflow leads to chemical irritation and inflammation of the gallbladder wall, for several reasons. Phospholipases from epithelial cells hydrolyze biliary lecithin to lysolecithin, which is toxic to the mucosa. The normally protective glycoprotein mucous layer is disrupted, exposing the mucosal epithelium to the detergent action of bile salts, and prostaglandins released within the wall of the distended gallbladder promote inflammation. Bacterial infection may be superimposed later, exacerbating the inflammation.

Morphology. The gallbladder usually is enlarged and tense, with bright red or blotchy, violaceous discoloration due to subserosal hemorrhages. The serosa frequently is covered by a fibrinous or, in severe cases, a fibrinopurulent exudate. The gallbladder is filled with turbid bile that may contain fibrin, blood, and pus. In advanced cases, the entire gallbladder is necrotic (*gangrenous cholecystitis*).

Clinical Features. Patients present with upper abdominal pain, often with fever, nausea, leukocytosis, and prostration. Conjugated hyperbilirubinemia, due to "back flux" of obstructed bile, is a frequent laboratory finding. Between 5% and 12% of cases with a clinical picture of acute cholecystitis do not have gallstones; these cases of acute acalculous cholecystitis tend to occur in the setting of major surgery, severe trauma, burns, or sepsis. Dehydration, gallbladder stasis, vascular compromise, and bacterial infection seem to be common underlying conditions.

Chronic Cholecystitis. This disease is also usually associated with gallstones. It may follow attacks of acute cholecystitis but more commonly develops without a prior history of acute attacks. The favored proposed etiology is chemical irritation of the mucosa by supersaturated bile, which may injure the mucosa even in the absence of stones. In line with this idea, both calculus and acalculous chronic cholecystitis are associated with similar morphologic findings and clinical symptoms.

Morphology. The morphologic changes are variable and can be subtle. In the absence of superimposed acute cholecystitis, collections of lymphocytes in the wall are the only sign of inflammation. Outpouchings of mucosal epithelium through the wall of the gallbladder (*Rokitansky-Aschoff sinuses*) may be quite prominent (Supplemental eFig. 13.13).

Clinical Features. The typical clinical presentation is recurrent attacks of abdominal pain with nausea, vomiting, and intolerance of fatty foods. The long-term risk of chronic cholecystitis is the association of gallstones and chronic inflammation with carcinoma of the gallbladder.

Tumors of the Biliary System

Cholangiocarcinoma

Cholangiocarcinoma is a malignant tumor of the intrahepatic or extrahepatic bile ducts. In recent classifications, the term *cholangiocarcinoma* is applied to tumors of the intrahepatic bile ducts, and tumors of the extrahepatic ducts are called *biliary adenocarcinoma*.

Pathogenesis. Cholangiocarcinoma often arises in the setting of chronic inflammation (e.g., primary sclerosing cholangitis). In areas of Asia where infestation by parasitic liver flukes *(Fasciola hepatica)* is endemic, the prevalence of the tumor is 30 to 40 times higher than in other parts of the world. As with hepatocellular carcinoma, rates of cholangiocarcinoma also are elevated in patients with hepatitis B and C and nonalcoholic fatty liver disease.

> *Morphology.* Extrahepatic cholangiocarcinomas are generally small lesions at the time of diagnosis, as they cause obstruction of the biliary tract early in their course. Intrahepatic cholangiocarcinomas occur in noncirrhotic livers and may track along the intrahepatic portal tract system or produce a single massive tumor. Fifty percent to 60% of all cholangiocarcinomas are perihilar *(Klatskin tumors),* and 20% to 30% are distal tumors, arising in the common bile duct where it lies posterior to the duodenum. The remaining 10% are intrahepatic. The tumors typically are mucin-producing adenocarcinomas that elicit a strong fibrotic (desmoplastic) reaction. Lymphovascular invasion and perineural invasion are both common (Supplemental eFig. 13.14).

Clinical Features. The prognosis is dismal, regardless of the site of origin: Survival rates are about 15% at 2 years after diagnosis for extrahepatic tumors. For intrahepatic tumors, which are often detected at an advanced stage, the median time to death from time of diagnosis is 6 months, even following surgical treatment. Typical presentations include signs and symptoms of biliary obstruction, cholangitis, and right upper quadrant pain.

Carcinoma of the Gallbladder

This is a rare tumor that is almost always associated with gallstones, presumably because the chronic inflammation promotes carcinogenesis. Primary sclerosing cholangitis is also a risk factor. It is slightly more common in women and occurs most frequently in the seventh decade of life. Tumors may be infiltrating or exophytic, and most are adenocarcinomas (Supplemental eFig. 13.15). Symptoms are insidious, so tumors are often detected at an advanced stage; the mean 5-year survival rate has remained unchanged over many years, at about 5% to 12%.

DISORDERS OF THE PANCREAS

The pancreas is composed of two anatomically discrete sets of cells, each with distinct functions. The *exocrine pancreas,* which makes up the bulk of the organ, produces enzymes that are essential for digestion. The *endocrine pancreas,* which consists of the islets of Langerhans, is the source of insulin and other hormones. Diabetes, the major endocrine disorder of insulin production and action, is discussed in Chapter 16. Here we consider inflammatory and neoplastic diseases of the exocrine pancreas.

The exocrine pancreas consists of glands lined with epithelial (acinar) cells, which secrete digestive enzymes into ducts that drain via the pancreatic duct and the common bile duct into the duodenum.

Most of the enzymes are produced as inactive precursors *(zymogens)* that are converted in the duodenum into their active forms.

Pancreatitis

Inflammation of the pancreas may be acute or chronic and has a number of consequences, some of which may be life-threatening.

Acute Pancreatitis

Acute pancreatitis results from autodigestion and inflammation of the pancreas caused by inappropriately activated pancreatic enzymes.

Pathogenesis. Almost 80% of cases are associated with gallstones or alcoholism.

* *Obstruction of the common bile duct by impacted gallstones* blocks the pancreatic duct and impedes the flow of pancreatic enzymes. These enzymes are activated within the body of the pancreas and autodigest the gland.
* *Excessive alcohol consumption* triggers pancreatitis, perhaps by stimulating the secretion of pancreatic enzymes and contraction of the sphincter through which the common bile duct drains, thus leading to functional obstruction.
* The remaining cases may be associated with various drugs, infections, vascular diseases, metabolic diseases, or genetic causes (such as mutations that lead to hyperactivation of trypsin, which activates other enzymes). In many cases, the underlying cause is unknown.

> *Morphology.* Classic morphologic features include acute inflammation, fat necrosis caused by lipases, enzymatic destruction of the parenchyma, and, in the most severe cases, destruction of blood vessels leading to hemorrhage (Fig. 13.15).

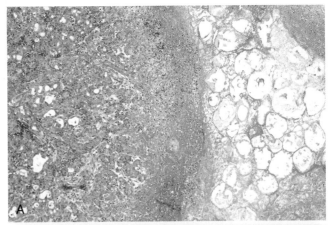

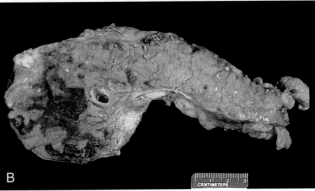

Fig. 13.15 Acute pancreatitis. (A) The microscopic field shows a region of fat necrosis *(right)* and focal pancreatic parenchymal necrosis *(center).* (B) The pancreas has been sectioned longitudinally to reveal dark areas of hemorrhage in the pancreatic substance and a small area of pale fat necrosis in the peripancreatic fat *(upper left).*

Clinical Features. Patients present with abdominal pain that may be severe and referred to the upper back. Laboratory findings include elevated serum lipase and amylase levels within the first 24 hours. Hypocalcemia can result from precipitation of calcium in areas of fat necrosis; if persistent, it is a poor prognostic sign. In 80% of cases, the inflammation is mild and resolves spontaneously; pancreatic pseudocyst (see the following) is one sequela. In other patients, the systemic release of digestive enzymes may lead to serious consequences, such as the systemic inflammatory response syndrome with shock and disseminated intravascular coagulation (see Chapter 3), acute respiratory distress syndrome (see Chapter 10), and systemic fat necrosis. In such cases, acute pancreatitis is a dire medical emergency.

Chronic Pancreatitis

Chronic inflammation of the pancreas is associated with long-term alcoholism and may lead to destruction of the organ.

Pathogenesis. About 50% of cases of chronic pancreatitis, especially in men, are associated with prolonged and excessive alcohol consumption; the association is weaker in women. How alcohol triggers chronic pancreatic injury and inflammation is not known; it may alter the activation of digestive enzymes, increase the production of oxygen-derived free radicals, or exert direct toxic effects on acinar cells. Other predisposing factors include functional or anatomic duct obstruction. It also is increasingly recognized that many "idiopathic" cases are associated with germ line mutations in genes such as *CFTR* (the affected gene in cystic fibrosis; see Chapter 6) and the gene encoding trypsin, one of the major pancreatic enzymes.

Morphology. There is patchy scarring (fibrosis), a reduced number and size of acini, variable dilation of the pancreatic ducts, and relative sparing of the islets of Langerhans (at least initially) (Fig. 13.16). Acinar loss is a constant feature, usually with a chronic inflammatory infiltrate around remaining lobules and ducts. The ductal epithelium may be atrophied or hyperplastic or exhibit squamous metaplasia, and ductal concretions may be noted. *Autoimmune pancreatitis* is a distinct form of chronic pancreatitis characterized by infiltration of the pancreas by lymphocytes and plasma cells, many of which are positive for IgG4, accompanied by a "swirling" fibrosis. It is part of so-called IgG4-related disease.

Clinical Features. The disease may be asymptomatic or may present as bouts of jaundice, indigestion, or abdominal and back pain. In some cases, the disease is silent until the appearance of diarrhea and malabsorption secondary to pancreatic insufficiency, or diabetes secondary to destruction of the islets of Langerhans. Although not common, the most feared long-term complication is pancreatic cancer.

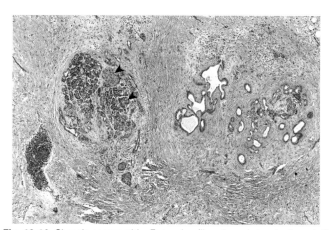

Fig. 13.16 Chronic pancreatitis. Extensive fibrosis and atrophy have left only residual islets *(left)* and ducts *(right)*, with a sprinkling of chronic inflammatory cells and acinar tissue.

Pseudocyst

A pseudocyst is an encapsulated collection of fluid that may occur in the pancreas, but more commonly is outside the pancreas. It arises weeks after a bout of acute pancreatitis, when liquefied areas of a necrotic pancreas become walled off by inflammatory and fibrous tissue that lacks an epithelial lining (hence a "pseudo," or false, cyst) (Fig. 13.17). Most resolve spontaneously, but some persist and may lead to complications such as infection, compression, obstruction of adjacent structures, rupture, and hemorrhage.

Tumors of the Pancreas

Cystic Tumors

Cystic tumors range from benign cysts to invasive cancers.

Pancreatic cysts are being detected with increasing frequency because of the use of imaging techniques, but only 5% to 15% are neoplastic. Cystic tumors are of two types.

- *Serous cystadenomas* are small cysts containing clear fluid and lined with cuboidal epithelial cells (Fig. 13.18A and B). Most of these lesions carry somatic loss-of-function mutations in the von Hippel-Lindau *(VHL)* tumor suppressor gene, which regulates angiogenesis and responses to hypoxia (see Chapter 5). Nevertheless, the lesions are almost always benign. The tumors typically manifest in the seventh decade of life with nonspecific symptoms such as abdominal pain; the female-to-male ratio is 2:1.
- *Mucinous cystadenomas* are lined by columnar mucin-producing epithelial cells with a dense cellular stroma, and are filled with thick, tenacious mucin (Fig. 13.18C,D). Most of these lesions carry gain-of-function mutations in the *RAS* oncogene. The tumors usually arise in the tail or body of the pancreas in women (95%) and manifest as painless, slow-growing masses. The cells display varying degrees of dysplasia, and up to a third of the tumors are associated with invasive adenocarcinoma.

Adenocarcinoma

Pancreatic adenocarcinoma is an aggressive tumor associated with very high mortality.

Although pancreatic cancer is less common than cancers of the lung, colon, and other tissues, it is a major killer, the 5-year survival rate being a dismal 8%.

Pathogenesis. Adenocarcinomas arise from precursor lesions in small ducts by the acquisition of sequential mutations in oncogenes and tumor suppressor genes. The precursor lesion is called *pancreatic intraepithelial neoplasia (PanIN).* The accumulation of genetic changes is similar to that described for colon cancer, and involves well-known tumor-causing genes (Fig. 13.19), particularly *RAS,* which is mutated in more than 90% of these cancers, and the tumor suppressor gene *CDKN2A,* which encodes the cell-cycle regulator p16 and is mutated in 95% of cases. The functions of these genes are described in Chapter 5.

Morphology. About 60% of pancreatic cancers arise in the head of the gland, 15% in the body, 5% in the tail, and the rest diffusely throughout. The typical tumor is a highly invasive, moderately to poorly differentiated adenocarcinoma. The cells form abortive glands that infiltrate a dense fibrotic stroma (Fig. 13.20). The tumors are hard and poorly defined. Cancers in the head of the pancreas tend to obstruct the common bile duct.

Clinical Features. The vast majority of pancreatic cancers occur between the ages of 60 and 80 years. These tumors often remain silent until they impinge on some other structure. Pain is often the first symptom, caused by entrapment of nerves by infiltrating tumor cells. Tumors of the head of the pancreas cause obstructive jaundice, usually late in the course. About 10% of patients develop migratory thrombophlebitis (*Trousseau syndrome*) caused by procoagulants released from tumor cells. These clinical manifestations virtually always appear too late for cure, which is confined to a small minority of tumors that become symptomatic at stages where the tumor can be completely resected surgically. Serum levels of many enzymes and antigens (e.g., carcinoembryonic antigen and CA19-9 protein) are elevated, but these markers are neither specific nor sensitive enough to be useful for screening or diagnosis. They are useful in following the response to therapy.

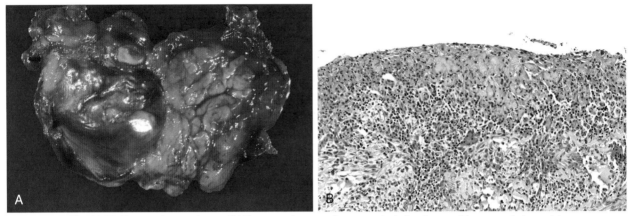

Fig. 13.17 Pancreatic pseudocyst. (A) Cross section revealing a poorly defined cyst with a necrotic brownish wall. (B) Histologically, the cyst lacks an epithelial lining and instead is lined by fibrin and granulation tissue, with typical changes of chronic inflammation.

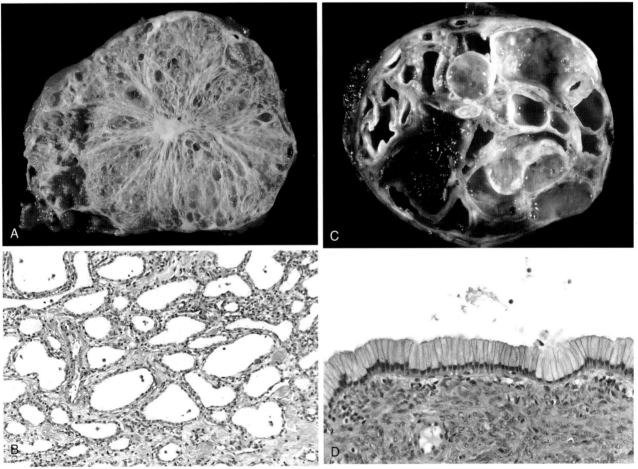

Fig. 13.18 Cystic tumors of the pancreas. Serous cystadenoma. (A) Cross section through a serous cystadenoma. Only a thin rim of normal pancreatic parenchyma remains. The cysts are relatively small and contain clear, straw-colored fluid. (B) The cysts are lined by cuboidal epithelium without atypia. Mucinous cystic neoplasm. (C) Cross section through a mucinous multiloculated cyst in the tail of the pancreas. The cysts are large and filled with tenacious mucin. (D) The cysts are lined by columnar mucinous epithelium, with a densely cellular stroma.

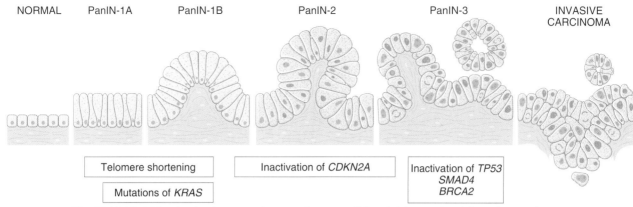

Fig. 13.19 Model for the development of pancreatic cancer. Although it is postulated that telomere shortening and mutations of the *KRAS* oncogene occur at early stages, inactivation of the *CDKN2A* tumor suppressor gene occurs at intermediate stages, and inactivation of the *TP53*, *SMAD4*, and *BRCA2* tumor suppressor genes occurs at late stages, the accumulation of multiple mutations is more important than their occurrence in a specific order. PanIN, Pancreatic intraepithelial neoplasm. The numbers following the labels on the top refer to stages in the development of PanINs. (Modified from Maitra A, Hruban RH: Pancreatic cancer, Annu Rev Pathol Mech Dis 3:157, 2008.)

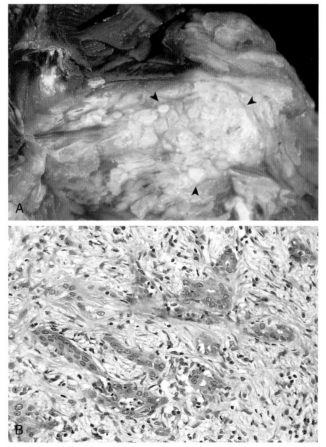

Fig. 13.20 Pancreatic adenocarcinoma. (A) Cross section through the head of the pancreas and adjacent common bile duct showing an ill-defined mass in the pancreatic substance (delineated by the *arrowheads*) and the green discoloration of the duct resulting from obstruction of bile flow. (B) Poorly formed glands are present in a densely fibrotic (desmoplastic) stroma within the tumor.

14

Male Genital Tract, Prostate, and Bladder

OUTLINE

Penis, 240
    Malformations and Inflammatory Lesions, 240
    Neoplasms, 240
Scrotum, Testis, and Epididymis, 240
    Cryptorchidism, 240
    Infections, 241
    Testicular Neoplasms, 241
Prostate, 242
    Benign Prostatic Hyperplasia, 243
    Carcinoma of the Prostate, 243

Ureter, Bladder, and Urethra, 245
    Ureter, 245
    Urinary Bladder, 245
Sexually Transmitted Diseases, 246
    Syphilis, 246
    Gonorrhea, 248
    Nongonococcal Urethritis and Cervicitis, 249
    Trichomoniasis, 249
    Genital Herpes Simplex, 249
    Human Papillomavirus (HPV) Infection, 249

Disorders of the male genital tract manifest mainly as inflammation (often related to sexually transmitted diseases), urinary obstruction, or testicular pain or swelling, and include diseases such as syphilis and testicular and prostate cancer that may have far-reaching systemic effects.

PENIS

Malformations and Inflammatory Lesions

- *Hypospadias.* In hypospadias (1 in 300 live male births), the urethral opening is on the ventral aspect of the penis along the shaft. This anomalous orifice is sometimes constricted, resulting in urinary tract obstruction and an increased risk for urinary tract infections.
- *Inflammatory/infectious lesions* are often caused by poor hygiene in uncircumcised males. *Balanitis* and *balanoposthitis* are local infections of the glans penis and of the overlying prepuce, respectively. Common agents include *Candida albicans* and several types of bacteria.
- *Phimosis* is a condition in which the prepuce cannot be retracted easily over the glans penis. It may be a congenital anomaly, but most cases stem from scarring caused by balanoposthitis.

Neoplasms

Virtually all penile neoplasms arise from squamous epithelium. In the United States, squamous cell carcinoma of the penis is uncommon, but in lower-income countries penile carcinoma occurs at higher rates, mainly in uncircumcised males older than 40 years of age. Poor hygiene, smoking, and infection with human papillomavirus (HPV; particularly the high-risk types 16 and 18) are implicated in the pathogenesis. In some cases, there is a precursor lesion called squamous cell carcinoma in situ *(Bowen disease)* that presents as a solitary plaque on the penis; approximately 10% of these lesions progress to invasive carcinoma (Supplemental eFig. 14.1). Invasive squamous cell carcinoma of the penis appears as an indurated, ulcerated lesion, most commonly on the glans penis (Supplemental eFig. 14.2). Its prognosis depends on the stage of the tumor at diagnosis.

SCROTUM, TESTIS, AND EPIDIDYMIS

Several inflammatory processes affect the skin of the scrotum, including fungal infections and systemic dermatoses such as psoriasis. Scrotal *squamous cell carcinoma* was the first human malignancy associated with environmental exposures, dating from Sir Percival Pott's observation in 1785 of a high incidence of the disease in chimney sweeps. This also led to a remarkably successful public health measure: Frequent bathing virtually eliminated these tumors by washing away the carcinogens in soot. Several disorders unrelated to the testes and epididymis may present as scrotal enlargement. In extreme cases of lymphatic obstruction, caused, for example, by filariasis, the scrotum and the lower extremities may enlarge to enormous sizes, a condition termed *elephantiasis*.

Cryptorchidism

Cryptorchidism is a failure of testicular descent into the scrotum by the age of 1 year.

Normally, the testes descend from the abdominal cavity into the pelvis by the third month of gestation, and then through the inguinal canals into the scrotum during the last 2 months of intrauterine life, but this passage may be delayed, particularly in premature infants. Cryptorchidism affects 1% of males and is of unknown etiology in most cases. It is bilateral in approximately 10% of affected patients. Cryptorchidism has two major consequences:

- *Testicular atrophy and loss of function* occurs in undescended testes. Tubular atrophy begins to appear by 5 to 6 years of age and is usually advanced by puberty (Supplemental eFig. 14.3). Unilateral cryptorchidism may be associated with atrophy of the contralateral descended gonad. Thus, even unilateral cryptorchidism may lead to sterility.
- Failure of testicular descent is associated with a 3- to 5-fold increased risk for *testicular cancer*. Notably, patients with unilateral cryptorchidism are at increased risk for the development of cancer in the contralateral, normally descended testis, again suggesting that cryptorchidism reflects some intrinsic gonadal abnormality.

Infections

Infections more commonly involve the epididymis than the testis proper. Sexually transmitted infectious disorders are discussed later.

- *Mumps orchitis* is rare in children but occurs in roughly 20% of infected adults. Severe mumps orchitis may lead to extensive necrosis of the seminiferous epithelium and atrophy of the seminiferous tubules, fibrosis, and sterility.
- *Tuberculosis* is the most common cause of granulomatous epididymitis. Histologically, there is granulomatous inflammation and caseous necrosis identical to that seen in active tuberculosis in other sites.

Testicular Neoplasms

Testicular neoplasms, mostly arising from germ cells, are the most common neoplasms in males from 15 to 34 years of age.

Testicular neoplasms occur in roughly 6 per 100,000 males. In postpubertal males, 95% of these tumors arise from germ cells and almost all are malignant. The remainder of this discussion is focused on testicular germ cell tumors.

Pathogenesis. The cause of testicular germ cell neoplasms is poorly understood. They are more common in Caucasians than in patients of African descent, and the incidence has increased in Caucasians in recent decades. Approximately 10% of cases are associated with cryptorchidism, with both the undescended and descended testis being at increased risk. Intersex syndromes, including androgen insensitivity syndrome and gonadal dysgenesis, also are associated with an increased frequency of testicular cancer. Brothers of affected males have an 8- to 10-fold increased risk, presumably owing to inherited factors. The development of cancer in one testis also is associated with an increased risk for neoplasia in the contralateral testis.

Most testicular germ cell tumors arise from *germ cell neoplasia in situ*. This precursor lesion is present in conditions associated with a high risk for developing germ cell tumors and is found in "normal" testicular tissue adjacent to germ cell tumors in virtually all cases. Germ cell neoplasia in situ and established neoplasms usually have extra copies of the short arm of chromosome 12 owing to the presence of an isochromosome 12 [i(12p)], but how this abnormality contributes to malignant transformation remains unknown.

Morphology. Testicular germ cell tumors are subclassified into seminomas and nonseminomatous germ cell tumors (Table 14.1). Nonseminomatous germ cell tumors include *embryonal carcinoma, yolk sac tumor, choriocarcinoma,* and *teratoma,* which may occur in "pure" or mixed histologies. These tumors resemble their ovarian homologues (see Chapter 15).

- *Seminoma* is most common, accounting for about 50% of testicular germ cell neoplasms. It presents as a soft, well-demarcated, gray-white tumor composed of large, uniform cells with distinct cell borders, clear cytoplasm, round nuclei, and conspicuous nucleoli (Figs. 14.1 and 14.2). A lymphocytic infiltrate usually is present and some tumors also elicit a granulomatous reaction. In 10%-15% of cases, syncitiotrophoblasts are present that may release sufficient human choriogonadotropin to minimally elevate serum levels.
- *Embryonal carcinoma* presents as an ill-defined, invasive mass containing foci of hemorrhage and necrosis. The neoplastic cells may be arrayed in undifferentiated, solid sheets or form primitive glandular structures and irregular papillae (Fig. 14.3). Embryonal carcinoma is a frequent component of mixed tumors; "pure" embryonal carcinoma accounts for only 2% to 3% of testicular tumors.

Table 14.1 Summary of Testicular Tumors and Associated Serum Markers

Tumor	Peak Patient Age (years)	Tumor Marker(s)
Seminoma	40–50	10% of patients have elevated hCG
Embryonal carcinoma	20–30	Negative (pure embryonal carcinoma)
Spermatocytic tumor	50-60	Negative
Yolk sac tumor	3	90% of patients have elevated AFP
Choriocarcinoma	20–30	100% of patients have elevated hCG
Teratoma	All ages	Negative (pure teratoma)
Mixed tumor	15–30	90% of patients have elevated hCG and AFP

AFP, Alpha-fetoprotein; hCG, human chorionic gonadotropin.

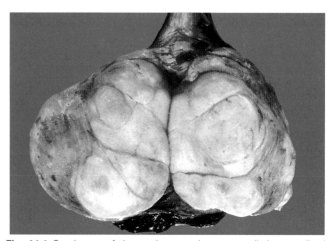

Fig. 14.1 Seminoma of the testis appearing as a well-circumscribed, pale, fleshy, homogeneous mass.

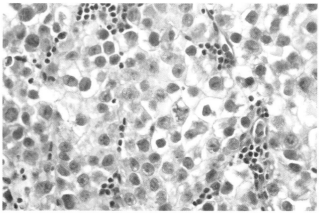

Fig. 14.2 Seminoma of the testis. Microscopic examination reveals large cells with distinct cell borders, pale nuclei, prominent nucleoli, and a sparse lymphocytic infiltrate.

- *Yolk sac tumor* may occur in children or adults; in the latter population, it is often admixed with embryonal carcinoma. Yolk sac tumor is composed of low cuboidal to columnar epithelial cells that form microcysts, lacelike patterns, sheets, glands, and

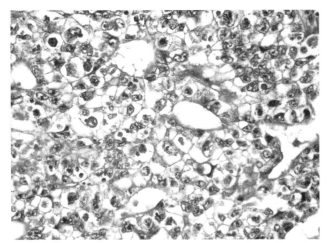

Fig. 14.3 Embryonal carcinoma. Note the sheets of undifferentiated cells forming primitive gland-like structures. The nuclei are large and hyperchromatic.

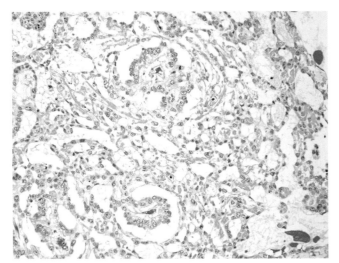

Fig. 14.4 Yolk sac tumor demonstrating areas of loosely textured, microcystic tissue and papillary structures resembling a developing glomerulus (Schiller-Duval bodies).

papillae (Fig. 14.4). These tumors often contain hyaline globules in which α_1-antitrypsin and alpha-fetoprotein are found.

- *Choriocarcinoma* is a tumor in which the pluripotent neoplastic germ cells differentiate into cells resembling placental trophoblasts. The tumor is composed of sheets of small cuboidal cytotrophoblast-like cells that are irregularly intermingled with or capped by large syncytiotrophoblast-like cells containing multiple dark, pleomorphic nuclei (Fig. 14.5). Human chorionic gonadotrophin can be identified in the syncytiotrophoblast-like cells by immunohistochemical staining.
- *Teratoma* is a tumor in which the neoplastic germ cells differentiate along multiple somatic cell lineages. These tumors may occur at any age from infancy to adult life. "Pure" teratoma is fairly common in children, in whom it pursues a benign course. By contrast, in adults pure teratoma is rare (constituting 2% to 3% of germ cell tumors) and is capable of metastasis, regardless of the extent of immature tissue present (in contrast with ovarian teratomas, in which prognosis correlates with the amount of immature tissue present; most are benign). It is composed of a heterogeneous collection of variably differentiated cells or organoid structures, such as neural

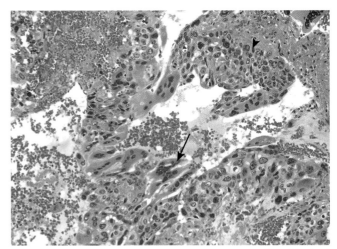

Fig. 14.5 Choriocarcinoma. Both cytotrophoblastic cells with single central nuclei *(arrowhead, upper right)* and syncytiotrophoblastic cells with multiple dark nuclei embedded in eosinophilic cytoplasm *(arrow, middle)* are present. Hemorrhage and necrosis are prominent.

tissue, islands of cartilage, and squamous epithelium, embedded in a fibrous or myxoid stroma (Supplemental eFig. 14.4).
- *Spermatocytic tumor,* formerly called spermatocytic seminoma, is a rare tumor that predominantly affects men over 50 years of age. It is composed of polygonal cells that are arranged in nodules or sheets.

Clinical Features. Testicular germ cell neoplasms most frequently present as painless, solid testicular masses. Because biopsy may lead to tumor seeding along the needle track, solid testicular masses are diagnosed and treated by radical orchiectomy, based on a presumption of malignancy. In other instances, germ cell neoplasms present with widespread metastases, sometimes in the absence of a palpable testicular lesion, particularly in cases of nonseminomatous tumors. Germ cell neoplasms often secrete proteins (summarized in Table 14.1, along with salient clinical features) that are useful in establishing the diagnosis and following the response of the tumor to therapy.

Seminomas and nonseminomatous tumors differ in their behavior and clinical course. Seminomas often remain confined to the testis for long periods and may reach a considerable size before diagnosis. Metastases occur first in abdominal lymph nodes, and hematogenous metastases occur late in the course. Nonseminomatous germ cell neoplasms tend to metastasize earlier by both lymphatic and hematogenous routes. Common sites of metastasis include the liver and lungs.

The treatment of testicular germ cell neoplasms is a remarkable success story: Approximately 95% of affected men are cured. Seminoma, which is extremely radiosensitive and tends to remain localized, has the best prognosis. Of patients with nonseminomatous germ cell tumors, approximately 90% achieve complete remission with conventional chemotherapy, and most are cured. The exception is choriocarcinoma, which has a poor prognosis.

PROSTATE

The prostate can be divided into distinct anatomic regions, the most important of which are the peripheral and transition zones (Fig. 14.6). Most hyperplastic lesions arise in the inner transition zone, and most carcinomas arise in the peripheral zones. As a result, carcinomas are often detected by rectal examination, whereas hyperplasias are more likely to come to attention because of urinary obstruction. The prostate is involved by infectious, inflammatory,

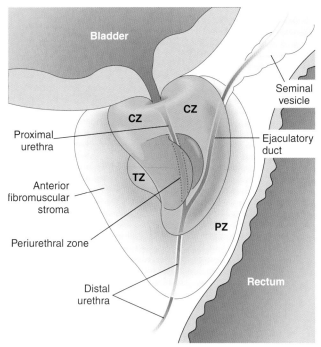

Fig. 14.6 Adult prostate. The normal prostate contains several distinct regions, including a central zone (CZ), a peripheral zone (PZ), a transitional zone (TZ), and a periurethral zone. Most carcinomas arise from the peripheral glands of the organ, whereas nodular hyperplasia arises from more centrally situated glands.

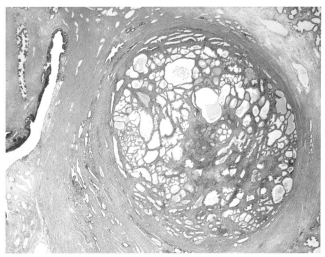

Fig. 14.7 Nodular hyperplasia of the prostate. Low-power photomicrograph demonstrates a well-demarcated nodule at the right of the field, with a portion of urethra seen to the left. In other cases of nodular hyperplasia, the nodularity is caused predominantly by stromal, rather than glandular, proliferation.

hyperplastic, and neoplastic disorders, of which benign prostatic hyperplasia and prostate cancer are the most important clinically.

Benign Prostatic Hyperplasia

Benign prostatic hyperplasia is a common cause of prostatic enlargement and often causes symptoms related to obstruction of the urinary tract.

Benign prostatic hyperplasia (BPH) is present in a significant number of men by 40 years of age, and its frequency increases progressively thereafter, reaching 90% by the eighth decade of life.

Pathogenesis. Although the cause of BPH is incompletely understood, excessive androgen-dependent growth of stromal and glandular elements has a central role. Dihydrotestosterone (DHT), the mediator of prostatic growth, is synthesized in the prostate from circulating testosterone by the enzyme *5α-reductase*. DHT binds and activates nuclear androgen receptors, which regulate the expression of genes that support the growth and survival of prostatic epithelial and stromal cells. However, DHT levels in the prostates of men with and without BPH do not differ significantly; thus, while androgens are needed for BPH to occur, other unknown factors also have key roles.

Morphology. BPH occurs in the inner transition zone of the prostate. The affected prostate is enlarged and contains well-circumscribed nodules that bulge from the cut surface. The urethra is usually compressed, often to a narrow slit, by the hyperplastic nodules, which are composed of variable proportions of glandular elements and fibromuscular stroma (Fig. 14.7).

Clinical Features. The most common manifestations of BPH are related to lower urinary tract obstruction, often in the form of difficulty in starting the stream of urine and intermittent interruption of the urinary stream while voiding. These symptoms frequently are accompanied by urgency, frequency, and nocturia, all indicative of bladder irritation. There is an increased risk of urinary tract infection due to incomplete voiding. In some men, BPH produces complete urinary obstruction, resulting in painful distention of the bladder and, if chronic, hydronephrosis (see Chapter 11). Initial treatment is with drugs that inhibit the formation of DHT (such as 5α-reductase inhibitors) or that relax prostatic smooth muscle by blocking α_1-adrenergic receptors. Various surgical techniques are available for cases that are unresponsive to medical therapy.

Carcinoma of the Prostate

Adenocarcinoma of the prostate is the second most common form of cancer in men, after skin cancer.

Prostate cancer is a disease of older men, and its incidence increases steadily after the age of 50 years. Over the past several decades, mortality rates from prostate cancer have decreased: It currently causes 10% of cancer deaths in American men. The relatively low mortality rate is related in part to increased detection of prostate cancer through screening, but how effective screening is at saving lives is controversial (discussed later).

Pathogenesis. Androgens, heredity, environmental factors, and acquired somatic mutations all have roles in the pathogenesis and progression of prostate cancer.

- *Androgens.* Cancer of the prostate does not develop in males who are castrated before puberty. The dependence on androgens extends to established cancers, which often regress in response to surgical or chemical castration. Moreover, tumors that initially respond to antiandrogen therapy often acquire androgen receptor gene amplifications or mutations that permit signals from androgen receptors to stimulate the expression of various target genes.
- *Heredity.* There is an increased risk among first-degree relatives of patients with prostate cancer. Prostate cancer is uncommon in Asians, and its incidence is highest among men of African descent and in Scandinavian countries. Aggressive disease is more common in African-Americans than in Caucasians.
- *Environment.* One measure of the role of environment is seen in Japanese immigrants to the United States, in whom the incidence of the disease rises. Also, as the diet in Asia becomes more westernized, the incidence of prostate cancer in this region of the world is

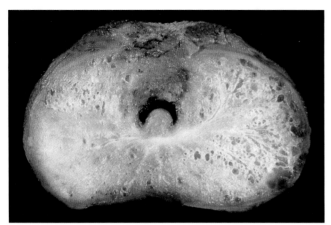

Fig. 14.8 Adenocarcinoma of the prostate. Carcinomatous tissue is seen on the posterior aspect *(lower left)*. Note the solid whiter tissue of cancer, in contrast with the spongy appearance of the benign peripheral zone on the contralateral side.

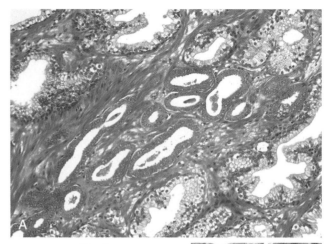

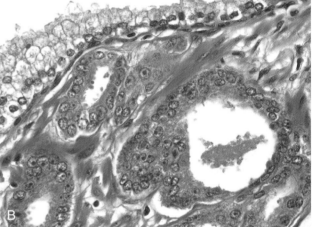

Fig. 14.9 (A) Adenocarcinoma of the prostate demonstrating small glands crowded between larger benign glands. (B) Higher magnification shows several small malignant glands with enlarged nuclei, prominent nucleoli, and dark cytoplasm, as compared with the larger, benign gland *(top)*.

increasing. However, the relationship between specific dietary components and prostate cancer risk is unclear.

- *Acquired genetic aberrations,* as in other cancers, are the actual drivers of cellular transformation. The most common gene rearrangements in prostate cancer create fusion genes consisting of the androgen-regulated promoter of the *TMPRSS2* gene (which contributes only a noncoding regulatory region) and the coding sequence of ETS family transcription factors. These rearrangements drive overexpression of ETS factors in androgen-responsive cells, leading to oncogenic changes in gene expression. Other mutations commonly lead to activation of the PI3K/AKT signaling pathway (see Chapter 5).

Morphology. Advanced cancers are firm, infiltrative lesions with ill-defined margins (Fig. 14.8). Most are moderately differentiated adenocarcinomas that produce well-defined glands lined by a single uniform layer of cuboidal or low columnar epithelium that lack the basal cell layer seen in benign glands (Fig. 14.9). In less differentiated tumors, the glands may have a cribriform appearance or gland formation may be absent altogether. The glandular patterns of growth are the basis for grading tumors using the *Gleason system,* which gives tumors scores of 2 (best) to 10 (worst).

Advanced cancers often infiltrate the seminal vesicles and periurethral zones of the prostate and may invade the adjacent soft tissues, the wall of the urinary bladder, or the rectum. Bone metastases, particularly to the axial skeleton, are frequent late in the disease and typically cause osteoblastic (bone-producing) lesions that can be detected on radionuclide bone scans or other types of imaging studies.

In approximately 80% of cases, prostatic tissue removed for carcinoma also harbors a presumptive precursor lesion referred to as *high-grade prostatic intraepithelial neoplasia (hPIN).* Many of the molecular changes seen in invasive cancers also are present in hPIN.

Clinical Features. In the United States, most prostate cancers are asymptomatic lesions discovered on needle biopsy performed to investigate an elevated serum *prostate-specific antigen* (PSA) level. A subset is detected on digital rectal examination as irregular hard nodules, and others are discovered unexpectedly during histologic examination of prostate tissue removed for BPH.

PSA is a product of normal and neoplastic prostatic epithelium. The PSA serum assay is widely used in the diagnosis and management of prostate cancer but suffers from several limitations. PSA screening can detect prostate cancers early in their course, but many prostate cancers do not cause significant morbidity, even over decades. Overtreatment of these indolent cancers may cause erectile dysfunction and incontinence. A second limitation of PSA is that it is not cancer-specific; BPH, prostatitis, prostatic infarcts, and ejaculation may all increase serum PSA levels. Furthermore, up to 40% of patients with early-stage prostate cancer have PSA values below the cutoffs that are used to identify those who are likely to have prostate cancer. Because of these issues, PSA assays are being reappraised as screening tests. By contrast, once cancer is diagnosed, serial PSA measurements have a clear value in assessing the response to therapy.

Common treatments for localized prostate cancer include radical prostatectomy and radiotherapy. The prognosis after radical prostatectomy depends on the pathologic stage, whether the margins of the resected specimen are free of tumor, and the Gleason score. The Gleason score, clinical stage, and PSA values are important predictors of the outcome after radiotherapy. Because many prostate cancers never cause disease, "watchful waiting" is an appropriate approach for older men, patients with significant comorbidity, and even younger men with low serum PSA values and small, low-grade cancers. Metastatic carcinoma is treated by androgen deprivation, often by administration of gonadotropin–releasing hormone agonists or drugs that interfere with androgen synthesis.

URETER, BLADDER, AND URETHRA

The renal pelves, ureters, bladder, and urethra are lined by a specialized multilayer transitional epithelium called urothelium. Beneath the mucosa lie the lamina propria and the muscularis propria (detrusor muscle), which makes up the bladder wall. Clinically significant disorders involving these organs include congenital aberrations, infectious and other inflammatory diseases, and neoplasms.

Ureter

Disorders of the ureter are uncommon and include congenital disorders, neoplasms, and reactive conditions. Several merit brief mention.
- *Vesicoureteral reflux* is defined as retrograde flow of urine from the bladder into the renal pelvis during bladder contraction. It is most often due to congenital absence or shortening of the intravesical portion of the ureter, such that it is not compressed during micturition, and is estimated to affect 1% to 2% of children. There is an increased risk of kidney infection due to incomplete voiding of urine.
- *Ureteropelvic junction obstruction*, a congenital disorder, is the most frequent cause of hydronephrosis in infants and children. It usually manifests in infancy or childhood and is much more common in boys than in girls.
- *Retroperitoneal fibrosis* is an uncommon cause of ureteral narrowing or obstruction characterized by an inflammatory process associated with fibrosis that encases the retroperitoneal structures and causes hydronephrosis in middle-aged and older adults. A proportion of cases are caused by *IgG4-related disease,* characterized by fibroinflammatory lesions rich in IgG4-secreting plasma cells. Other cases are associated with exposure to drugs (e.g., ergot derivatives, adrenergic blockers), radiation, infection, prior surgery, or malignant disease (lymphomas, urinary tract carcinomas).

Urinary Bladder

The bladder may be affected by nonneoplastic conditions or neoplasms. The most important nonneoplastic condition involving the bladder is cystitis, which may be inflammatory or infectious in origin.
- *Bacterial cystitis* is common, particularly in women. The most common etiologic agents are enteric bacteria.
- *Hemorrhagic cystitis* may occur in patients receiving cytotoxic antitumor drugs, such as cyclophosphamide, and sometimes complicates adenovirus infection.

- *Malakoplakia* is an uncommon inflammatory disease that most commonly occurs in the bladder. It results from defects in the phagocytic or degradative function of macrophages, often in the setting of some type of acquired immune deficiency (e.g., HIV infection). Undigested bacterial products accumulate within distended phagosomes, which are seen in histologic sections as abundant granular material within the cytoplasm of macrophages (Supplemental eFig. 14.5).

Bladder Cancer

Bladder cancer accounts for approximately 5% of cancers and 3% of cancer deaths in the United States. The vast majority are urothelial carcinomas occurring in adults older than the age of 50 years. Environmental risk factors include cigarette smoking, various occupational carcinogens, and prior cyclophosphamide or radiation therapy. A family history of bladder cancer also is a risk factor.

Squamous cell carcinomas make up about 5% of bladder cancers in the United States but are much more common in countries such as Egypt, where *Schistosoma haematobium* infection is endemic. The resultant squamous metaplasia and chronic cystitis predispose to cancer development (see Chapter 5).

Pathogenesis. Two different molecular pathways leading to the development of urothelial carcinoma have been described, one in tumors

Morphology. Invasive urothelial carcinoma often arises from precursor lesions with papillary or flat growth patterns, the latter corresponding to *carcinoma in situ*. The most important prognostic factor in noninvasive papillary urothelial neoplasms is the tumor grade, which is based on both architectural and cytologic features (Fig. 14.10). Carcinoma in situ is defined by the presence of cells in the epithelium that appear overtly malignant (Fig. 14.11). It often is multifocal (Supplemental eFig. 14.6) and sometimes involves most of the bladder surface or extends into the ureters and urethra. In both high-grade papillary urothelial carcinoma and carcinoma in situ, the cells lack cohesiveness and are shed into the urine, where they can be detected by cytology.

Invasive urothelial carcinoma may superficially invade the lamina propria or extend more deeply into underlying muscle. The extent of invasion and spread (tumor stage) at the time of initial diagnosis is the most important prognostic factor.

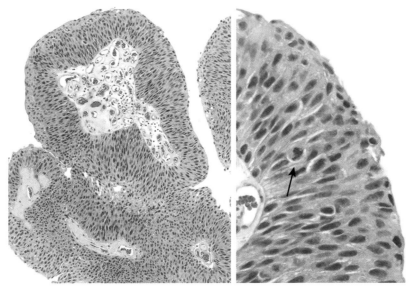

Fig. 14.10 Noninvasive low-grade papillary urothelial carcinoma. Higher magnification *(right)* shows slightly irregular nuclei with scattered mitotic figures *(arrow).*

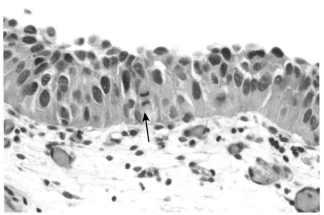

Fig. 14.11 Carcinoma in situ (CIS) of urinary bladder with enlarged hyperchromatic nuclei and a mitotic figure *(arrow).*

with a papillary growth pattern and the second in tumors that arise from carcinoma in situ. Acquired loss-of-function mutations in *TP53* and deletion of an unidentified tumor suppressor gene on chromosome 9 play central roles in both.

Clinical Features. Bladder carcinoma most commonly presents with painless hematuria. Urothelial tumors, whatever their grade, have a strong tendency to recur. Many recurrent tumors arise at sites different from that of the original lesion, yet share many of the exact same clonal abnormalities as those of the initial tumor. This finding suggests that these recurrences are produced by tumor cells that shed from the primary tumor and implant at distant sites.

Treatment depends on the tumor grade, stage, and growth pattern. For small, localized papillary tumors that are not of a high grade, transurethral resection is sufficient. Patients with tumors that are at high risk for recurrence or progression typically are treated with intravesical instillation of an attenuated strain of the tuberculosis bacillus called *Bacillus Calmette-Guérin (BCG),* sometimes followed by intravesical

chemotherapy. BCG elicits a granulomatous inflammatory reaction that triggers an effective local antitumor immune response. Radical cystectomy is reserved for tumors that invade the muscularis propria and those that are refractory to BCG. Metastatic bladder cancer is treated using chemotherapy, which is palliative but not curative.

SEXUALLY TRANSMITTED DISEASES

Globally, approximately 15 million new cases of sexually transmitted diseases occur every year and include infections caused by viruses, bacteria, and protozoans. Women are more likely to become infected and to be asymptomatic. In the United States, genital herpes and genital HPV infection are the most common STDs, but several other types merit discussion because they cause significant morbidity. Although these infections affect both men and women, they are discussed here together (Table 14.2).

Syphilis

Syphilis is a chronic venereal infection caused by the spirochete *Treponema pallidum.*

In the United States, the incidence of primary and secondary syphilis has risen at least three-fold since the year 2000, mostly due to an increased incidence among men who have sex with men. A strong racial disparity is evident; people of African descent are affected six times more often than Caucasians. Syphilis also is more common in HIV-infected patients, in whom it is more likely to progress to organ involvement and neurosyphilis.

Pathogenesis. The usual source of infection is contact with a cutaneous or mucosal lesion in a sexual partner in the early (primary or secondary) stages of syphilis. The organism is transmitted from such lesions during sexual activity through breaks in the skin or mucous membranes of the uninfected partner. In congenital cases, *T. pallidum* is transmitted across the placenta from mother to fetus, particularly during the early stages of maternal infection.

Once introduced, the organisms rapidly disseminate through lymphatics and the blood, even before the appearance of lesions at the

Table 14.2 Sexually Transmitted Diseases

Pathogen	Males	Both	Females
		Associated Disease(s)—Distribution by Gender	
Viruses			
Herpes simplex virus		Primary and recurrent herpes, neonatal herpes	
Hepatitis B virus		Hepatitis	
Human papillomavirus	Cancer of penis (some cases)	Condyloma acuminatum, anal cancer, oropharyngeal carcinoma	Cervical dysplasia and cancer, vulvar cancer
Human immunodeficiency virus		Acquired immunodeficiency syndrome	
Bacteria			
Neisseria gonorrhoeae	Epididymitis, prostatitis, urethral stricture	Urethritis, proctitis, pharyngitis, disseminated gonococcal infection	Cervicitis, endometritis, bartholinitis, salpingitis, and sequelae (infertility, ectopic pregnancy, recurrent salpingitis)
Chlamydia trachomatis	Urethritis, epididymitis, proctitis		Urethral syndrome, cervicitis, bartholinitis, salpingitis, and sequelae
Ureaplasma urealyticum	Urethritis		Cervicitis
Treponema pallidum		Syphilis	
Protozoa			
Trichomonas vaginalis	Urethritis, balanitis		Vaginitis

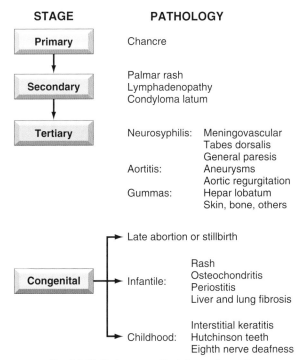

STAGE **PATHOLOGY**

Primary — Chancre

Secondary — Palmar rash
Lymphadenopathy
Condyloma latum

Tertiary — Neurosyphilis: Meningovascular
Tabes dorsalis
General paresis
Aortitis: Aneurysms
Aortic regurgitation
Gummas: Hepar lobatum
Skin, bone, others

Congenital —
Late abortion or stillbirth

Infantile: Rash
Osteochondritis
Periostitis
Liver and lung fibrosis

Childhood: Interstitial keratitis
Hutchinson teeth
Eighth nerve deafness

Fig. 14.12 Protean manifestations of syphilis.

primary inoculation site. This widespread dissemination accounts for the protean manifestations of the disease (Fig. 14.12), which in adults can be divided into primary, secondary, and tertiary stages.

- *Primary syphilis.* Several weeks after infection, a primary lesion, termed a *chancre,* appears at the point of spirochete entry. During systemic dissemination of organisms, the host mounts an immune response. The organism elicits antibodies specific for treponemal antigens and others that cross-react with host constituents (nontreponemal antibodies), but the humoral response fails to eradicate the organism.
- *Secondary syphilis.* The chancre of primary syphilis resolves over a period of 4 to 6 weeks and is followed in approximately 25% of untreated patients by the development of secondary syphilis, characterized by mucocutaneous lesions and generalized lymphadenopathy. The mucocutaneous lesions of both primary and secondary syphilis are teeming with spirochetes and thus are highly infectious.
- *Tertiary syphilis.* The lesions of secondary syphilis also resolve spontaneously, and untreated patients enter an asymptomatic *latent* phase, defined as being more than 1 year after the initial infection. In about one third of cases, symptoms develop anew over the next 5 to 20 years. This late symptomatic phase, or tertiary syphilis, is marked by the development of lesions in the cardiovascular system, central nervous system, or, less frequently, other organs. Spirochetes are much more difficult to detect during the later stages of disease, and patients are accordingly unlikely to be infectious.

T. pallidum also may be transmitted across the placenta from an infected mother to the fetus at any time during pregnancy, leading to the development of *congenital syphilis.* The likelihood of transmission is greatest during the primary and secondary stages of disease in the mother, when spirochetes are numerous. Manifestations of maternal disease may be subtle, mandating routine serologic testing for syphilis in all pregnancies. Many infected infants die *in utero,* typically after the fourth month of gestation, while those who survive present at birth or in infancy with a variety of findings related to chronic infection and inflammation (described next). The incidence of congenital syphilis is expected to rise due to increased maternal infection rates.

Morphology. The pathognomonic lesion is a *proliferative endarteritis* of small arterioles accompanied by an inflammatory infiltrate rich in plasma cells. It is thought that the host immune response is responsible for the endothelial cell activation and proliferation that are the hallmark of the endarteritis, which eventually leads to perivascular fibrosis, luminal narrowing, and ischemic tissue damage.

Both primary and secondary syphilis are associated with characteristic lesions. The *primary chancre* is usually on the glans, corona, or perianal region in males, whereas in females, multiple chancres may be present, usually on the labia or vagina as well as the perianal region. The lesion develops 2 to 4 weeks after sexual exposure as a small, firm papule that enlarges to produce a painless ulcer with well-defined, indurated margins and a "clean," moist base (Fig. 14.13). Microscopic examination reveals the typical lymphocytic and plasmacytic inflammatory infiltrate and endarteritis. Spirochetes are readily demonstrable with silver stains or immunohistochemical stains specific for spirochetes (Supplemental eFig. 14.7).

Within approximately 2 months of resolution of the chancre, the lesions of secondary syphilis appear. The manifestations are varied but typically include a variety of *mucocutaneous lesions.* Skin lesions usually are symmetrically distributed; may be maculopapular, scaly, or pustular; and characteristically involve the palms of the hands and soles of the feet. In moist skin areas, such as the anogenital region, inner thighs, and axillae, broad-based, elevated lesions termed *condylomata lata* may appear. Similar mucosal lesions may also occur in the oral cavity and pharynx. The mucocutaneous lesions also show the characteristic proliferative endarteritis and abundant spirochetes.

Lesions associated with tertiary syphilis develop in approximately one third of untreated patients, usually after a latent period of 5 years or more. These fall into three major categories, which may occur singly or in combination: cardiovascular syphilis, neurosyphilis, and so-called "benign" tertiary syphilis. Cardiovascular syphilis takes the form of *syphilitic aortitis* and accounts for more than 80% of cases of tertiary disease. *Neurosyphilis* accounts for 10% of cases of tertiary syphilis overall and occurs at a higher frequency in those with HIV. There are two clinical manifestations of neurosyphilis: *general paresis,* characterized by dementia; and *tabes dorsalis,* characterized by involvement of the posterior columns of the spinal cord and dorsal nerve roots. In benign tertiary syphilis, there is the formation of *gummas* in multiple organs. Gummas have a zone of coagulative necrosis surrounded by dense fibrous tissue and a mixed inflammatory infiltrate suggestive of a delayed hypersensitivity reaction (Supplemental eFig. 14.8). Once common, gummas are now rare due to the use of effective antibiotics such as penicillin and occur mainly in patients with AIDS.

Manifestations of congenital syphilis include stillbirth, infantile syphilis, and late (tardive) congenital syphilis. Infantile syphilis refers to congenital syphilis in infants that manifests at birth or within the first few months of life. Affected infants present with rhinitis (snuffles) and mucocutaneous lesions similar to those seen in adults with secondary syphilis. Visceral and skeletal changes also may be present. Late congenital syphilis is an untreated case of congenital syphilis of more than 2 years' duration. Classic manifestations include the *Hutchinson triad:* notched central incisors, blindness from corneal inflammation, and deafness from eighth cranial nerve injury. Other changes include "saber shin" deformity caused by chronic inflammation of the periosteum of the tibia, deformed molar teeth, meningitis, chorioretinitis, and gummas of the nasal bone and cartilage resulting in "saddlenose" deformity.

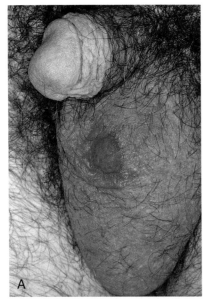

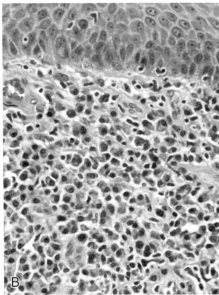

Fig. 14.13 (A) Syphilitic chancre of the scrotum. Such lesions typically are painless despite the presence of ulceration. (B) Histologic features of the chancre include a diffuse plasma cell infiltrate beneath squamous epithelium of skin.

Clinical Features. Serology is the mainstay of diagnosis and includes tests for nontreponemal and treponemal antibodies. *Nontreponemal antibody tests* measure antibody to cardiolipin, an antigen that is present in both host tissues and the treponemal cell wall. These tests are usually positive by 4 to 6 weeks of infection and are strongly positive in the secondary phase of infection. Up to 15% of positive nontreponemal antibody tests are unrelated to syphilis. These false-positive results increase in frequency with age and are associated with a variety of conditions, including the antiphospholipid syndrome (see Chapter 3). *Treponemal antibody tests* also become positive by 4 to 6 weeks after an infection. As with all serologic tests for infection, certain pitfalls must be considered, such as the confounding influence of defective immunity, particularly in those who are HIV-infected.

Gonorrhea

Gonorrhea is second only to chlamydial infection among reportable communicable diseases in the United States.

Coinfection of gonorrhea with other STDs is common, particularly infection with *Chlamydia trachomatis*, which is found in 30% of males with gonorrhea. The gravity of gonococcal infections has increased with the emergence of strains of *Neisseria gonorrhoeae* that are resistant to multiple antibiotics.

Pathogenesis. Humans are the only natural reservoir for *N. gonorrhoeae*. The organism is highly fastidious, and spread of infection requires direct contact with the mucosa of an infected individual, usually during sexual activity. The bacteria first attach to mucosal epithelium using structures termed pili. Such attachment prevents the organism from being flushed away by body fluids such as urine or endocervical mucus. The attached organism then penetrates through the epithelial cells to invade the deeper tissues of the host.

Morphology. *N. gonorrhoeae* provokes an intense acute inflammatory reaction. In males, this manifests most often as a purulent urethral discharge associated with an inflamed urethral meatus. Gram-negative diplococci, some within neutrophils, are identified in Gram stains of the purulent exudate. Ascending infection may lead to prostatitis, epididymitis, or orchitis (Supplemental eFig. 14.9). In females, infection of the Bartholin glands is fairly common. Infection may ascend through the uterus to produce salpingitis, sometimes complicated by tuboovarian abscesses. The inflammatory process leads to the development of granulation tissue and scarring, resulting in strictures and other deformities and giving rise to *pelvic inflammatory disease* (see Chapter 15).

Clinical Features. In infected males, gonorrhea is manifested by dysuria, urinary frequency, and a mucopurulent urethral exudate within 2 to 14 days of initial infection. Treatment with antibiotics eradicates the organism and leads to prompt resolution of symptoms. Untreated infections may ascend to involve the prostate, seminal vesicles, epididymis, and testis, or give rise to an asymptomatic carrier state, which is seen in less than 5% of infected males.

Among female patients, acute infections acquired by vaginal intercourse may be asymptomatic or may be associated with dysuria, lower pelvic pain, and vaginal discharge. Scarring of the fallopian tubes may produce infertility and increase the risk for ectopic pregnancy. Infection may spread to the peritoneal cavity. Other sites of primary infection in both males and females include the oropharynx and the anorectal area.

Disseminated infection occurs in 0.5% to 3% of cases of gonorrhea, particularly with strains resistant to the lytic effects of complement. It is more frequent in females than in males. Manifestations include tenosynovitis, arthritis, and pustular or hemorrhagic skin lesions, and (rarely) endocarditis and meningitis.

Gonococcal infection also may be transmitted to infants during passage through the birth canal. The affected neonate may develop purulent infection of the eyes *(ophthalmia neonatorum)*, an important historic cause of blindness. The routine application of antibiotic ointment to the eyes of newborns has markedly reduced this disorder.

Both culture and molecular tests that detect organism-specific nucleic acids can be used to diagnose gonococcal infections. The advantage of culture is that it permits determination of antibiotic sensitivity. Nucleic acid–based tests are more rapid and somewhat more sensitive than culture, and are being used increasingly.

Nongonococcal Urethritis and Cervicitis

Nongonococcal urethritis and cervicitis are the most common forms of STD.

In the United States, most cases with known causes are attributed to *Chlamydia trachomatis,* with *Mycoplasma genitalium* running a close second, but in almost 50% of cases no pathogen is identified. As discussed earlier, chlamydial and gonorrheal coinfections are common.

Pathogenesis. *C. trachomatis* is a gram-negative bacterium that exists in two forms. The infectious form, the elementary body, is capable of survival in the extracellular environment. The elementary body has tropism for columnar epithelial cells and is taken up by receptor-mediated endocytosis into host cells, where it differentiates into a metabolically active form, termed the reticulate body. Using the energy sources of the host cell, the reticulate body replicates and ultimately forms new infectious elementary bodies, which propagate the infection.

Clinical Features. *C. trachomatis* infections are associated with a range of findings that are virtually indistinguishable from those of infections with *N. gonorrhoeae.* Patients typically present 1 to 5 weeks after exposure with dysuria with or without urethral discharge. *C. trachomatis* may give rise to epididymitis, prostatitis, pelvic inflammatory disease, pharyngitis, conjunctivitis, peritoneal inflammation, and, among individuals who engage in anal sex, proctitis. A large percentage of both men and women, however, are asymptomatic (but capable of spreading the infection). The infection may be transmitted to newborns during vaginal birth. Up to 15% of exposed newborns develop chlamydial pneumonia and 50% develop chlamydial conjunctivitis. Another important manifestation of chlamydial infection is *reactive arthritis* (formerly Reiter syndrome), discussed further in Chapter 18. The diagnosis is made by a nucleic acid amplification test on voided urine.

Trichomoniasis

***Trichomonas vaginalis* is a sexually transmitted protozoan that is a frequent cause of vaginitis.**

The trophozoite form adheres to the mucosa, where it causes superficial lesions. In women, *T. vaginalis* infection often is associated with loss of acid-producing commensal lactobacilli (e.g., due to treatment with antibiotics), which allows the pathogenic organisms to become established. The incubation period is 4 to 28 days and may be asymptomatic or associated with pruritus and a frothy, yellow vaginal discharge. Urethral colonization may cause urinary frequency and dysuria. *T. vaginalis* infection typically is asymptomatic in males but in some cases may manifest as nongonococcal urethritis. The organism usually is demonstrable in smears of vaginal scrapings.

Genital Herpes Simplex

Genital infections caused by herpes simplex virus (HSV) are a very common form of STD. There are two types, HSV-1 and HSV-2. One in six persons between the ages of 14 and 49 years has HSV-2 infection in the United States. Most cases of anogenital herpes are caused by HSV-2, but recent years have seen a rise in the number of genital infections caused by HSV-1 because of the increasing practice of oral sex.

Pathogenesis. As with other STDs, the risk for infection is directly related to the number of sexual contacts. Up to 95% of HIV-positive men who have sex with men are seropositive for HSV-1 and/or HSV-2. HSV is transmitted when the virus comes into contact with a mucosal surface or broken skin of a susceptible host. Such transmission requires direct contact with an infected individual, because the virus is readily inactivated at room temperature, particularly if dried.

Morphology. The lesions of genital HSV infection appear as erythematous vesicles on the mucosa or skin of the lower genitalia and adjacent extragenital sites. The vesicles contain necrotic cellular debris, neutrophils, and cells harboring characteristic intranuclear viral inclusions. Infected cells commonly fuse to form multinucleate syncytia. The inclusions stain with antibodies to HSV, permitting a rapid, specific diagnosis of HSV infection in histologic sections or smears.

Clinical Features. HSV-1 and HSV-2 produce indistinguishable primary or recurrent mucocutaneous lesions. Primary infection may be asymptomatic or may produce a variety of signs and symptoms. Painful vesicular lesions may be accompanied by dysuria, urethral discharge, lymph node enlargement and tenderness, and systemic manifestations, such as fever, muscle aches, and headache, all of which may last for several weeks. HSV is shed during this period and may continue for as long as 3 months after the initial infection. Recurrences are milder and of shorter duration than in the primary episode. The diagnosis is most often made by viral culture or nucleic acid amplification testing of fluid collected after "unroofing" of a vesicular lesion. In immunocompetent adults, genital herpes generally is not life threatening. However, HSV is a major threat to immunosuppressed patients, in whom disseminated, even fatal, disease may develop. Also life threatening is *neonatal herpes infection,* which occurs in about half of infants delivered vaginally of mothers with either primary or recurrent genital HSV infection. Its incidence has risen in parallel with the rise in genital HSV infection. The manifestations of neonatal herpes vary from infection of superficial sites (skin, eyes, and mouth) to involvement of the CNS, with or without infection of other organs such as the liver and lungs. Approximately 60% of affected infants die of the disease, and half of the survivors have substantial morbidity.

Human Papillomavirus (HPV) Infection

Human papillomavirus causes squamous proliferations in the genital tract, including genital warts and precancerous lesions at risk for transformation to carcinoma.

Condylomata acuminata, also known as *venereal warts,* are caused by low-risk HPV types 6 and 11. These lesions occur on the penis and the female genitalia. Genital HPV infection may be transmitted to neonates during vaginal delivery. Recurrent, potentially life-threatening papillomas of the upper respiratory tract may develop subsequently in affected infants. Precancerous lesions most commonly involve the cervix (see Chapter 15) but also occur in the penis, vulva, oropharyngeal tonsil, and conjunctiva. They are caused by high-risk HPV types, such as types 16 and 18.

Morphology. In males, condylomata acuminata usually occur on the coronal sulcus or inner surface of the prepuce, where they range in size from small, sessile lesions to large, papillary proliferations measuring several centimeters in diameter (Supplemental eFig. 14.10). In females, they commonly occur on the vulva (Supplemental eFig. 14.11). Examples of the microscopic appearance of these lesions are presented in Chapter 15.

15

Female Genital Tract and Breast

OUTLINE

Vulva, 250
  Vulvitis, 250
  Tumors, 250
Vagina, 250
  Vaginitis, 251
Cervix, 251
  Cervicitis, 251
  Neoplasia of the Cervix, 251
Uterus, 253
  Endometritis, 253
  Endometriosis, 253
  Abnormal Uterine Bleeding, 254
  Proliferative Lesions of the Endometrium and Myometrium, 254

Fallopian Tubes, 256
Ovaries, 256
  Tumors of the Ovary, 256
Diseases of Pregnancy, 258
  Placental Inflammations and Infections, 258
  Ectopic Pregnancy, 258
  Gestational Trophoblastic Disease, 258
  Preeclampsia and Eclampsia, 259
Breast, 260
  Inflammatory Processes, 260
  Stromal Neoplasms, 260
  Benign Epithelial Lesions, 260
  Carcinoma, 261

VULVA

The vulva is the external female genitalia, including the hair-bearing skin (labia majora) and mucosa (labia minora). Most disorders of the vulva are inflammatory or infectious. Malignant tumors of the vulva occur and may be life threatening but are rare.

Vulvitis

A common cause of vulvitis is an inflammatory reaction to irritants or allergens. Both manifest as erythematous weeping and crusting papules and plaques. Vulvitis is also often caused by sexually transmitted infections, particularly those due to human papillomavirus (HPV, discussed later), herpes simplex virus (HSV-1 or HSV-2), *Neisseria gonorrhoeae,* and *Treponema pallidum,* the cause of syphilis (see Chapter 14). *Candida* is also a cause of vulvitis, but it is not sexually transmitted. An important complication of vulvitis, particularly that caused by gonorrhea, is obstruction of the excretory ducts of the Bartholin glands. This blockage may result in painful dilation of the glands *(Bartholin cyst)* and abscess formation.

Tumors

Condyloma Acuminatum

Condyloma acuminatum is a warty vulvar lesion caused by human papillomavirus infection.

These lesions may be papillary and elevated or flat and rough-surfaced (Fig. 15.1A). They occur anywhere on the anogenital surface, usually as multiple lesions. Identical lesions occur in men on the penis. The characteristic cellular feature is *koilocytosis,* a cytopathic change marked by perinuclear cytoplasmic vacuolization and a wrinkled nuclear contour (Fig. 15.1B). More than 90% of condylomata acuminata are positive for HPV subtypes 6 or 11, which are transmitted sexually. HPV 6 and 11 are low-risk types, and vulvar condylomas do not progress to cancer. HPV vaccines afford protection against the development of condyloma acuminatum.

Carcinoma of the Vulva

Carcinoma of the vulva is uncommon and mainly occurs in women older than 60 years of age. Most are squamous cell carcinomas. Clear cell adenocarcinoma is rare; historically, it was associated with in utero exposure to diethylstilbestrol, a treatment for threatened miscarriage that is no longer in use.

Pathogenesis. Two types of vulvar squamous cell carcinoma with differing pathogenesis are recognized. The HPV-associated type is caused by infection with high-risk HPV (especially HPV type 16); it occurs in middle-aged women and is preceded by precancerous changes. Progression to invasive carcinoma is more likely in the setting of immunodeficiency (e.g., HIV infection). HPV-negative squamous carcinoma occurs in older women, sometimes in the setting of lichen sclerosus, an inflammatory skin condition of uncertain etiology that also produces vulvar epithelial atrophy and fibrosis.

> *Morphology.* Precursor lesions and early vulvar squamous cell carcinomas commonly manifest as smooth whitish plaques *(leukoplakia).* HPV-positive tumors are often multifocal and warty and tend to be poorly differentiated, whereas HPV-negative tumors usually are solitary and well differentiated (Supplemental eFig. 15.1).

Clinical Features. Both forms of vulvar carcinoma tend to remain confined to their site of origin for a few years but ultimately invade and spread, usually to regional lymph nodes. The risk of metastasis correlates with the depth of invasion. As with most carcinomas, the outcome is dependent on the tumor stage.

VAGINA

Congenital anomalies of the vagina are uncommon and include entities such as total absence of the vagina or a septate or double vagina.

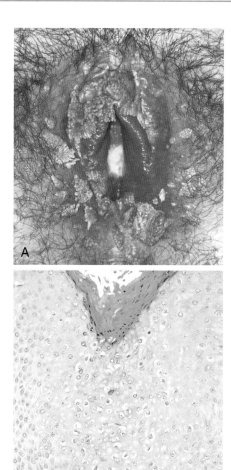

Fig. 15.1 (A) Numerous condylomas of the vulva. (B) Histopathologic features of condyloma acuminatum include acanthosis (thickening of the squamous layer), hyperkeratosis, and cytoplasmic vacuolization (koilocytosis, *center*). (A, Courtesy Dr. Alex Ferenczy, McGill University, Montreal, Quebec, Canada.)

Acquired disorders are most likely to be due to secondary spread of cancers or infections involving nearby organs. A few infections of the vagina occur with some frequency and are discussed next.

Vaginitis

Vaginitis is common but is usually transient and of little clinical consequence. A variety of organisms have been implicated. Many are normal commensals that become pathogenic in the setting of diabetes, systemic antibiotic therapy (which disrupts the normal microbial flora), immunodeficiency, pregnancy, or recent abortion. The most frequent offenders are *Candida albicans* and *Trichomonas vaginalis*. Symptomatic *Candida* infection usually occurs in the setting of one of the predisposing influences listed above and is characterized by a thick white discharge *(leukorrhea)*. *T. vaginalis* is sexually transmitted and produces a watery, gray-green discharge in which parasites can be identified by microscopy.

CERVIX

The most common cervical lesions are inflammatory or infectious (cervicitis). One of these infectious agents, HPV, is the central actor in the development of cancer of the cervix.

Cervicitis

The most important causes of cervicitis are sexually transmitted diseases, including infections caused by *Chlamydia trachomatis, Ureaplasma urealyticum, T. vaginalis, N. gonorrhoeae,* HSV-2 (the agent of genital herpes), and HPV. *C. trachomatis* is the most common agent, accounting for as many as 40% of cases of cervicitis. Although less common, HSV infections are noteworthy because maternal–infant transmission during childbirth may result in serious, sometimes fatal, systemic herpetic infection in the newborn. Cervicitis commonly comes to attention on routine examination or because of leukorrhea. It often is treated empirically with antibiotics that are active against *Chlamydia* and gonococci.

Neoplasia of the Cervix

Most tumors of the cervix are caused by oncogenic strains of HPV.

HPV is detectable in squamous intraepithelial lesions (SILs), which are precancerous lesions, and in nearly all cervical carcinomas. Important risk factors for the development of SILs and carcinoma are directly related to HPV exposure and include early age at first intercourse, multiple sexual partners, a male partner with multiple sexual partners, and persistent infection by high-risk strains of HPV.

Pathogenesis. HPV has a tropism for the immature squamous cells of the transformation zone, an area of squamous metaplasia at the junction of the cervical squamous mucosa and the columnar mucosa of the endocervical canal (Fig. 15.2). Most HPV infections are transient and are eliminated by the host immune response. A subset of infections persists, however, and some cause SILs, from which invasive cervical carcinoma may develop.

High-risk strains of HPV (e.g., types 16 and 18) encode two oncoproteins, E6 and E7, that inhibit the functions of the p53 and RB tumor suppressor proteins, respectively (see Chapter 5). They promote cell survival in the presence of DNA breaks (by inhibiting p53) and enhance epithelial cell proliferation and delaying squamous cell maturation (by inhibiting RB). High-risk HPV variants are more likely to cause persistent infections and to integrate into the genome of host cells, two features that correlate with progression to cancer. Viral integration contributes to transformation by disrupting an HPV gene that negatively regulates E6 and E7, increasing their expression. By contrast, low-risk HPV variants (e.g., types 6 and 11) associated with the development of condylomas of the lower genital tract (Fig. 15.3) express E6 and E7 variants with different or weaker activities and do not integrate into the host genome.

Squamous Intraepithelial Lesion

HPV-related carcinogenesis begins with precancerous epithelial changes termed squamous intraepithelial lesions.

Squamous intraepithelial lesions (SILs) peak in incidence at about 30 years of age, roughly 15 years before the peak incidence of cervical carcinomas. The lesions are subclassified into two types:
- Low-grade SIL (LSIL), previously called cervical intraepithelial neoplasia (CIN) I, is associated with productive HPV infection and does not progress directly to invasive carcinoma. Most LSILs regress, and only a small percentage progress to HSIL.
- High-grade SIL (HSIL), previously designated CIN II and CIN III, demonstrates increased proliferation, arrested epithelial maturation, and lower levels of viral replication. HSIL has a relatively high risk for progression to carcinoma.

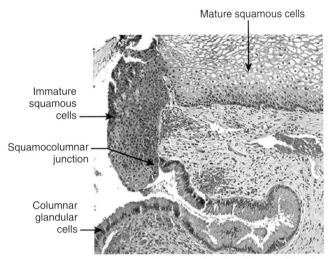

Fig. 15.2 Cervical transformation zone showing the transition from mature glycogenated squamous epithelium, to immature metaplastic squamous cells, to columnar endocervical glandular epithelium. This is the region where human papillomavirus (HPV) infection occurs and cervical neoplasia originates.

Clinical Features. SIL is asymptomatic and is diagnosed following an abnormal cytologic finding detected by a Pap test. In the United States, Pap screening has sharply lowered the incidence of invasive cervical tumors, but the observed incidence of SIL has increased, probably owing to increased detection. Tests to identify HPV DNA

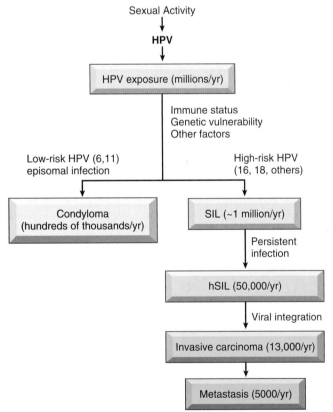

Fig. 15.3 Consequences of human papillomavirus (HPV) infection. Progression is associated with integration of virus and acquisition of additional mutations, as discussed in the text. SIL, Squamous intraepithelial lesion; hSIL, high-grade squamous intraepithelial lesion.

Morphology. Fig. 15.4 illustrates the histologic stages of SIL. LSIL is characterized by dysplastic changes in the lower third of the mucosa and koilocytic change superficially, and HSIL shows dysplasia (variation in cell and nuclear size) and mitoses, some atypical, in upper layers of the epithelium; koilocytic change is usually absent. When dysplasia affects the entire thickness of the epithelium, it is called *carcinoma in situ.* Supplemental eFigure 15.2 shows the cytologic appearance of normal cervical squamous cells, LSIL, and HSIL in cervical Papanicolau smears. Note the reduction in cytoplasm and the increase in the nucleus-to-cytoplasm ratio that occurs as the grade of the lesion increases, reflecting the progressive loss of cellular differentiation on the surface of the lesions.

from cervical scrapings are highly sensitive but not as specific for SIL as cytologic examination, because most HPV infections do not progress to SIL. Therefore, HPV DNA screening is recommended for women older than 30 years; a positive test in this population is more likely to identify a persistent infection that may lead to neoplasia.

Positive Pap tests typically lead to cervical biopsy, performed to subclassify the lesion. Women with biopsy-documented LSIL are managed with observation, whereas HSILs and persistent LSILs are treated with surgical excision (cone biopsy). The recently introduced 9-valent HPV vaccine is effective in protecting against types 6, 11, 16, 18, 31, 33, 45, 52, and 58 and is expected to greatly lower the incidence of genital warts and cervical cancers associated with these HPV genotypes, especially if the vaccine is administered before infection occurs. However, vaccination does not supplant the need for cervical cancer screening; many at-risk women are already infected, and current vaccines protect against only some of the oncogenic HPV genotypes.

Invasive Carcinoma of the Cervix

Progression of SIL to invasive carcinoma results from the effects of the HPV-encoded E6 and E7 oncoproteins and the progressive accumulation of mutations in host cell tumor suppressor genes and oncogenes.

Morphology. Cervical carcinomas range from small foci of stromal invasion to conspicuous exophytic tumors. Most are squamous cell carcinomas (75%; Supplemental eFigure 15.3), followed by adenocarcinoma (20%) and small cell (neuroendocrine) carcinoma (<5%), all of which are associated with HPV. Extension into the parametrial soft tissues may affix the uterus to the surrounding pelvic structures. The likelihood of metastasis correlates with the depth of tumor invasion and the presence of tumor cells in vascular spaces (lymphovascular invasion). Squamous tumors and adenocarcinomas are graded based on the degree of differentiation, but all small cell carcinomas are considered high grade.

Clinical Features. Cervical cancer is now uncommon in the Western world and most often occurs in women who have never had a Pap test or who have not been screened for many years. Patients come to medical attention for vaginal bleeding, leukorrhea, painful coitus (dyspareunia), or dysuria. The primary treatment is surgical, with adjuvant chemotherapy and radiation when necessary. The outcome is predicted by the tumor stage and, in the case of small cell carcinoma (which pursues an aggressive course), by the cell type.

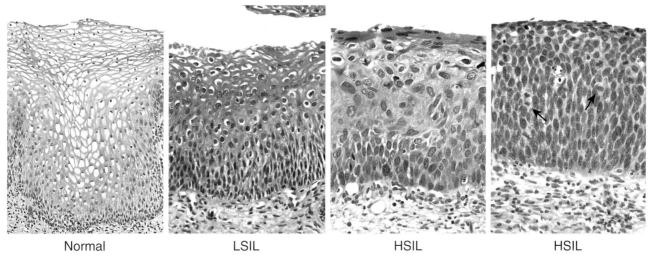

| Normal | LSIL | HSIL | HSIL |

Fig. 15.4 Spectrum of squamous intraepithelial lesions (SILs) with normal squamous epithelium for comparison: LSIL with koilocytotic atypia; HSIL with progressive atypia in all layers of the epithelium; and HSIL with diffuse atypia, mitotic figures above the basal zone (*arrows*), and loss of maturation (carcinoma in situ, *far right image*).

UTERUS

The body (corpus) of the uterus is composed of the endometrium, consisting of glands and stroma, and the myometrium, made up of smooth muscle. It may be involved by inflammatory, infectious, and neoplastic disorders.

Endometritis

Endometritis is a component of pelvic inflammatory disease. It is frequently a result of *N. gonorrhoeae* or *C. trachomatis* infections, which lead to acute and chronic inflammation. Tuberculosis causes granulomatous endometritis, frequently with associated tuberculous salpingitis and peritonitis; it is rare in the United States and seen mainly in immunocompromised women, but is common in countries in which tuberculosis is endemic. Endometritis also may result from retained products of conception or the presence of a foreign body, such as an intrauterine device, which acts as a nidus for ascending infection. Endometritis manifests with fever, abdominal pain, and menstrual abnormalities, and is associated with an increased risk of infertility and ectopic pregnancy due to scarring of the fallopian tubes.

Endometriosis

Endometriosis is defined by the presence of endometrial glands and stroma in a location outside the uterus.

It occurs in up to 10% of women in their reproductive years and in nearly half of women with infertility. It is frequently multifocal and often involves pelvic structures. Less commonly, distant areas of the peritoneal cavity or sites such as the lymph nodes, lungs, or other tissues are affected. Adenomyosis refers to the presence of endometrial glands and stroma deep in the myometrium. It can coexist with endometriosis.

Pathogenesis. Theories about the origin of endometriosis include regurgitation of endometrial cells shed during menstruation, metaplasia of peritoneal mesothelium into endometrium, and differentiation of circulating stem cells into endometrial cells. Endometriotic tissue is not just misplaced but also is abnormal (Fig. 15.5). Compared with normal endometrium, it expresses higher levels of inflammatory mediators, possibly because factors made by endometrial stromal cells recruit and activate macrophages. Stromal cells also

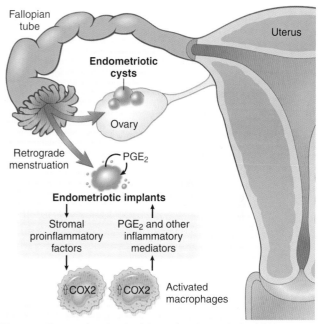

Fig. 15.5 Proposed pathophysiology of endometriosis. COX2, cyclooxygenase 2; PGE$_2$, prostaglandin E$_2$.

make aromatase, leading to the local production of estrogen, which may enhance the survival and persistence of the endometriotic tissue within an ectopic location.

Morphology. Endometriotic lesions are composed of endometrial stroma and glands that undergo cyclic bleeding and appear as red-brown nodules or implants (Supplemental eFig. 15.4). Ovarian lesions may form large, blood-filled cysts that turn brown as the blood ages (*chocolate cysts*) (Supplemental eFig. 15.5). Complications, all due to scarring, include pelvic adhesions, fallopian tube obstruction, and distortion of the ovaries.

Table 15.1 Causes of Abnormal Uterine Bleeding by Age Group

Age Group	Cause(s)
Prepuberty	Precocious puberty (e.g., hypothalamic, pituitary, or ovarian origin)
Adolescence	Anovulatory cycle
Reproductive age	Complications of pregnancy (e.g., abortion, trophoblastic disease, ectopic pregnancy)
	Proliferations (e.g., leiomyoma, adenomyosis, polyps, endometrial hyperplasia, carcinoma)
	Anovulatory cycle
	Ovulatory dysfunctional bleeding (e.g., inadequate luteal phase)
Perimenopause	Anovulatory cycle
	Irregular shedding
	Proliferations (e.g., carcinoma, hyperplasia, polyps)
Postmenopause	Proliferations (e.g., carcinoma, hyperplasia, polyps)
	Endometrial atrophy

Clinical Features. Dysmenorrhea and pelvic pain are nearly constant features of endometriosis, but are not specific. Other manifestations depend on the distribution of the lesions. Scarring of the fallopian tubes and ovaries often produces discomfort in the lower abdomen and sterility. Rectal wall involvement may produce pain on defecation, whereas involvement of the uterine or bladder serosa can cause dyspareunia and dysuria, respectively. Antiinflammatory drugs (e.g., COX-2 inhibitors) and estrogen antagonists (aromatase inhibitors) provide symptomatic relief.

Abnormal Uterine Bleeding

Abnormal uterine bleeding, such as *menorrhagia* (profuse or prolonged bleeding with menstruation), *metrorrhagia* (irregular bleeding between periods), or postmenopausal bleeding, commonly occur. The probable cause varies with patient age (Table 15.1). Abnormal bleeding in the absence of a uterine lesion is called *dysfunctional uterine bleeding*, which often is due to failure to ovulate (anovulation) due to hormonal imbalances; it is most common at menarche and in the perimenopausal period. Less commonly, dysfunctional uterine bleeding is caused by:

- *Endocrine disorders*, such as thyroid disease, adrenal disease, or pituitary tumors
- *Ovarian lesions*, such as a functioning ovarian tumor (e.g., granulosa cell tumors)
- *Metabolic disturbances*, such as obesity and malnutrition
- An *inadequate luteal phase*, due to insufficient progesterone production by the corpus luteum

Proliferative Lesions of the Endometrium and Myometrium

The most common proliferative lesions of the uterine corpus are endometrial hyperplasia, endometrial carcinomas, and smooth muscle tumors. All tend to produce abnormal uterine bleeding as their earliest manifestation.

Endometrial Hyperplasia

An excess of estrogen relative to progestin, if prolonged or marked, induces endometrial proliferation (hyperplasia).

Common causes of estrogen excess are obesity (adipose tissue converts steroid precursors into estrogens), failure of ovulation (e.g.,

perimenopause), estrogen therapy, and estrogen-producing ovarian lesions (e.g., ovarian granulosa cell tumors). Endometrial hyperplasia is categorized as hyperplasia without cellular atypia (Supplemental eFig. 15.6A) and hyperplasia with atypia (Supplemental eFig. 15.6B). The former rarely progresses to endometrial carcinoma, whereas the latter, also called *endometrial intraepithelial neoplasia*, progresses to carcinoma in 20% to 50% of cases. Lesions with atypia share loss of the tumor suppressor gene *PTEN* with endometrial cancers (see the following).

Endometrial Carcinoma

In the United States and many other Western countries, endometrial carcinoma is the most frequent cancer occurring in the female genital tract.

Endometrial carcinoma generally manifests between the ages of 55 and 65 years and is uncommon before age 40 years. There are two pathogenically distinct categories: endometrioid and serous carcinoma.

Pathogenesis. The *endometrioid type* accounts for 80% of cases of endometrial carcinoma and is associated with estrogen exposure and a history of endometrial hyperplasia. Mutations in mismatch repair genes and the tumor suppressor gene *PTEN* are early events in the stepwise development of endometrioid carcinoma. The *serous type* of endometrial carcinoma is less common but more aggressive. It is associated with endometrial atrophy and arises mainly in older postmenopausal women. Nearly all cases have mutations in the *TP53* tumor suppressor gene.

> *Morphology.* **Endometrioid carcinoma** closely resembles normal endometrium and may be exophytic or infiltrative into the myometrium (Fig. 15.6A,B). Lymphovascular invasion is associated with metastasis to regional lymph nodes. Grade is based on the degree of differentiation. **Serous carcinoma** typically grows in small tufts and papillae and exhibits marked cytologic atypia (Fig. 15.6C,D); by definition, it is high grade. It is an aggressive tumor that often spreads to the peritoneal cavity and to other sites.

Clinical Features. Endometrial carcinomas typically manifest with irregular or postmenopausal bleeding. Endometrioid carcinoma is usually slow to metastasize, but if left untreated, eventually disseminates to regional nodes and more distant sites. The 5-year survival rate for early-stage endometrioid carcinoma is high, but survival drops precipitously in higher-stage tumors. Tumors with mutations in mismatch repair genes have a high burden of passenger mutations that generate tumor neoantigens; such tumors may respond to immune checkpoint inhibitors. The prognosis with serous carcinomas is dependent on staging, but because of its aggressive behavior, it often presents as high-stage disease and has a poor prognosis.

Leiomyoma

Leiomyomas are common benign tumors arising from smooth muscle cells in the myometrium.

Because of their fibrous tissue-like firmness, leiomyomas often are referred to as *fibroids*. Leiomyomas affect up to half of women of reproductive age and are more frequent in women of African descent. These tumors are associated with several recurrent chromosomal abnormalities, including rearrangements of chromosomes 6 and 12 that are found in other benign neoplasms, such as lipomas. Estrogens stimulate the growth of leiomyomas; predictably, these tumors shrink after menopause.

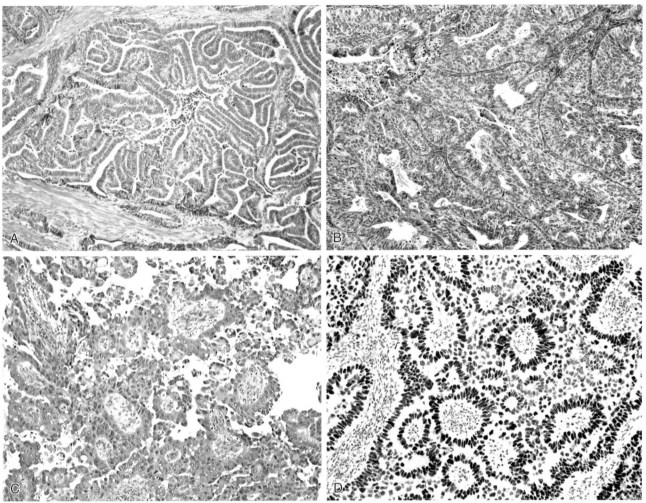

Fig. 15.6 Endometrial carcinoma. (A) Endometrioid type, grade 1, infiltrating myometrium and growing in a glandular pattern. (B) Endometrioid type, grade 3, has a predominantly solid growth pattern. (C) Serous carcinoma of the endometrium, with papilla formation and marked cytologic atypia. (D) Immunohistochemical staining of serous carcinoma shows accumulation of p53, a finding associated with *TP53* mutation.

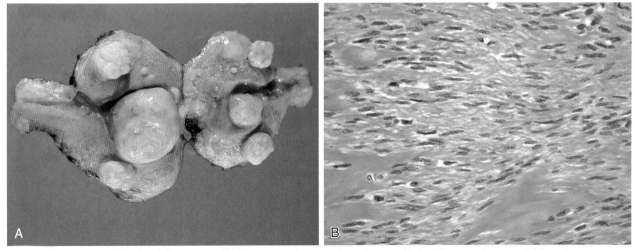

Fig. 15.7 Uterine leiomyomas. (A) The uterus is opened to show multiple submucosal, myometrial, and subserosal gray-white tumors, each with a characteristic whorled appearance on cut section. (B) Microscopic appearance of leiomyoma shows bundles of normal-looking smooth muscle cells.

Morphology. Leiomyomas are sharply circumscribed, firm gray-white masses with a whorled cut surface. They are often multiple (Fig. 15.7A). On histologic examination, the tumors are composed of bundles of smooth muscle cells similar to normal myometrium (Fig. 15.7B).

Clinical Features. Uterine leiomyomas often are asymptomatic and discovered incidentally on pelvic examination, but they may present with menorrhagia, with or without metrorrhagia. Tumors causing severe or refractory symptoms are treated with surgical excision or tumor ablation by a variety of chemical or physical methods, such as exposure to microwaves.

Leiomyosarcoma

Leiomyosarcomas of the uterus are aggressive tumors that arise de novo from myometrial mesenchymal cells.

Morphology. Leiomyosarcomas are usually solitary hemorrhagic masses. They may be well-differentiated to highly anaplastic tumors. Features that distinguish leiomyosarcoma from leiomyoma include necrosis, cytologic atypia, and mitotic activity (Supplemental eFig. 15.7A,B).

Clinical Features. Leiomyosarcomas most often occur in postmenopausal women. Recurrence after surgical resection is common, and many tumors metastasize, typically to the lungs. The outlook with anaplastic tumors is less favorable than with well-differentiated tumors.

FALLOPIAN TUBES

The most common disorder of the fallopian tubes is inflammation (salpingitis), usually occurring in the context of pelvic inflammatory disease. Other important disorders of the fallopian tubes are ectopic pregnancy and endometriosis.

    Salpingitis is almost always caused by infection. *Gonococcus, Chlamydia, Mycoplasma,* enteric bacteria, and (in the postpartum setting) streptococci and staphylococci are the major offenders. Coliforms, streptococci, and staphylococci can give rise to a blood-borne infection that seeds distant sites. Tuberculous salpingitis is less common and usually encountered in combination with tuberculous endometritis. All forms of salpingitis produce fever, lower abdominal or pelvic pain, and pelvic masses due to distention of the tubes with exudate and inflammatory debris, a process referred to as *pelvic inflammatory disease* (Fig. 15.8). Adherence of the inflamed tube to the ovary and adjacent tissues may produce a tuboovarian abscess. More serious are adhesions of the tubal plicae, which are associated with an increased risk of tubal ectopic pregnancy (discussed later).

OVARIES

Tumors of the Ovary

The most important ovarian disorders are neoplasms. In the United States, ovarian cancer is the fifth leading cause of cancer deaths in women. Ovarian tumors are remarkably varied; they may arise from the multipotent surface (coelomic) epithelium, germ cells, or sex cord–stromal cells, or may be metastatic from other sites. Here we focus on the relatively common epithelial ovarian tumors. Other rare types and the most common metastatic lesions are summarized in Table 15.2.

Surface Epithelial Tumors

"Ovarian" epithelial neoplasms have several distinct origins. Some subtypes appear to arise from ovarian epithelial cells or from ovarian

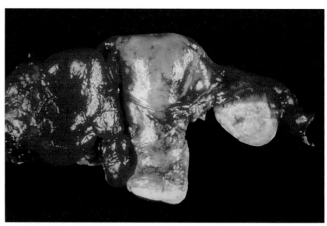

Fig. 15.8 Pelvic inflammatory disease, bilateral and asymmetric. The tube and ovary to the left of the uterus are totally obscured by a hemorrhagic inflammatory mass. The tube is adherent to the adjacent ovary on the other side.

inclusion cysts, which are lined by epithelium that may be of ovarian or extraovarian origin (Fig. 15.9). Aggressive serous carcinomas, by contrast, may arise from the fallopian epithelium or other extraovarian sites. These neoplasms have traditionally been lumped together with other ovarian cancers, and we will follow this convention.

    Based on histologic features, ovarian epithelial neoplasms are classified as benign, malignant, or borderline, a gray zone within which tumors usually pursue a benign course but sometimes progress to malignancy. The most common and important ovarian epithelial neoplasms are serous and mucinous tumors. About 60% of serous tumors are benign, 25% are malignant, and 15% are borderline. By contrast, 80% of mucinous tumors are benign, 10% are malignant, and 10% are borderline.

Pathogenesis. Serous carcinomas are categorized as low grade or high grade. The former arise from benign or borderline lesions, progress slowly, and are commonly associated with mutations in genes encoding signaling proteins such as RAS, which is also frequently mutated in *mucinous carcinomas.* High-grade serous tumors develop rapidly and often arise from the fallopian tube rather than from ovarian epithelium; *TP53* mutations are present in over 95% of cases. Familial cases are often associated with germline mutations in the *BRCA1* or *BRCA2* tumor suppressor genes, which also are often mutated in familial breast cancer (described later). Other frequently mutated genes in aggressive serous cancers include the tumor suppressor genes *NF1* and *RB.*

Morphology. Most ovarian tumors are cystic, and they are often large in size. In benign tumors, the cystic spaces are smooth and are lined by a single layer of epithelial cells, which are ciliated in serous tumors and mucin-secreting in mucinous tumors (Supplemental eFig. 15.9). Malignant tumors are recognized by serosal invasion and exuberant papillary projections lined by markedly atypical multilayered epithelial cells (Fig. 15.10 and Supplemental eFig. 15.10). Borderline tumors lie between these extremes (Supplemental eFig. 15.11). Malignant tumors spread by implanting throughout the peritoneal cavity and through lymphatics to regional lymph nodes. Mucin-secreting gastrointestinal carcinomas can spread to the ovary and may mimic primary mucinous tumors. These tumors, so-called *Krukenberg tumors,* are more likely to be bilateral than primary tumors.

Table 15.2 Salient Features of Ovarian Germ Cell and Sex Cord Neoplasms

Neoplasm	Peak Incidence	Usual Location	Morphologic Features	Behavior
Germ Cell Origin				
Dysgerminoma	Second to third decade of life Occur with gonadal dysgenesis	Unilateral in 80% to 90%	Counterpart of testicular seminoma Sheets or cords of large clear cells Stroma may contain lymphocytes and occasional granulomas	All malignant but only one third metastasize; all radiosensitive; 80% cure rate
Choriocarcinoma	First 3 decades of life	Unilateral	Identical to placental tumor Two types of epithelial cells: cytotrophoblast and syncytiotrophoblast	Metastasizes early and widely Primary focus may degenerate, leaving only metastases Resistant to chemotherapy
Sex Cord Tumors				
Granulosa–theca cell	Most postmenopausal, but may occur at any age	Unilateral	Composed of mixture of cuboidal granulosa cells and spindled or plump lipid-laden theca cells Granulosa elements may recapitulate ovarian follicle (Call-Exner bodies)	May elaborate large amounts of estrogen Granulosa element may be malignant (5% to 25%)
Thecoma–fibroma	Any age	Unilateral	Yellow (lipid-laden) plump thecal cells	Most hormonally inactive About 40% produce ascites and hydrothorax (Meigs syndrome) Rarely malignant
Sertoli-Leydig cell	All ages	Unilateral	Recapitulates development of testis with tubules or cords and plump pink Sertoli cells	Often hormonally active, many masculinizing or defeminizing Rarely malignant
Metastases to Ovary				
	Older ages	Mostly bilateral	Anaplastic tumor cells, cords, glands, dispersed through fibrous background Cells may be "signet-ring" mucin-secreting	Primaries are gastrointestinal tract (Krukenberg tumors), breast, and lung

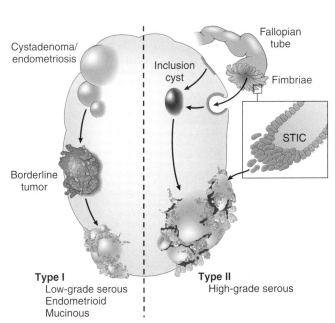

Fig. 15.9 Derivation of various ovarian neoplasms. Type I tumors progress from benign tumors through borderline tumors that may give rise to a low-grade carcinoma. Type II tumors arise from inclusion cysts/fallopian tube epithelium via intraepithelial precursors that are often not identified. They demonstrate high-grade features and are most commonly of serous histology. STIC, serous tubal intraepithelial carcinoma.

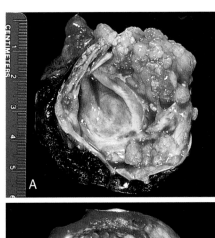
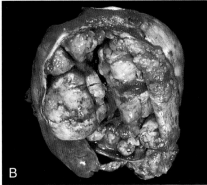

Fig. 15.10 Ovarian serous tumors. (A) Borderline serous cystadenoma opened to display a cyst cavity lined by delicate papillary tumor growths. (B) Cystadenocarcinoma. The cyst is opened to show a large, bulky tumor mass. (Courtesy Dr. Christopher Crum, Brigham and Women's Hospital, Boston.)

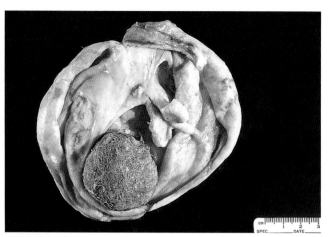

Fig. 15.11 Mature cystic teratoma (dermoid cyst) of the ovary. A ball of hair *(bottom)* and a mixture of tissues are evident. (Courtesy Dr. Christopher Crum, Brigham and Women's Hospital, Boston.)

Clinical Features. Prognosis is poor because tumors are usually advanced at presentation. Symptoms are vague and include pain and gastrointestinal complaints. About 30% of all ovarian neoplasms are discovered incidentally on gynecologic examination, often following an increase in abdominal girth. Malignant serous tumors frequently cause ascites.

Targeted treatments and effective screening methods for ovarian cancers are limited. CA-125 protein is a serum marker that is elevated in 75% to 90% of cases, but it lacks both specificity and sensitivity; while not useful for screening or diagnosis, it can be valuable in monitoring the response to therapy. The prognosis correlates with the stage. In contrast to overtly malignant tumors, borderline tumors are associated with nearly 100% survival rates.

Other Ovarian Tumors

Many other types of tumors of germ cell and sex cord–stromal origin also arise in the ovary. Sex cord tumors are of interest because some, such as granuloma-theca cell tumors, secrete estrogens and cause endometrial hyperplasia (Table 15.2). *Teratoma* constitutes 15% to 20% of ovarian tumors. They often arise in the first two decades of life and are more likely to be malignant in the very young. Overall, more than 90% are benign.

- *Benign teratomas* are marked by the presence of mature tissues derived from all three germ cell layers: ectoderm, endoderm, and mesoderm. Usually these tumors contain cysts lined by epidermis replete with adnexal appendages—hence the common designation *dermoid cysts.* They may also produce hair, teeth, bone, cartilage, and other tissues (Fig. 15.11 and Supplemental eFig. 15.12). Most are discovered in young women as ovarian masses or are found incidentally on abdominal imaging studies; infertility may be a presenting sign. Torsion occurs in 10% to 15% of cases and is an acute surgical emergency.
- *Malignant teratomas* arise early in life; the mean age at detection is 18 years. They typically are bulky and solid, with areas of necrosis. The presence of immature elements or minimally differentiated tissues is required for diagnosis (Supplemental eFig. 15.13). The grade is based on the proportion of immature neuroepithelium.
- *Specialized teratomas* are comprised of only one specialized differentiated tissue type, most commonly mature thyroid tissue (struma ovarii), which may produce hyperthyroidism.

DISEASES OF PREGNANCY

Diseases of pregnancy and pathologic conditions of the placenta are important contributors to morbidity and mortality for both mother and child. Discussed in this section are a limited number of relatively common placental disorders.

Placental Inflammations and Infections

Infections may reach the placenta by (1) ascension through the birth canal (more common) or (2) hematogenous (transplacental) spread. *Ascending infections* are usually bacterial and associated with premature rupture of the fetal membranes. Rarely, placental infections arise by *hematogenous spread* of bacteria and other organisms. Transplacental infections can affect the fetus and, based on similar clinical presentations, have been grouped under the TORCH complex (*toxo-plasmosis, other infections [e.g., syphilis], rubella, cytomegalovirus infection, herpes*). Each of these infections produces changes that are typically associated with infections at other sites.

Ectopic Pregnancy

Ectopic pregnancy is defined as implantation of a fertilized ovum in any site other than the uterus.

As many as 1% of pregnancies occur in ectopic locations, most commonly (~50% of cases) the fallopian tube (tubal pregnancy) because of obstruction from chronic inflammation and scarring of the oviduct, as may occur in pelvic inflammatory disease. Other sites include the ovaries and the abdominal cavity. Ovarian pregnancies probably result from rare instances in which the ovum is fertilized just as the follicle ruptures. Gestation within the abdominal cavity occurs when the fertilized egg drops from the fallopian tube to implant on the peritoneum.

> *Morphology.* With tubal pregnancies, the invading placenta burrows through the wall of the fallopian tube, causing *intratubal hematoma* (hematosalpinx) or *intraperitoneal hemorrhage,* or both. The tube is usually distended by freshly clotted blood containing bits of gray placental tissue and fetal parts. Histologically, chorionic villi and decidualized stroma are seen.

Clinical Features. Until rupture occurs, an ectopic pregnancy may be indistinguishable from a normal pregnancy, with cessation of menstruation and elevation of serum and urinary placental hormones. Rupture of an ectopic pregnancy may be fatal, with the sudden onset of abdominal pain and signs of an acute abdomen, often followed by shock. Prompt surgical intervention is necessary.

Gestational Trophoblastic Disease

Gestational trophoblastic disease refers to abnormal proliferations arising from fetal trophoblast cells.

The World Health Organization broadly divides these diseases into two categories: molar lesions and nonmolar lesions. The molar lesions are further divided into partial, complete, and invasive hydatidiform moles. The nonmolar category consists of choriocarcinoma and other uncommon types of trophoblast-derived malignancies. All elaborate human chorionic gonadotropins (hCGs), which are detected in the blood and urine at levels considerably higher than those found during normal pregnancy. In addition to aiding in the diagnosis, hCG levels in the blood or urine can be used to monitor treatment efficacy.

Hydatidiform Mole: Complete and Partial

Hydatidiform mole consists of a mass of swollen, cystically dilated, chorionic villi.

Varying amounts of normal to highly atypical chorionic epithelium cover the swollen villi. There are two distinctive subtypes of hydatidiform moles: *complete* and *partial.* Complete hydatidiform moles are not compatible with embryogenesis. All of the chorionic villi are abnormal, and the chorionic epithelial cells are diploid (46,XX or, uncommonly,

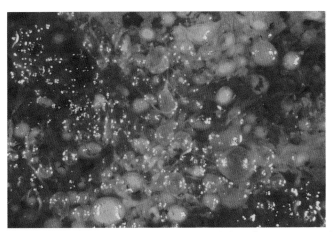

Fig. 15.12 Complete hydatidiform mole, consisting of numerous swollen (hydropic) villi.

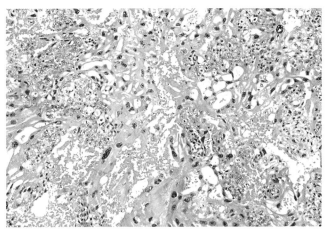

Fig. 15.13 Choriocarcinoma. This field contains both neoplastic cytotrophoblasts and multinucleate syncytiotrophoblasts. (Courtesy Dr. David R. Genest, Brigham and Women's Hospital, Boston.)

46,XY). Partial hydatidiform moles can result in early embryo formation and may contain fetal parts, have some normal chorionic villi, and are almost always triploid (e.g., 69,XXY). Both types result from an abnormal fertilization event involving two sperm or a single abnormal diploid sperm. In a complete mole, the entire genetic content is paternal, yielding diploid cells containing only paternal chromosomes, whereas in a partial mole, a normal egg is fertilized by two sperm equivalents, resulting in a triploid karyotype with a preponderance of paternal genes.

The incidence of complete hydatidiform mole is about 1 to 1.5 per 2000 pregnancies in the United States and other Western countries, but it has a much higher incidence in Asian countries. In both complete and partial moles, elevation of hCG in the maternal blood (higher than appropriate for the duration of pregnancy) and absence of fetal heart sounds are typical.

Morphology. In advanced cases, the uterine cavity is expanded by a friable mass of thin-walled, translucent cystic structures (Fig. 15.12). *Complete mole* shows swollen, poorly vascularized chorionic villi with a loose, myxomatous, edematous stroma (Supplemental eFig. 15.14). There is a proliferation of both cytotrophoblasts and syncytiotrophoblasts. In *partial moles,* edema involves only a subset of the villi, the trophoblastic proliferation is focal, and fetal tissue may be present.

Clinical Features. Most moles do not recur after curettage, but 10% of complete moles are invasive and may require treatment with chemotherapy. Another 2% to 3% give rise to choriocarcinoma, described next.

Gestational Choriocarcinoma

Choriocarcinoma, an aggressive malignant tumor, arises from gestational chorionic epithelium or, less frequently, from germ cells in the gonads.

These tumors are rare in the Western hemisphere but are much more common in Asian and African countries. Approximately 50% of choriocarcinomas arise from complete hydatidiform moles. In most cases, choriocarcinoma presents as a bloody, brownish discharge accompanied by a rising titer of hCG in blood and urine.

Morphology. Choriocarcinoma usually appears as a hemorrhagic, necrotic uterine mass (Supplemental eFig. 15.15). Sometimes the primary lesion regresses completely, leaving only metastases. The tumor is composed of anaplastic cytotrophoblasts and syncytiotrophoblasts (Fig. 15.13). By the time it is discovered, widespread vascular spread usually has occurred to the lungs (50%) and other tissues.

Clinical Features. Despite its aggressive nature, placental choriocarcinomas are sensitive to chemotherapy, and nearly all affected patients are cured. By contrast, the response of gonadal choriocarcinomas to chemotherapy is relatively poor. This difference may be related to the presence of paternal antigens on placental but not gonadal choriocarcinomas, making the placental tumors more susceptible to host antitumor immunity, which cooperates with the effects of chemotherapy to enhance tumor cell killing.

Preeclampsia and Eclampsia

The development of hypertension accompanied by proteinuria and edema in the third trimester of pregnancy is referred to as preeclampsia.

This syndrome is particularly common in first pregnancies in women older than 35 years. In severely affected women, seizures may occur, and the symptom complex is then termed *eclampsia.*

Pathogenesis. Although the etiology remains unknown, a common feature is insufficient maternal blood flow to the placenta. In normal pregnancy, the musculoelastic walls of the spiral arteries are invaded by trophoblasts and dilate into wide vascular sinusoids. In preeclampsia and eclampsia, this vascular remodeling is impaired, the musculoelastic walls are retained, and the channels remain narrow. Decreased uteroplacental blood flow results in placental hypoxia and dysfunction, causing the release of several circulating factors that interfere with angiogenesis. Several serious consequences may be associated with these alterations:

- *Placental infarction,* stemming from chronic hypoperfusion
- *Hypertension,* resulting from reduced endothelial production of the vasodilators prostacyclin and prostaglandin E_2 and from increased production of the vasoconstrictor thromboxane A2
- *Hypercoagulability,* due to endothelial dysfunction and release of tissue factor from the placenta
- *End-organ failure.* Approximately 10% of the patients with severe preeclampsia develop the so-called HELLP syndrome (*h*emolysis, *e*levated *l*iver enzymes, *l*ow *p*latelets), characterized by liver abnormalities, microangiopathic hemolytic anemia, thrombocytopenia due to platelet consumption, and sometimes disseminated intravascular coagulation.

Morphology. Placental abnormalities include infarcts, which are much more numerous in severe preeclampsia or eclampsia than in normal placentas; retroplacental hemorrhages; and fibrinoid necrosis of decidual vessels.

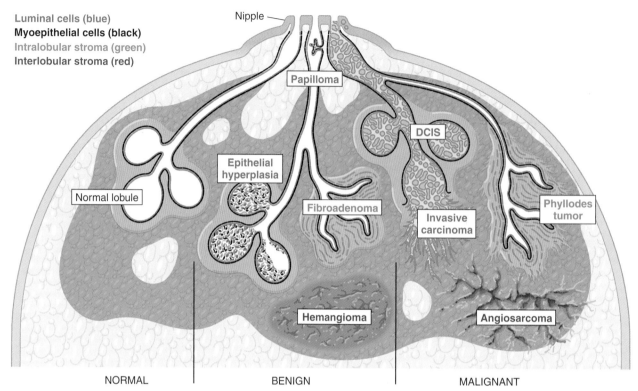

Luminal cells (blue)
Myoepithelial cells (black)
Intralobular stroma (green)
Interlobular stroma (red)

Nipple

Papilloma

DCIS

Epithelial hyperplasia

Normal lobule

Fibroadenoma

Invasive carcinoma

Phyllodes tumor

Hemangioma

Angiosarcoma

NORMAL · BENIGN · MALIGNANT

Fig. 15.14 Origins of breast disorders. Benign epithelial lesions include intraductal papillomas that grow in sinuses below the nipple and epithelial hyperplasia that arises in lobules. Malignant epithelial lesions are mainly breast carcinomas, which may remain in situ or invade the breast and spread by metastasis. Specialized intralobular stroma *(green)* cells may give rise to fibroadenomas and phyllodes tumors, whereas interlobular stroma *(red)* may give rise to a variety of rare benign and malignant tumors. DCIS, ductal carcinoma in situ.

Clinical Features. Preeclampsia presents during weeks 24 to 25 of gestation with edema, proteinuria, and rising blood pressure. Evolution to eclampsia results in impaired renal function, worsening hypertension, and convulsions. Antihypertensive therapy prevents these complications, and the condition resolves promptly after delivery.

BREAST

The functional unit of the breast is the lobule, which is supported by a specialized intralobular stroma. Breast lobules expand after menarche, undergo periodic remodeling during adulthood, especially during and after pregnancy, and ultimately involute and regress. During lactation, the inner luminal epithelial cells produce milk, which is ejected by contractile myoepithelial cells through the ducts to the nipple. The size of the breast is determined by interlobular stroma, which increases during puberty and involutes with age.

Each of these normal constituents is a source of benign and malignant lesions (Fig. 15.14). Clinically, the most important of these disorders is carcinoma of the breast (discussed later). The main significance of benign breast disorders is they frequently simulate the mammographic appearance of breast cancer or produce local symptoms that mimic carcinoma.

Inflammatory Processes

Inflammatory breast diseases are rare and may be caused by infections, autoimmune disease, or foreign body–type reactions. *Staphylococcus aureus* is the most common pathogen; it typically gains entry via fissures in nipple skin during breastfeeding, and "lactational abscesses" may develop. Most cases are treated adequately with antibiotics and continued expression of milk. Rarely, surgical incision and drainage is required.

Stromal Neoplasms

The most common stromal tumors, *fibroadenoma* and *phyllodes tumor*, share driver mutations and have a similar pathogenesis. Both are derived from intralobular stroma. Fibroadenomas are benign; phyllodes tumors may recur and occasionally metastasize. Other rare soft tissue tumors derived from interlobular stromal cells also occur in the breast, most notably angiosarcoma (see Chapter 5), which is associated with breast irradiation, usually in the setting of breast cancer therapy.

Morphology. Fibroadenoma and phyllodes tumors are composed of neoplastic intralobular fibroblasts and entrapped nonneoplastic epithelial cells. The proliferating fibroblasts distort the epithelial cells, forming elongated slit-like structures. Fibroadenoma has circumscribed borders and low cellularity (Fig. 15.15A); mitoses are rare. By contrast, the stromal cells of phyllodes tumors are more proliferative and form bulbous nodules lined by epithelium (Fig. 15.15B), the characteristic "phyllodes" (Greek for "leaflike") growth pattern.

Benign Epithelial Lesions

The majority of benign epithelial lesions are incidental findings detected by mammography. Their major clinical significance is the subsequent risk of malignant transformation. Benign changes are divided into three groups, nonproliferative disease, proliferative disease without atypia, and proliferative disease with atypia, each associated with a different degree of breast cancer risk.

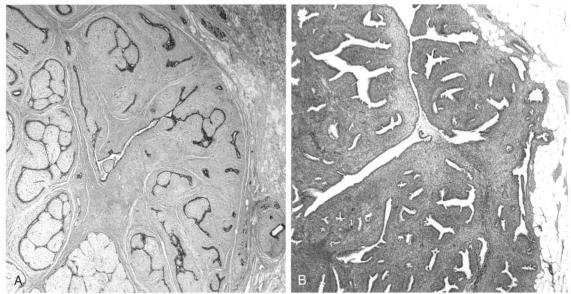

Fig. 15.15 Intralobular stromal neoplasms. (A) Fibroadenoma. This benign tumor has an expansile growth pattern with pushing circumscribed borders. (B) Phyllodes tumor. Proliferating stromal cells distort the glandular tissue, forming cleft-like spaces, and bulge into surrounding stroma.

Morphology. The most common *nonproliferative* breast lesions are simple cysts lined by a layer of luminal cells that often undergo apocrine metaplasia (Supplemental eFig. 15.16). The apocrine secretions may calcify, leading to detection by mammography. When cysts rupture, chronic inflammation and fibrosis in response to the spilled debris may produce palpable nodularity of the breast (so-called *fibrocystic changes*). *Proliferative disease without atypia* is associated with epithelial cell proliferation that expands the ductal and lobular spaces (Supplemental eFig. 15.17). *Proliferative disease with atypia* resembles lobular carcinoma in situ or ductal carcinoma in situ (described later), but is more limited in extent (Supplemental eFig. 15.18A,B).

Carcinoma

Breast carcinoma includes several molecular subtypes, each with different pathologic features and treatment approaches.

The worldwide incidence of breast cancer and related deaths is increasing, possibly due to behavioral changes that increase breast cancer risk—particularly delayed childbearing and fewer pregnancies—combined with a lack of access to optimal health care.

The lifetime risk of breast cancer is 12% for women living to age 90 years in the United States. The mortality rate for breast cancer is second only to that for lung cancer. Almost all breast malignancies are adenocarcinomas (>95%). For clinical management, breast cancers are classified based on hormone receptor expression—estrogen receptor (ER) and progesterone receptor (PR)—and the expression of the human epidermal growth factor receptor 2 (HER2, also known as ERBB2) into three major groups (Table 15.3):

- *ER positive cancers* (HER2 negative; 50% to 65% of cases), which occur in older women, tend to follow a prolonged course, and are responsive to antiestrogen therapies
- *HER2 positive cancers* (ER positive or negative; 10% to 20% of cases), which are aggressive but respond to HER2 inhibitors
- *Triple negative cancers* (ER, PR, and HER2 negative; 10% to 20% of cases), which are aggressive and often respond poorly to therapy

Epidemiology

A large number of risk factors for breast cancer have been identified. The most important are the following:

Table 15.3 Summary of the Major Subtypes of Breast Cancer

Feature	ER-Positive/HER2-Negative	HER2-Positive (ER-Positive or Negative)	Triple-Negative (ER-, PR-, and HER2-Negative)
Overall frequency	50% to 65%	20%	15%
Typical patient groups	Older women; cancers detected by screening; germline *BRCA2* mutation carriers	Young women; germline *TP53* mutation carriers	Young women; germline *BRCA1* mutation carriers
Race/ethnicity	Caucasian women of European descent	None	Hispanic women, women of African descent
Grade	Mainly grade 1 and 2	Mainly grade 2 and 3	Mainly grade 3
Timing of relapse	May be late (>10 years after diagnosis)	Usually < 10 years after diagnosis	Usually < 8 years after diagnosis
Metastatic sites	Bone, viscera,	Bone , viscera, brain	Bone, viscera, brain
Common somatic mutations	PI3K gene, *TP53*	*TP53*, PI3K gene	*TP53*

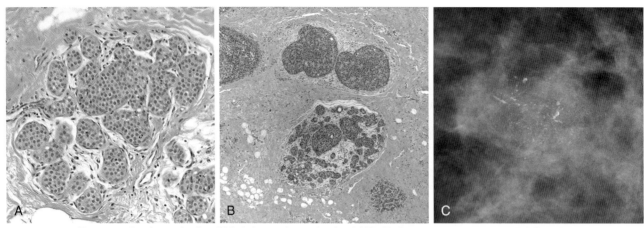

Fig. 15.16 Carcinoma in situ. (A) Lobular carcinoma in situ (LCIS). (B) Ductal carcinoma in situ (DCIS). DCIS partially involves the lobule in the lower half of this photo and has completely effaced the upper lobules, producing a duct-like appearance. (C) Mammographic detection of calcifications associated with DCIS.

- *Age and gender.* Breast cancer is rare in women younger than age 25 years, but it increases in incidence rapidly after age 30 years; 75% of women with breast cancer are older than 50 years of age. The incidence in men is only 1% of that in women.
- *Family history.* In most families, an increased risk is likely due to low-penetrance "weak" cancer risk genes. Approximately 5% to 10% of breast cancers are due to highly penetrant germline mutations in tumor suppressor genes (discussed later).
- *Geographic factors.* The risk is significantly higher in the Americas and Europe compared to Asia and Africa. As Western habits are adopted, breast cancer rates appear to be rising in these developing countries.
- *Race and ethnicity.* The highest rate of breast cancer is in women of European descent, who typically develop ER-positive cancers; Hispanic women and women of African descent tend to develop aggressive tumors at a younger age. Such disparities may be due to a combination of differences in genetics, social factors, and access to health care.
- *Reproductive history.* An early age of menarche, nulliparity, the absence of breastfeeding, and an older age at first pregnancy are associated with increased risk, due to increased estrogen exposure.
- *Oral contraceptives.* There is a small (~1.2-fold) increased risk of breast cancer in women using oral contraceptives. The risk of endometrial and ovarian cancers is lower, however, so the overall risk of cancer in this population is slightly decreased.
- *Radiation exposure.* Chest radiation, particularly high doses at a young age, is associated with an increased risk of breast cancer.
- *Other factors.* Moderate to heavy alcohol use increases breast cancer risk. Exercise has a small protective effect.

Pathogenesis. Factors that contribute directly to the development of breast cancer can be grouped into genetic, hormonal, and environmental categories.
- *Genetic factors.* Driver mutations in cancer genes may be acquired or inherited. *BRCA1* and *BRCA2* are two commonly mutated tumor suppressor genes that encode proteins that are required for repair of certain kinds of DNA damage. Thirty percent to 90% of patients with *BRCA1* or *BRCA2* mutations develop breast cancer by the age of 70 years. Somatic mutations in these genes are rare in sporadic cancers, but epigenetic inactivation of *BRCA1* occurs in up to 50% of triple-negative cancers. Somatic mutations in *TP53* are common in breast cancer, particularly triple-negative tumors, whereas mutations that activate PI3K-AKT signaling are frequent in ER-positive

breast cancers. *HER2* gene amplification is also an important driver in a subset of cancers. HER2 is a receptor tyrosine kinase that promotes cell proliferation and opposes apoptosis. Therapeutic agents that specifically target HER2 are highly active in this class of breast cancer and have markedly improved the prognosis for patients with HER2-amplified tumors.
- *Estrogen exposure.* Estrogen-receptor signaling stimulates the production of growth factors and regulates the expression of genes that are important for the growth and survival of normal and transformed breast epithelial cells. Blockade of estrogen receptors is therapeutic in these tumors.

Morphology. Most tumors arise in the upper outer quadrant (50%), followed by the central portion (20%). About 4% of women with breast cancer have bilateral primary tumors or sequential lesions in the same breast.

Carcinoma in situ is an epithelial proliferation with all of the morphologic features of cancer that is limited by the basement membrane. There are two morphologic subtypes: ductal carcinoma in situ (DCIS) and lobular carcinoma in situ (LCIS). LCIS usually expands involved lobules (Fig. 15.16A), whereas DCIS distorts lobules into duct-like spaces (Fig. 15.16B). Necrotic debris or secretory material associated with DCIS produces calcifications (Fig. 15.16C), which can be detected by mammography. LCIS is usually an incidental finding because it rarely produces calcifications.

Invasive carcinoma has several histologic subtypes. *Invasive ductal carcinoma* induces a desmoplastic response that results in a mammographic density (Fig. 15.17A,B) and eventually produces a hard, palpable irregular mass. *Invasive lobular carcinoma* makes up 10% to 15% of invasive carcinomas and consists of linear cords of infiltrating cells similar to the tumor cells seen in LCIS (Fig. 15.17C). Most of these tumors manifest as palpable masses or mammographic densities, but others invade without a desmoplastic response, making them difficult to detect by imaging (Fig. 15.17D). Almost all lobular carcinomas express hormone receptors, whereas HER2 overexpression is rare. Lobular carcinoma often spreads to cerebrospinal fluid, serosal surfaces, or the gastrointestinal tract, ovary, and uterus.

Several other subtypes of invasive breast cancer are recognized, including *carcinoma with medullary features,* a subtype of triple-negative cancer with pushing borders that consists of sheets of large anaplastic cells associated with lymphocytic infiltrates

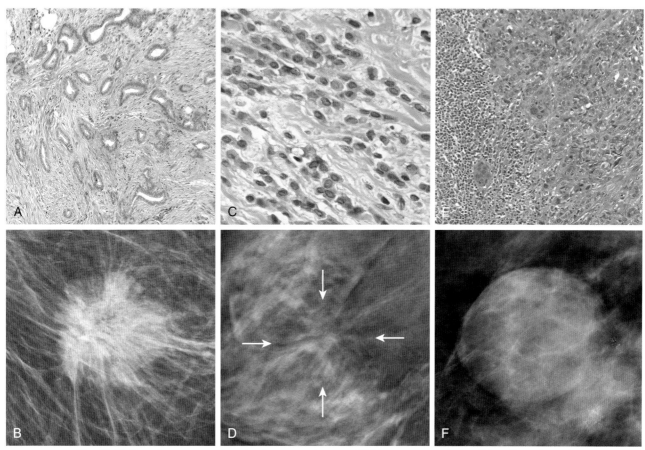

Fig. 15.17 Growth patterns of invasive breast carcinomas. (A) Most grow as tubules ("ductal" carcinoma) and stimulate a reactive desmoplastic stromal proliferation. In mammograms (B), these carcinomas appear as dense masses with spicular margins resulting from invasion of adjacent radiolucent breast tissue. (C) Lobular carcinomas are composed of noncohesive tumor cells that invade as linear cords of cells and induce little stromal response. Accordingly, in mammograms (D), lobular carcinomas often appear as relatively subtle, irregular masses *(arrows)*. (E) Uncommonly, carcinomas consist of tightly adhesive clusters of cells, as in this carcinoma with medullary features, or when there is abundant extracellular mucin production. (F) Such tumors may appear as well-circumscribed masses in mammograms, mimicking the appearance of a benign lesion.

composed predominantly of T cells (Fig. 15.17E), and *inflammatory carcinoma*, which invades and obstructs dermal lymphatic spaces, causing an "inflamed" appearance with reddening, thickening, and fine pitting of the skin *(peau d'orange)*.

Invasive breast carcinoma is graded based on nuclear pleomorphism, tubule formation, and proliferation. Most low-grade carcinomas form well-defined tubules, whereas high-grade carcinomas invade as solid sheets or single cells. Proliferation is evaluated by counting mitotic figures or by staining for cell cycle markers.

Clinical Features. In unscreened populations, most breast cancers are detected as a palpable mass. Almost all are invasive, and at least half of these have metastasized to regional lymph nodes when they are detected. In older, screened populations, approximately 60% of breast cancers discovered are asymptomatic and about 20% are in situ carcinomas; the invasive carcinomas detected are small, and only 15% will have metastasized to the lymph nodes at the time of discovery.

The prognosis of a woman with breast cancer depends on the molecular and morphologic features of the tumor and its stage at diagnosis:

- *Proliferation rate* correlates with the responsiveness to cytotoxic chemotherapy

- *Expression of estrogen or progesterone receptors* predicts the response to antiestrogen therapy
- *Overexpression of HER2* predicts the response to HER2 antagonists
- *RNA expression profiling* can be used to identify cancers that do not require treatment with chemotherapy
- *Tumor stage,* which is based on features of the primary tumor (T), involvement of regional lymph nodes (N), and the presence of distant metastases (M); the majority of breast cancers first metastasize to regional nodes; nodal involvement is a strong prognostic factor; sentinel lymph node biopsy (see Chapter 5) is frequently performed at the time of surgery

Historically, virtually all women with untreated breast cancer died within 3 to 4 years; currently, 80% of women with optimally treated breast cancer survive. Endocrine therapy, by blockade of estrogen receptor with tamoxifen and suppression of estrogen synthesis with aromatase inhibitors, is very effective for ER-positive cancers. HER2 antagonists markedly improve survival times in women with HER2-positive carcinomas. Other targeted therapies and immunotherapies in development may improve outcomes in subtypes that currently have a poor prognosis, such as triple-negative breast cancer.

16

Endocrine System

OUTLINE

Overview of the Endocrine System, 264
Pituitary Gland, 264
   Hyperpituitarism, 265
   Hypopituitarism, 266
   Posterior Pituitary Syndromes, 267
   Craniopharyngioma, 267
Thyroid, 267
   Clinical Syndromes of Thyroid Dysfunction, 267
   Autoimmune Thyroid Disease, 268
   Other Forms of Inflammatory Thyroid Disease, 269
   Goiter, 269
   Tumors of the Thyroid Gland, 269
Parathyroid Glands, 272

Endocrine Pancreas: Diabetes, 272
   Overview of Diabetes, 272
   Insulin Physiology, 272
   Pathogenesis of Diabetes, 273
   Clinicopathologic Features of Diabetes, 274
Adrenal Glands, 276
   Cushing Syndrome: Hypercortisolism, 276
   Hyperaldosteronism, 276
   Adrenogenital Syndromes, 276
   Adrenal Cortical Insufficiency, 277
   Tumors of the Adrenal Medulla, 278
Multiple Endocrine Neoplasia Syndromes, 279

OVERVIEW OF THE ENDOCRINE SYSTEM

Hormone production occurs in response to physiologic demands and is regulated by negative feedback loops.

The body's metabolic balance is maintained by the actions of hormones, molecules secreted by glands of the endocrine system that are carried in the blood to their target tissues. Hormone production is tightly regulated by two properties of the endocrine system.

- Most hormones are produced only in response to specific needs. For instance, insulin, which increases glucose utilization, is produced following a glucose-containing meal. The production of most hormones is stimulated by other so-called trophic hormones that are produced by organs other than the hormone-producing gland.
- Secretion of a hormone downregulates the production of the trophic hormone, creating a negative feedback loop that limits hormone production to the precise amount that is needed.

Hormones act by binding to specific receptors on target cells and activating various biochemical signaling pathways.

The receptors fall into two broad groups.

- *Cell surface receptors.* Hormones that bind to cell surface receptors include proteins, such as insulin and growth hormone, and small molecules, such as epinephrine. These receptors activate signaling pathways that lead to the production of so-called second messengers, which include cyclic adenosine monophosphate (cAMP), inositol(3,4,5)triphosphate (IP3), and calcium. The second messengers have diverse effects depending on the target tissue, including stimulation of cell growth and differentiation, alteration of

cellular metabolism, and changes in contractility (in the case of cardiac muscle).
- *Intracellular receptors.* Lipid-soluble hormones, such as steroids and thyroxine, diffuse through cellular membranes and bind to intracellular receptors. Following binding of the hormone, the hormone-receptor complex migrates into the nucleus and alters transcription of particular target genes.

Endocrine disorders are diverse but are caused by a limited set of underlying abnormalities.

Most endocrine diseases are attributable to one or more of the following.

- Underproduction or overproduction of a hormone
- Resistance of target cells to the actions of a hormone
- Tumors, which may be nonfunctional and produce mass effects (such as pituitary tumors causing impaired vision and headaches) or may be associated with underproduction or overproduction of hormones

The diagnosis of endocrine diseases relies on the clinical presentation and biochemical measurement of the levels of hormones and other metabolites. Morphologic examination is of value primarily for diagnosing endocrine tumors.

PITUITARY GLAND

The pituitary is composed of two morphologically and functionally distinct components: the anterior lobe (adenohypophysis) and the posterior lobe (neurohypophysis).

The anterior pituitary produces trophic hormones that stimulate the production of hormones from the thyroid, adrenal, and other endocrine glands. It is composed of cell populations that produce different hormones and have morphologically distinct staining characteristics in tissue sections. The major cell types are lactotrophs (producers of prolactin), somatotrophs (growth hormone), corticotrophs (adrenocorticotrophic hormone [ACTH], which acts on the adrenal gland), thyrotrophs (thyroid-stimulating hormone [TSH]), and gonadotrophs (follicle-stimulating hormone [FSH] and luteinizing hormone [LH]). All pituitary hormones are under tight feedback control. For instance, ACTH and TSH stimulate production of adrenal and thyroid hormones, respectively, which in turn inhibit production of these hormones by the pituitary. Functioning tumors derived from each pituitary cell type cause clinical syndromes related to overproduction of particular hormones. Also, pituitary hormones are produced in response to hypothalamic factors, so in rare cases, pituitary disease results from alterations in the hypothalamus. Although most hypothalamic factors are stimulatory, some such as somatostatin and dopamine are inhibitory.

The posterior pituitary produces two hormones: antidiuretic hormone (ADH), which stimulates water resorption in the kidney, and oxytocin, which stimulates muscle contraction in the pregnant uterus and the lactating breast.

Hyperpituitarism

The major cause of hyperpituitarism is a hormone-producing benign tumor (adenoma) of the anterior pituitary.

Hyperpituitarism refers to a syndrome caused by overproduction of an anterior pituitary hormone. The clinical findings reflect the activity of the tumor-derived hormones, which are produced in excess and independent of feedback control (Table 16.1). Some pituitary adenomas are nonfunctional and their clinical manifestations are related mainly to mass effects. Among the genetic alterations believed to give rise to pituitary adenomas, the most common ones

dysregulate G-protein signaling, leading to persistent generation of cAMP and unchecked cell growth. The role of this pathway in pituitary tumors is not surprising because many of the hypothalamic trophic hormones that normally activate pituitary endocrine cells do so via G protein–coupled receptors.

Morphology. Pituitary adenomas are classified on the basis of several properties:
- The hormones produced
- Whether they are functional (hormone producing) or nonfunctional
- Size: They may be small (<1 cm, called microadenomas) or large (>1 cm, macroadenomas). Nonfunctional tumors, most commonly gonadotroph adenomas, grow to a larger size before they are detected, often because of a mass effect. They may destroy the functional cells of the pituitary and cause hypopituitarism.

Pituitary adenomas are typically solitary, well-circumscribed lesions composed of homogeneous cells with little supporting stroma (Fig. 16.1). The hormones produced by tumors can be identified by immunohistochemical stains. Small tumors are usually confined to the sella turcica, whereas large tumors may cause compression of the optic chiasma and extend to the cavernous or sphenoid sinuses. Compression of the optic nerves produces characteristic visual field defects in one or both eyes.

We next summarize the salient features of the most common pituitary adenomas.

Lactotroph Adenoma

Lactotroph adenomas account for about 30% of hyperfunctioning pituitary adenomas, overproduce prolactin, and cause amenorrhea and infertility.

These tumors come to attention relatively quickly in women of reproductive age because the symptoms are obvious, but in older

Table 16.1 Pituitary Adenomas

Pituitary Cell Type	Hormone	Adenoma Subtypes	Associated Syndrome[a]
Lactotroph	Prolactin	Lactotroph adenoma	Galactorrhea and amenorrhea (in females) Sexual dysfunction, infertility
Somatotroph	GH	Somatotroph adenoma	Gigantism (children) Acromegaly (adults)
Mammosomatotroph	Prolactin, GH	Mammosomatotroph adenoma	Combined features of GH and prolactin excess
Corticotroph	ACTH and other POMC-derived peptides	Corticotroph adenoma	Cushing syndrome
Thyrotroph	TSH	Thyrotroph adenoma	Hyperthyroidism
Gonadotroph	FSH, LH	Gonadotroph adenoma	Hypogonadism

[a]These syndromes are confined to functional adenomas. Note that nonfunctional (silent) adenomas in each category express the corresponding hormone(s) within the neoplastic cells, as determined by special immunohistochemical staining on tissues, but do not produce the associated clinical syndrome, and typically present with mass effects and hypopituitarism due to destruction of normal pituitary parenchyma.
ACTH, Adrenocorticotrophic hormone; FSH, follicle-stimulating hormone; GH, growth hormone; LH, luteinizing hormone; POMC, pro-opiomelanocortin; TSH, thyroid-stimulating hormone.
Partially adapted from Asa SL, Ezzat S: The pathogenesis of pituitary tumors. *Annu Rev Pathol* 4:97, 2009.

women and in men they may not be detected until they become large. The cells contain abundant prolactin; even small microadenomas can produce sufficient amounts of hormone to cause symptoms. However, any suprasellar mass can interrupt the hypothalamic inhibitory fibers, leading to increases in prolactin release (the stalk effect); thus, elevation of prolactin in the blood does not always indicate the presence of a functional adenoma.

Somatotroph Adenoma

Somatotroph adenomas secrete growth hormone and cause gigantism in children or acromegaly in adults.

Persistent growth hormone excess stimulates hepatic secretion of insulin-like growth factor-1 (IGF-1), which acts together with growth hormone to cause overgrowth of bones and muscles. If this happens before the epiphyses of long bones close at puberty, the result is *gigantism,* characterized by an increased body size and disproportionately long limbs. If the growth hormone excess develops after the epiphyses have closed, it leads to *acromegaly,* in which the bones of the face, hands, and feet show the greatest enlargement. Enlargement of the jaw results in its protrusion *(prognathism).* In addition to its growth-promoting actions, growth hormone induces insulin resistance in tissues, leading to diabetes. Growth hormone levels are dynamic and under normal circumstances are markedly suppressed by an oral glucose load (a glucose tolerance test). High IGF-1 levels and the failure of an oral load of glucose to suppress growth hormone levels are useful for diagnosing this type of pituitary adenoma.

Corticotroph Adenoma

Corticotroph adenomas secrete ACTH, which stimulates excessive production of cortisol from the adrenal glands, leading to a disorder called Cushing syndrome.

Cushing syndrome also may result from abnormalities other than a pituitary adenoma, such as adrenal tumors. When caused by an ACTH-secreting pituitary adenoma, the disorder is called Cushing disease. Corticotroph adenomas are usually small (microadenomas) at the time of diagnosis. The manifestations of Cushing syndrome are described later, in the discussion of diseases of the adrenal glands.

Other Pituitary Adenomas

Gonadotroph adenomas produce LH and FSH, which act on reproductive organs. Because hormone production by these tumors is variable and limited in amount, they usually do not cause a clinical syndrome but are recognized because of mass effects. Thyrotroph (TSH-producing) adenomas are rare and can cause hyperthyroidism (discussed later under diseases of the thyroid gland). About 25% of pituitary adenomas are nonfunctional and are identified due to mass effects, including visual field abnormalities and hypopituitarism.

Hypopituitarism

Deficiencies of pituitary hormones are uncommon and have several underlying causes.

- *Ischemic necrosis of the pituitary (Sheehan syndrome)* is a rare postpartum complication. The anterior pituitary enlarges during pregnancy because of an increased demand for prolactin. The blood supply does not increase proportionally, making the gland susceptible to ischemia. Ischemic necrosis of the pituitary may occur in women who develop hypotension during delivery and, less commonly, due to shock in other settings, sickle cell disease, and other conditions that compromise the blood supply.
- *Nonfunctional tumors of the pituitary* can compress the normal pituitary
- *Iatrogenic causes,* such as surgery and radiation

Hypofunction of the anterior pituitary can cause growth failure (dwarfism) in children because of growth hormone deficiency, amenorrhea and infertility in women because of gonadotropin deficiency, and hypothyroidism and hypoadrenalism due to reduced production of the relevant trophic hormones, TSH and ACTH, respectively.

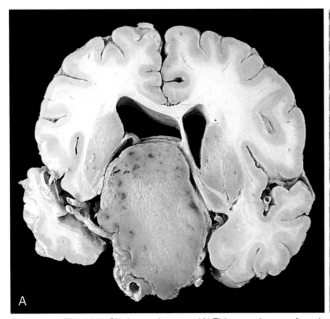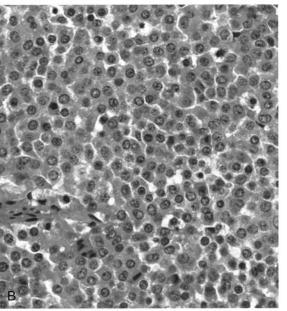

Fig. 16.1 Pituitary adenoma. (A) This massive, nonfunctioning adenoma has grown far beyond the confines of the sella turcica and has distorted the overlying brain. Nonfunctioning adenomas tend to be larger at the time of diagnosis than those that secrete a hormone. (B) The monomorphism of these cells and the absence of a reticulin network contrast with the admixture of cells seen in the normal anterior pituitary gland.

Posterior Pituitary Syndromes

The most common syndrome resulting from a posterior pituitary abnormality is diabetes insipidus, caused by deficiency of ADH.

The posterior pituitary may be damaged by head trauma, tumors, or surgical procedures involving the hypothalamus or pituitary. The result of ADH deficiency is inadequate resorption of water in the kidney, producing *polyuria*. The excessive renal water loss elevates the sodium concentration and osmolality in the blood, inducing thirst and frequent drinking of water (*polydipsia*). This constellation of symptoms in the presence of normal blood glucose is characteristic of *diabetes insipidus*. Affected patients who are bedridden and unable to drink enough water can develop life-threatening dehydration.

Excess secretion of ADH (*syndrome of inappropriate ADH secretion [SIADH]*) is seen most often as a paraneoplastic syndrome with cancers, such as small cell cancer of the lung, which produce this hormone ectopically. The excessive resorption of water reduces plasma sodium levels and can lead to cerebral edema and neurologic dysfunction.

Craniopharyngioma

This tumor arises from Rathke pouch and may induce hypofunction or hyperfunction of the anterior pituitary, diabetes insipidus, or combinations of these manifestations.

Craniopharyngiomas are epithelial neoplasms that originate from vestigial remnants of Rathke pouch. Most are suprasellar, but intrasellar extension can occur. A bimodal age distribution is observed, with one peak in childhood (5 to 15 years) and a second peak in adults 65 years or older. Adults typically present with headaches and visual disturbances, whereas children may present with growth retardation due to pituitary hypofunction and growth hormone deficiency. There are two subtypes, one with *BRAF* mutations, characterized by papillary architecture, and a second with β-catenin mutations, recognized by compact, lamellar ("wet") squamous epithelium with peripheral palisading that is known as the adamantinomatous type (Supplemental eFig. 16.1). Treatment consists of surgical resection, often followed by local radiation for unresectable or recurrent disease. The prognosis is generally excellent, but endocrine and neurologic complications related to the tumor and its treatment are common and often irreversible.

THYROID

Thyroid hormones regulate the body's metabolism.

The thyroid gland, located in the neck adjacent to the larynx, is composed of follicles that are lined with hormone-producing epithelial cells. Thyroid-stimulating hormone (TSH, or thyrotropin) is released from the pituitary in response to hypothalamic signals, which in turn respond to sympathetic nervous stimulation, exposure to cold, and other alterations requiring metabolic adaptation. TSH binds to its G protein–coupled receptor on thyroid follicular epithelial cells and activates signaling pathways that lead to the synthesis and secretion of two hormones, thyroxine (T_4) and triiodothyronine (T_3). These small molecules are stored in the gland lumens bound to proteins such as thyroglobulin in a viscous fluid called colloid. Once released from colloid, the hormones circulate bound to plasma proteins and reach peripheral tissues, where most of the T_4 is converted to the more potent T_3. Both hormones can pass through the plasma membrane of cells and bind to the nuclear thyroid hormone receptor. The hormone-receptor complex stimulates the transcription of target genes, whose products are responsible for the metabolic effects of the hormones, including increased catabolism of carbohydrates and lipids (to provide energy) and increased protein synthesis. The net result of these processes is an increase in the basal metabolic rate.

Clinical Syndromes of Thyroid Dysfunction

Hyperthyroidism

Increased production of thyroid hormones causes hyperthyroidism (thyrotoxicosis), and decreased production causes hypothyroidism, both producing significant clinical manifestations.

Hyperthyroidism refers to increased activity of the thyroid gland, resulting in increased production of T_3 and T_4. Elevated levels of these hormones are most often caused by a primary thyroid abnormality but may result from a TSH-producing pituitary adenoma. Strictly speaking, the term *thyrotoxicosis* is used for the clinical syndrome caused by increased thyroid hormone levels, regardless of the cause, and *hyperthyroidism* is the syndrome caused by an intrinsic abnormality of the thyroid, but the two terms are used interchangeably.

The most common causes of hyperthyroidism are
- *Graves disease,* an autoimmune disorder that causes diffuse hyperplasia of the thyroid (~85% of cases of hyperthyroidism)
- *Hyperfunctioning (so-called toxic) multinodular goiter*
- *Hyperfunctioning (toxic) adenoma*

The clinical manifestations of hyperthyroidism are attributable to a hypermetabolic state and overactivity of the sympathetic nervous system. The major symptoms include:
- *Systemic:* warm skin because of increased blood flow; heat intolerance and sweating; weight loss
- *Gastrointestinal:* hypermotility, resulting in malabsorption and steatorrhea
- *Cardiac:* tachycardia with palpitations
- *Neuromuscular:* tremor, irritability, and, in almost half of patients, muscle weakness (thyroid myopathy)
- *Ocular:* wide staring gaze and lid lag due to sympathetic overstimulation of ocular muscles (Supplemental eFig. 16.2); full-blown ophthalmopathy is seen only in Graves disease, discussed later
- Acutely elevated catecholamine levels may synergize with increased thyroid hormones to severely exacerbate the manifestations of hyperthyroidism, a rare medical emergency seen during times of stress (e.g., infection, surgery, trauma) called thyroid storm.

The diagnosis of hyperthyroidism is confirmed by biochemical measurements of TSH (typically decreased) and T_4 (typically elevated). The TSH level is the single most important screening test for hyperthyroidism because levels are decreased even at the earliest stages. As discussed later, radioactive iodine uptake is valuable in determining the cause of thyroid hyperfunction.

Hypothyroidism

Hypothyroidism is the clinical syndrome resulting from deficiency of thyroid hormones. Its main causes are
- *Dietary deficiency of iodine,* which is required for the synthesis of T_3 and T_4. This condition is more common in lower-income countries than in higher-income countries related to iodine supplementation in salt.
- *Autoimmune thyroid disease,* primarily *Hashimoto thyroiditis*
- *Congenital defects* (rare)
- *Iatrogenic,* due to damage caused by surgery or radiation

The manifestations of hypothyroidism vary depending on whether it develops during childhood or in adults. Congenital hypothyroidism is the form in infancy and early childhood. It usually results from iodine deficiency and is therefore endemic in regions of the world where such deficiency is common, such as the foothills of the Himalayas and Andes. Development of the skeletal and nervous systems is impaired, leading to short stature, intellectual disability, and coarse facial features. By contrast, *myxedema* is the form in older children and adults. Its manifestations reflect a reduced basal metabolic rate and include fatigue, apathy, sluggishness, cool skin (due to decreased blood flow), and reduced cardiac output leading to shortness of breath. In addition, extracellular matrix proteins accumulate in connective tissues, causing nonpitting edema (the basis for the name of the disease), enlarged tongue, and coarse facial features. Constipation is an early sign resulting from decreased sympathetic nervous system activity. Laboratory tests reveal increased serum TSH and reduced T_4.

Our discussion of thyroid diseases now turns to the major immunologic, metabolic, and neoplastic disorders affecting the gland.

Autoimmune Thyroid Disease

The major autoimmune diseases of the thyroid cause hypothyroidism (Hashimoto thyroiditis) or hyperthyroidism (Graves disease).

Although both disorders are the result of autoimmune responses against thyroid antigens, their pathogenesis is completely different: Hashimoto thyroiditis is a destructive inflammatory disease caused mainly by T cells, whereas Graves disease is due to excessive stimulation of the gland by autoantibodies.

Chronic Lymphocytic (Hashimoto) Thyroiditis

In Hashimoto thyroiditis, T cells reactive with unknown thyroid antigens destroy follicular epithelial cells, resulting in reduced production of thyroid hormones.

Pathogenesis. As in most autoimmune diseases, the initiating events are unknown. The disease has a genetic predisposition, as evidenced by the high concordance rate in identical twins and the identification of associated polymorphisms in genes involved in immune regulation. The immune response is directed against follicular epithelial cells; the target antigens may include thyroglobulin and the TSH receptor. Autoreactive CD8+ cytotoxic T cells directly kill epithelial cells, and CD4+ T cells secrete cytokines that cause inflammation and damage to follicles. Antibodies against thyroid antigens are also present, but their pathogenic role is unclear.

Morphology. The thyroid is enlarged and contains dense mononuclear cell infiltrates, composed of lymphocytes, plasma cells, and even well-formed germinal centers (Fig. 16.2A). The thyroid follicles are atrophic. Some injured follicular cells undergo a metaplastic response that converts them to large, granular eosinophilic cells called Hürthle cells.

Clinical Features. Hashimoto thyroiditis is the most common cause of hypothyroidism in higher-income countries. It is most prevalent between 45 and 65 years of age and is much more common in women (female to male ratio, 10:1 to 20:1). Although it is primarily a disease of older adults, it can occur at any age, including childhood. Patients present with painless, usually diffuse and symmetric enlargement of the thyroid and varying degrees of hypothyroidism, which progresses gradually. In some cases, there is transient thyrotoxicosis early in the course because of release of hormones from injured follicular epithelial cells. There is an increased risk for developing B-cell lymphoma within the affected thyroid gland, another example of the association between chronic inflammation and cancer (see Chapter 5).

Graves Disease

Graves disease is caused by autoantibodies that bind to the TSH receptor on thyroid follicular epithelial cells and stimulate uncontrolled hormone production from these cells.

Pathogenesis. Multiple antibodies have been described, of which the most important are directed against the TSH receptor expressed on thyroid epithelial cells. They stimulate the epithelial cells, thus mimicking the actions of the trophic hormone TSH. Because the antibodies are not subject to feedback control (as is TSH), the stimulation is constant and unrestrained. A consistent feature is ophthalmopathy, involvement of the eye that is likely caused by T cell–mediated inflammation of the retroorbital space.

Morphology. The thyroid gland is enlarged due to diffuse hypertrophy and hyperplasia of follicular epithelial cells (Fig 16.2B). The proliferating thyroid epithelial cells are thrown into folds. Lymphoid infiltrates are present but are usually not as prominent as in Hashimoto thyroiditis. In patients with ophthalmopathy, retroorbital tissues show edema, deposition of extracellular matrix, and T-cell infiltrates.

Clinical Features. Most patients are women in the 20- to 40-year-old age group. Patients present with signs of hyperthyroidism, discussed earlier. The telltale features of Graves disease are diffuse enlargement of the thyroid, protrusion of the eyes (*exophthalmos*; Supplemental eFig. 16.2), and induration of the skin, especially over the tibia (*pretibial myxedema*). Radioiodine uptake shows a diffuse pattern because the entire gland is involved. By contrast, focal lesions (such as functional adenomas) show localized uptake of radioiodine.

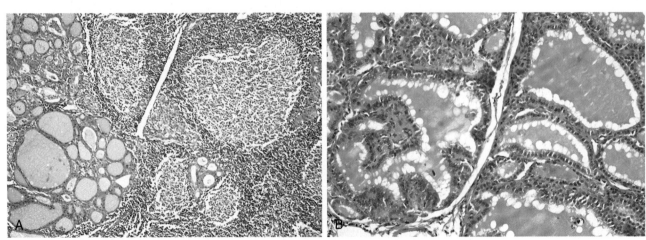

Fig. 16.2 (A) Hashimoto thyroiditis. The thyroid parenchyma contains a dense lymphocytic infiltrate with germinal centers. (B) Graves disease. The follicles are lined by tall, hyperplastic columnar epithelial cells that are actively resorbing the colloid in the follicles, resulting in a "scalloped" appearance.

Other Forms of Inflammatory Thyroid Disease

Several other less common types of thyroiditis are recognized.

- *Subacute granulomatous (de Quervain) thyroiditis* is self-limited and may be caused by an as yet unidentified viral infection. It is most common between 30 and 50 years of age and, like other forms of thyroiditis, is more common in women. The onset is acute, often with neck pain, fever, and thyroid enlargement. There may be transient hyperthyroidism. Histologic examination reveals disrupted follicles and inflammatory infiltrates (Supplemental eFig. 16.3). The condition typically resolves within 6 to 8 weeks.
- *Subacute lymphocytic thyroiditis* occurs mostly in women, sometimes following pregnancy. It may be an autoimmune disorder. Patients present with a painless neck mass or signs of hyperthyroidism. The initial phase of thyrotoxicosis is followed by a return to a euthyroid state within a few months. Histologically, there are lymphocytic infiltrates with germinal centers in the gland, but unlike Hashimoto thyroiditis, Hürthle cell change is not prominent.
- *Riedel thyroiditis* is characterized by fibrosis replacing the thyroid, producing a firm mass. It may be part of IgG4-related disease, a syndrome characterized by fibrosis of multiple organs and elevated levels of serum IgG4 (which is of uncertain pathogenic significance).

Goiter

Goiter (enlargement of the thyroid), the most common clinical manifestation of thyroid disease, is caused by impaired synthesis of thyroid hormone, elevated levels of TSH, and a resultant hyperplasia of follicular epithelial cells.

Pathogenesis. The fundamental abnormality that leads to goiter development is defective synthesis of T_3 and T_4. Because of the failure of negative feedback, TSH production is sustained, driving proliferation of epithelial cells. There are two forms of goiter that differ mechanistically.

- *Endemic goiter* is caused by dietary iodine deficiency, and is therefore seen in only some regions of the world. Its incidence has decreased greatly due to dietary iodine supplementation.
- *Sporadic goiter* is most common in women and has a peak incidence in puberty and young adulthood (when the demand for thyroid hormone is greatest). Other causes include excessive dietary intake of substances that interfere with thyroid hormone synthesis (e.g., calcium and cruciferous vegetables such as cabbage and cauliflower), and inherited defects in enzymes involved in the synthesis of thyroid hormones.

Morphology. The TSH-induced proliferation of follicular epithelial cells produces a diffusely enlarged gland initially (diffuse goiter). The cells may involute if the demand for thyroid hormones goes down. Over time, multiple cycles of proliferation and involution lead to irregular enlargement of the gland, so diffuse goiter tends to evolve into multinodular goiter (Fig. 16.3).

Clinical Features. The typical presentation is a neck mass, which may become so large that it compresses other structures and causes airway obstruction, dysphagia, and vascular compromise (Supplemental eFig. 16.4). Multinodular goiters usually are functionally silent, but a minority (~10% over 10 years) manifest with thyrotoxicosis secondary to the development of autonomous nodules that produce thyroid hormone independent of TSH stimulation. This condition, known as *toxic multinodular goiter,* lacks the infiltrative ophthalmopathy and dermopathy of Graves disease–associated thyrotoxicosis. The incidence of malignancy in long-standing multinodular goiters is low (<5%); concern for malignancy increases with goiters that demonstrate sudden changes in size or symptoms caused by compression (e.g., hoarseness).

Tumors of the Thyroid Gland

The majority of thyroid nodules are benign, either adenomas or dominant nodules in a goiter, and only about 1% are carcinomas. But this distinction is so important clinically that all thyroid nodules are routinely examined by fine-needle aspiration and pathologic study of a biopsy, if needed. The following clinical characteristics increase the probability that a nodule is malignant:

- If the nodule is solitary
- Age less than 20 years or older than 70 years
- History of radiation exposure
- Failure to take up radioactive iodine in imaging studies (cold nodule)
- Ultrasonographic evidence of extrathyroidal extension or enlargement of cervical lymph nodes

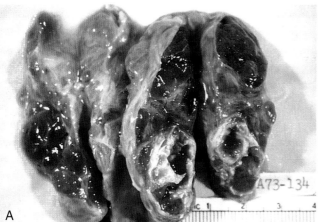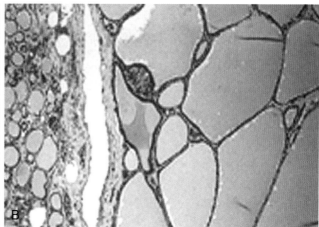

Fig. 16.3 Multinodular goiter. (A) Gross morphologic appearance. The coarsely nodular gland contains areas of fibrosis and cystic change. (B) Photomicrograph of a specimen from a hyperplastic nodule, with compressed residual thyroid parenchyma on the periphery. The hyperplastic follicles contain abundant pink "colloid" within their lumina. Note the absence of a prominent capsule, a feature distinguishing such lesions from neoplasms of the thyroid. (B, Courtesy Dr. William Westra, Department of Pathology, Johns Hopkins University, Baltimore.)

Thyroid Adenoma

Thyroid adenomas are benign, usually solitary, tumors derived from follicular epithelium.

The vast majority are nonfunctional; a small subset secretes thyroid hormones and causes hyperthyroidism.

Pathogenesis. About 50% of functional adenomas harbor gain-of-function mutations in the TSH receptor pathway, either in the receptor itself or in downstream G protein–coupled signaling. The result is increased proliferation and hormone production by follicular epithelial cells, independent of TSH stimulation. This leads to the development of benign hormone-producing tumors (so-called toxic adenomas). Such mutations also are observed in a subset of autonomous nodules that give rise to toxic multinodular goiters, discussed earlier. A minority of nonfunctioning follicular adenomas (<20%) exhibits mutations in the *RAS* or other genes, genetic alterations that are shared with follicular thyroid carcinomas (discussed later).

Morphology. The typical adenoma is a solitary lesion composed of colloid-filled follicles lined with uniform-appearing epithelial cells, surrounded by a capsule (Fig. 16.4). Sometimes, adenomas show cellular atypia, but a diagnosis of malignancy requires demonstration of capsular invasion. Therefore, evaluation of the integrity of the capsule is critical. In general, follicular adenomas are not precursors of carcinomas.

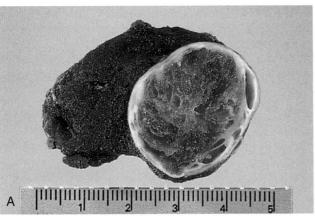

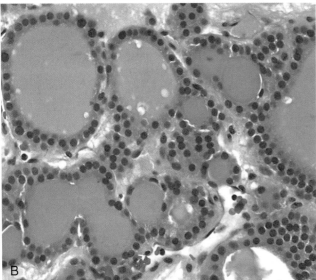

Fig. 16.4 Follicular adenoma of the thyroid. (A) A solitary, well-circumscribed nodule is visible in this gross specimen. (B) The photomicrograph shows well-differentiated follicles resembling those of normal thyroid parenchyma.

Clinical Features. Patients typically present with a painless nodule, often detected incidentally during a routine physical examination. As mentioned earlier, toxic adenomas produce thyroid hormones. Scanning with radioactive iodine is useful in the management of thyroid nodules. Nodules that take up less iodine than the adjacent normal thyroid tissue are called cold nodules, and approximately 10% of them prove to be malignant. Hot nodules (toxic adenomas) are positive by scanning and are rarely malignant.

Thyroid Carcinoma

There are four main types of thyroid carcinoma, each with unique pathogenesis, morphologic features, and clinical course.

- *Papillary carcinoma* accounts for more than 85% of cases and can present at any age. Exposure of the neck to ionizing radiation is a well-known risk factor. Most of these tumors are associated with activation of the MAP-kinase pathway, caused either by rearrangements of the gene encoding the receptor tyrosine kinase RET or by activating mutations involving *BRAF* (Chapter 5). Lesions may be solitary or multiple and may infiltrate the adjacent parenchyma. Their microscopic hallmark is the presence of branching papillae covered by well-differentiated epithelial cells with finely dispersed chromatin, which makes them look clear or empty in the center (Fig. 16.5). *Psammoma bodies* (concentrically calcified structures) are often present within the lesion; these structures are almost never found in follicular and medullary carcinomas. Clinically, the tumors present as neck masses, either within the thyroid or as metastatic deposits in draining cervical lymph nodes. Of interest, the presence of isolated cervical lymph node metastases does not have a significant influence on the prognosis. Unlike follicular carcinomas, described next, hematogenous spread is uncommon. Papillary carcinomas are nonfunctional, and their course is indolent, with a 10-year survival rate of more than 95%.

- *Follicular carcinoma* accounts for 5% to 15% of cases. They are more common in women (by a ratio of 3:1) and manifest at older ages than papillary carcinomas, with a peak incidence between 40 and 60 years of age. The most common oncogenic drivers are mutations that activate RAS and a translocation that fuses portions of two genes, *PAX8* (important in thyroid development) and *PPARγ* (which encodes a nuclear hormone receptor). Histologically, the tumors are composed of uniform cells forming small follicles (Fig. 16.6) that resemble follicular adenomas; the presence of capsular invasion, vascular invasion, or metastases distinguishes follicular carcinoma from follicular adenoma. The tumors usually present as solitary cold nodules. Distant metastases via the bloodstream are much more frequent than in papillary cancers. Lymph node metastases are uncommon. The prognosis is much worse than that of papillary carcinomas: Survival at 10 years is approximately 50%.

- *Anaplastic carcinoma* accounts for less than 5% of thyroid cancers. It is an aggressive tumor that is almost always fatal. Patients are older than those with other variants of thyroid cancer, with a mean age of 65 years. Approximately 50% develop from a preexisting papillary or follicular carcinoma. The most common mutations associated with acquisition of the aggressive, anaplastic phenotype are loss-of-function mutations in *TP53*. Anaplastic carcinomas are composed of poorly differentiated, rapidly growing cells. The tumor expands and metastasizes rapidly, and may be fatal within 1 year of detection.

- *Medullary carcinoma* makes up less than 5% of cases of thyroid cancer and is derived from calcitonin-producing neuroendocrine cells. The most common oncogenic events are mutations in the *RET* oncogene that lead to constitutive activation of the encoded

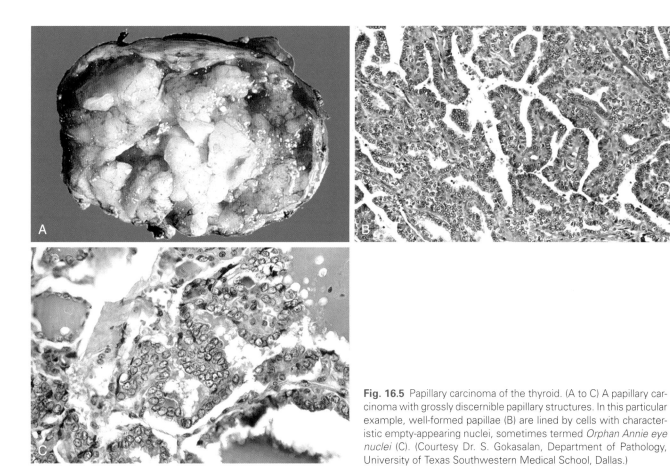

Fig. 16.5 Papillary carcinoma of the thyroid. (A to C) A papillary carcinoma with grossly discernible papillary structures. In this particular example, well-formed papillae (B) are lined by cells with characteristic empty-appearing nuclei, sometimes termed *Orphan Annie eye nuclei* (C). (Courtesy Dr. S. Gokasalan, Department of Pathology, University of Texas Southwestern Medical School, Dallas.)

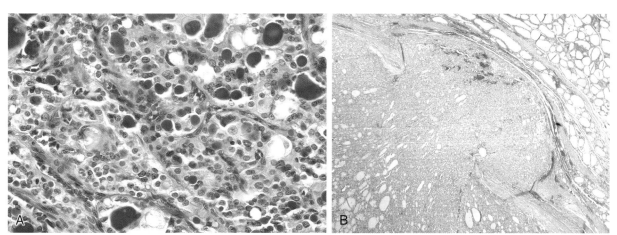

Fig. 16.6 Follicular carcinoma of the thyroid. (A) A few of the glandular lumina contain recognizable colloid. (B) Capsular invasion may be minimal, as in this case, or widespread, with extension into local structures of the neck.

tyrosine kinase receptor. Medullary carcinomas arise sporadically in about 70% of cases; the remaining 30% are familial, occurring in the setting of multiple endocrine neoplasia (MEN) syndrome 2A or 2B, discussed later, or familial medullary thyroid carcinoma without an associated MEN syndrome. Tumors may be solitary or multiple, composed of nests of spindle-shaped or polygonal cells.

The tumors frequently contain deposits of amyloid derived from the large amounts of calcitonin that are produced by the tumor cells (Supplemental eFig. 16.5). The clinical presentation is of a neck mass. Most patients have increased levels of serum calcitonin.

PARATHYROID GLANDS

The main function of the parathyroid glands is to regulate calcium levels in the body. Reduced concentrations of blood calcium stimulate the production of parathyroid hormone (PTH), which has multiple actions: It increases renal tubular reabsorption of calcium; increases urinary phosphate excretion, thereby releasing calcium from its phosphate-bound form; increases conversion of vitamin D to its active form in the kidneys, which increases calcium uptake in the gastrointestinal tract; and increases the breakdown of bone, releasing sequestered calcium. All these activities serve to elevate blood calcium levels, which inhibit further PTH production. Diseases of the parathyroids are associated with excessive or deficient PTH activity.

Hyperparathyroidism may stem from a primary abnormality of the glands or may be secondary to chronic renal failure.

- *Primary hyperparathyroidism* is a common endocrine disorder and the most frequent cause of clinically silent hypercalcemia, usually detected during routine blood tests. It is much more common in women than in men (by nearly 4:1). In most instances, it is caused by a parathyroid adenoma that secretes excessive PTH (Supplemental eFig. 16.6). Less commonly, it is caused by multiglandular parathyroid hyperplasia or parathyroid carcinoma. Abnormalities in two genes are commonly associated with parathyroid tumors: cyclin D1 gene rearrangements and mutations of the tumor suppressor gene *MEN1*.
- *Secondary hyperparathyroidism* occurs in the setting of chronic renal failure, which depresses blood calcium levels, in part owing to decreased phosphate excretion and hyperphosphatemia. This in turn triggers overactivity of the parathyroid glands (diffuse hyperplasia). Compensatory increases in PTH levels restore blood calcium levels, and the clinical problems are related mainly to the renal disease.

Hypercalcemia is also seen in cancers with bony metastases and as a paraneoplastic syndrome associated with lung cancer and other tumors, resulting from ectopic production of PTH-related protein (PTHrP) by the tumor cells. The clinical manifestations of hypercalcemia include gastrointestinal disturbances, depression and lethargy, muscle weakness, and polyuria. Hypercalcemia also can give rise to renal stones and metastatic calcification.

Hypoparathyroidism is rare and is most often caused by inadvertent removal of parathyroid glands during thyroid or other neck surgery. The most frequent clinical manifestations are increased neuromuscular irritability (tetany) and cardiac arrhythmias.

ENDOCRINE PANCREAS: DIABETES

Most of the pancreas is composed of exocrine glands, which secrete digestive enzymes into the duodenum (see Chapter 13). The endocrine component of the pancreas is the *islets of Langerhans,* which contain cells that produce the hormones insulin, glucagon, somatostatin, and pancreatic polypeptide, each secreted by a distinct population of cells. Deficient insulin production or function causes diabetes, which is one of the great medical scourges of the modern world and the focus of the discussion that follows.

Overview of Diabetes

Diabetes is a metabolic disorder characterized by hyperglycemia, resulting from defective production or inadequate action of insulin.

The incidence of this disease has risen alarmingly in recent years, because one of the two major forms of diabetes (type 2 diabetes, discussed later) is associated with obesity, an increasing problem worldwide. More than a million new cases are diagnosed each year in the United States; it is estimated that almost 10% of the population is diabetic, and that one third of these people are unaware of their disease. Many more may be prediabetic (elevated blood glucose level that is not high enough for a diagnosis of diabetes) and at high risk for developing diabetes. Long-standing diabetes results in abnormalities in many organs. In the United States, diabetes is the leading cause of end-stage renal disease, adult-onset blindness, and lower extremity amputation (due to diabetes-associated peripheral vascular disease).

The World Health Organization criteria for the diagnosis of diabetes include one or more of the following test results:
- A fasting plasma glucose > 126 mg/dL
- A 2-hour plasma glucose > 200 mg/dL during an oral glucose tolerance test with a loading dose of 75 g
- A glycated hemoglobin (HbA1c) level > 6.5%. HbA1c is formed by nonenzymatic addition of glucose to hemoglobin in red cells in a reaction that depends only on glucose concentration. Because of the long life span of red cells (~120 days), the level of HbA1c reflects glucose levels over a sustained period of time, unlike a single blood glucose level, which may vary widely due to superimposed infection, trauma, and other acute stresses. Thus, measurement of the HbA1c level is a reliable test for diabetes; it is also useful in judging the efficacy of therapy.

Insulin Physiology

Insulin is produced by pancreatic islet β cells; it increases the rate of glucose transport principally into muscle and to a lesser extent into adipose cells and reduces the production of glucose from glycogen in the liver.

Glucose is the body's principal fuel. In muscle cells, it is stored as glycogen, and when needed, the glycogen is converted to glucose, which is oxidized in mitochondria to generate ATP, providing energy for cellular functions (Fig. 16.7). Glucose metabolism also generates intermediates needed for synthesis of cellular building blocks that are required for cell growth. In adipose tissues, glucose is metabolized to lipids, which are stored as fat.

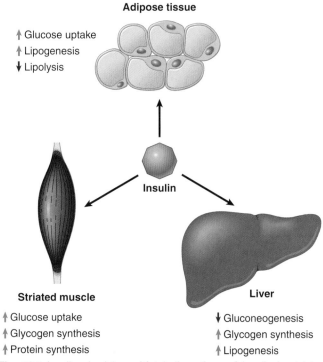

Adipose tissue

↑ Glucose uptake
↑ Lipogenesis
↓ Lipolysis

Insulin

Striated muscle

↑ Glucose uptake
↑ Glycogen synthesis
↑ Protein synthesis

Liver

↓ Gluconeogenesis
↑ Glycogen synthesis
↑ Lipogenesis

Fig. 16.7 Insulin physiology. Metabolic actions of insulin in striated muscle, adipose tissue, and liver.

Oral intake of food raises the level of glucose in the blood and stimulates insulin production from islet β cells, an effect that is augmented by certain hormones *(incretins)* released from intestinal cells. Insulin acts via the insulin receptor to increase glucose uptake into muscle and fat, thus providing the substrate for generating energy and reducing blood glucose. It also stimulates the uptake of amino acids and inhibits the degradation of lipids and proteins, so its net effects are anabolic. In addition, insulin reduces the generation of glucose from glycogen stores in the liver, further reducing blood glucose levels. Many of the effects of insulin are counteracted by glucagon, a hormone that is produced by α cells in pancreatic islets. The major function of glucagon is to stimulate glycogen breakdown (glycogenolysis) in the liver, leading to an increase in blood glucose. During fasting states, low insulin and high glucagon levels facilitate hepatic glycogen breakdown while decreasing glycogen synthesis, in an attempt to maintain normal blood glucose.

Pathogenesis of Diabetes

The two major forms of diabetes, type 1 (accounting for 5% to 10% of cases) and type 2 (90% of cases), are caused by different mechanisms.

Type 1 Diabetes

Type 1 diabetes (T1D) is an autoimmune disease in which T cells attack and destroy β cells, resulting in a deficiency of insulin.

As in other autoimmune diseases, the reason why tolerance fails and the immune system attacks the individual's own islet β cells is unknown. Many different variants in genes involved in immune regulation are associated with an increased risk for the disease, foremost among these being HLA class II genes. Defective regulation by regulatory T cells is a popular hypothesis, but why this affects only the islets is not known. A role for environmental factors, including infections and the microbiome (commensal microbes), is suspected but not established. Regardless of the underlying mechanism, it is clear that T and B cells that react with islet antigens are present in patients. Much of the β cell damage is caused by CD8+ cytotoxic T lymphocytes, which kill islet cells, and by CD4+ T cells, which induce destructive inflammation. Antibodies specific for islet cell antigens are useful markers for the disease, but their contribution to β cell destruction is uncertain.

Type 2 Diabetes

Type 2 diabetes (T2D) is a complex disease resulting from insulin resistance in peripheral tissues (failure to respond to insulin) and β cell dysfunction manifested as insulin secretion that is inadequate for the plasma glucose level.

T2D remains a poorly understood disease in which genetics, environmental factors, and inflammation all seem to play a role (Fig. 16.8).

- *Genetics.* Genetic factors are clearly involved, as evidenced by the 80% to 90% concordance in identical twins (even more than in T1D). Despite many studies and the identification of dozens of genetic polymorphisms that are statistically associated with T2D, an understanding of how genetic variants cause insulin resistance or β cell dysfunction remains elusive.
- *Obesity.* Obesity is associated with the development of insulin resistance, even in the absence of hyperglycemia. The amount of body fat and its location (central more than peripheral) influence the risk of developing T2D. This association has led to the term *metabolic syndrome* for the combination of visceral obesity, glucose intolerance, cardiovascular disease, and abnormal lipid profiles. Individuals with metabolic syndrome are at high risk for T2D. Obesity may promote insulin resistance by multiple mechanisms: (1) intracellular triglycerides and products of fatty acid metabolism inhibit

insulin signaling; (2) adipose tissue secretes cytokines, some of which (adiponectin and leptin) promote the insulin sensitivity of tissues; adiponectin levels are reduced in obesity and while leptin levels are increased, there is a state of leptin resistance; and (3) free fatty acids that accumulate in cells activate the sensing pathway called the inflammasome (see Chapter 2), stimulating the production of cytokines (such as interleukin-1), which induce insulin resistance.

- *β cell dysfunction.* β cell function may increase early in the development of T2D, in response to increased blood glucose, but ultimately, defective β cell function is an essential contributor to the development of overt diabetes. This dysfunction may be due to excess free fatty acids (lipotoxicity) or glucose itself (glucotoxicity); defects in the production of insulin-releasing hormones from the intestine; poorly defined genetic defects; or replacement of islets with amyloid (which may be an effect of long-standing islet dysfunction rather than its cause).

Other Forms of Diabetes

About 5% of cases are attributable to single gene defects with high penetrance and expressivity that follow Mendelian inheritance. The most common of these is *maturity-onset diabetes of the young (MODY)*, which may result from mutations in one of several genes involved in β cell function. *Congenital early-onset diabetes,* which is usually detected in the neonatal period, is caused by mutations in the insulin or insulin receptor gene or genes that affect receptor expression or signaling. Diabetes may also appear during pregnancy *(gestational diabetes),* especially in women

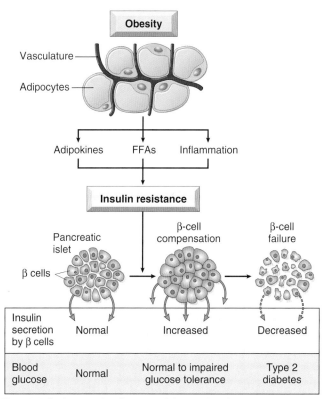

Fig. 16.8 Pathogenesis of type 2 diabetes. Insulin resistance associated with obesity is induced by adipokines, free fatty acids, and chronic inflammation in adipose tissue. Pancreatic β cells compensate for insulin resistance by hypersecretion of insulin. However, at some point, β-cell compensation is followed by β-cell failure, and diabetes ensues. FFA, free fatty acids. (Reproduced with permission from Kasuga M: Insulin resistance and pancreatic β-cell failure. *J Clin Invest* 116:1756, 2006.)

who are already prediabetic; pregnancy-associated hormones favor insulin resistance. In rare cases, diabetes may result from destruction of the pancreas by chronic pancreatitis or hemochromatosis, or a tumor in the exocrine pancreas that secondarily affects the islets.

Clinicopathologic Features of Diabetes

The morbidity associated with diabetes is mainly due to chronic complications of hyperglycemia and the resulting vascular injury.

The classic clinical presentation of T1D is the triad of polyuria (frequent urination, due to the osmotic effect of glucose in the urine), polydipsia (frequent drinking, due to dehydration from urinary losses), and polyphagia (excessive eating, due to tissue "starvation" in the midst of plenty). By contrast, most individuals with T2D are asymptomatic; hyperglycemia is discovered on routine laboratory testing. The morbidity of both forms results from the chronic complications of poorly controlled blood sugar, particularly damage to small and medium-sized arteries; small blood vessels develop diffuse basement membrane thickening, whereas larger arteries develop accelerated atherosclerosis. The most severely affected organs are those that are particularly sensitive to disruption of the blood supply (Fig. 16.9). The development of the tissue injury involves at least three pathogenic pathways.

- *Advanced glycation end-products (AGEs)* are formed by interactions between glucose-derived molecules such as glyoxal and cellular proteins, a process that is accelerated by hyperglycemia. AGEs bind to a receptor called RAGE (receptor for AGE) that is expressed on inflammatory cells (macrophages and T cells), endothelium, and vascular smooth muscle cells. Binding for AGEs to RAGE leads to the production of cytokines and growth factors, generation of reactive oxygen species, increased procoagulant activity of endothelium, proliferation of smooth muscle cells, and synthesis of extracellular matrix. It is not known if these activities serve a physiologic role, but in diabetes they are major contributors to the vascular pathology, described later.

- *In some tissues, intracellular concentrations of glucose increase and have toxic consequences.* This is because some tissues (nerve, lens, kidney, blood vessels) do not require insulin for glucose uptake, and, in the setting of hyperglycemia, intracellular glucose levels rise. Intracellular glucose is metabolized to sorbitol in a reaction that depletes NADPH, a cofactor that is required for the regeneration of reduced glutathione, an important antioxidant (see Chapter 1). These cells therefore have increased susceptibility to damage caused by oxidative stress.

- *Intracellular glucose is also converted to diacylglycerol, which activates the enzyme protein kinase C.* This enzyme stimulates several signaling pathways, leading to increased production of growth factors such as vascular endothelial growth factor (which stimulates endothelial proliferation, contributing to the neovascularization seen in diabetic retinopathy) and TGF-β (which stimulates production of extracellular matrix proteins).

In the next section we discuss some of the most serious and well-defined lesions affecting different organs. In addition to these, diabetics show an increased susceptibility to infections. It is not clear if this reflects reduced host defenses due to reduced tissue blood supply or an undefined immunological abnormality.

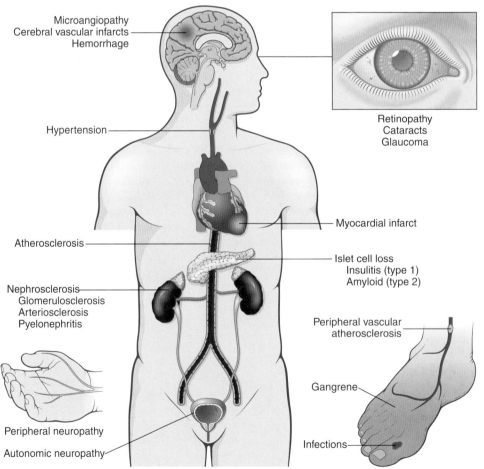

Fig. 16.9 Chronic complications of diabetes.

Vascular Lesions

The hallmarks of diabetic vascular disease are accelerated atherosclerosis and hyalinization of small and medium-sized arteries.

Pathogenesis. The hyperglycemia-associated abnormalities described above lead to proliferation of vascular endothelial and smooth muscle cells, deposition of extracellular matrix proteins in the vessel wall and arterial basement membrane, a propensity for small thrombi to form, and chronic inflammation. Collectively, these processes narrow the lumens of vessels and accelerate aging-associated atherosclerosis, leading to vascular compromise and ischemia.

Clinical Features. The consequences of the vascular lesions are evident in numerous tissues.
- *Myocardial infarction* is the most common cause of death in diabetics.
- *Ischemic necrosis of the legs* (gangrene) is 100 times more common in diabetics than in the general population.
- *Small-vessel disease (microangiopathy)* characterized by diffuse thickening of the capillary basement membranes underlies lesions of the kidney, eyes, and nerves, described next.

Diabetic Nephropathy

Renal complications of diabetes include glomerular disease (see Chapter 11), leading to scarring (glomerulosclerosis), as well as vascular and other lesions.

Pathogenesis. AGEs may stimulate the production of cytokines and growth factors that lead to the increased synthesis of matrix proteins in the glomerular mesangium. Microvascular disease leads to reduced blood flow and activation of the renin–angiotensin system, which compensates by increasing flow through the glomeruli. The resulting glomerular hyperfiltration and increase in vascular pressure in the glomeruli may have deleterious effects on the glomerular permeability barrier. Many other abnormalities in signaling pathways in glomerular epithelial cells (podocytes) and proteins of the slit diaphragm have been reported, but their contribution to the lesions remains unclear.

Morphology. The histologic hallmarks of diabetic glomerular disease are deposits of matrix material in the mesangium and capillary wall, diffuse glomerular basement membrane thickening, and progressive scarring (Fig. 16.10). Sometimes, the matrix material deposited in the glomerulus appears nodular, giving rise to the term *nodular glomerulosclerosis* (Kimmelstiel-Wilson lesions). In addition to glomerular lesions, narrowing of arterioles caused by microvascular disease may result in nephrosclerosis, with tubular atrophy and interstitial fibrosis. Hyaline arteriolosclerosis, a vascular lesion associated with hypertension, is both more prevalent and more severe in diabetics than in nondiabetics; it is characterized by amorphous, hyaline thickening of the wall of the arterioles. Patients are also prone to infections and have a higher incidence of pyelonephritis (see Chapter 11) than do normoglycemic individuals.

Clinical Features. The glomerular disease presents with proteinuria that may progress to full-blown nephrotic syndrome. About 40% of patients develop end-stage renal disease from a combination of glomerular scarring and vascular lesions causing widespread ischemic damage.

Diabetic Retinopathy

Retinopathy is the result of lesions affecting retinal blood vessels, and can seriously compromise vision.

Diabetic retinopathy is the principal cause of visual impairment between the ages of 25 and 75. There may be a genetic predisposition, because some patients with uncontrolled hyperglycemia never develop retinopathy whereas others with reasonable blood glucose control do.

Pathogenesis. The pathogenesis of diabetic retinopathy is complex and incompletely understood. The chief risk factor is sustained hyperglycemia, which is believed to damage vessels due to alterations in blood flow, formation of AGEs, and possibly other mechanisms. These vascular changes initially lead to minute hemorrhages, ischemia, small infarcts (cotton wool spots), and macular edema, all of which impair vision. If ischemia is severe, local production of VEGF induces neoangiogenesis (proliferative retinopathy), which is often associated with more extensive retinal and vitreous hemorrhages. These may organize and undergo fibrosis, placing traction on the retina that leads to retinal detachment, impaired vision, and even blindness.

Morphology. Retinal disease may be nonproliferative or proliferative. Nonproliferative retinopathy is characterized by thickening of capillaries, aneurysms, hemorrhages, edema, and exudates of leaked plasma proteins and lipids. Proliferative retinopathy is a process of new vessel formation and fibrosis.

Clinical Features. Visual impairment, sometimes even total blindness, can result from proliferative retinopathy, especially if the macula is

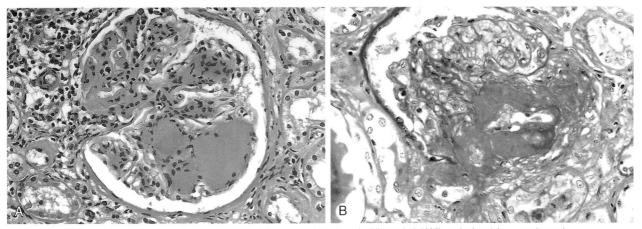

Fig. 16.10 Diabetic nephropathy. (A) Nodular glomerulosclerosis (Kimmelstiel-Wilson lesions) in a renal specimen from a patient with long-standing diabetes. (B) Severe renal hyaline arteriolosclerosis. Note the markedly thickened, tortuous afferent arteriole. The amorphous nature of the thickened vascular wall is evident. (A, Courtesy Dr. Lisa Yerian, Department of Pathology, University of Chicago, Chicago. B, Courtesy Dr. M.A. Venkatachalam, Department of Pathology, University of Texas Health Science Center, San Antonio, Texas.)

affected. Organization and fibrosis of vitreous hemorrhages from the newly formed vessels can cause retinal detachment. In addition to the retinal disease, patients are prone to developing cataracts and glaucoma.

Diabetic Neuropathy

This is typically a symmetric peripheral neuropathy of the legs that affects mainly sensory nerves but may also impair motor function. Autonomic neuropathy also occurs, resulting in bowel and urinary disturbances. These changes are probably the result of microangiopathy affecting vessels supplying the nerves, but may also have a component of direct axonal damage.

Acute Diabetic Ketoacidosis and Nonketotic Hyperosmolar Coma

Although chronic complications constitute the major clinical problems in diabetics, acute ketoacidosis is the leading cause of morbidity and mortality in type 1 diabetes (and often how the disease presents in this patient population) and occasionally complicates type 2 diabetes, particularly in the obese. Unrecognized type 1 diabetes or altered diet, infection, and other types of stress superimposed on known diabetes may worsen the metabolic imbalance, leading to sudden increases in blood glucose to levels as high as 500 to 700 mg/dL. This level of hyperglycemia markedly worsens the osmotic diuresis, resulting in severe dehydration. Insulin deficiency triggers lipolysis, generating acidic ketones, which are an alternative source of energy (particularly for the brain) during states of starvation. Excessive ketosis leads to a metabolic acidosis and increases the risk for developing cerebral edema, which can be fatal if it is not recognized and treated immediately. Dehydration and electrolyte imbalances must be carefully corrected if the patient is to survive. Type 2 diabetics may develop hyperosmolar nonketotic coma. This syndrome results from severe dehydration due to sustained osmotic diuresis in individuals whose water intake is inadequate. Affected patients are typically older adults who have been disabled by stroke or some other debilitating illness.

ADRENAL GLANDS

Each adrenal gland consists of two distinct regions, the cortex and medulla. The cortex produces three types of steroid hormones: glucocorticoids (mainly cortisol), mineralocorticoids (aldosterone), and sex steroids (estrogens and androgens). The medulla produces catecholamines, mainly epinephrine. Most of the known diseases of the adrenal glands are related to excessive or defective function of the adrenal cortex.

Cushing Syndrome: Hypercortisolism

This syndrome is caused by increased levels of glucocorticoids, resulting in metabolic and other abnormalities.

Pathogenesis. In clinical practice, the most common cause of Cushing syndrome is the administration of steroids to treat inflammatory diseases. Endogenous Cushing syndrome may be caused by increased ACTH production by a pituitary adenoma (also called Cushing disease, ~70% of cases), a tumor or hyperplasia of the adrenal cortex (15% to 20%), or ectopic ACTH production by some other tumor, such as small cell lung cancer (~10%). In all forms, urinary free cortisol concentration is increased. In pituitary Cushing disease and Cushing syndrome caused by ectopic ACTH secretion, serum ACTH levels are elevated due to loss of negative feedback control by cortisol. When Cushing syndrome is caused by a tumor or primary hyperplasia of the adrenal cortex, ACTH levels are below normal because feedback inhibition is intact.

Morphology. Patients with ACTH-dependent Cushing syndrome show diffuse hyperplasia of the adrenal cortex (Fig. 16.11A). Primary cortical hyperplasia is typically associated with nodular lesions, which are often dark in appearance due to accumulation of lipofuscin

(Fig. 16.11B). By contrast, functional adenomas are solitary lesions composed of normal-appearing cells surrounded by a capsule (Fig. 16.11C, D). Carcinomas are uncommon; in these malignancies, cells show more atypia and have a tendency to invade veins and lymphatics. With functioning adrenal tumors, both benign and malignant, the adjacent adrenal cortex and that of the contralateral adrenal gland are atrophic as a result of suppression of endogenous ACTH production by high cortisol levels. Carcinomas of other organs metastatic to the adrenals are much more common than primary adrenal cancers, but usually cause hypoadrenalism, not Cushing syndrome.

Clinical Features. Patients with hypercortisolism present with hypertension and centripetal redistribution of adipose tissue, manifested as truncal obesity, "moon facies," and accumulation of fat in the posterior neck and back (buffalo hump). Hypercortisolism causes selective atrophy of fast-twitch (type II) myofibers, with a resultant decreased muscle mass and proximal limb weakness. Glucocorticoids induce gluconeogenesis and inhibit the uptake of glucose by cells, resulting in secondary diabetes. The skin becomes thin and fragile and is easily bruised, leading to cutaneous hemorrhages (striae), particularly in the abdominal area (Supplemental eFig. 16.7). Cortisol increases the resorption of bone and consequent osteoporosis. Because glucocorticoids suppress the immune response, patients are at increased risk for a variety of infections. Additional manifestations include hirsutism, menstrual abnormalities, and a number of psychiatric symptoms, including mood swings, depression, and frank psychosis. Extraadrenal Cushing syndrome caused by pituitary or ectopic ACTH secretion usually is associated with increased skin pigmentation secondary to melanocyte-stimulating activity of the ACTH precursor molecule.

Hyperaldosteronism

Excessive, chronic overproduction of aldosterone causes hypertension.

- *Primary hyperaldosteronism* is caused most often by bilateral nodular hyperplasia of the adrenal glands or an adrenal tumor, most commonly a solitary adenoma. Aldosterone increases sodium reabsorption in the kidney, leading to fluid retention and increased blood pressure. Because renal blood flow increases, the production of renin in the kidney is reduced. Patients present with hypertension, and up to a third have reduced serum potassium (because of reduced reabsorption in the kidneys). Diagnostic laboratory findings are increased serum aldosterone and reduced renin activity.
- *Secondary hyperaldosteronism* is caused by aldosterone production in response to activation of the renin–angiotensin system, seen in conditions of reduced renal perfusion, as in vascular diseases of the kidney and congestive heart failure. It also is a basis for hypertension.

Adrenogenital Syndromes

Excessive production of androgenic hormones causes changes in genital organs.

Androgens are produced in the gonads and adrenal cortex. The adrenal cortex produces precursors that are converted to testosterone in peripheral tissues. Unlike gonadal androgens, adrenal androgens are regulated by ACTH. Excessive adrenal androgens may be produced under the influence of ACTH, by adrenal tumors, or in an uncommon genetic disease called *congenital adrenal hyperplasia (CAH)*. CAH is an autosomal recessive disease in which enzymes involved in cortisol biosynthesis, most often 21-hydroxylase, are defective. Because cortisol production is reduced, there is a compensatory increase in ACTH release from the pituitary that secondarily increases the production of adrenal androgens. The adrenal glands are hyperplastic, sometimes to

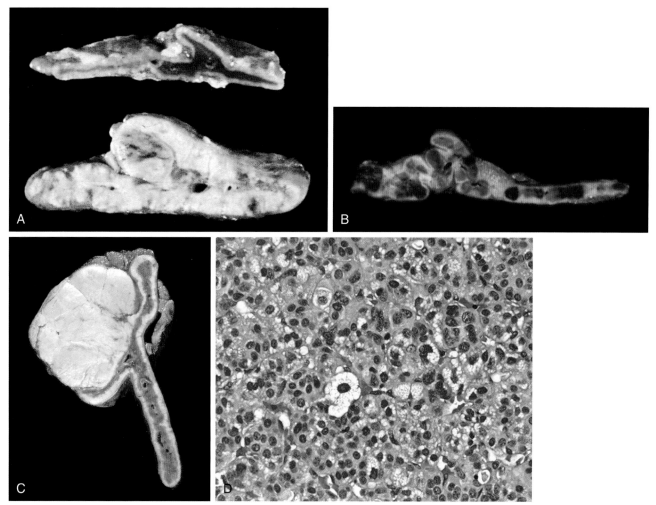

Fig. 16.11 Cushing syndrome. (A) Diffuse hyperplasia of the adrenal gland *(bottom)* contrasted with a normal adrenal gland *(top)*. In a cross section, the adrenal cortex is yellow and thickened, and a subtle nodularity is evident. The abnormal gland was from a patient with ACTH-dependent Cushing syndrome, in whom both adrenal glands were diffusely hyperplastic. (B) Primary pigmented nodular adrenocortical hyperplasia showing prominent pigmented nodules in the adrenal gland. (C) Adrenocortical adenoma. The adenoma is distinguished from nodular hyperplasia by its solitary, circumscribed nature. (D) Histologic features of an adrenal cortical adenoma. The neoplastic cells are vacuolated because of the presence of intracytoplasmic lipid. There is mild nuclear pleomorphism. Mitotic activity and necrosis are not seen. (B, Courtesy Dr. Aidan Carney, Department of Medicine, Mayo Clinic, Rochester, Minnesota.)

enormous size. If the disease is present from birth, girls present with ambiguous genitalia. In postpubertal children, hirsutism and acne are prominent. Males present with precocious puberty and enlarged genitals. Patients respond well to steroid treatment, which replaces the deficient glucocorticoids and suppresses ACTH production.

Adrenal Cortical Insufficiency

Chronic Adrenal Insufficiency (Addison Disease)

In Addison disease, progressive destruction of the adrenal cortex leads to deficiency of multiple hormones.

Pathogenesis. In higher-income countries, 60% to 70% of chronic adrenocortical insufficiency (also known as Addison disease) is due to autoimmune adrenalitis, most commonly as part of a disorder called the autoimmune polyglandular syndrome. One subtype of this syndrome results from loss of function mutations in the gene *AIRE,* which controls the expression of self antigens in the thymus and hence the elimination of self-reactive T cells. Other endocrine glands that are subject to autoimmune attack in affected patients include the thyroid, parathyroid, pituitary, and pancreas. In lower-income

countries, tuberculosis and fungal infections are important causes of Addison disease.

Morphology. In autoimmune adrenalitis, the adrenal glands are shrunken due to atrophy of the cortex, which contains a variable lymphocytic infiltrate. In infections, granulomatous or other types of inflammatory reactions to the pathogen may be present.

Clinical Features. Clinical manifestations become apparent only after more than 90% of the glands are destroyed. Patients present with weakness, gastrointestinal symptoms, electrolyte imbalances, and hypotension. The skin is hyperpigmented because the precursor polypeptide that gives rise to ACTH also is processed to release melanocyte-stimulating hormone, which rises in response to the low cortisol levels.

Acute Adrenal Insufficiency

In contrast to Addison disease, which is chronic and progressive, acute adrenal insufficiency may be a medical emergency. The most common cause is adrenal hemorrhage due to coagulation disorders. In the setting of disseminated sepsis, this condition is referred to as the *Waterhouse-Friderichsen syndrome*. The most life-threatening manifestation of adrenal crisis is hypotension and shock, but a variety of systemic signs and symptoms related to the underlying cause of sepsis are common. Acute adrenal insufficiency also occurs upon sudden withdrawal of steroid treatment (which suppresses ACTH and, therefore, endogenous steroid production) or stress in patients with underlying adrenal insufficiency.

Tumors of the Adrenal Medulla

The two most common primary tumors of the adrenal medulla are pheochromocytoma and neuroblastoma.

Pheochromocytoma

Pheochromocytomas are tumors of chromaffin cells that produce catecholamine and other hormones.

These rare tumors arise from catecholamine-producing cells in the adrenal medulla (90%) and sympathetic ganglia (10%, also called *paragangliomas*). Their chief clinical significance lies in the fact that they produce a surgically correctable form of hypertension.

Pathogenesis. Most tumors have mutations in one of several oncogenes, including *RET, NF1* (the cause of neurofibromatosis), and *VHL* (the cause of von Hippel-Lindau syndrome). How these genes may contribute to tumorigenesis was discussed in Chapter 5.

Morphology. The tumors are usually well-defined masses that compress the adrenal. They range from small, circumscribed lesions to large, hemorrhagic, cystic masses (Fig. 16.12A). They are composed of nests of polygonal or spindle-shaped cells, containing catecholamines in their granules, surrounded by a vascular network (Fig. 16.12B). Benign lesions may show capsular and vascular invasion, so the defining characteristic of malignancy is distant metastasis.

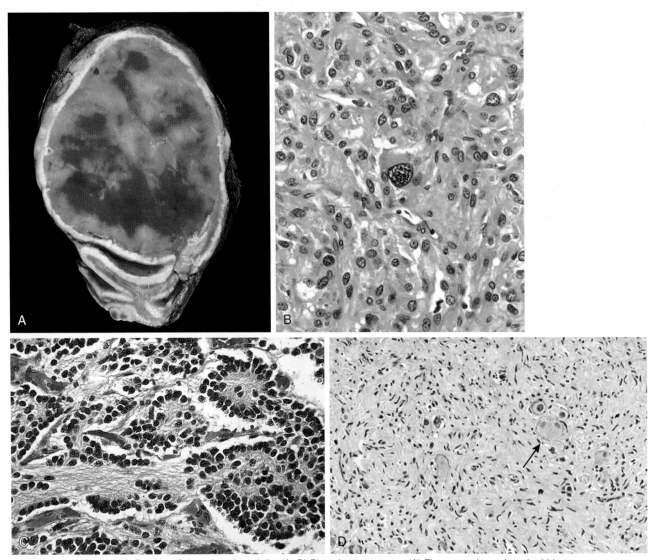

Fig. 16.12 Tumors of the adrenal medulla. (A, B) Pheochromocytoma. (A) The tumor is enclosed within an attenuated cortex and demonstrates areas of hemorrhage. The comma-shaped residual adrenal gland is seen *(lower portion)*. (B) Photomicrograph demonstrating characteristic nests of cells with abundant cytoplasm. Granules containing catecholamine are not visible in this preparation. It is not uncommon to find bizarre cells (such as the one in the center of this image), even in pheochromocytomas that are benign. (C) Neuroblastoma. The tumor cells form psuedorosettes around a central core of fibrillary material. (D) Ganglioneuroma, a tumor showing extensive neuronal differentiation. The *arrow* points to a neuron.

Clinical Features. The "rule of ten" is often used to characterize pheochromocytoma: 10% are extraadrenal, 10% are bilateral, and 10% are malignant. The majority of patients present with hypertension which may be episodic, presenting as an abrupt and precipitous increase in blood pressure, associated with tachycardia, headache, sweating, and tremors. These paroxysms are attributable to the periodic release of catecholamines from the tumor. In severe cases, the sudden production of the hormone may cause heart failure, myocardial infarction, and ventricular fibrillation, so-called catecholamine cardiomyopathy.

Neuroblastoma

Neuroblastoma is a tumor of children arising from primordial neural crest cells in the adrenal medulla and sympathetic ganglia.

It is the second most common tumor of children (following brain tumors), accounting for almost 10% of pediatric tumors and 50% of tumors diagnosed in infancy.

Pathogenesis. Most of these tumors are sporadic, but 1% to 2% are familial. The familial tumors are associated with germline mutations in the *ALK* (anaplastic lymphoma kinase) gene, and somatic gain-of-function mutations in *ALK* are present in 8% to 10% of the sporadic tumors. Amplification of the *MYCN* gene, which encodes a transcription factor that is functionally identical to the oncoprotein MYC (Chapter 5), is present in 25% to 30% of tumors and portends a poor prognosis.

Morphology. In about 40% of cases, the tumor arises in the adrenal medulla. The remaining cases arise in sympathetic ganglia, most frequently in the paravertebral region of the abdomen (25%) and mediastinum (15%). They range in size from clinically silent small nodules (in situ lesions) to huge masses. They may be encapsulated or infiltrate adjacent tissues. The tumors are composed of small, primitive-appearing cells with dark nuclei, sometimes arranged around fibrillary material, forming "pseudorosettes" (Fig. 16.12C). Some cells may show features of ganglion cells (neurons), reflecting partial differentiation. Tumors with extensive neuronal differentiation are called ganglioneuromas (Fig. 16.12D).

Clinical Features. The most common presentation in children under 2 years of age is an abdominal mass. The clinical course varies widely, from spontaneous regression to development of extensive metastatic disease. Many of the tumors produce elevated levels of catecholamines, and measurement of catecholamine metabolites in blood and urine is useful for the diagnosis, but these hormones do not cause hypertension as often as in pheochromocytoma. The prognosis depends on several factors, including age of onset (better in children < 18 months of age), stage, histology (evidence of neuronal differentiation indicating a better prognosis), *MYCN* amplification (worse prognosis), and DNA ploidy (hyperdiploid tumors have a better prognosis).

MULTIPLE ENDOCRINE NEOPLASIA SYNDROMES

Multiple endocrine neoplasia (MEN) syndromes are inherited, autosomal dominant diseases characterized by proliferative or neoplastic lesions affecting multiple endocrine glands.

The tumors usually develop at a young age, may arise in multiple glands at the same or different times, are usually multifocal (even if only a single gland is affected), and tend to be aggressive and recur after resection. Tumors are usually preceded by an asymptomatic stage of endocrine hyperplasia involving the cell of origin of the tumor (e.g., patients with MEN-2 almost universally demonstrate hyperplasia of calcitonin-producing C cells in the thyroid parenchyma adjacent to medullary thyroid carcinomas).

MEN syndromes are divided into two major types.

- *MEN-1 is caused by germline mutations in the MEN1 tumor suppressor gene,* which encodes a protein called menin that is a component of several transcription factor complexes. Organs most commonly involved are the "three Ps": parathyroids (hyperplasia and adenomas causing hyperparathyroidism), pancreas (including gastrin- and insulin-producing tumors, causing Zollinger-Ellison syndrome and hypoglycemia, respectively), and pituitary (most often a prolactin-secreting microadenoma). *Primary hyperparathyroidism* is the most common manifestation of MEN-1 (80% to 95% of patients), appearing in almost all by 40 to 50 years of age, whereas endocrine tumors of the pancreas are the leading cause of death. These tumors usually are aggressive and present with metastatic disease.

- *MEN-2 is caused by gain-of-function mutations of the RET oncogene.* MEN type 2A consists of medullary thyroid carcinoma, adrenal pheochromocytoma, and parathyroid hyperplasia. MEN type 2B presents with medullary thyroid carcinoma, pheochromocytoma, and lesions outside the endocrine organs, including mucosal ganglioneuromas and a marfanoid appearance of the skeleton; parathyroid lesions are not seen. Affected individuals carrying germline *RET* mutations are advised to have a prophylactic thyroidectomy to prevent the inevitable development of medullary carcinoma.

17

Disorders of the Nervous System

OUTLINE

Congenital Malformations of the CNS, 280
Cerebral Edema, Herniation, and Hydrocephalus, 280
Cerebrovascular Diseases, 281
   Cerebral Artery Thrombosis, Embolism, and Brain
     Infarction, 281
   Intracranial Hemorrhage, 282
   Other Vascular Diseases, 283
CNS Trauma, 283
   Parenchymal Brain Injury, 283
   Chronic Traumatic Encephalopathy, 284
   Perinatal Brain Injury, 284
CNS Infections, 284
Prion Diseases, 286
Demyelinating Diseases, 287
   Multiple Sclerosis, 287
   Other Acquired Demyelinating Disorders, 287
   Leukodystrophies, 287

Neurodegenerative Diseases, 288
   Alzheimer Disease, 289
   Frontotemporal Lobar Degeneration (FTLD), 289
   Parkinson Disease, 290
   Huntington Disease, 291
   Spinocerebellar Ataxias, 291
   Amyotrophic Lateral Sclerosis, 291
CNS Tumors, 292
   General Features and Pathogenesis of Astrocytoma, 292
   Classification of Astrocytomas, 292
   Other CNS Tumors, 293
   Inherited Syndromes Associated with CNS Tumors, 294
   Retinoblastoma, 294
Disorders of Peripheral Nerves, 295
   Peripheral Neuropathy, 295
   Peripheral Nerve Tumors, 295
   Diseases of Neuromuscular Junctions, 295

Diseases of the central nervous system (CNS) have characteristics distinct from disorders of other organ systems. These stem from features unique to the CNS, including the tight physical constraints within the skull, the extreme sensitivity of neurons to hypoxia and other injurious stimuli, and the inability of neurons to regenerate. This chapter focuses on diseases of the brain. Spinal cord involvement is mentioned when relevant. We conclude with a brief discussion of the major diseases of peripheral nerves.

CONGENITAL MALFORMATIONS OF THE CNS

Congenital malformations of the CNS may result from genetic abnormalities, neonatal or perinatal trauma, or other insults.

CNS malformations giving rise to intellectual disability, cerebral palsy, or neural tube defects are seen in an estimated 1% to 2% of births. The underlying cause can be established in only a minority of cases. The malformations may affect different regions of the brain or spinal cord, and are usually associated with severe functional deficits (Table 17.1). Neural tube defects are associated with folate deficiency during the first month of pregnancy. Because this time period precedes the detection of most pregnancies, reduction of risk requires folate supplementation throughout a woman's reproductive years.

CEREBRAL EDEMA, HERNIATION, AND HYDROCEPHALUS

These disorders are usually complications of some underlying disease. Their severity reflects the anatomic constraints on the brain. *Cerebral edema* is the accumulation of fluid in the brain parenchyma. It may

Table 17.1 Congenital Malformations of the Brain and Spinal Cord

Defect	Features
Neural Tube Defects	
Spina bifida	Outpouching of disorganized segment of spinal cord covered by meninges due to failure of closure of posterior segment of neural tube
Myelomeningo-cele	Extension of spinal cord through defect in vertebral column, usually lumbosacral
Anencephaly	Absence of the forebrain caused by malformation of anterior end of neural tube
Encephalocele	Outpouching of CNS tissue, usually the occipital region, through a cranial defect
Forebrain Malformations	
Microcephaly	Small brain in a small cranium; associated with chromosomal abnormalities, fetal alcohol syndrome, Zika virus infection acquired in utero
Defects in neuronal migration or differentiation	Examples include disruption of normal midline patterns *(holoprosencephaly)*, loss of gyri *(lissencephaly)*, increased numbers of improperly formed gyri *(polymicrogyria)*
Posterior Fossa Abnormalities	
Arnold-Chiari malformation	Small posterior fossa causing misshapen cerebellum and extension of vermis through foramen magnum
Dandy-Walker malformation	Enlarged posterior fossa, absence of the cerebellar vermis, and a large midline cyst.

result from inflammation, ischemic or toxic injury to neurons and glia, or space-filling lesions (e.g., tumors), and typically stems from increased vascular permeability. In the setting of generalized edema, the gyri are swollen and flattened, the sulci are narrowed, and the ventricles are compressed (Supplemental eFig. 17.1). The clinical manifestations range from subtle neurologic defects to loss of consciousness and are usually dictated by the underlying condition. When severe, edema may lead to herniation.

Herniation is the displacement of brain tissue from one compartment to another because of increased intracranial pressure. It may damage tissue directly or indirectly by compressing blood vessels. There are three types of herniation (Fig. 17.1):

- *Subfalcine (cingulate) herniation* occurs when expansion of one cerebral hemisphere pushes the cingulate gyrus under the falx. It may compress the anterior cerebral artery.
- *Transtentorial (uncinate) herniation* occurs when the temporal lobe is compressed against the free margin of the tentorium. Pressure on the third cranial nerve causes pupillary dilation (blown pupil) due to impaired ocular reflexes on the side of the lesion. The posterior cerebral artery may also be compressed, leading to ischemic injury to the primary visual cortex. With progressive herniation, pressure on the midbrain may compress the contralateral cerebral peduncle against the tentorium, resulting in hemiparesis ipsilateral to the side of the herniation. Brain stem compression causes loss of consciousness. Linear or flame-shaped hemorrhages in the midbrain and pons, termed *Duret hemorrhages*, may occur because of tearing of the vessels in this region (Supplemental eFig. 17.2).
- *Tonsillar herniation* is displacement of the cerebellar tonsils through the foramen magnum. It causes brain stem compression, resulting in respiratory and cardiac failure.

Hydrocephalus is an increase in volume of the cerebrospinal fluid (CSF) within the ventricles of the brain, usually due to obstruction of CSF outflow. When obstruction results in dilation of only the ventricles upstream of the block, it is called noncommunicating hydrocephalus (Supplemental eFig. 17.3). If the accumulation of CSF occurs secondary to defective absorption (or, rarely, excessive production), all the ventricles are affected (communicating hydrocephalus). If the ventricles enlarge because of atrophy of the brain parenchyma, it is called hydrocephalus ex vacuo. When hydrocephalus develops in infancy before closure of the cranial sutures it produces enlargement of the head. Obstruction of CSF outflow may be caused by congenital malformations, tumors, and some infections. It is more common in children than in adults, and may present with headache, behavioral changes, lethargy, and delayed development.

CEREBROVASCULAR DISEASES

The major cerebrovascular disorders are caused by thromoembolic diseases, which lead to infarction, and hemorrhage.

Clinically, these conditions are called *stroke*. They are a leading cause of death and the most preventable cause of neurologic morbidity and mortality. The brain is highly dependent on oxygen. Although the brain constitutes only about 2% of the body weight, it receives 15% of the resting cardiac output and is responsible for 20% of the body's oxygen consumption. Therefore, compromise of the blood supply to the brain has devastating consequences. In this section, we discuss the common causes of stroke and some of the downstream consequences, such as cerebral edema and herniation.

Cerebral Artery Thrombosis, Embolism, and Brain Infarction

Occlusion of the arterial supply to any region of the brain results in liquefactive necrosis, creating an infarct.

Pathogenesis. Arterial occlusion may be caused by
- *Embolism,* which may be from the heart (e.g., thrombi formed following myocardial infarction, atrial fibrillation, and in valvular diseases), or from a deep vein thrombus (*paradoxical embolism* in a patient with a patent foramen ovale). The territory of the middle cerebral artery is the most common site of embolic occlusion.
- *Thrombosis* superimposed on an atherosclerotic plaque in an artery, for example, at the carotid bifurcation, the origin of the middle cerebral artery, or either end of the basilar artery

Occlusions may cause infarction of significant areas of the brain. Thrombotic occlusions of small penetrating arteries are usually associated with hypertension and lead to small, so-called *lacunar infarcts*.

Ischemic injury to the brain may also be the result of global ischemia without a focal vascular obstruction. Global ischemia results from severe hypotension (blood pressure < 50 mm Hg), as may occur with cardiac arrest and various types of shock.

Morphology. Infarcts are typically nonhemorrhagic at the outset, but can evolve into hemorrhagic lesions, especially if the blood supply to the infarcted region is restored (Fig. 17.2). Hemorrhagic infarcts are associated with petechial hemorrhages, whereas nonhemorrhagic infarcts evolve from initial edema to gelatinous, friable tissue followed by liquefaction, leaving a cystic cavity. Microscopically, the earliest changes result from ischemic injury in neurons (cytoplasmic eosinophilia, producing so-called *red neurons* [Supplemental eFig. 17.4], and edema), followed by infiltration of neutrophils (Supplemental eFig. 17.5) and then monocytes (Supplemental eFig. 17.6). Surrounding astrocytes are activated (reactive gliosis). Global ischemia produces similar microscopic changes that are typically widespread. Hypotensive episodes may cause focal infarcts in the most distal areas of the arterial supply (so-called *watershed infarcts*).

Clinical Features. The clinical manifestations depend on the anatomic location of the infarct, together with the effects of cerebral edema,

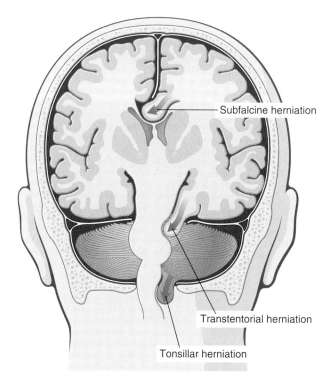

Fig. 17.1 Herniation. Displacement of brain parenchyma across fixed barriers can be subfalcine, transtentorial, or tonsillar (into the foramen magnum).

Subfalcine herniation

Transtentorial herniation

Tonsillar herniation

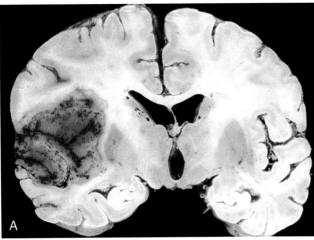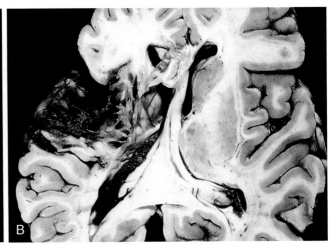

Fig. 17.2 Cerebral infarction. (A) Section of the brain showing a large, discolored, focally hemorrhagic region in the distribution of the left middle cerebral artery (hemorrhagic, or red, infarction). (B) Old cystic infarct shows destruction of cortex and surrounding gliosis.

described earlier. Treatment of thrombotic occlusions with fibrinolytic agents within 4.5 hours of the onset of symptoms can reduce or prevent permanent brain injury; thus, rapid clinical and radiological evaluation and diagnosis is critical in patients with suspected stroke.

Intracranial Hemorrhage

Hemorrhages in different compartments of the brain may result from traumatic injury of vessels, vascular injury due to hypertension, or structural abnormalities of vessels such as aneurysms and arteriovenous malformations.

Pathogenesis. Hemorrhages may occur in the epidural, subdural, or subarachnoid spaces or within the brain parenchyma (Table 17.2). Each has different underlying causes and distinct clinical manifestations. Trauma is a major cause of vascular injury in the brain because physical displacement of the brain tends to tear vessels.

- *Epidural and subdural hematomas* are almost always secondary to trauma.
- *Subarachnoid hemorrhage* is most often due to rupture of a saccular (berry) aneurysm (described below). Less commonly, the bleed is from a ruptured arteriovenous malformation (AVM). AVMs may be present at birth, but aneurysms usually develop over time.
- *Parenchymal hemorrhages* are usually associated with hypertension causing rupture of small arteries.

Morphology. Epidural and subdural hematomas are collections of blood in the cranial space that do not extend into the brain (Fig. 17.3A,B). If the patient survives the acute episode, the hematoma resolves like other collections of blood (see Chapter 3). Hypertensive parenchymal bleeds typically involve the basal ganglia, thalamus, pons, and cerebellum. They compress the adjacent tissue (Fig. 17.3C) and, over time, are converted into cavities with residual hemosiderin around the edges. *Aneurysms* are thin-walled outpouchings of arteries. The vast majority are in the anterior cerebral circulation near arterial branch points (Fig. 17.4). They lack a muscular wall and are lined only by intima, so they are prone to rupture, especially during acute increases in intracranial pressure (e.g., when straining at stool or during sexual intercourse). AVMs are tangled networks of vascular tissue, often involving subarachnoid vessels.

Clinical Features. The manifestations of different types of hemorrhage are summarized in Table 17.2. Some distinctive features are the lucid interval that may follow a traumatic epidural bleed before the abrupt appearance

Table 17.2 Brain Hemorrhages

Location	Etiology	Additional Features
Epidural space	Trauma	Usually associated with a skull fracture (in adults); rapidly evolving neurologic symptoms require prompt surgical intervention
Subdural space	Trauma	Level of trauma may be mild; slowly evolving neurologic symptoms, often with a delay from the time of injury
Subarachnoid space	Vascular abnormalities (AVM or aneurysm)	Sudden onset of severe headache, often with rapid neurologic deterioration; secondary injury may emerge due to vasospasm
	Trauma	Typically associated with underlying contusions
Intraparenchymal	Trauma (contusions)	Selective involvement of the crests of gyri where the brain contacts the skull (frontal and temporal tips, orbitofrontal surface)
	Hemorrhagic conversion of an ischemic infarction	Petechial hemorrhages in an area of previously ischemic brain, usually following the cortical ribbon
	Cerebral amyloid angiopathy	"Lobar" hemorrhage, involving cerebral cortex, often with extension into the subarachnoid space
	Hypertension	Centered in the deep white matter, thalamus, basal ganglia, or brain stem; may extend into the ventricular system
	Tumors (primary or metastatic)	Associated with high-grade gliomas and certain metastases (e.g., melanoma, choriocarcinoma, renal cell carcinoma)

AVM, arteriovenous malformation.

of neurologic signs; and the sudden, excruciating headache that follows an aneurysm rupture (thunderclap headache) followed by rapid loss of consciousness due to subarachnoid bleeding. Localizing symptoms may also be seen and are related to the area of brain that is affected.

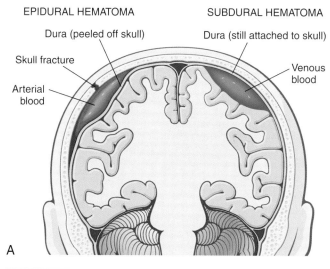

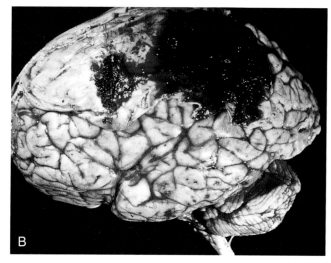

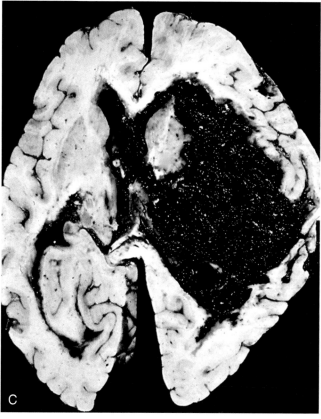

Fig. 17.3 Intracranial hemorrhage. (A) Epidural hematoma *(left)* in which rupture of a meningeal artery, usually associated with a skull fracture, has led to accumulation of arterial blood between the dura and the skull. In a subdural hematoma *(right),* damage to bridging veins between the brain and the superior sagittal sinus has led to the accumulation of blood between the two layers of dura. (B) Epidural hematoma covering a portion of the dura. (C) Massive hypertensive cerebral (parenchymal) hemorrhage rupturing into a lateral ventricle.

Other Vascular Diseases

Hypertension and amyloid deposition may lead to clinically significant vascular abnormalities in the CNS.

With sustained hypertension, small arteries and arterioles show hyaline sclerosis and their walls are weakened. Rupture of affected vessels may result in small or large parenchymal hemorrhages or lacunar infarcts. Sudden severe increases in blood pressure may cause the syndrome of *acute hypertensive encephalopathy,* in which there is an increase in intracranial pressure and global dysfunction manifested by headaches, confusion, convulsions, and coma. The brain may show edema, necrosis of arterioles, and petechiae.

In *cerebral amyloid angiopathy,* deposits of amyloid in small- and medium-sized arteries weaken their walls, resulting in small hemorrhages that often occur in the lobes of the cerebral cortex (lobar hemorrhages). The amyloid is derived from amyloid precursor protein (APP),

the same protein that gives rise to amyloid deposits within the brain in Alzheimer disease (described later). Some, but not all, individuals with cerebral amyloid angiopathy also have dementia.

CNS TRAUMA

Trauma to the brain may injure the parenchyma or blood vessels.

Vascular trauma was described earlier in the context of cerebral hemorrhage. In this section, we discuss parenchymal injury and two forms of traumatic injury that are unique to the brain.

Parenchymal Brain Injury

When an object impacts the head, brain injury may occur at the site of impact (a *coup injury*) or opposite the site of impact on the other side of the brain (a *contrecoup injury*). The latter occurs when the brain

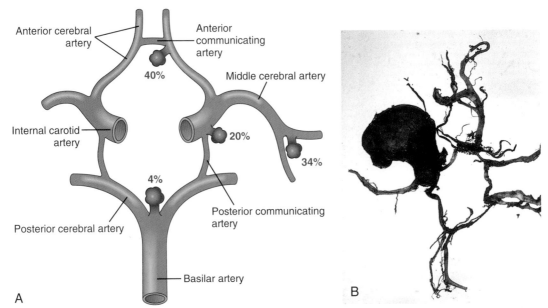

Fig. 17.4 Cerebral aneurysms. (A) Common sites of saccular aneurysms. (B) The circle of Willis is dissected to show a large aneurysm.

strikes the opposite inner surface of the skull after sudden deceleration. Both coup and contrecoup lesions are *contusions,* hemorrhagic foci of tissue injury and edema caused by rapid tissue displacement, most common in regions of the brain overlying rough and irregular inner skull surfaces (i.e., the orbitofrontal regions and the temporal lobe tips). Grossly, contusions are wedge shaped, with the widest aspect closest to the point of impact. Microscopically, the lesions show evidence of neuronal injury (cytoplasmic eosinophilia, nuclear pyknosis) and hemorrhage. Older lesions typically involve the crests of gyri and appear as depressed, yellowish-brown patches with gliosis and residual hemosiderin-filled macrophages.

Trauma may also cause more subtle but widespread injury to axons within the brain (called *diffuse axonal injury*) that can result in coma. The movement of one region of brain relative to another is thought to disrupt axonal integrity and function. This form of injury may underlie some of the CNS dysfunction seen in individuals exposed to explosive blast waves, such as soldiers and victims of terror attacks.

Concussion is a clinical term for a reversible change in brain function, with or without loss of consciousness, resulting from head trauma. The characteristic transient neurologic dysfunction includes loss of consciousness, temporary respiratory arrest, and loss of reflexes.

Chronic Traumatic Encephalopathy

Repeated head trauma may lead to cognitive defects, parkinsonism, and neurodegeneration.

Chronic traumatic encephalopathy is now recognized as a distinct disorder in individuals involved in contact sports, and has thus captured the attention of physicians and the lay public. Many of the features seen in neurodegenerative diseases (discussed later) are present in this condition as well, including cortical atrophy and accumulation of neurofibrillary tangles. Patients present with slowly developing dementia, typically years after the trauma. The pathogenesis is not understood.

Perinatal Brain Injury

Cerebral hemorrhages and infarcts in the perinatal period can lead to long-term neurologic deficits.

Premature infants are especially susceptible to parenchymal hemorrhages and infarcts. These are mostly in the germinal matrix and may extend to the ventricles. Infarcts typically occur in supratentorial periventricular white matter and when extensive can cause massive destruction and formation of residual cystic lesions. Perinatal injury may lead to the clinical condition called *cerebral palsy,* which refers to nonprogressive neurologic deficits characterized by spasticity, dystonia, ataxia, and paresis. However, in most cases of cerebral palsy, no specific injuries are identified.

CNS INFECTIONS

A wide range of bacteria, viruses, and fungi can infect the brain parenchyma, causing *encephalitis,* or the leptomeninges covering the brain, causing *meningitis.* The host responses to these infectious agents are similar to the reactions in other tissues. Here we discuss the general principles of CNS infections, and then the group of prion diseases that are unique to the CNS.

Pathogenesis. Infectious pathogens enter the brain through one of four routes:
- *Hematogenous spread* from a distant site: Predisposing conditions include bacterial endocarditis, in which infected vegetations are prone to embolization; congenital heart disease associated with right-to-left shunts and pulmonary arteriovenous shunts, in both instances because of a lack of pulmonary "filter" function; and chronic lung infections, which provide a source of organisms.
- *Direct implantation* of microbes as a result of trauma or (uncommonly) a surgical procedure or lumbar puncture.
- *Local extension* from infected sinuses, osteomyelitis, or an infected malformation, such as a meningomyelocele.
- *Retrograde spread* from peripheral nerves, the major route of infection with rabies and varicella zoster viruses.

Both generalized neurologic manifestations (headaches, seizures, coma) and localizing signs may be seen. The analysis of CSF obtained by lumbar puncture is an important part of the diagnostic workup, especially in suspected cases of meningitis. In bacterial infections, the CSF shows increased pressure, increased protein, decreased glucose, and abundant neutrophils. By contrast, in viral infections, there is an early neutrophilic pleocytosis that rapidly converts to a lymphocytosis; the protein concentration is elevated, but the glucose is normal and the pressure is normal or only slightly elevated.

Table 17.3 CNS Infections

	Common Organisms	Pathology and Clinical Features
Meningitis		
Bacterial (acute pyogenic) meningitis	*Neisseria, Streptococcus*	Headache, neurologic signs, often fulminant Lumbar puncture shows neutrophils, increased protein, reduced glucose; culture may be positive Neutrophil-rich meningeal exudate
Aseptic (viral) meningitis	Presumptive viral agent, usually not identified	Less fulminant clinical course Lumbar puncture shows lymphocytosis, moderate protein elevation, normal glucose; bacterial cultures negative No or mild meningeal lymphocytic infiltrate
Chronic meningitis	Neurosyphilis Tuberculosis Fungi	Tertiary stage of syphilis; may involve small blood vessels, parenchyma, or dorsal nerve roots Diffuse inflammation or localized mass Usually opportunistic infections in immunosuppressed patients; common organisms are *Cryptococcus* (meningitis and encephalitis), *Histoplasma* (basal meningitis), *Coccidioides* (meningitis)
Encephalitis		
Brain abscess	Various bacteria	Discrete destructive lesions with central necrosis surrounded by granulation tissue and gliosis
Viral encephalitis	Arboviruses (West Nile, equine encephalitis)	Cause epidemic encephalitis, especially in tropical countries; perivascular and parenchymal mononuclear inflammation with microglial nodules; neurologic symptoms include seizures, delirium, stupor
	Herpesviruses	Necrotizing, hemorrhagic lesions preferentially involving temporal lobes; behavioral changes
	Varicella zoster	Latent infection of dorsal root ganglia; reactivation in adults leads to shingles (skin eruptions) and severe pain due to nerve involvement
	Poliovirus	Damages motor neurons in spinal cord and brain stem (paralytic polio)
	Rabies	Encephalitis manifested by extreme sensitivity to touch, including seizures, and aversion to water
	JC virus	Infects oligodendrocytes, causing demyelination and progressive multifocal leukoencephalopathy; immunosuppressed patients (deficient cell-mediated immunity)
	HIV	Poorly understood encephalopathy
Fungal encephalitis	*Candida, Mucor, Aspergillus*	Granulomatous inflammation or abscesses
Parasitic infections	*Toxoplasma*	Congenital infection acquired from mother during birth; causes chorioretinitis, hydrocephalus, intracranial calcifications. Immunodeficient adults also affected
	Ameba	Meningoencephalitis

The features of common infections are summarized in Table 17.3. Selected examples of meningitis and encephalitis are discussed briefly in the following and are illustrated in Fig. 17.5.

- *Acute pyogenic meningitis* is caused by bacterial infection, most often streptococcus and *Escherichia coli* in neonates, streptococcus and *Neisseria* in older children and young adults, and streptococcus and *Listeria* in older adults. Patients present with headache, neck stiffness, and systemic signs of inflammation. Grossly, an exudate is evident within the leptomeninges on the surface of the brain (Fig. 17.5A). Microscopic features are typical of acute inflammation.
- *Aseptic (viral) meningitis* presents with signs of meningitis but an absence of neutrophils and bacteria in the CSF. A viral origin is presumed, but the specific agent is not identified in most cases. The disease is often self-limited.
- *Chronic meningitis* may be associated with tuberculosis, syphilis, or fungal infections. The fungus *Cryptococcus neoformans* causes meningitis that may spread into the brain parenchyma to produce meningoencephalitis. As these mucin-producing organisms spread through perivascular Virchow-Robin spaces and proliferate, they create a typical "soap bubble" histologic appearance (Fig. 17.5B).
- *Brain abscesses* (Fig. 17.5C) are discrete lesions with central liquefactive necrosis surrounded by granulation tissue. They may eventually be replaced by gliosis. They are usually caused by bacterial infections. Predisposing conditions include bacterial endocarditis, congenital heart disease with right-to-left shunt, and lung infections.

Abscesses may produce a mass effect leading to increased intracranial pressure and even herniation.
- *Viral encephalitis* has many causes. The typical lesions show mononuclear cell infiltrates, microglial nodules (collections of activated microglia), and neuronophagia (phagocytosis of damaged neurons).
  - *Herpes simplex virus* causes a destructive encephalitis affecting primarily the temporal lobes (Supplemental eFig. 17.7). Neurons and astrocytes often contain large intranuclear inclusions (Cowdry type A bodies).
  - *Varicella zoster* causes chickenpox and establishes latent infection in the neurons of dorsal root ganglia in the spinal cord. Reactivation of the virus may occur as immune defenses decline, associated with aging or immunodeficiencies. The disease manifests as a painful skin eruption called *shingles* affecting one or a few dermatomes supplied by those neurons.
  - *Poliovirus* is an enterovirus that infects and destroys motor neurons in the spinal cord and brain stem, causing a flaccid paralysis.
  - *Rabies* is acquired from the bite of an infected animal (most often bats, and rarely dogs). The virus ascends along peripheral nerves, enters the CNS, and infects and damages neurons in the hypothalamus, cortex, and throughout the brain (Supplemental eFig. 17.8). The classic presentation is extreme CNS excitability, with convulsions and contracture of the pharyngeal muscles that create an aversion to swallowing water (hydrophobia).

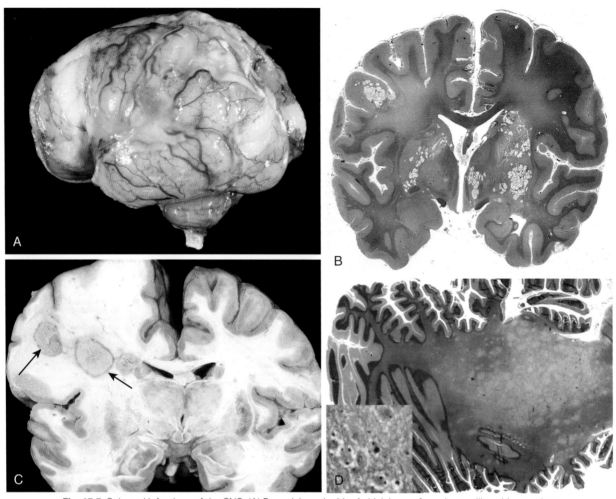

Fig. 17.5 Selected infections of the CNS. (A) Bacterial meningitis. A thick layer of purulent, milky white exudate covers the surface of the brain. (B) Cryptococcal infection. Whole-brain section showing the numerous areas of tissue destruction associated with the spread of organisms in the perivascular spaces. (C) Bacterial abscesses. Cerebral abscesses in the frontal lobe white matter *(arrows)*. (D) Progressive multifocal leukoencephalopathy caused by JC virus. Section stained for myelin showing irregular, poorly defined areas of demyelination, which become confluent in places. *Inset,* Enlarged oligodendrocyte nucleus represents the effect of viral infection.

- *HIV* causes an encephalopathy that has severe clinical consequences; the pathogenesis is poorly understood (see Chapter 4).
- *Progressive multifocal leukoencephalopathy* (PML) is caused by JC virus, a polyomavirus that latently infects many healthy people and is reactivated in states of immune deficiency. The virus infects oligodendrocytes and causes progressively enlarging foci of white matter destruction and demyelination (Fig. 17.5D).
- *Arboviruses (arthropod-borne viruses)* are more common in tropical regions of the world and include Eastern and Western equine encephalitis and West Nile virus infection. Patients develop generalized neurologic symptoms as well as focal signs.
- Other types of encephalitis are caused by fungi, parasites, and rickettsia, some of which produce distinctive lesions:
  - *Toxoplasmosis* is caused by the protozoan parasite *Toxoplasma gondii* in adults or neonates. The neonatal infection, which is acquired by transplacental passage and is called congenital toxoplasmosis, is characterized by chorioretinitis, hydrocephalus, and intracranial calcifications. In adults, it is an opportunistic infection seen in immune deficiency states, and is manifested by abscesses, often multiple (Supplemental eFig. 17.9).
  - *Cysticercosis* is infection by the tapeworm *Taenia solium*. Larvae are ingested and mature in the gastrointestinal tract, and exit to inhabit multiple tissues, where they may form cysts. In the brain,

these cysts form mass lesions that may produce convulsions and must be distinguished from tumors.
- *Malaria* is associated with severe CNS manifestations (cerebral malaria) believed to be caused by obstruction of small vessels by red cells infected with the protozoan parasites.

PRION DISEASES

Prions are abnormally folded proteins that self-propagate, accumulate in neural tissues, and cause progressive, often fatal, white matter damage.

Prion is an abbreviation of "proteinaceous infectious particle." Although prion diseases are rare (affecting 1 to 2 people per million each year), they illustrate a novel principle of disease development that may be relevant to many other diseases involving misfolded proteins.

Pathogenesis. Normal prion proteins (PrP^C) are membrane proteins found in all cells, and are abundant in neurons and probably glial cells. At some very low rate, PrP^C can undergo conversion to a protease-resistant, misfolded pathogenic conformation called PrP^{SC} (so named because it was identified in a disease of sheep and goats called scrapie, which laid the foundations for the elucidation of prion diseases). Remarkably, when PrP^{SC} interacts with PrP^C, it converts the

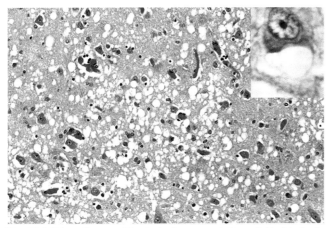

Fig. 17.6 Prion disease. Histologic features of Creutzfeldt-Jakob disease (CJD) include spongiform change in the cerebral cortex. *Inset,* High magnification of a neuron with vacuoles.

normal protein into PrP^SC, thus propagating itself like an infectious agent. Once this process commences, PrP^SC accumulates in neurons and white matter of the brain, forms aggregates, and induces cell injury by mechanisms that are not understood. It is also not known why normal PrP^C undergoes the initial conformational change; certain germline mutations in the gene encoding PrP^C accelerate the process, but in many cases the disease develops without an identified mutation.

The prototypic prion disease is *Creutzfeldt-Jakob disease* (CJD), which is sporadic in the majority of cases. It may be initiated by the spontaneous misfolding of PrP^C, possibly in a cell that has acquired a PrP^C mutation. Once the process starts, PrP^C misfolding can spread to other cells, even those that express normal PrP^C. The disease can also be acquired: *bovine spongiform encephalopathy* (so-called mad cow disease) can be transmitted to people by consumption of contaminated beef; the human counterpart is called *variant CJD*. In rare instances, the disease has been transmitted by transplantation of contaminated tissues (e.g., corneal transplants), or administration of contaminated medicines (e.g., growth hormone derived from human pituitary).

Morphology. The classic finding is multiple small vacuoles in the cerebral cortex and white matter (Fig. 17.6), giving the tissue a sponge-like appearance (hence the name *transmissible spongiform encephalopathies*).

Clinical Features. Patients with the sporadic form are typically over 70 years old, whereas those with forms of the disease stemming from genetic variants or consumption of contaminated food may become symptomatic at much younger ages. Whatever the cause, affected patients present with rapidly progressive dementia that leads to death within months.

DEMYELINATING DISEASES

Loss of myelin may result from an autoimmune process that destroys myelin or a genetic anomaly that affects the synthesis or turnover of myelin.

Within the CNS, axons are ensheathed by myelin, an electrical insulator that allows rapid propagation of neural impulses. Myelinated axons are the dominant component of white matter; therefore, diseases of myelin are referred to as white matter disorders. White matter disorders are separated into two broad groups: (1) acquired demyelinating diseases of the CNS, characterized by preferential damage to previously normal myelin (exemplified by multiple sclerosis); and (2) diseases in which myelin is not formed properly or has accelerated turnover (the leukodystrophies).

Multiple Sclerosis

Multiple sclerosis (MS) is an autoimmune disease in which myelin is destroyed by the immune system.

MS is characterized by episodes of disease activity, separated in time, resulting from white matter lesions that are separated in space. It is the most common demyelinating disorder, having a prevalence of approximately 1 per 1000 individuals in the United States and Europe; its incidence appears to be increasing, for unknown reasons.

Pathogenesis. The major culprits in MS are CD4+ Th1 and Th17 T-cells that recognize myelin proteins and activate macrophages, which destroy the myelin. Antibodies against myelin or oligodendrocytes, the cells that produce myelin, may contribute to the demyelination. It is not known why patients develop immune reactions against myelin. Certain genetic variants are linked to increased risk, the strongest association being with the HLA class II allele *HLA-DRB1*1501* (which increases the risk of developing the disease about 3-fold).

Morphology. The classic lesions (plaques) are areas of myelin loss that appear as small, gray or tan depressions in the white matter (Fig. 17.7). Macrophages containing myelin debris, as well as lymphocytes, are present in active plaques (Supplemental eFig. 17.10). Over time, the inflammation wanes, leaving behind inactive plaques consisting of areas of demyelination with gliosis.

Clinical Features. Young adults typically present with new onset vision loss (caused by optic neuritis), paresthesias or weakness of extremities, or abnormal gait and balance. The most common form of the disease is the relapsing-remitting form, in which there are unpredictable episodes of neurologic dysfunction followed by periods in which symptoms improve but do not return to baseline. A minority of patients have the progressive form, in which the disability gradually worsens without periods of remission. In both forms, the clinical features are attributable to white matter lesions that can be documented by MRI. CSF examination shows an elevated protein level due to increases in IgG antibodies that are apparently produced by a small number of B-cell clones, suggesting that MS is associated with immune responses to a limited number of self antigens.

Other Acquired Demyelinating Disorders

Immune-mediated demyelination can occur after a number of systemic infectious illnesses, including relatively mild viral diseases. Non-immune myelin loss in the basis pontis can occur after rapid correction of hyponatremia (termed *osmotic demyelination syndrome*); this may result in a rapidly evolving quadriplegia.

Leukodystrophies

Leukodystrophies are inherited dysmyelinating diseases caused by abnormal myelin synthesis or turnover. In contrast to MS, the neurologic defects present at an early age and are progressive. Imaging studies reveal diffuse and symmetric myelin loss.

There are three leukodystrophies that merit mention:
- *Krabbe disease,* an autosomal recessive leukodystrophy resulting from a deficiency of galactocerebroside β-galactosidase, presents between 3 to 6 months of age. Because of this enzyme defect, galactocerebroside is metabolized through an alternative pathway that forms a cytotoxic product, galactosylsphingosine. The brain shows loss of myelin and oligodendrocytes in the CNS and a similar process in peripheral nerves (Supplemental eFig. 17.11). Survival beyond 2 years is rare.

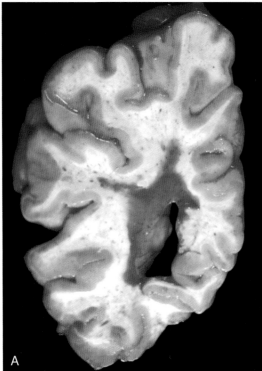

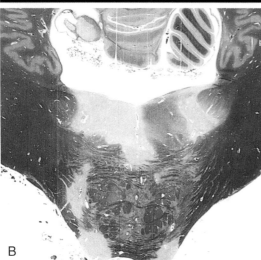

Fig. 17.7 Multiple sclerosis. (A) Section of brain showing a dark plaque around the occipital horn of the lateral ventricle. (B) Luxol fast blue–periodic acid–Schiff stain for myelin. Shows unstained regions of demyelination (MS plaques) around the fourth ventricle.

- *Metachromatic leukodystrophy* is an autosomal recessive disease that results from a deficiency of the lysosomal enzyme arylsulfatase A that causes a buildup of sulfatides within macrophages and other cells. Sulfatides have a range of biologic actions that contribute to damage to oligodendrocytes and Schwann cells, culminating in central and peripheral demyelination. The prognosis depends on the age at diagnosis, with earlier age of onset associated with more rapid progression.
- *Adrenoleukodystrophy* is an X-linked recessive disease caused by mutations in a member of the ATP-binding cassette transporter family of proteins (ABCD1), which is involved in the transport of molecules into the peroxisome. Very-long-chain fatty acids cannot be catabolized in peroxisomes, resulting in elevated levels in serum and accumulation in tissues, mainly the CNS and adrenal glands. The fatty acids may impair mitochondrial function or elicit inflammatory responses, both of which damage the involved tissues. Young boys present with behavioral changes and adrenal insufficiency. Death typically occurs 1 to 10 years after diagnosis.

Hematopoietic stem cell transplantation, which may allow repopulation of the CNS with enzymatically competent macrophages, has shown some benefit in Krabbe disease and metachromatic leukodystrophy.

NEURODEGENERATIVE DISEASES

Neurodegenerative diseases are characterized by accumulation of protein aggregates and progressive loss of neurons, typically affecting groups of neurons with shared functions located in particular regions of the CNS.

The identity of the aggregated proteins varies among different diseases, although there is some overlap (Table 17.4). At their outset, these diseases affect neurons in different areas, and therefore produce distinct neurologic deficits.

- *Diseases that affect the cerebral cortex and hippocampus,* such as Alzheimer disease, present with cognitive changes that progress to dementia.
- *Diseases that affect the basal ganglia* present with movement disorders, which may be hypokinetic (Parkinson disease) or hyperkinetic (Huntington disease).
- *Diseases that affect the cerebellum or its input or output,* such as the spinocerebellar ataxias, present with disorders of balance (ataxia).
- *Diseases that affect the motor system in the spinal cord,* such as amyotrophic lateral sclerosis, lead to limb weakness and difficulty with swallowing and breathing.

Pathogenesis. Various proteins form insoluble aggregates in cells, either because of mutations that render the protein prone to aggregation and resistant to proteolysis or because of defects in protein clearance. Large aggregates form inclusions that are visible by microscopy, but it is the smaller aggregates composed of only a few protein molecules that are thought to be neurotoxic. These oligomers injure cells in part by triggering

Table 17.4 Neurodegenerative Diseases

Disease	Region of CNS Mainly Affected	Proteins in Aggregates[a]	Neurologic Deficits
Alzheimer disease	Cerebral cortex, hippocampus	Aβ (plaques), Tau (tangles)	Dementia
Frontotemporal lobar degeneration	Frontal and temporal lobes	Tau, TDP-43	Behavioral changes
Parkinson disease	Substantia nigra	α-synuclein	Movement disorder (hypokinetic)
Huntington disease	Caudate nucleus, putamen, cortex	Huntingtin	Movement disorder (hyperkinetic)
Spinocerebellar ataxias	Cerebellar cortex, spinal cord, other regions	Various	Ataxia (balance disorder)
Amyotrophic lateral sclerosis	Anterior roots of spinal cord	SOD-1, TDP-43	Progressive weakness and paralysis

[a]The proteins involved in the formation of aggregates are described in the text.

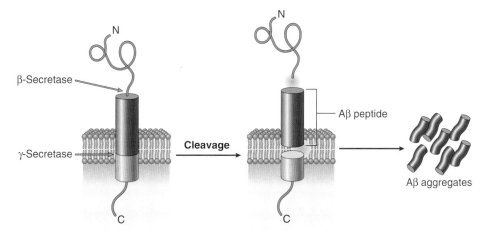

Fig. 17.8 Generation of beta-amyloid (Aβ) aggregates. Amyloid precursor protein cleavage by β-secretase, also called β-amyloid–converting enzyme (BACE), and γ-secretase releases Aβ peptides, which form pathogenic aggregates.

the unfolded protein response (see Chapter 1), which leads to apoptotic cell death if the protein misfolding cannot be corrected. Aggregation also leads to loss of function of the protein, and through other poorly understood mechanisms may impair gene transcription or protein synthesis. Interestingly, in several of these diseases, the conformationally altered proteins may be capable of spreading from cell to cell in a "prion-like" fashion, providing a possible mechanism of disease progression.

With this overview, we next discuss the major neurodegenerative diseases.

Alzheimer Disease

Alzheimer disease (AD) is the most common cause of dementia in older adults.

The incidence of AD increases with age and is estimated to be about 3% in individuals 65 to 74 years of age, 19% in those 75 to 84 years of age, and 47% in those older than 84. With our aging population, the disease is taking a terrible toll on patients and their families, and is a major problem for the health care system.

Pathogenesis. **The fundamental abnormality in AD is the accumulation of two proteins (Aβ and Tau) in specific brain regions.**

These proteins accumulate in the form of plaques (Aβ) and tangles (Tau) and lead to secondary effects, including neuronal dysfunction, neuronal death, and inflammation.

Aβ is a peptide produced by cleavage of the transmembrane amyloid precursor protein (APP) (Fig. 17.8). The peptide self-associates into oligomers that propagate into fibrils and large aggregates, which persist as extracellular *plaques* after neurons die. The oligomers and small fibrils are believed to disrupt synapses, altering learning and memory, and eventually cause neuronal death, leading to progressive neurologic deficits. Aβ is also recognized by the innate immune system, leading to low-level inflammation that, over time, may further injure neurons. Mutations in an enzyme that cleaves APP or in the *APP* gene itself are associated with a familial form of early-onset AD, presumably because of increased Aβ generation early in life. Notably, *APP* is located on chromosome 21, and the increased risk and occurrence of AD at young ages in those with trisomy 21 (Down syndrome; see Chapter 6) may stem from the presence of an extra copy of this gene. The risk for AD is also increased with inheritance of particular alleles of the gene encoding apolipoprotein E (ApoE), and mutations in some ApoE alleles may be protective, but how this protein influences the development of AD is not known.

Tau is a microtubule-associated protein in axons. In AD, it is hyperphosphorylated and aggregates, forming structures called *tangles* and

dystrophic neurites. These aggregates may damage neurons by eliciting a stress response or by disrupting microtubule function. Tau aggregates initially form inside cells and may persist in the extracellular tissue if affected neurons die.

Morphology. There is variable cortical atrophy that increases over time (Supplemental eFig. 17.12). The morphologic hallmarks of the disease are plaques and tangles, detected microscopically.

- Neuritic plaques are extracellular collections of dilated, tortuous processes (dystrophic neurites) that contain hyperphosphorylated Tau aggregates and surround a central amyloid core containing Aβ aggregates (Fig. 17.9A). They are found in the hippocampus, cortex, and some subcortical structures. Aβ deposition precedes other neuropathologic changes, possibly by many years.
- Neurofibrillary tangles are bundles of fibrils formed of hyperphosphorylated Tau in the cytoplasm of cortical neurons, as well as neurons in other regions (see Fig. 17.9B).

Clinical Features. The disease usually manifests with the insidious onset of impaired higher intellectual function, memory loss, and altered mood and behavior. Over time, disorientation and aphasia (findings indicative of severe cortical dysfunction) develop; those in the final phases of AD are profoundly disabled, often mute, and immobile. Death usually occurs from pneumonia or other infections. At present, a definitive distinction between AD and other forms of dementia can only be made at autopsy; it is hoped that new imaging approaches that permit identification of amyloid in the brain will improve the ability to diagnose AD during life.

Frontotemporal Lobar Degeneration (FTLD)

FTLD is a group of diseases characterized pathologically by neuronal loss and atrophy in the frontal and/or temporal lobes and clinically by behavioral changes or language problems.

The dominant clinical manifestation is related to the site of neuronal loss, with changes in behavior being more prominent in cases with frontal lobe involvement, while language difficulties predominate in those with primarily temporal lobe disease. The term *degeneration* refers to the neuropathologic changes; clinically, this disease is called *frontotemporal dementia (FTD).* Global dementia may occur with progressive disease, but unlike AD, behavioral changes precede memory loss and the disease onset is at a younger age. FTLD may be sporadic or heritable. Pathologic subgroups may be distinguished based on the

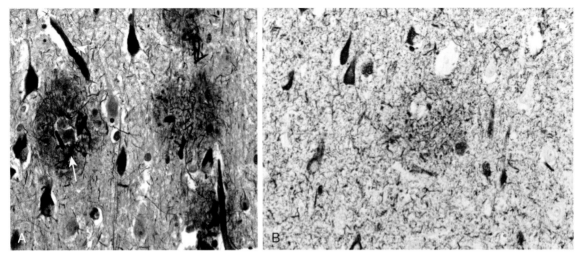

Fig. 17.9 Alzheimer disease. (A) Silver stain highlights both neuritic plaques (which consist of β amyloid core surrounded by dystrophic neurites; *arrow*) and neurofibrillary tangles (black, flame-shaped inclusions in neuronal cell bodies; *arrowhead*). (B) Both neurofibrillary tangles and dystrophic neurites (which surround the plaque amyloid core) consist of hyperphosphorylated and aggregated Tau protein, which in this image is highlighted by an anti-Tau immunostain. (Note that normal neurons without neurofibrillary tangles lack significant Tau immunopositivity in their cell bodies and are seen as areas devoid of staining in the image, whereas fine fibrillary staining in the background reflects normal Tau immunoreactivity in the axons and dendrites.)

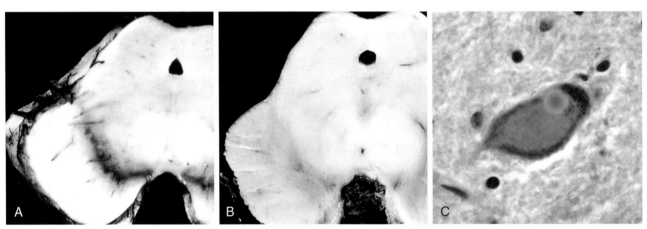

Fig. 17.10 Parkinson disease. (A) Normal substantia nigra. (B) Depigmented substantia nigra in Parkinson disease. (C) Lewy body in a neuron from the substantia nigra stains pink.

composition of characteristic neuronal inclusions, which contain Tau or TDP-43, a DNA/RNA binding protein. Regardless of the type of inclusion, there is neuronal loss and gliosis in the frontal and/or temporal lobes, with varying degrees of cortical atrophy (Supplemental eFig. 17.13).

Parkinson Disease

Parkinson disease (PD) is characterized by α-synuclein aggregates throughout the brain and a loss of dopamine-producing neurons in the substantia nigra that leads to a hypokinetic movement disorder.

Pathogenesis. The best-characterized inclusions of PD contain aggregates of the protein α-synuclein, which is involved in synaptic transmission. These intracytoplasmic aggregates are found predominantly in dopaminergic neurons of the substantia nigra; they also occur in other regions of the brain, including various brain stem nuclei, the cerebral cortex, and the sympathetic ganglia. Although most cases are sporadic, mutations and duplication of the gene encoding α-synuclein,

as well as mutations affecting autophagic degradation, which may be involved in clearance of the protein, are associated with familial forms of PD. As discussed earlier, these protein aggregates may damage neurons either by loss of function of the protein or by the toxic effects of accumulated misfolded proteins. Certain familial forms of PD are associated with mutations in genes that are involved in mitochondrial function, implicating mitochondrial abnormalities in the disease.

Morphology. The substantia nigra shows loss of pigmented dopamine-producing neurons, resulting in grossly apparent pallor (Fig. 17.10). Residual neurons may contain cytoplasmic inclusions composed of α-synuclein called *Lewy bodies*.

Clinical Features. The typical presentation is gradual and progressive slowing of movement (bradykinesia), tremors, and rigidity, causing postural instability and gait difficulties. Cognitive dysfunction and dementia

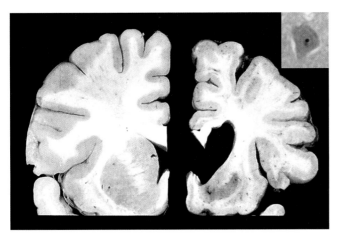

Fig. 17.11 Huntington disease. Normal hemisphere *(left)* compared with a hemisphere with Huntington disease *(right)* showing atrophy of the striatum and ventricular dilation. *Inset,* An intranuclear inclusion in a cortical neuron is strongly immunoreactive for ubiquitin. (Gross photo courtesy of Dr. J-P. Vonsattel, Columbia University, New York.)

may occur late in the course. The initial stages of the disease respond to replacement therapy with L-dopa (a precursor of dopamine), but during later stages the benefits of L-dopa fade.

Huntington Disease

Huntington disease (HD) is an autosomal dominant movement disorder caused by degeneration of the caudate and putamen.

Pathogenesis. HD is caused by a glutamine-encoding CAG trinucleotide repeat expansion in the gene encoding a protein called Huntingtin. The normal gene contains 11 to 34 copies of the repeat; in patients, this number is increased, sometimes into the hundreds. Larger numbers of repeats result in earlier-onset disease. Further expansions of the CAG repeats occur during spermatogenesis, so paternal transmission is associated with an earlier onset of disease in the next generation, a phenomenon referred to as *anticipation* (see Chapter 6). Larger numbers of repeats result in earlier-onset disease. Huntingtin is expressed in many cell types, but is abundant in the brain and is believed to serve signaling and transport functions in neurons. The mutant protein undergoes proteolysis to generate fragments that form intranuclear aggregates, which may injure neurons through several poorly defined mechanisms, including sequestration of transcription factors and disruption of mitochondrial function.

Morphology. The brain shows striking atrophy of the caudate nucleus and sometimes the putamen (Fig. 17.11). There is a loss of neurons from affected regions, especially neurons that produce neurotransmitters such as γ-amino butyric acid (GABA) and enkephalin. Surviving neurons contain intranuclear inclusions composed of ubiquitinated Huntingtin.

Clinical Features. HD is characterized by involuntary, jerky, writhing movements (chorea) of all parts of the body, especially the extremities. It is relentlessly progressive, resulting in death after an average course of about 15 years. Early cognitive symptoms include forgetfulness and thought and affective disorders, and there may be progression to severe dementia. These behavioral changes are associated with an increased risk for suicide.

Spinocerebellar Ataxias

This group of diseases is caused by trinucleotide repeat expansions in various genes, leading to degeneration of neurons in different regions of the brain.

Pathogenesis. More than 30 forms of the disease are known, all of which include cerebellar ataxia as a clinical feature. Most are caused by polyglutamine expansions affecting different proteins in the brain and other tissues. The abnormal proteins form intranuclear inclusions. One subtype, *Friedreich ataxia,* is an autosomal recessive disease that is caused by GAA repeat expansions in a gene called frataxin. The encoded protein is involved in regulating mitochondrial function. Repeat expansions result in decreased synthesis of frataxin, leading to mitochondrial dysfunction and increased oxidative damage.

Morphology. The disease is dominated by degeneration of neurons. Different regions of the brain may be affected, and the site influences the clinical manifestations. Cerebellar involvement is associated with ataxia, and spinal cord and peripheral nerve involvement with motor defects and/or ataxia.

Clinical Features. Most spinocerebellar ataxias show autosomal dominant inheritance and present in middle age; the age of onset and rate of progression are influenced by the number of trinucleotide repeats. The typical manifestations are progressive ataxia and diverse other neurologic symptoms.

Amyotrophic Lateral Sclerosis

Amyotrophic lateral sclerosis (ALS) is caused by degeneration of motor neurons in the spinal cord, brain stem, and motor cortex, resulting in muscle weakness and spasticity.

Pathogenesis. More than 90% of ALS cases are sporadic, and their pathogenesis is unknown. Possible mechanisms have been suggested based on the identification of genes associated with familial forms of the disease. A hexanucleotide repeat expansion in *C9orf72* is the most common genetic cause of ALS, accounting for approximately 40% of familial cases; it is present in about 7% of sporadic cases. Mutations in superoxide dismutase *(SOD-1)* account for about 12% of familial cases. The abnormal SOD-1 protein is believed to misfold, trigger the unfolded protein response, and cause apoptotic death of neurons. Less common pathogenic mutations affect the genes encoding FUS and TDP-43. The genetic overlap with FTLD suggests a similar pathogenesis, the difference being the principal sites affected: neurons in the frontal and temporal lobes in FTLD and anterior horn motor neurons in the spinal cord in ALS.

Morphology. The characteristic findings are degeneration of motor neurons and reactive gliosis. There is loss of neurons in the anterior horns of the spinal cord, and in severe cases, there may also be loss of neurons in the motor cortex (Supplemental eFig. 17.14). The result is anterograde axonal loss and gliosis in the corticospinal tracts in the lateral portions of the spinal cord (lateral sclerosis). The spinal cord is atrophic, with thin ventral roots and loss of myelinated fibers in motor nerves. Intracellular inclusions of TDP-43 are seen in a subset of cases.

Clinical Features. The loss of lower motor neurons results in denervation of muscles, muscular atrophy (amyotrophy), weakness, and fasciculations, while the loss of upper motor neurons results in paresis, hyperreflexia, and spasticity. Sensation usually is unaffected, but a degree of cognitive impairment is not infrequent.

CNS TUMORS

The most common primary tumors of the CNS are *gliomas*, which arise from glial cells such as astrocytes, oligodendrocytes, and ependymal cells, and *meningiomas*, which arise from arachnoid cells of the meninges lining the brain.

Gliomas have some important general characteristics.

- Gliomas do not have any recognizable premalignant or in situ stages, unlike carcinomas (see Chapter 5).
- Even low-grade gliomas can produce major clinical abnormalities because they are not encapsulated, infiltrate the brain parenchyma, and produce mass effects.
- Gliomas rarely spread outside the CNS (i.e., there are no distant metastases).

Patients present with focal or generalized symptoms and signs, including headaches, seizures, aphasia, vomiting, visual disturbances, and cognitive dysfunction (memory and mood disorders). Intracranial pressure may be increased. A glioma may be suspected on the basis of imaging studies (MRI), but tissue biopsy is required to confirm the diagnosis. The classification of gliomas is based on morphology and, increasingly, on molecular abnormalities, both of which have prognostic implications.

General Features and Pathogenesis of Astrocytoma

Astrocytomas account for about 80% of adult gliomas and most often arise in the fourth through sixth decades of life. They usually occur in the cerebral hemispheres. Low-grade tumors can be static for several years but inevitably progress. Progression often is marked by rapid clinical deterioration due to transformation to aggressive high-grade glioblastoma. Other patients present with glioblastoma from the outset. Once glioblastoma appears, the prognosis is very poor; with treatment (resection, radiotherapy, and chemotherapy), the median survival time is 15 months.

All astrocytomas contain cells with elongated or irregular, hyperchromatic nuclei and eosinophilic cytoplasm that stain positively for the glial marker *glial fibrillary acidic protein*. Higher-grade tumors show greater morphologic evidence of malignancy, such as mitoses, microvascular proliferation, and necrosis.

As with all cancers, astrocytomas are caused by driver mutations in cancer genes, some of which are also mutated in other cancers. One genetic abnormality that seems to be especially important in astrocytic tumors is mutation of the gene *IDH1* (or, less commonly, its homologue, *IDH2*). The mutated genes encode forms of isocitrate dehydrogenase with a new enzymatic activity that converts α-ketoglutarate to 2-hydroxyglutarate, discussed in Chapter 5 as a classic example of an "oncometabolite." The presence of *IDH1/2* mutations predicts a better prognosis in all grades of astrocytic tumors.

Classification of Astrocytomas

Astrocytomas are divided into several groups based on their morphology and are subclassifed within each group based on molecular alterations.

- *Diffuse astrocytoma* (also known as WHO grade II tumors) is most common in young adults. It arises in the cerebral hemispheres, and as with other astrocytomas, tends to infiltrate diffusely, sometimes well away from the main mass (Fig. 17.12A). The tumors are cellular, and the tumor cells often show signs of atypia, but mitoses are rare. Endothelial (microvascular) proliferation and necrosis (features of higher-grade tumors) are not seen (Fig. 17.12B). The transition between neoplastic and normal tissues is not distinct. Most tumors are associated with *IDH1* mutations.
- *Anaplastic astrocytoma* (grade III tumors) is more cellular and more mitotically active and displays greater cytologic atypia than grade II

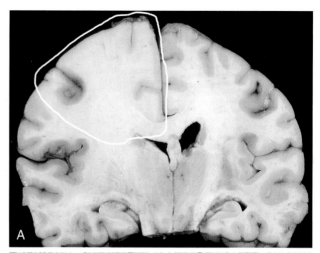

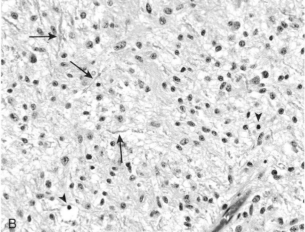

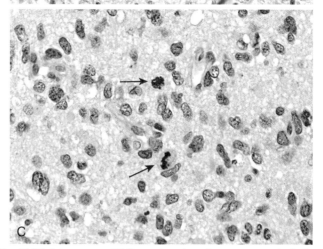

Fig. 17.12 Astrocytoma. (A) Coronal section of a postmortem brain from a patient with a diffuse astrocytoma involving the frontal lobe, roughly outlined within the white borders. Note the larger size of the involved frontal lobe compared with the opposite side, the ill-defined borders of the tumor, the mass effect with compression of the superior frontal horn of the lateral ventricle, and the whitish discoloration of cortex with patchy blurring of the gray-white borders due to intracortical tumoral infiltration. (B) In this biopsy specimen, the majority of the nuclei represent infiltrating astrocytoma cells, characterized by nuclear enlargement, irregular contours, and hyperchromasia (dark chromatin), set against a fibrillary background (pink meshwork of glial fibers). The linear bright-red structures are entrapped axons *(arrows)*, whereas the small rounded nuclei *(arrowheads)* represent entrapped oligodendrocytes. (C) In this diffuse astrocytoma, mitotic figures were also found *(arrows)*, qualifying this tumor as an "anaplastic astrocytoma, WHO grade III." (Courtesy Dr. Arie Perry, Department of Pathology, University of California San Francisco.)

tumors. However, endothelial proliferation and necrosis are not present (Fig. 17.12C). Approximately 80% have *IDH1* mutations.

- *Glioblastoma* (grade IV tumor) is the most common and most malignant primary brain tumor of adults. The tumors are densely cellular, the cells are highly pleomorphic, mitoses are easily found, and there are extensive endothelial proliferation and areas of necrosis (Fig. 17.13). The majority do not have *IDH1* mutations, except for a subset that arises by progression from lower-grade astrocytomas.

- *Pilocytic astrocytoma* (grade I tumor) is a slow-growing tumor that usually occurs in the cerebellum in children and young adults. The tumors are often cystic (Supplemental eFig. 17.15). Tumor cells are elongated and have extended processes that create a fibrillary background. Most pilocytic astrocytomas have bright-red corkscrew-shaped inclusions called Rosenthal fibers. Many cases have mutations involving the kinase BRAF, which functions in the RAS signaling pathway; *IDH1* mutations are not typically seen.

Other CNS Tumors

- *Oligodendroglioma* accounts for 5 to 15% of glial tumors and shares with its astrocytic counterparts a predisposition for extensive infiltration. It arises mostly in the frontal or temporal lobe. The cells have round nuclei and perinuclear haloes (a "fried-egg" appearance), reminiscent of normal oligodendrocytes (Supplemental eFig. 17.16). The stroma includes a dense network of branching capillaries. Calcification is seen in the vast majority of tumors. Anaplastic variants have more pleomorphic cells with mitoses and endothelial proliferation. A defining set of genetic alterations consists of deletions leading to loss of chromosomes 1p and 19q, often because of an unbalanced translocation, in association with an *IDH1/2* mutation. Grade for grade, oligodendrogliomas have a better prognosis than astrocytic tumors.

- *Ependymoma* arises from the ependymal cells lining the ventricular system, and is most often found adjacent to these channels. In the first two decades of life, it occurs near the fourth ventricle, but in adults, it is located primarily in the spinal cord. Tumor cells may form rosettes or canals that resemble the embryonic ependymal canal (Supplemental eFig. 17.17).

- *Medulloblastoma* is a tumor of children that is thought to arise from cerebellar stem cells; it accounts for almost 20% of pediatric tumors. Most tumors are located in the midline of the cerebellum (Fig. 17.14). They are densely cellular, with sheets of undifferentiated small cells that stain blue because of the hyperchromatic nuclei and scant cytoplasm. They thus belong to the family of "small blue cell tumors," which includes neuroectodermal tumors such as Ewing sarcoma. The cells often form rosettes with central neuronal processes (neuropil). Driver mutations that result in hyperactivation of the Hedgehog pathway or the WNT pathway or overexpression of the *MYC* oncogene are seen in a subset of cases. Tumors with WNT pathway activation have the best prognosis, followed by those with Hedgehog pathway activation or *MYC* overexpression.

- *Meningioma* is a usually benign tumor that occurs in adults. It arises from arachnoid meningothelial cells and is often attached to the dura. It may compress the underlying brain but only rarely infiltrates it (Fig. 17.15). Numerous morphologic variants have been described, including tumor cells with an epitheliod, fibroblastic, or secretory appearance. Higher-grade variants are called atypical (WHO grade II) or anaplastic (WHO grade III); these are considered malignant. Patients with neurofibromatosis type 2, described later, frequently have multiple meningiomas, and about 50% of sporadic meningiomas have loss-of-function mutations of the *NF2* gene.

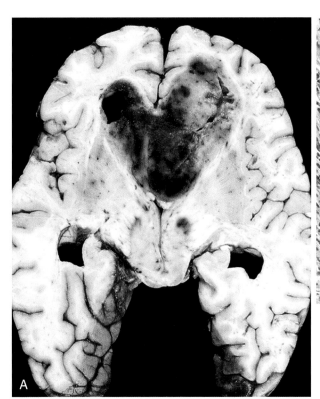
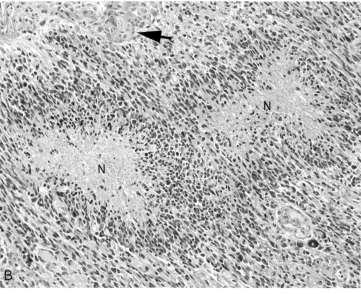

Fig. 17.13 Glioblastoma. (A) Glioblastoma appearing as a necrotic, hemorrhagic, infiltrating mass. (B) Histopathologic features of glioblastoma, WHO grade IV, include the presence of microvascular proliferation *(arrow)* and tumor necrosis *(N)*, often associated with palisading (lining up) of tumor cells adjacent to the necrosis. (B, Courtesy Dr. Arie Perry, Department of Pathology, University of California San Francisco.)

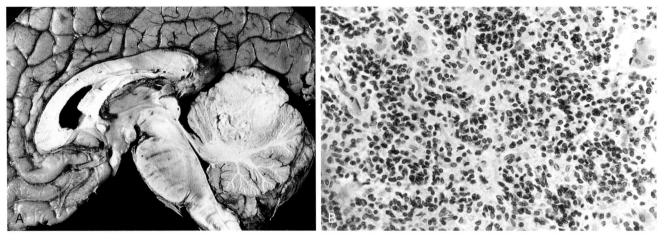

Fig. 17.14 Medulloblastoma. (A) Sagittal section of a brain showing medulloblastoma involving the superior vermis of the cerebellum. (B) Microscopic appearance of medulloblastoma, showing mostly small, blue, primitive-appearing tumor cells.

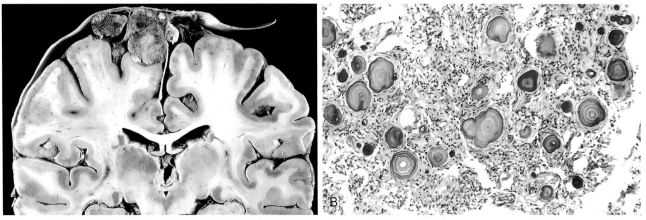

Fig. 17.15 Meningioma. (A) Parasagittal multilobular meningioma attached to the dura with compression of underlying brain. (B) Meningioma with a whorled pattern of cell growth and psammoma bodies (calcified remnants of epithelial cells).

Inherited Syndromes Associated with CNS Tumors

Several autosomal dominant syndromes are frequently associated with proliferations involving the CNS:

- *Tuberous sclerosis* is an autosomal dominant hereditary cancer syndrome associated with multiple benign hamartomas of the brain, eyes, kidneys, heart, and other organs. The syndrome is caused by mutations in one of two *TSC* genes (*TSC1* and *TSC2*) that encode the proteins hamartin and tuberin, respectively. The two TSC proteins form a dimeric complex that negatively regulates mTOR. Upregulation of mTOR leads to increased cell growth.
- *von Hippel-Lindau disease* is an autosomal dominant hereditary cancer syndrome associated with the development of hemangioblastomas, most commonly in the cerebellar hemispheres and retina. Patients may have cysts involving the pancreas, liver, and kidneys and have an increased risk of renal cell carcinoma and pheochromocytoma. The affected gene, the tumor suppressor *VHL*, encodes a protein that is part of a ubiquitin–ligase complex that degrades the transcription factor hypoxia-inducible factor (HIF).

Retinoblastoma

Retinoblastoma is an intraocular tumor of children. It is discussed here because of the anatomic and physiologic connections between the eyes and CNS.

Pathogenesis. The tumor is associated with loss-of-function mutations in the *RB* (retinoblastoma) tumor suppressor gene, which as discussed in Chapter 5 encodes a key regulator of the cell cycle. About 40% of cases are familial, caused by germline *RB* mutations, and usually present as multiple bilateral tumors. In familial cases, one mutant copy is inherited and the other is lost somatically in retinoblasts. Sporadic tumors, which are unilateral and solitary lesions, usually have somatic mutations in one allele of *RB* and an acquired deletion leading to loss of the other *RB* allele.

Morphology. The tumors are nodular masses usually arising from the posterior retina. They consist of small round cells with hyperchromatic nuclei, resembling undifferentiated retinoblasts (Supplemental eFig. 17.18). Many tumors contain more differentiated cells, sometimes forming "pseudorosettes" around a central lumen. The tumors may spread through the optic nerve and may metastasize to the CNS, bones, and lymph nodes.

Clinical Features. The tumor usually presents before 2 years of age with visual disturbances and pain and tenderness in the affected eye. The tumor may be fatal if untreated, but can be cured with radiation, chemotherapy, and, if necessary, enucleation. Rarely, the tumors regress spontaneously.

DISORDERS OF PERIPHERAL NERVES

Peripheral nerves are made up of axons surrounded by an insulating myelin sheath, which is synthesized by lining cells called Schwann cells. Sensory nerves detect signals from the surroundings and provide the brain with information about the environment, and motor nerves stimulate muscle movement. Motor nerves contact muscles through the neuromuscular junction, through which neurotransmitters (mainly acetylcholine) are secreted from nerve endings and act on muscles to stimulate contraction; these structures form the motor units. Diseases of nerves lead to atrophy of the muscles supplied by those nerves (see Chapter 18).

Peripheral Neuropathy

Peripheral neuropathy refers to any disorder of the peripheral nervous system that affects multiple or single nerves.

Nerves are susceptible to injury by a variety of agents and disorders, such as many types of vasculitis, diabetes, various therapeutic drugs, toxins (e.g., alcohol), infections (e.g., varicella zoster and leprosy), uremia, and rare congenital anomalies. Here we discuss two illustrative examples.

- *Diabetic neuropathy* is the most common cause of peripheral neuropathy, reflecting the high incidence of diabetes. It is usually seen with long-standing and poorly controlled diabetes. The pathogenesis is complex and poorly understood; it may involve advanced glycation end-products, reactive oxygen species, and microvascular injury (see Chapter 16). Diabetic neuropathies include several forms that occur singly or together: *distal sensorimotor neuropathy* (the most common, in which sensory involvement is prominent and leads to paresthesias and numbness), *autonomic neuropathy* (which affects bowel and bladder function), and *lumbosacral disease* (which causes back pain and lower extremity weakness).
- *Guillain-Barre syndrome* is an acute demyelinating disorder affecting motor neurons that causes ascending weakness. The disease is presumed to be caused by an autoimmune attack against peripheral nerve myelin or Schwann cells. An association with viral infections (e.g., EBV, HIV, Zika virus, and cytomegalovirus [CMV]) has led to the suggestion that the disease may be triggered by a viral infection that provokes the generation of microbe-specific T cells and antibodies, which then cross-react with antigens in the nerve sheath. Injury to nerve roots and proximal nerve segments is accompanied by infiltrates of macrophages and lymphocytes. In the majority of patients, the disease progresses for two to four weeks after onset and then remits. In about 30% of patients, the disease may progress rapidly, leading to respiratory failure that requires mechanical ventilation. In severe cases, removal of offending antibodies by plasmapheresis can be lifesaving.

Peripheral Nerve Tumors

Peripheral nerve sheath tumors are uncommon neoplasms that often arise in individuals with neurofibromatosis type 1 and neurofibromatosis type 2.

- *Schwannoma* is a benign tumor arising from the cells lining nerve axons, most often within spinal nerve roots but also in soft tissues or various organs. They are encapsulated tumors composed of spindle-shaped cells (Supplemental eFig. 17.19A,B). Cellularity characteristically varies from densely cellular areas to sparsely cellular areas with myxoid stroma. Most schwannomas are sporadic, but about 10% are associated with *familial neurofibromatosis type 2 (NF2)*. These patients have a dominant loss-of-function mutation of *NF2*, which encodes merlin, a cytoskeletal protein that acts as a tumor suppressor. Loss of merlin is also seen in sporadic schwannomas.
- *Neurofibromatosis type 1 (NF1)* is an autosomal dominant disease caused by mutations in the tumor suppressor gene *NF1*. Loss of function of this gene results in overactivity of RAS. The most common tumors that develop in individuals with NF1 are benign *neurofibromas* of peripheral nerves, which may be multiple and lead to disfigurement (Supplemental eFig. 17.19C,D). Affected individuals are at high risk for malignant peripheral nerve sheath tumors, optic gliomas, and other CNS tumors. These patients also may exhibit a number of developmental abnormalities, such as skeletal abnormalities, arterial stenoses, pigmented nodules of the iris *(Lisch nodules),* pigmented skin lesions (axillary freckling and café-au-lait spots), learning disabilities, and seizure disorders.
- *Neurofibromatosis type 2 (NF2)* is also an autosomal dominant disease. NF2 patients are at risk of developing multiple schwannomas, meningiomas, and ependymomas. The presence of bilateral vestibular schwannomas is a hallmark of NF2; despite the name, neurofibromas are not found in NF2 patients.

Diseases of Neuromuscular Junctions

As mentioned earlier, the neuromuscular junction transmits nerve impulses to the muscle and converts them into muscle contractions.

- *Myasthenia gravis* is an autoimmune disease caused by autoantibodies that target the neuromuscular junction, most commonly the acetylcholine receptor (AChR). It has a bimodal age distribution: Onset before age 50 years is more common in females, whereas late-onset cases show a more equal sex distribution. The causative AChR antibodies block neuromuscular transmission and decrease expression of the receptor by causing its endocytosis. Myasthenia gravis is sometimes associated with thymic abnormalities. These may take the form of so-called *thymic hyperplasia,* marked by increased numbers of reactive B cells within the thymus, or *thymoma,* a neoplasm of thymic epithelium. Patients typically present with drooping eyelids (ptosis) and double vision (diplopia) because of weak extraocular muscles. The severity of the weakness fluctuates, getting worse with repeated movements. Administration of cholinesterase inhibitors increases the amount of acetylcholine and thus ameliorates the symptoms. Effective treatments include cholinesterase inhibitors, immunosuppression, plasmapheresis, and (in patients with thymoma) thymectomy.
- *Lambert-Eaton syndrome* is caused by autoantibodies that inhibit the function of presynaptic calcium channels, thereby reducing the release of acetylcholine into the synaptic cleft. It may arise as a paraneoplastic disorder, particularly in patients with small cell lung carcinoma. In contrast to myasthenia gravis, repeated stimulation improves strength by allowing the buildup of sufficient intracellular calcium to facilitate acetylcholine release. Cholinesterase inhibitors are not effective, and therapy is therefore directed toward reducing the titer of causative antibodies, through either plasmapheresis or immunosuppression.

18

Musculoskeletal System and Skin

OUTLINE

Bones, 296
    Congenital Disorders, 296
    Metabolic Diseases, 297
    Fractures and Avascular
        Necrosis, 298
    Osteomyelitis, 298
    Tumors, 299
Joints, 301
    Arthritis, 301

Skeletal Muscle, 305
    Muscular Dystrophies, 305
    Myositis, 306
    Tumors of Muscle and Soft Tissue, 306
Skin, 307
    Acute Inflammatory Dermatoses, 307
    Chronic Inflammatory Dermatoses, 308
    Blistering (Bullous) Disorders, 309
    Tumors, 310

The musculoskeletal system consists of bones, joints, and skeletal muscles. Diseases of bones and joints are becoming increasingly common as the mechanical stresses of daily life accumulate over time and take their toll on an aging population. Bones and muscles are also frequent victims of accidental trauma. Much of this chapter is focused on disorders of bones and joints. At the end, we discuss some common diseases of the skin.

BONES

The functions of bone include mechanical support, transmission of forces generated by muscles, protection of viscera, calcium homeostasis, and providing a protected niche for production of blood cells. The constituents of bone include a specialized extracellular matrix that is produced and maintained by several types of resident cells. These include osteoblasts and osteocytes, which synthesize the matrix of the bone, and osteoclasts, specialized macrophages that dissolve bone. Bone remodeling refers to the continuous synthesis and dissolution of bone matrix by these various cells. Bone is made up of an organic part called osteoid, composed of mainly type I collagen, and an inorganic component, hydroxyapatite, that is mainly a form of calcium phosphate and is unique to bone.

Congenital Disorders

Congenital diseases of bone are classified into two types:
- *Dysostoses* refer to defects in the formation of the cartilage anlage that gives rise to bone, so that the shapes or numbers of bone are abnormal. These include an absence of or extra numbers of digits and the fusion of bones that are normally separate.
- *Dysplasias* are abnormalities of bone development or remodeling, in which bone is formed but does not grow or is not maintained normally.

Hundreds of congenital disorders have been described. Most are exceedingly rare, and the features of only a few relatively common ones are outlined here.

Dwarfism

Congenital short stature is of two major types, both caused by different mutations in the same FGF pathway.
- *Achondroplasia,* the most common skeletal dysplasia and a major cause of dwarfism, is an autosomal dominant disorder resulting from diminished elongation of long bones. It is caused by gain-of-function mutations that activate the tyrosine kinase activity of the fibroblast growth factor-3 (FGF-3) receptor, which normally functions to suppress endochondral bone growth. Affected individuals have shortened proximal extremities, a relatively normal trunk length, and an enlarged head with a bulging forehead and conspicuous depression of the root of the nose.
- *Thanatophoric dysplasia,* the most common lethal form of dwarfism, is caused by different gain-of-function mutations in the FGF-3 receptor, which appear to cause greater increases in FGFR3 signaling than those that produce achondroplasia, thus resulting in a more severe phenotype. Affected individuals have shortening of the limbs, frontal bossing, macrocephaly, and a small chest cavity. The underdeveloped thoracic cavity leads to respiratory insufficiency, and these individuals usually die at birth or soon thereafter.

Osteogenesis Imperfecta

Osteogenesis imperfecta, the most common inherited disorder of connective tissue, is manifested by reduced bone formation and skeletal fragility due to deficient synthesis of type I collagen.

This autosomal dominant disease usually results from mutations in the genes that encode the α1 or α2 chain of type I collagen. Because mature collagen is a triple helix, abnormalities in one chain interfere with assembly of the complete molecule (an example of a dominant negative mutation). The disease affects tissues rich in type I collagen, such as bone (causing fragility), eyes (blue, transparent sclera), middle ear (hearing loss), and teeth (abnormal shapes). The severity of the disease ranges from mild to lethal depending on the mutation (Supplemental eFig. 18.1).

Osteopetrosis

Osteopetrosis is a group of diseases characterized by excessive bone formation due to defective osteoclast function and reduced bone resorption.

Osteopetrosis is a genetic disorder with variable inheritance patterns that is caused by mutations in several genes, most of which encode proteins that are needed for osteoclasts to generate acidic secretions, which are necessary for bone resorption. The resulting defect in bone resorption leads to bones that are "chalk-like" and prone to fracture (Supplemental eFig. 18.2). Other clinical effects are due to (1) reduction of the marrow cavity, resulting in decreased intramedullary hematopoiesis and consequent extensive extramedullary hematopoiesis in the spleen, liver, and elsewhere, and (2) compression of nerves exiting the foramens in the skull and vertebral column.

Metabolic Diseases

Metabolic abnormalities may affect bone formation or resorption and result in skeletal defects of different types.

Osteoporosis

Osteoporosis is characterized by clinically significant decrease in bone mass, most commonly associated with aging and postmenopausal hormonal changes in women, that leads to increased fracture risk.

The term *osteopenia* refers to decreased bone mass, and osteoporosis is defined as osteopenia that is severe enough to significantly increase the risk of fracture (at least 2.5 standard deviations less than the normal peak bone mass).

Pathogenesis. The peak bone mass is achieved during young adulthood, and its level is influenced by heredity, physical activity, diet, and hormonal state. The most common forms of primary osteoporosis are the senile and postmenopausal types, which may coexist (Fig. 18.1). Osteoporosis can also be secondary to endocrine disorders (e.g., hyperthyroidism), gastrointestinal disorders (e.g., malnutrition), or drugs (e.g., corticosteroids).

The development of osteoporosis is the result of several factors.
- *Aging:* Osteoblast proliferation and synthetic activity is reduced *(senile osteoporosis).*
- *Reduced physical activity:* Mechanical forces stimulate bone remodeling.
- *Reduced dietary intake of calcium and vitamin D*
- *Decreased levels of hormones,* especially estrogens. Bone resorption increases owing to the increased production by osteoclasts of RANK-ligand (the ligand for receptor activator of NF-κB), a protein that stimulates bone resorption, and the decreased production of its competitive antagonist osteoprotegerin (OPG). It has been postulated that estrogens alter the production of cytokines that regulate levels of RANKL and OPG. Prolonged steroid administration also leads to increased bone resorption, by unknown mechanisms.
- *Smoking* accelerates osteoporosis, possibly through effects on estrogen metabolism as well as other mechanisms.
- *Genetics:* Numerous genes have been linked to the development of osteoporosis, but their individual contributions are unclear.

Morphology. Histologically, the bone appears normal, but of decreased quantity (Fig. 18.2; Supplemental eFig. 18.3). The entire skeleton is involved in postmenopausal and senile osteoporosis, but some bones are more severely affected. In postmenopausal osteoporosis, increased osteoclastic activity primarily affects trabecular bone; by contrast, senile osteoporosis predominantly affects cortical bone.

Clinical Features. Individuals are susceptible to fractures, especially of the vertebrae (postmenopausal) and femoral neck (senile). Multiple vertebral fractures may lead to deformities, such as lumbar lordosis (forward bowing of the spine) and kyphoscoliosis (lateral bowing). The immobility following fractures of the femoral neck, pelvis, or spine results in complications such as pulmonary embolism and pneumonia, which can be lethal. The prevention and treatment of senile and postmenopausal osteoporosis includes exercise, appropriate calcium and vitamin D intake, smoking cessation, and pharmacologic agents that decrease bone resorption (bisphosphonates).

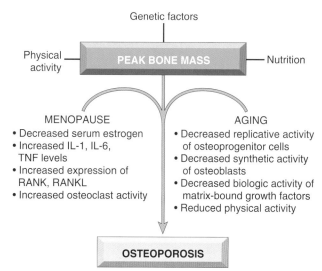

Fig. 18.1 Osteoporosis. Mechanisms that contribute to postmenopausal and senile osteoporosis. *RANK,* receptor activator of NF-κB; *RANKL,* RANK ligand; *TNF,* tumor necrosis factor.

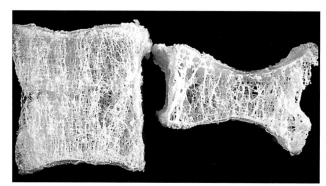

Fig. 18.2 Osteoporosis. Osteoporotic vertebral body (*right*) shortened by compression fractures compared with a normal vertebral body (*left*). The osteoporotic vertebra has a characteristic loss of horizontal trabeculae and thickened vertical trabeculae.

Rickets and Osteomalacia

Deficiency of vitamin D causes hypocalcemia, resulting in defective bone formation, manifested as rickets in children and osteomalacia in adults.

Both rickets and osteomalacia are manifestations of vitamin D deficiency or its abnormal metabolism (detailed in Chapter 19). *Rickets* refers to the disorder in children, in whom it interferes with the deposition of bone in the growth plates. *Osteomalacia* is the adult counterpart, in which bone formed during remodeling is undermineralized, resulting in a predisposition to fractures.

Hyperparathyroidism

Excess production of parathyroid hormone (PTH) leads to increased osteoclast activity, bone resorption, and osteopenia.

The actions of PTH and the causes of primary hyperparathyroidism (adenoma or hyperplasia of the glands) and secondary hyperparathyroidism (response to renal disease) were discussed in Chapter 16. Primary hyperparathyroidism causes generalized osteoporosis by mobilizing calcium from bone and increasing urinary phosphate excretion. The bone loss predisposes to microfractures that elicit a vascular and macrophage-rich repair response, forming masses of reactive tissue called "brown tumors" that exhibit hemorrhage, vascularity, and hemosiderin deposition (Supplemental eFigs. 18.4 and 18.5).

These lesions may undergo cystic degeneration. The combination of increased osteoclastic activity, peritrabecular fibrosis, and cystic brown tumors is the hallmark of severe hyperparathyroidism and is known as *generalized osteitis fibrosa cystica*.

Paget Disease of Bone

Paget disease is characterized by the formation of increased but disordered and structurally unsound bone.

Pathogenesis. The etiology of Paget disease is unknown; both genetic and infectious causes have been proposed. Uncommon familial forms of the disease are associated with mutations that increase RANKL activity and decrease OPG activity, resulting in uncontrolled activation of osteoclasts. Viral infections are suspected as contributors, but no causative agent has been identified.

> *Morphology.* The skeletal changes progress from an early osteolytic phase characterized by bone resorption due to increased numbers of activated, abnormally large osteoclasts, to a mixed sclerotic and lytic phase, ending with an osteosclerotic stage. By the time the disease comes to clinical attention, the bone is sclerotic and lamellar bone shows a striking mosaic pattern reflecting disordered remodeling, with prominent cement lines haphazardly joining units of bone (Fig. 18.3).

Clinical Features. Paget disease most frequently (~85% of cases) affects multiple bones (polyostotic); less commonly only one bone is affected (monostotic). The axial skeleton or proximal femur is involved in the vast majority of cases (Supplemental eFig. 18.6). The incidence of the disease increases with age. It is most common in Caucasians in parts of northern Europe, North America, and Australia and New Zealand. The disease is usually asymptomatic and discovered as an incidental radiographic finding. Less often, Paget disease presents with pain, caused by fractures or nerve compression by the expanded bone. Skull deformities and bowing of the femurs are frequently seen. Complications include fractures, osteoarthritis, and the development of bone tumors; secondary osteosarcoma is the most common tumor, occurring in 5% to 10% of cases with severe polyostotic disease.

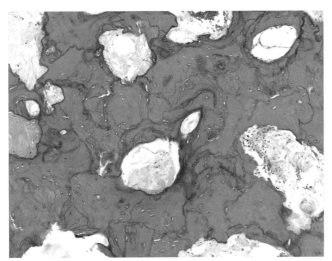

Fig. 18.3 Paget disease. Mosaic pattern of lamellar bone pathognomonic of Paget disease.

Fractures and Avascular Necrosis

Fractures

Fractures are the most common pathologic condition affecting bone. There are several types:

- *Simple* fractures, which leave the overlying skin intact
- *Compound* fractures, in which the broken bone reaches to or through the skin
- *Comminuted* fractures, characterized by bone fragmentation
- *Stress* fractures, which develop slowly, usually as a result of physical activity in which the bone is subjected to repetitive loads
- *Greenstick* fractures, which extend only partway through the bone, are usually seen in infancy or early childhood, when the bones are soft
- *Pathologic* fractures, which occur in bones that are weakened by an underlying disease process, such as a tumor

The healing of fractures involves much the same sequence of events as the repair of other injured vascularized tissues (see Chapter 2).

- Formation of a *hematoma* that fills the fracture gap
- Formation of a platelet–fibrin *clot*
- *Ingrowth of macrophages and fibroblasts and increased osteoblastic and osteoclastic activity* in the adjacent bone, in response to cytokines and growth factors released from macrophages, platelets, and other cells
- Within a week, bridging of the ends of the fractured bone by newly formed uncalcified tissue called a *soft callus*
- Within 2 weeks, deposition of bone, converting the soft callus into a mineralized *bony callus*
- *Gradual remodeling* in response to movement and weight bearing, reducing the size of the callus and replacing it with lamellar bone

Inadequate immobilization may permit movement of the callus and result in delayed union. If this persists, the malformed callus may acquire a lining of synovial cells, forming a pseudoarthrosis. Infection of the site, which is rare except with compound fractures, is a serious obstacle to normal healing.

Avascular Necrosis of Bone

This condition, also called *osteonecrosis,* refers to infarction (ischemic necrosis) of the bone and marrow cavity.

Pathogenesis. The etiology of avascular necrosis may be traumatic (most commonly fracture of the femoral neck) or because of bone ischemia secondary to vascular injury (e.g., vasculitis), drugs (e.g., corticosteroids and bisphosphonates), radiation, or systemic diseases that lead to vascular obstruction (e.g., sickle cell disease). The underlying etiology is unknown in about 25% of cases.

> *Morphology.* Typically, infarcts of the femoral head are wedge shaped and subchondral and involve the bone plate and marrow but spare the cortex and overlying cartilage, which receive nutrients from the collateral blood supply or synovial fluid (Fig. 18.4).

Clinical Features. Subchondral infarcts may cause pain that is initially associated only with activity but then becomes constant. These infarcts often collapse and may lead to severe, secondary osteoarthritis.

Osteomyelitis

Infection of the bone, most often caused by bacteria, and the attendant inflammation may cause destructive acute and chronic lesions.

Acute Pyogenic Osteomyelitis

Pathogenesis. Pyogenic osteomyelitis is most often caused by *Staphylococcus aureus* (accounting for 80% to 90% of cases). These bacteria express

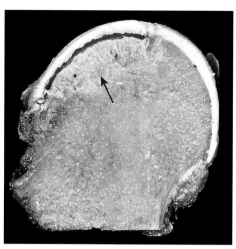

Fig. 18.4 Avascular necrosis. Femoral head with a subchondral, wedge-shaped pale yellow area of osteonecrosis *(arrow)*. The space between the overlying articular cartilage and bone is caused by trabecular compression fractures without repair.

cell wall proteins that bind to bone matrix components and facilitate adherence to bone. *Escherichia coli, Pseudomonas,* and *Klebsiella* are more frequently isolated from individuals with genitourinary tract infections or who are intravenous drug users. Individuals with sickle cell disease are prone to *Salmonella* osteomyelitis. Mixed bacterial infections are seen in the setting of direct spread, inoculation of organisms during surgery, or open fractures. In neonates, streptococci are often the causative agent. In almost 50% of suspected cases, no organisms can be identified.

Infection may be acquired by hematogenous spread (more common in children) or by extension from an adjacent infection (such as an infected foot ulcer in diabetics), or occur as a complication of an open fracture or surgical procedure (more often in adults). Even with hematogenous spread, there is often only a single focus of disease.

Morphology. Pyogenic osteomyelitis shares pathologic features with other pyogenic infections, including necrosis and acute inflammation. The dead bone is called a *sequestrum* (Fig. 18.5). The extension of infection within the bone depends on the pattern of vascular connections. In infants and adults, the bacteria can spread from the

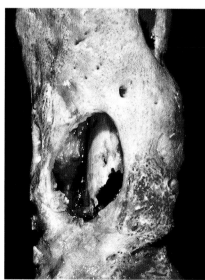

Fig. 18.5 Osteomyelitis. Resected femur in a person with draining osteomyelitis. The drainage tract in the subperiosteal shell of viable new bone (involucrum) shows the inner native necrotic cortex (sequestrum).

metaphysis to the epiphysis. In children, the avascular growth plate prevents the infection from extending into the epiphysis, but the periosteum is loosely attached to the cortex, and hence abscesses may form under the periosteum and spread into the adjacent connective tissue. Over time, the dead bone is resorbed, fibrous tissue grows in, and a shell of reactive bone, called the *involucrum*, is deposited around the sequestrum. Eventually, the dead bone is absorbed.

Clinical Features. Osteomyelitis may present as an acute febrile illness or with subtle systemic signs of inflammation and local pain. X-ray reveals a lytic focus surrounded by a sclerotic reaction. The combination of antibiotics and surgical drainage is usually curative, but in 5% to 25% of cases, the acute infection does not resolve and the disease becomes chronic. Complications of chronic osteomyelitis include pathologic fracture, secondary amyloidosis, endocarditis, sepsis, and the development of squamous cell carcinoma in the draining sinus tracts.

Tuberculous Osteomyelitis

Chronic osteomyelitis caused by *Mycobacterium tuberculosis* is largely confined to lower-income countries, where the infection is endemic. About 1% to 2% of patients with tuberculosis in the lungs or elsewhere develop bone infection. The vertebral column is involved in almost 40% of cases. Spine infections may spread through intervertebral disks to multiple vertebrae and into surrounding soft tissues (Pott disease); destruction of the vertebrae may cause kyphosis or scoliosis. The histopathology and clinical features are similar to those of tuberculosis affecting other organs.

Tumors

Bone tumors are often classified on the basis of the normal cell they resemble or the type of matrix they produce (Table 18.1). Benign tumors are much more frequent than malignant ones. Here we discuss only selected examples of relatively common tumors.

Osteochondroma

Osteochondroma, known clinically as *exostosis,* is a benign cartilage-capped tumor that is attached to the underlying skeleton by a bony stalk (Supplemental eFig. 18.7). It is the most common benign bone tumor. About 85% are solitary and arise in late adolescence and early adulthood; men are affected three times more often than women. Osteochondromas arise from the metaphysis near the growth plate of the long tubular bones, especially near the knee. They can be sessile or pedunculated. In the latter, the cortex of the stalk merges with the cortex of the host bone with continuity of the medullary cavity. Rarely, osteochondromas progress to chondrosarcoma.

Giant Cell Tumor

This tumor arises in the epiphyses of long bones in adults, affecting typically the distal femur and proximal tibia. Histologically, the tumor consists of two components. The tumor cells are osteoblast-derived small mononuclear cells that express high levels of RANKL, which stimulates osteoclast differentiation and proliferation. The activated osteoclasts develop into large, multinucleate giant cells, which give the tumor its name (Supplemental eFig. 18.8). The tumors are locally aggressive and tend to recur after surgery, but distant metastases are unusual.

Osteosarcoma

Osteosarcoma is a malignant bone-producing tumor.

This tumor (also called osteogenic sarcoma) is the most common primary malignant tumor of the bone. It shows a bimodal age distribution, with approximately 75% occurring in individuals younger than 20 years of age and the remainder in adults over 65. Risk factors include prior radiation therapy for another solid tumor, Paget disease, and inheritance of germline *RB* mutations (familial retinoblastoma).

Table 18.1 Primary Bone Tumors

Category	Behavior	Tumor Type	Common Locations	Age (yr)	Morphology
Cartilage forming	Benign	Osteochondroma	Metaphysis of long bones	10–30	Bony excrescence with cartilage cap
		Chondroma	Small bones of hands and feet	30–50	Circumscribed hyaline cartilage nodule in medulla
	Malignant	Chondrosarcoma (conventional)	Pelvis, shoulder	40–60	Extends from medulla through cortex into soft tissue, chondrocytes with increased cellularity and atypia
Bone forming	Benign	Osteoid osteoma	Metaphysis of long bones	10–20	Cortical, interlacing microtrabeculae of woven bone
		Osteoblastoma	Vertebral column	10–20	Posterior elements of vertebra, histology similar to osteoid osteoma
	Malignant	Osteosarcoma	Metaphysis of distal femur, proximal tibia	10–20	Extends from medulla to lift periosteum, malignant cells producing woven bone
Unknown origin	Benign	Giant cell tumor	Epiphysis of long bones	20–40	Destroys medulla and cortex, small mono-nuclear tumor cells and multinucleate osteoclasts
		Aneurysmal bone cyst	Proximal tibia, distal femur, vertebra	10–20	Vertebral body, hemorrhagic spaces separated by cellular, fibrous septae
	Malignant	Ewing sarcoma	Diaphysis of long bones	10–20	Sheets of primitive small round cells

Adapted from Unni KK, Inwards CY: *Dahlin's Bone Tumors,* ed 6. Philadelphia, 2010, Lippincott-Williams & Wilkins; by permission of Mayo Foundation.

Pathogenesis. Most of these tumors have mutations in the tumor suppressor genes *RB* and *TP53* and in regulators of the cell cycle, most commonly the tumor suppressor *CDKN2A* or the oncogene *CDK4* (see Chapter 5). Interestingly, the incidence peaks at the time of the adolescent growth spurt and the tumors develop most often in the region of the growth plate in rapidly growing long bones (distal femur, proximal tibia), suggesting that proliferation of osteoblasts predisposes to tumor development.

Morphology. The tumors are bulky masses with areas of hemorrhage and necrosis (Fig. 18.6). Extension into soft tissue is common. Tumor cells are pleomorphic and anaplastic, and mitoses are abundant. The hallmark of these tumors is production of osteoid matrix that can be mineralized to produce bone.

Clinical Features. Osteosarcoma typically presents as a painful expanding mass that comes to attention due to an injury or a pathologic fracture. Most are localized to the metaphyseal region of long bones around the knee joints (lower femur or upper tibia). Imaging is helpful for diagnosis. They are aggressive tumors with early hematogenous spread to the lungs. Osteosarcoma is treated with a multimodality approach that consists of neoadjuvant chemotherapy followed by surgery and additional chemotherapy. The amount of chemotherapy-induced necrosis found at surgical resection is an important prognostic finding.

Chondrosarcoma

This cartilage-producing tumor is the second most common malignant bone tumor after osteosarcoma and usually occurs in adults over 50 years of age. Unlike osteosarcoma, it occurs most often in the axial skeleton in the bones of the pelvis, shoulder, and ribs. It usually appears within the center of bones (the medullary cavity) (Supplemental eFig. 18.9A) but also may arise in the cortex or in chondral cartilage. The tumors are usually bulky and contain nodules of cartilaginous material that may be calcified, but bone formation does not occur. The cells vary in atypia and mitotic activity (see Supplemental eFig. 18.9B). A high histologic grade predicts a worse outcome. Chondrosarcomas are genetically heterogeneous;

approximately 40% harbor mutations in *IDH1* or *IDH2* genes. They present as painful, progressively enlarging masses. Treatment consists of surgical resection.

Ewing Sarcoma

Ewing sarcoma is a malignant tumor composed of primitive-appearing cells showing varying degrees of neuroectodermal differentiation.

The tumor most often presents in children, in whom it is the second most common malignant bone tumor after osteosarcoma. Almost 20% arise outside the skeleton. It belongs to the group of "small round blue cell tumors," including neuroblastoma, embryonal rhabdomyosarcoma, and Wilms tumor, all of which occur in children and are grouped together because of similar histologic features. In some of these tumors there is neuroectodermal differentiation, and they were previously called primitive neuroectodermal tumors.

Pathogenesis. The vast majority (85%) of Ewing sarcomas contain a balanced (11;22) (q24;q12) translocation generating in-frame fusion of the *EWSR1* gene on chromosome 22 to the *FLI1* gene on chromosome 11. The encoded fusion protein binds chromatin and influences gene expression, but precisely how it contributes to transformation is unclear. The cell of origin for the tumor also remains a mystery.

Morphology. The tumor usually arises in the marrow cavity and invades the cortex, periosteum, and adjacent soft tissue. It is composed of uniform small, round cells with dark blue staining nuclei and scant cytoplasm (Fig. 18.7). The cytoplasm is often clear because of the presence of glycogen, which can be identified with special stains.

Clinical Features. The tumor presents as a painful, enlarging mass, most often in the proximal long bone and some flat bones such as the pelvis. Imaging studies reveal a diaphyseal lytic lesion with a periosteal reaction. It is an invasive, aggressive tumor usually associated with occult metastases, most commonly to the lung, at the time of diagnosis. Surgical resection combined with chemotherapy is curative in most patients without overt metastases; the overall cure rate is about 50%.

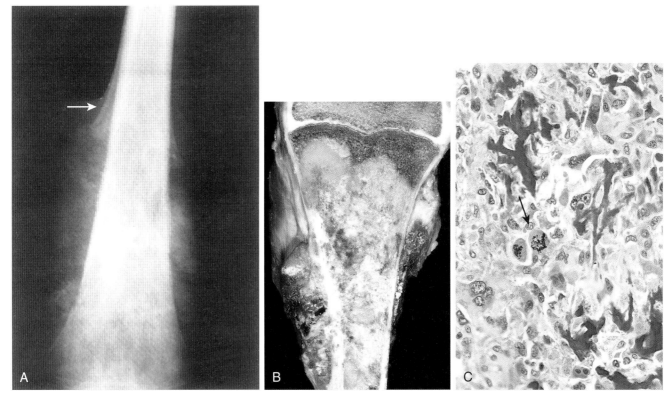

Fig. 18.6 Osteosarcoma. (A) Distal femoral osteosarcoma with prominent bone formation extending into the soft tissues. The periosteum, which has been lifted, has laid down a triangular shell of reactive bone known as a Codman triangle *(arrow)*. (B) Osteosarcoma of the proximal tibia. The tan-white tumor fills most of the medullary cavity of the metaphysis and proximal diaphysis. It has infiltrated through the cortex, lifted the periosteum, and formed soft tissue masses on both sides of the bone. (C) Fine, lacelike pattern of neoplastic bone produced by anaplastic malignant tumor cells in an osteosarcoma. Note the abnormal mitotic figure *(arrow)*.

Metastatic Tumors

Tumors metastatic to bone greatly outnumber primary bone cancers.

The pathways of tumor spread to bone include direct extension, lymphatic or hematogenous dissemination, and intraspinal seeding (via the Batson plexus of veins). In adults, more than 75% of skeletal metastases originate from cancers of the prostate, breast, kidney, and lung. In children, metastases to bone most frequently originate from neuroblastoma, Wilms tumor, and rhabdomyosarcoma. Skeletal metastases are typically multifocal and involve the axial skeleton, especially the vertebral column. The radiographic appearance of metastases may be *osteo-lytic* (bone destroying), *osteoblastic* (bone forming), or *mixed*. Some tumors, such as those arising in the prostate, typically produce osteoblastic lesions whereas others, such as renal, pulmonary, and gastrointestinal tumors, tend to give rise to lytic metastases.

JOINTS

Bones that form synovial joints are lined by hyaline cartilage, which functions as an elastic shock absorber and wear-resistant surface. The type II collagen in the articular cartilage resists tensile stress and transmits vertical loads. Unlike bone, cartilage has a limited capacity for repair. Consequently, processes that destroy cartilage (such as infection, inflammation, and trauma) usually lead to permanent damage.

Arthritis

The two main forms of arthritis differ in pathogenesis, morphology, and clinical features: osteoarthritis is an age-related degeneration of joint cartilage, whereas rheumatoid arthritis is an autoimmune disease that destroys cartilage.

Although both diseases present with joint pain and loss of mobility, their underlying biology is very different (Table 18.2). Together, they are major causes of morbidity and enormous burdens on the health care system. Most of our discussion focuses on these diseases. We also mention some related forms of arthritis and conclude with a brief consideration of gout.

Osteoarthritis

Osteoarthritis is caused by degeneration and disordered repair of articular cartilage in synovial joints, with superimposed inflammation.

Osteoarthritis is the most common disease of joints. Its incidence increases dramatically after the age of 50, and about 40% of individuals older than 70 are affected. Associated risk factors include obesity, female sex (possibly due to the association with osteoporosis), and occupations that place mechanical stresses on joints.

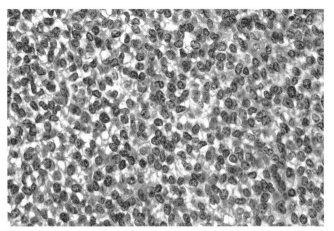

Fig. 18.7 Ewing sarcoma. The tumor is composed of sheets of small round cells with minimal amounts of clear cytoplasm.

Pathogenesis. Multiple factors contribute to the disease.

- *Degeneration of articular cartilage* resulting from repeated biomechanical stress is the likely initiating abnormality. Whether genetic polymorphisms contribute to the cartilage loss is unclear. The cartilage loss further increases biomechanical stress on the joint, leading to additional chondrocyte injury and inadequate production of type II collagen and proteoglycans.
- *Chronic, low-level inflammation* seems to be important in disease progression. Although inflammation is typically minimal in the joints when they are removed surgically (the end stage of the

disease), it is believed that cytokines such as interleukins (IL)-1 and IL-6 reduce proteoglycan production and increase its degradation, creating an imbalance that contributes to cartilage loss. Whether these cytokines are produced as a result of joint damage or are a cause remains unclear.

- *Genetic factors,* shown most clearly by twin studies documenting a high concordance rate among identical twins. The genes involved in pathogenesis are not defined.

Morphology. Initially, chondrocytes respond by proliferating, leading to the appearance of clusters of these cells. Eventually, the damage leads to fissuring of the articular surface and loss of pieces of cartilage and subchondral bone (forming "joint mice") (Fig. 18.8). This exposes the subchondral bone plate, damage of which causes small fractures and cysts and stimulates the outgrowth of bony protrusions (osteophytes). The synovium may show scattered inflammatory cells.

Clinical Features. Osteoarthritis usually develops after the age of 50 and mostly affects the weight-bearing synovial joints, including the knees, hips, and vertebral joints. For some reason, small joints of the hand and first tarsometatarsal joint are also affected. Prominent osteophytes at the distal interphalangeal joints, called Heberden nodes, are common in women. Patients present with joint pain and a progressive decrease in the range of movement. Compression of the spinal nerves may cause pain, spasm, muscle atrophy, and motor weakness. Treatment consists of antiinflammatory drugs and, in advanced cases, joint replacement.

Table 18.2 Comparative Features of Osteoarthritis and Rheumatoid Arthritis

	Osteoarthritis	Rheumatoid Arthritis
Primary pathogenic abnormality	Mechanical injury to articular cartilage	Autoimmunity
Role of inflammation	May be secondary; inflammatory mediators exacerbate cartilage damage	Primary: cartilage destruction is caused by T cells and antibodies reactive with joint antigens
Joints involved	Primarily weight bearing (knees, hips)	Often begins with small joints of fingers; progression leads to multiple joints involved
Pathology	Cartilage degeneration and fragmentation, bone spurs, subchondral cysts; minimal inflammation	Inflammatory pannus invading and destroying cartilage; severe chronic inflammation; joint fusion (ankylosis)
Serum antibodies	None	Various, including ACPA, rheumatoid factor
Involvement of other organs	No	Yes (lungs, heart, other organs)

ACPA, Anti–citrullinated peptide antibody.

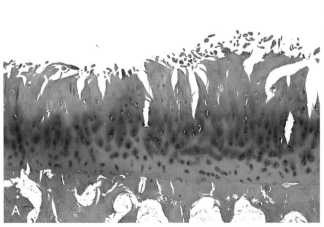
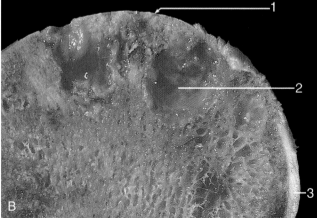

Fig. 18.8 Osteoarthritis. (A) Characteristic fibrillation of the articular cartilage. (B) Eburnated articular surface exposing subchondral bone (1), subchondral cyst (2), and residual articular cartilage (3).

Rheumatoid Arthritis

Rheumatoid arthritis is an autoimmune disease in which CD4+ T cells reactive with self antigens in the synovium induce destructive joint inflammation and antibodies reactive with joint antigens exacerbate the injury.

Rheumatoid arthritis (RA) is one of the most common autoimmune diseases, believed to affect 1% of the population.

Pathogenesis. As in other autoimmune diseases, the etiology is not known, but genetic and environmental factors are believed to contribute. The disease shows linkage to particular class II HLA alleles, and polymorphisms in many other genes have been identified by genome-wide association studies. Almost 70% of smokers who develop RA have serum antibodies specific for citrullinated peptides. One possibility is that in genetically susceptible individuals, smoking or oral infections lead to the posttranslational modification of arginine to citrulline in many self proteins, thus creating "neoantigens" that trigger immune responses. These antigens may be present in joints, so the result is joint inflammation. CD4+ Th1 and Th17 cells react with synovial antigens and produce cytokines that induce inflammation and cartilage destruction:

- *IFN-γ* from Th1 cells activates macrophages and synovial cells.
- *IL-17* from Th17 cells recruits neutrophils and monocytes.
- *RANKL* expressed on activated T cells stimulates osteoclasts and bone resorption.
- *TNF* and *IL-1* from macrophages stimulate resident synovial cells to secrete proteases that destroy hyaline cartilage.

Of various cytokines, tumor necrosis factor (TNF) seems to play a central role as evidenced by the beneficial effects of treatment with TNF antagonists. Antibodies produced by plasma cells in the synovium lead to further damage.

Morphology. The arthritis is symmetric and mainly affects the small joints of the hands and feet. The synovium is thickened and edematous, because of synovial cell hyperplasia and inflammatory infiltrate (Fig. 18.9). The inflammation consists of CD4+ helper T cells, B cells, macrophages, and other immune cells such as plasma cells, and sometimes germinal centers form in the synovium. A mass of edematous synovium and inflammatory cells, referred to as a *pannus*, grows over and erodes the articular cartilage. In advanced cases, the pannus can bridge the bones and fuse them (*ankylosis*), with ultimate ossification, completely destroying the joint space. Inflammation in the tendons, ligaments, and occasionally the adjacent skeletal muscle frequently accompanies the arthritis and produces the characteristic radial deviation of the wrist, ulnar deviation of the fingers, and flexion–hyperextension of the fingers (swan-neck deformity). Rheumatoid nodules are necrotizing granulomas that can be present in subcutaneous tissue (especially the forearm, elbows, occiput, and lumbosacral area) but also the heart, spleen, and other organs (Supplemental eFig. 18.10). Acute necrotizing vasculitis of small and large blood vessels can also occur.

Clinical Features. Symptoms usually develop in the hands (metacarpophalangeal and proximal interphalangeal joints) and feet, followed by the wrists, ankles, elbows, and knees. Involved joints are swollen, warm, painful, and particularly stiff when rising in the morning or following inactivity. Serum rheumatoid factor, an antibody that reacts with self IgG, is seen in about 80% of patients (but is not specific), and detection of serum anti-citrullinated peptide antibody (ACPA) is a diagnostic test. The elucidation of the pathogenic mechanisms has led to the development of novel therapies, such as antagonists of the inflammatory cytokine TNF (see Chapter 2) and antibodies that deplete B cells, which have dramatically altered the course of the disease. Long-term complications include *systemic amyloidosis* (see Chapter 4) in 5% to 10% of patients and infection with opportunistic organisms in patients who receive long-term anti-TNF or other immunosuppressive agents.

Other Forms of Arthritis

Features of some other important forms of arthritis are summarized in the following.

- *Juvenile idiopathic arthritis* (JIA) is similar to RA but occurs before the age of 16. In contrast to RA, in JIA (1) oligoarthritis is more common; (2) systemic disease is more frequent; (3) large joints are affected more often than small joints; (4) rheumatoid nodules and rheumatoid factor are usually absent; and (5) antinuclear antibody (ANA) seropositivity is common.
- *Ankylosing spondylitis* (AS) is one of the seronegative spondyloarthropathies that are characterized as a group by (1) the absence of rheumatoid factor; (2) pathologic changes in the ligamentous

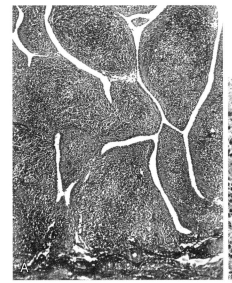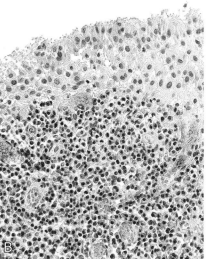

Fig. 18.9 Rheumatoid arthritis. (A) Low magnification shows marked synovial hypertrophy with formation of villi. (B) Higher magnification shows subsynovial tissue containing a dense infiltrate of lymphocytes and plasma cells.

attachments rather than the synovium; (3) the involvement of sacroiliac joints, with or without other joints; (4) association with HLA-B27; and (5) bony proliferation leading to ankylosis (fusion of joints). AS affects the vertebral column, especially the sacroiliac joints, and patients usually do not have serum autoantibodies, in particular rheumatoid factor. Approximately 90% of individuals are HLA-B27 positive.

- *Reactive arthritis* may follow infection with certain microbes such as *Chlamydia, Shigella, Yersinia,* and *Campylobacter* and is characterized by the triad of nongonococcal urethritis, conjunctivitis, and arthritis. It may be caused by an autoimmune reaction that is initiated by an infectious agent. It is also associated with HLA-B27.

- *Lyme arthritis* is the leading arthropod-borne disease in the United States and is caused by infection with the tick-borne spirochete *Borrelia burgdorferi.* The disease can affect the skin, heart, and meninges, in addition to the joints. The pathogenesis is not understood but is postulated to involve immune reactions against the infectious agent that cross-react with antigens in the joint. Lyme disease progresses through three phases and involves multiple organs.

  - The *early localized phase* is characterized by a skin rash at the site of the tick bite, which may spread to other sites and is known as erythema migrans.

  - In the *early disseminated phase,* spirochetes spread via the blood and inflammatory lesions are seen in the skin, cranial nerves, meninges, and heart.

  - The *late phase* manifests as arthritis affecting large joints, especially the knees. Rare cases develop neurologic problems, including encephalopathy and polyneuropathy. Spirochetes are not detectable in the joints, suggesting that the arthritis is caused by an immune response and not the infection itself. The synovium shows synoviocyte hyperplasia, an infiltrate of CD4+ T cells, and thickening of vessel walls.

  The disease usually responds well to antibiotic treatment.

- *Septic (infectious) arthritis* is infection of the joints most often by pyogenic bacteria. *S. aureus* is the main agent in older children and adults, and gonococcus is prevalent during late adolescence and young adulthood. The infection may be acquired hematogenously, by direct extension from another infectious focus, or by inoculation through the skin. The classic presentation is the abrupt onset of joint pain and swelling, with systemic signs of acute inflammation. In the vast majority of cases, the infection involves only a single joint, most commonly the knee, followed in decreasing frequency by the hip, shoulder, elbow, wrist, and sternoclavicular joints. The axial joints are more often involved in drug users. Joint aspiration is diagnostic if it yields purulent fluid in which the causative agent can be identified. Because cartilage has a limited repair potential, early detection and antibiotic treatment are necessary to prevent permanent joint damage.

Gout

Gout is an inflammatory arthritis caused by a reaction to urate crystals deposited in joints.

Pathogenesis. Gout may be primary (idiopathic, ~90% cases) or secondary to disorders associated with extensive cell death, as may occur in cancer patients undergoing chemotherapy. Uric acid is the end product of catabolism of purine nucleotides; therefore, its levels increase when cell death and DNA breakdown increase. Uric acid, regardless of its source, is filtered through the glomerulus, and most of it is reabsorbed in tubules. In primary gout, plasma uric acid levels are increased, probably because of reduced excretion, for unknown reasons, rather than increased production. The uric acid is converted to monosodium urate, and when the concentration of urate exceeds its saturation point, it forms crystals that deposit in joints and other soft tissues. Because most individuals with hyperuricemia do not form crystals, there may be other, as yet unknown, factors that predispose to crystal deposition. The crystals are

phagocytosed by neutrophils and macrophages; in macrophages, urate activates the inflammasome, leading to release of the proinflammatory cytokine IL-1 and the influx of more leukocytes (see Chapter 2). Crystals also may damage lysosomal membranes of the phagocytes, leading to the release of lysosomal enzymes and other mediators. The net result is acute inflammation at the site of urate deposition.

> *Morphology.* In acute gouty arthritis, there is severe acute inflammation in the synovium with urate crystals in the fluid and inside neutrophils. Repeated attacks may lead to deposits of urate which evoke an inflammatory response, forming nodules called *tophi* (Fig. 18.10).

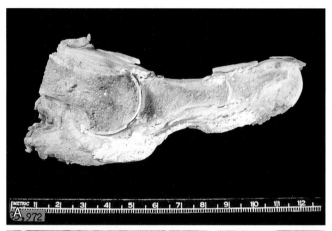

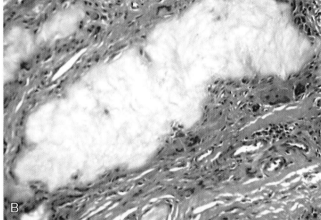

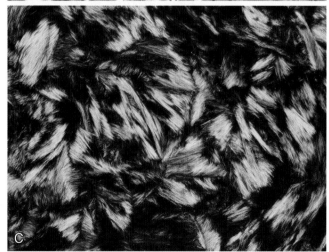

Fig. 18.10 Gout. (A) Amputated great toe with white tophi involving the joint and soft tissues. (B) Gouty tophus: An aggregate of dissolved urate crystals is surrounded by reactive fibroblasts, mononuclear inflammatory cells, and giant cells. (C) Urate crystals are needle shaped and negatively birefringent under polarized light.

Tophi consist of amorphous deposits of urate crystals surrounded by mononuclear cells and foreign body giant cells. Tophi may deposit in the articular cartilage, ligaments, tendons, and renal medulla. Uric acid stones in the kidneys predispose to pyelonephritis.

Clinical Features. Gout is associated with male sex, obesity, metabolic syndrome, certain drugs (e.g., thiazides), and excess alcohol intake. Most affected individuals are older than 30 years. Acute arthritis is typically monoarticular; it presents with a sudden onset of excruciating pain and redness in a joint, most commonly (for unclear reasons) the first metatarsophalangeal joint of the big toe. The acute attack usually subsides but frequently recurs. Acute attacks are treated with antiinflammatory drugs, and the risk of recurrence is lowered by inhibitors of urate synthesis. Chronic tophaceous gout usually takes more than 10 years to develop after the initial attack.

Calcium Pyrophosphate Crystal Deposition Disease

Calcium pyrophosphate deposition disease, also known as *pseudogout*, arises in individuals over 50 years old. Though frequently asymptomatic, it may produce acute, subacute, or chronic arthritis. Crystals appear in the articular cartilage, menisci, and intervertebral discs; large deposits may rupture and seed the joint (Supplemental eFig. 18.11). The knee is the most commonly affected joint, followed by the wrists, elbows, and shoulders. Ultimately, approximately 50% of affected individuals experience significant joint damage. Its pathogenesis is not clear. It is thought that articular cartilage proteoglycans, which normally inhibit crystallization, are degraded, allowing calcium pyrophosphate crystals to form around chondrocytes. The crystals trigger inflammation presumably by inflammasome activation.

SKELETAL MUSCLE

In response to inputs from the central nervous system, skeletal muscles generate the force needed for both purposeful and involuntary movements. These inputs are organized into motor units composed of a lower motor neuron, its associated axon, the neuromuscular junction, and the muscle fibers innervated by that axon. Diseases of muscle may be primary, or secondary to nerve defects that disrupt the motor unit. Here we discuss primary myopathies; diseases of peripheral nerves that affect muscles are discussed in Chapter 17.

Muscular Dystrophies

Congenital diseases of muscle, called muscular dystrophies or myopathies, are caused by mutations in a variety of nuclear and mitochondrial genes, and present with involuntary contractions (myotonia) or weakness progressing to paralysis. In some of these disorders, the abnormalities are present almost from birth, whereas in others, the muscles are normal at birth and the disorder develops over time. Only the most common of these rare diseases are described here.

Duchenne Muscular Dystrophy and Becker Muscular Dystrophy

These are X-linked diseases caused by mutations that disrupt the function of the structural protein dystrophin.

Duchenne muscular dystrophy and Becker muscular dystrophy are, therefore, collectively called *dystrophinopathies;* they are the most common forms of muscular dystrophy, with an incidence of 1 in about 3500 births.

Pathogenesis. Dystrophin is a large cytoplasmic protein found in skeletal and cardiac muscle, the brain, and the nerves. In muscle cells, it tethers the cytoskeleton to a complex of several membrane proteins that binds to the extracellular matrix. This complex stabilizes the muscle cell during contraction and also may be involved in signaling. Mutations of the *dystrophin* gene, which is located on the X chromosome, disrupt this complex, leading to signaling defects and making muscle cells vulnerable to transient membrane tears during contraction. Duchenne muscular dystrophy is associated

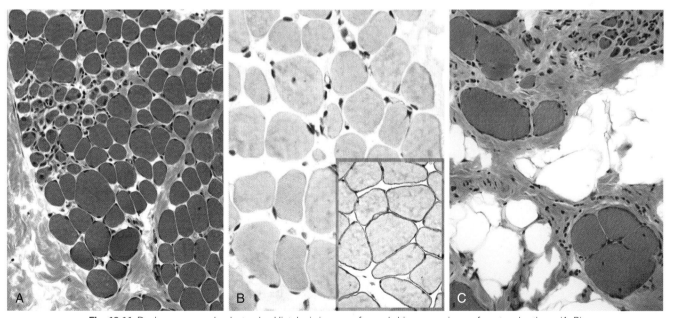

Fig. 18.11 Duchenne muscular dystrophy. Histologic images of muscle biopsy specimens from two brothers. (A–B) Specimens from a 3-year-old boy. (C) Specimen from his brother, 9 years of age. As seen in (A), at a younger age the fascicular muscle architecture is maintained, but myofibers show a variation in size. Additionally, there is a cluster of basophilic regenerating myofibers *(left side)* and slight endomysial fibrosis, seen as focal pink-staining connective tissue between myofibers. In (B), immunohistochemical staining shows a complete absence of membrane-associated dystrophin, seen as a brown stain in normal muscle *(inset)*. In (C), the biopsy from the older brother illustrates disease progression, which is marked by extensive variation in myofiber size, fatty replacement, and endomysial fibrosis.

with earlier and more severe manifestations than Becker muscular dystrophy, because in the former the causative mutations lead to the complete absence of the protein, whereas in the latter the mutations are such that they permit production of some functional dystrophin. The presence and type of dystrophin mutation can be confirmed by genetic studies.

> **Morphology.** The histologic changes in skeletal muscle are dominated by myofiber necrosis, leading to the progressive replacement of muscle by fibrous and adipose tissue (Fig. 18.11). There is also ongoing ineffectual muscle fiber regeneration, leading to the existence of fibers that vary in size and contain abnormally located nuclei. Cardiac muscle also may be affected.

Clinical Features. Boys with Duchenne muscular dystrophy present with progressive muscle weakness, usually between the ages of 3 and 5, often manifested by clumsiness and gait difficulties. The weakness usually starts in the pelvic girdle and then affects the shoulders. Muscles in the calf and other sites may appear to be enlarged, because of compensatory hypertrophy initially and replacement by fat and fibrous tissue as the disease progresses. Serum creatine kinase is markedly elevated during the first decade of life due to ongoing muscle damage, and then falls as the disease progresses and muscle mass is lost. Cardiac muscle damage may lead to heart failure and arrhythmias. Death results from respiratory and cardiac failure, often complicated by pneumonias. Becker muscular dystrophy becomes symptomatic later in childhood or adolescence and progresses more slowly and variably; life expectancy may be nearly normal. Cardiac involvement may be the dominant feature, sometimes in the absence of skeletal muscle weakness.

Myositis

These inflammatory myopathies are a heterogeneous group of diseases with diverse, and often poorly understood, underlying mechanisms.

Three principal forms of myositis are recognized, which may be distinguished based on morphology and have distinct clinical presentations.

- *Polymyositis* is an autoimmune disease in which CD8+ cytotoxic T lymphocytes attack and kill muscle cells. The specificity of the autoimmune reaction is undefined. The muscle shows myofiber

necrosis and regeneration (Fig. 18.12A). Of note, many cases that were called polymyositis in the past are now being reclassified as *immune-mediated necrotizing myopathy,* which shows sparse inflammation and some evidence of an immune mechanism, or as inclusion-body myositis (discussed below). Therefore, whether polymyositis is truly a distinct entity is uncertain.

- *Dermatomyositis* is the most common inflammatory myopathy in children, and may occur as a paraneoplastic disorder in adults. It is believed to be an autoimmune disorder; some patients have autoantibodies of particular specificities. It is associated with damage to small blood vessels with secondary injury to muscles and skin. Myofiber damage is prominent in the paraseptal or perifascicular regions, and may be accompanied by a mononuclear cell infiltrate (Fig. 18.12B). There is skin involvement in the form of a rash (Supplemental eFig. 18.12). Some cases have systemic manifestations such as pulmonary fibrosis.
- *Inclusion body myositis* is the most common inflammatory myopathy in individuals over 60 years old. Its morphologic hallmark is the presence of rimmed vacuoles (Fig. 18.12C) that contain aggregates of the same proteins that accumulate in the brains of patients with neurodegenerative diseases, such as beta-amyloid and Tau (see Chapter 17). Whether the inflammation seen in muscle is the cause or effect of the myofiber injury is not known.

Muscle injury also occurs as an idiosyncratic reaction to drugs or because of alcohol toxicity. Statins are the most significant cause of drug-induced myositis and rhabdomyolysis due to their widespread use. Almost 1.5% of patients receiving statin therapy develop muscle injury, which can be severe enough to require hospitalization.

Tumors of Muscle and Soft Tissue

The tumors of connective tissue and muscle are a diverse group of rare entities, including malignancies that are referred to as *sarcomas.* Their cellular origins are poorly understood, and precursor lesions have not been identified. Microscopically, they may produce recognizable types of tissue, such as muscle, or they may be poorly differentiated. We consider them here as a group because they share many features.

Pathogenesis. These tumors may arise from pluripotent mesenchymal stem cells. Most sarcomas in adults are genomically unstable and have complex chromosomal aberrations that produce aneuploidy and

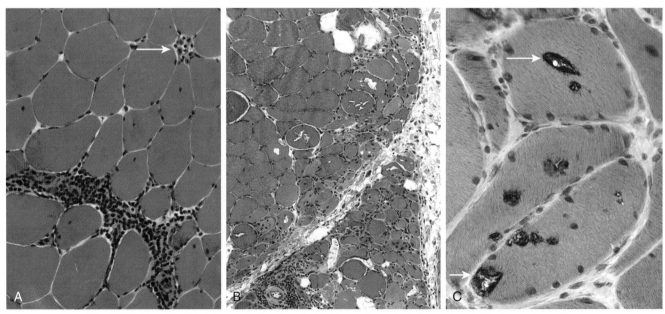

Fig. 18.12 Myositis. (A) Polymyositis is characterized by endomysial inflammatory infiltrates and myofiber necrosis *(arrow).* (B) Dermatomyositis often shows prominent perifascicular and paraseptal atrophy. (C) Inclusion body myositis, showing myofibers containing rimmed vacuoles *(arrows).* Modified Gomori trichrome stain.

Table 18.3 Tumors of Muscle and Soft Tissue

Tumor (Cell Type)	Morphology	Clinical Presentation	Unique Features
Benign Tumors			
Leiomyoma (smooth muscle)	Spindle cells in fascicles	Most common in uterus (Chapter 15)	
Lipoma (adipose cells)	Well-encapsulated collections of mature adipocytes	Most common soft tissue tumor in adults; painless mass that may be large	
Nodular fasciitis (fibroblasts)	Proliferation of mature fibroblasts	In deep dermis, sometimes at site of trauma; may regress spontaneously	Contains fusion of *USP6* gene to a myosin gene
Superficial fibromatosis (fibroblasts)	Locally infiltrating proliferation of fibroblasts	May cause local deformity; benign course; may be palmar, plantar, or penile	
Deep fibromatosis (fibroblasts); also called *desmoid tumor*	Locally infiltrating masses of proliferating fibroblasts	Mass may recur after excision, not metastatic	Mutations of *CTNNB1* (beta catenin) or *APC* gene
Malignant Tumors (Sarcomas)			
Rhabdomyosarcoma (skeletal muscle)	*Embryonal:* various stages of maturation *Alveolar:* clusters of cells separated by fibrous septae *Pleomorphic:* anaplastic cells	Local mass; may spread to distant sites; most common soft tissue sarcoma of children and adolescents	Alveolar type contains fusions of *FOXO1* to *PAX* genes
Liposarcoma (adipose cells)	May be well-differentiated, myxoid (abundant extracellular matrix) or pleomorphic	Local mass, may spread; most common sarcoma of adults	Well-differentiated: amplification of *MDM2* gene (encodes inhibitor of p53) Myxoid: t(12;16) translocation; encodes a fusion protein that inhibits adipose differentiation
Synovial sarcoma (unknown; not synovial cells)	Spindle cells growing in fascicles may contain epithelial-like component or glands	Local mass, may metastasize	t(X;18) translocation; creates a fusion gene (*SS18-SSX*) which encodes a chromatin regulator that disrupts cell cycle control

polyploidy, and others have specific, often diagnostically useful, chromosomal translocations that create oncogenic fusion genes. As a rule, soft tissue sarcomas are resistant to chemotherapy and are only curable when complete surgical resection is possible.

The features of the most common benign and malignant tumors of muscle and soft tissue are summarized in Table 18.3.

SKIN

Skin diseases are common and diverse. Many are intrinsic to the skin, but some are manifestations of diseases involving many tissues, such as systemic lupus erythematosus, or genetic syndromes such as neurofibromatosis. Here, we discuss several common and pathogenically illustrative inflammatory, immunologic, and neoplastic skin diseases.

Acute Inflammatory Dermatoses

The skin is exposed to a large number of potentially irritating or antigenic environmental agents, which frequently cause inflammatory reactions. In other instances, the source of the reaction is a circulating antigen or immune complexes that deposit in the skin. In general, acute inflammatory dermatoses are characterized by varying degrees of edema and leukocytic infiltrate, sometimes accompanied by epidermal, vascular, or subcutaneous injury. Some acute dermatoses persist, transitioning to a chronic phase, whereas others are self-limited.

Acute Eczematous Dermatitis

Eczema (meaning, to boil) refers to a group of acute dermatoses with diverse underlying etiologies that share a similar morphologic appearance. The causes of eczema can be divided into "inside jobs," or reactions to an internal circulating antigen (such as from ingested food or drug), and "outside jobs", diseases resulting from contact with an external antigen (such as poison ivy). There are several subtypes:

- *Allergic contact dermatitis* is the most common form of eczema. It stems from topical exposure to an allergen that leads to a T cell–mediated delayed hypersensitivity reaction. ("Allergic" in the name implies immediate hypersensitivity but is actually a misnomer.) A classic trigger is urushiol, a chemical found in poison ivy that reacts with self proteins to form neoantigens that are recognized by T cells. Reexposure to poison ivy activates memory T cells in the skin, which release cytokines, producing the classic itchy rash.
- *Atopic dermatitis* is thought to stem from inherited defects in keratinocyte barrier function, causing increased permeability to substances such as potential antigens, which elicit a Th2 reaction typical of allergy. It usually appears in early childhood and often remits spontaneously as patients mature into adults. Because it is caused by an intrinsic defect in barrier function, it is the only form that may cause persistent, chronic eczematous dermatitis.
- *Drug-related eczematous dermatitis* stems from a hypersensitivity reaction to a drug.
- *Photoeczematous dermatitis* is an abnormal reaction to UV or visible light.
- *Primary irritant dermatitis*, also called *irritant contact dermatitis*, results from exposure to substances that chemically, physically, or mechanically damage the skin, without evidence of a hypersensitivity reaction.

Morphology. Contact dermatitis is limited to sites of direct contact with the triggering agent (Fig. 18.13A), whereas in other forms of eczema, lesions may be widely distributed. Epidermal edema (*spongiosis*) characterizes all forms and often is severe enough to splay apart keratinocytes and produce vesicles (Fig. 18.13B). There typically are perivascular lymphocytic infiltrates, sometimes accompanied by eosinophils, and edema of the dermal papillae.

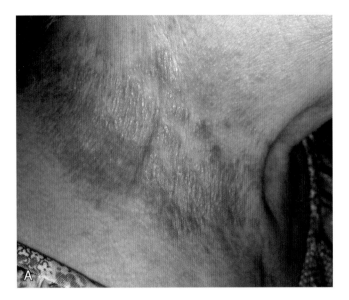

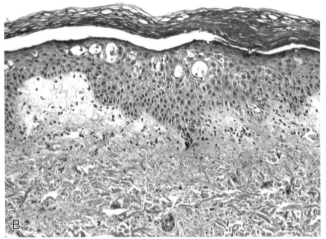

Fig. 18.13 Eczematous dermatitis. (A) Patterned erythema and scale stemming from a nickel-induced contact dermatitis produced by a necklace. (B) Microscopically, there is accumulation of fluid (spongiosis) between epidermal cells, which may progress to frank blister formation.

Clinical Features. New lesions take the form of erythematous papules, often with overlying vesicles, which ooze and become crusted. Pruritus is characteristic. With persistence, these lesions coalesce into raised, scaling plaques. Treatment consists of avoidance of triggering agents and antiinflammatory drugs such as steroids given topically or systemically.

Erythema Multiforme

Erythema multiforme is characterized by epithelial injury mediated by skin-homing CD8+ cytotoxic T lymphocytes. It is an uncommon, usually self-limited, disorder that appears to be a hypersensitivity reaction to certain infections and drugs, including sulfonamides, penicillin, and salicylates. Affected individuals present with a wide array of lesions, which may include macules, papules, vesicles, and bullae (hence the term *multiforme*). Erythema multiforme caused by medications may progress to more serious eruptions, such as Stevens-Johnson syndrome or toxic epidermal necrolysis, which can be life-threatening because of sloughing of large portions of the epidermis.

Chronic Inflammatory Dermatoses

Chronic inflammatory dermatoses are skin conditions that develop and persist over many months to years; sometimes, they begin with an acute stage.

The skin surface in some chronic inflammatory dermatoses is roughened as a result of excessive or abnormal hyperkeratosis (scale formation) and shedding of squamous cells.

Psoriasis

Psoriasis is a common chronic inflammatory skin disease, affecting 1% to 2% of individuals in the United States. In up to 10% of patients, it is associated with arthritis, which may be severe.

Pathogenesis. The pathogenesis of psoriasis is incompletely understood, but it involves an immune stimulus that results in the homing of activated T cells to the dermis, where they release cytokines that recruit neutrophils and stimulate the hyperproliferation of overlying keratinocytes. IL-17 produced by Th17 cells plays a central role, as shown by the therapeutic efficacy of agents that block the development of these cells or the actions of IL-17. It is unclear whether the inciting antigens are self antigens or environmental antigens, or some combination of the two. Psoriatic lesions can be induced in susceptible individuals by local trauma, which may induce an inflammatory response that promotes lesion development.

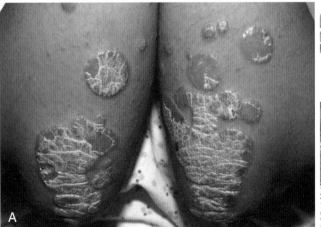

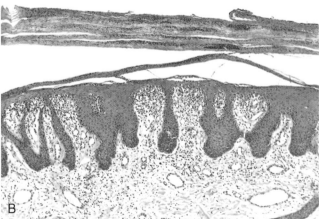

Fig. 18.14 Psoriasis. (A) Erythematous psoriatic plaques covered by silvery-white scale. (B) Microscopic examination shows marked epidermal hyperplasia, downward extension of rete ridges (psoriasiform hyperplasia), and prominent parakeratotic scale with infiltrating neutrophils.

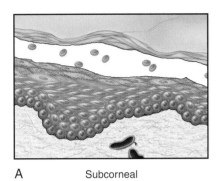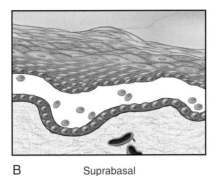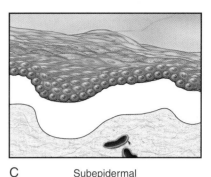

Fig. 18.15 Levels of blister formation. (A) Subcorneal (as in pemphigus foliaceus). (B) Suprabasal (as in pemphigus vulgaris). (C) Subepidermal (as in bullous pemphigoid or dermatitis herpetiformis).

A Subcorneal	B Suprabasal	C Subepidermal

Morphology. Psoriasis most frequently affects the skin of the elbows, knees, scalp, lumbosacral areas, intergluteal cleft, glans penis, and vulva. The typical lesion is a well-demarcated, pink to salmon–colored plaque covered by loosely adherent silver-white scale (Fig. 18.14A). There is epidermal thickening (acanthosis) and downward elongation of the rete ridges (Fig. 18.14B), producing a pattern likened to "test tubes in a rack." Increased epidermal cell turnover and lack of maturation result in loss of the stratum granulosum and extensive parakeratotic scale (retention of nuclei in stratum corneum). The epidermal cell layer is thinned overlying the tips of the dermal papillae, and dilated and tortuous blood vessels are present within the papillae. These vessels bleed readily when the scale is removed, giving rise to punctate bleeding points. Neutrophils are present in small aggregates within the superficial epidermis and the stratum corneum.

Clinical Features. In most cases, psoriasis is limited in distribution, but it can be widespread and severe. Treatment is aimed at preventing the release or actions of inflammatory mediators. Therapy includes topical corticosteroids; antibodies that block the actions of IL-17, TNF, and other cytokines; and phototherapy (which has immunosuppressive effects).

Blistering (Bullous) Disorders

Although vesicles and bullae (blisters) occur as secondary phenomena in several conditions (e.g., herpesvirus infection), there is a group of disorders in which blisters are the primary and most distinctive feature. Blistering tends to occur at specific levels within the skin in different diseases and is a helpful diagnostic feature (Fig. 18.15).

Pemphigus (Vulgaris and Foliaceus)

Pemphigus is an autoimmune blistering disorder resulting from loss of normal intercellular attachments within the epidermis and the squamous mucosal epithelium.

Pathogenesis. Pemphigus is caused by antibody-mediated (type II) hypersensitivity reactions (see Chapter 4). The pathogenic antibodies are IgG autoantibodies that bind to intercellular desmosomal proteins (desmoglein types 1 and 3) found in the skin and mucous membranes. The antibodies disrupt the adhesive function of desmosomes and may also activate proteases that further loosen intercellular connections.

Morphology. Two major variants are recognized. *Pemphigus vulgaris* involves both mucosa and skin and produces lesions consisting of flaccid vesicles and bullae that rupture easily, leaving erosions covered with a serum crust. By direct immunofluorescence study, lesional sites show a fishnet-like pattern

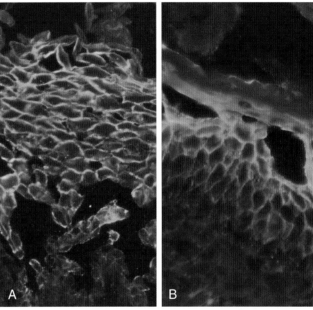

Fig. 18.16 Pemphigus: Immunofluorescence findings. (A) Pemphigus vulgaris. Note the uniform deposition of immunoglobulin *(green)* along keratinocyte cell membranes in a characteristic "fishnet" pattern. (B) Pemphigus foliaceus. Immunoglobulin deposits are confined to superficial layers of the epidermis.

of intercellular IgG deposits (Fig. 18.16). *Pemphigus foliaceus,* a less common, milder form, results in bullae that are mainly confined to the skin and produces blisters that are superficial and less likely to produce extensive erosions. The common feature in both forms is *acantholysis,* lysis of the intercellular adhesive junctions between neighboring squamous epithelial cells that results in the rounding up of the detached cells. In pemphigus vulgaris, the acantholysis selectively involves the layer of cells immediately above the basal cell layer (Fig. 18.17A), whereas in pemphigus foliaceus, acantholysis involves the superficial epidermis at the level of the stratum granulosum (Fig. 18.17B).

Clinical Features. Pemphigus vulgaris occurs more frequently in older adults, more commonly in women. Lesions are painful, particularly when ruptured, and frequently develop secondary infections. Most affected patients at some point have oropharyngeal involvement, which may be so severe as to interfere with eating. The mainstay of treatment is immunosuppressive therapy, sometimes for life. Pemphigus foliaceous is a mild form of the disease.

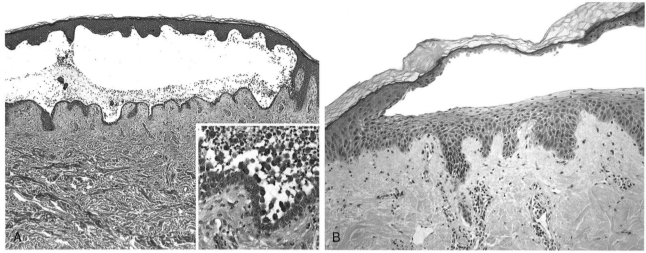

Fig. 18.17 Pemphigus. (A) Pemphigus vulgaris. Suprabasal intraepidermal blister in which rounded, dissociated (acantholytic) keratinocytes are plentiful *(inset)*. (B) Pemphigus foliaceus. Microscopic appearance of a characteristic subcorneal blister.

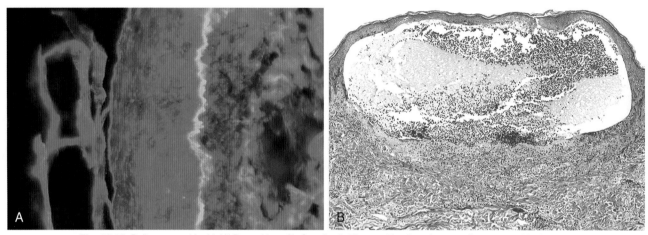

Fig. 18.18 Bullous pemphigoid. (A) Deposition of IgG antibody (detected by direct immunofluorescence) in the subepidermal basement membrane (epidermis is on the left side of the fluorescent band). (B) Subepidermal vesicle with an eosinophil-rich inflammatory infiltrate. (B, Courtesy Dr. Victor G. Prieto, MD Anderson Cancer Center, Houston.)

Bullous Pemphigoid

Bullous pemphigoid is an autoimmune blistering disorder caused by loss of anchoring interactions between the epidermis and the underlying basement membrane.

Pathogenesis. In bullous pemphigoid, blistering is caused by the linear deposition of autoreactive IgG antibodies and complement in the epidermal basement membrane and attachment plaques (hemidesmosomes) (Fig. 18.18A), where the target antigen (usually type XVII collagen) is located. IgG autoantibodies to hemidesmosome components fix complement and recruit neutrophils and eosinophils, which release proteases that may contribute to loosening of anchoring interactions.

> *Morphology.* Early lesions of bullous pemphigoid show variable numbers of eosinophils at the dermal-epidermal junction, occasional neutrophils, superficial dermal edema, and associated basal cell layer vacuolization. The vacuolated basal cell layer eventually gives rise to a fluid-filled blister (Fig. 18.18B).

Clinical Features. The lesions of bullous pemphigoid do not rupture as readily as in pemphigus and, if uncomplicated by infection, heal without scarring. The disease tends to follow a remitting and relapsing course and responds to topical or systemic immunosuppressive agents.

Dermatitis Herpetiformis

Dermatitis herpetiformis is an autoimmune blistering disorder associated with gluten sensitivity (in about 80% of cases) and celiac disease (Chapter 12) that is characterized by extremely pruritic, grouped vesicles and papules. The disease affects predominantly males, often in the third and fourth decades of life. Genetically predisposed individuals develop IgA antibodies to dietary gluten (derived from the wheat protein gliadin), as well as IgA autoantibodies that cross-react with endomysium and tissue transglutaminases, including epidermal transglutaminase expressed by keratinocytes. By direct immunofluorescence, the skin shows discontinuous, granular deposits of IgA selectively localized in the tips of dermal papillae (Supplemental eFig. 18.13). The resultant injury and inflammation produce a subepidermal blister.

Tumors

Squamous Cell Carcinoma

Squamous cell carcinoma is a common tumor that typically arises on sun-exposed sites in fair-skinned, older adults.

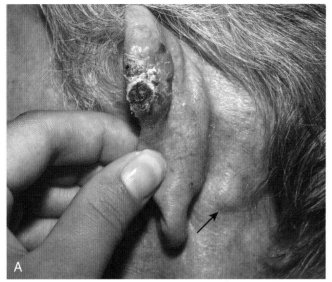

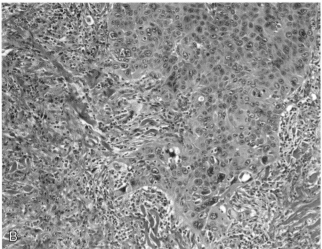

Fig. 18.19 Squamous cell carcinoma. (A) A nodular, hyperkeratotic lesion occurring on the ear, associated with metastasis to a prominent postauricular lymph node *(arrow)*. (B) Tumor invades the dermal soft tissue as irregular projections of atypical squamous cells.

Pathogenesis. **Cutaneous squamous cell carcinoma is mainly caused by UV light exposure and is associated with widespread DNA damage in keratinocytes.**

Patients with the rare disorder *xeroderma pigmentosum,* which disrupts repair of UV-induced DNA damage, develop multiple squamous cell carcinomas early in life. *TP53* mutations are common, as are mutations in Notch genes. Immunosuppression, particularly in organ transplant recipients, is associated with an increased incidence of cutaneous squamous cell carcinomas; a role for HPV infection in the setting of immunosuppression is suspected but not established.

Morphology. Early squamous cell carcinomas appear as sharply defined, red, scaling plaques. More advanced, invasive squamous cell carcinomas are nodular, often scaly lesions that may ulcerate (Fig. 18.19A). The tumors show variable degrees of differentiation (Fig. 18.19B).

Clinical Features. Invasive squamous cell carcinomas of the skin usually are discovered while small and resectable. Less than 1% will have metastasized to regional lymph nodes at diagnosis. The likelihood of metastasis is related to the thickness of the lesion and degree of invasion into the subcutis.

Basal Cell Carcinoma

Basal cell carcinoma is a common, slow-growing cancer that rarely metastasizes.

It tends to occur at sites subject to chronic sun exposure in lightly pigmented individuals.

Pathogenesis. Basal cell carcinomas are often associated with mutations that inactivate the tumor suppressor *PTCH1,* leading to excessive activity of the Hedgehog signaling pathway, which drives transformation. The central role of Hedgehog signaling in this tumor is emphasized by Gorlin syndrome, an autosomal dominant disorder caused by inherited defects in *PTCH1* that is associated with familial basal cell carcinoma. Mutations in *TP53* caused by UV light–induced damage also are common in both familial and sporadic tumors.

Morphology. Basal cell carcinomas manifest as pearly papules, often with prominent, dilated subepidermal blood vessels (telangiectasia) (Fig. 18.20A). The tumor cells grow downward from the epidermis into the dermis as cords and islands of basophilic cells with hyperchromatic nuclei (Fig. 18.20B). Peripheral tumor cell nuclei align (palisade) in the outermost layer, which often separates from the stroma, creating a characteristic cleft.

Clinical Features. More than 1 million basal cell carcinomas are treated in the United States annually. The most important risk factor is cumulative sun exposure. Individual tumors usually are cured by local excision, but approximately 40% of patients develop another basal cell carcinoma within 5 years. Advanced lesions may ulcerate, and extensive local invasion of bone or facial sinuses may occur if the lesions are neglected. Metastasis is exceedingly rare.

Melanoma

Melanoma is less common but much more deadly than basal or squamous cell carcinoma. Because of public awareness of the earliest signs of skin melanomas, most melanomas are cured surgically. Nonetheless, the incidence of these lesions has increased dramatically over the past several decades, at least in part as a result of increasing sun exposure.

Pathogenesis. **Melanoma is usually caused by UV light–induced mutations involving a characteristic set of cancer genes.**

Intense intermittent exposure to sunlight in fair-skinned people at an early age is particularly harmful. Hereditary predisposition also plays a role in an estimated 5% to 10% of cases. Early lesions tend to spread within the epidermis (radial growth), but with disease progression, a vertical growth phase supervenes. This event often is heralded by the development of a nodule in a previously flat lesion and correlates with the emergence of metastatic potential. DNA sequencing studies have shown that melanomas frequently have mutations involving tumor suppressor genes that regulate the cell cycle, cell growth, and apoptosis (e.g., *TP53*); in oncogenes that drive growth (e.g., *RAS* and components of the MAP-kinase [MAPK] pathway); and in telomerase. Activating mutations in *BRAF,* a serine/threonine kinase that is downstream of RAS in the MAPK pathway, are seen in 40% to 50% of melanomas, whereas activating mutations in *RAS* occur in an additional 15% to 20% of tumors. Melanomas with *BRAF* mutations also often show loss of the PTEN tumor suppressor, leading to heightened activation of the PI3K/AKT pathway. PTEN is also silenced in 20% of melanomas arising at sites that have not been exposed to the sun.

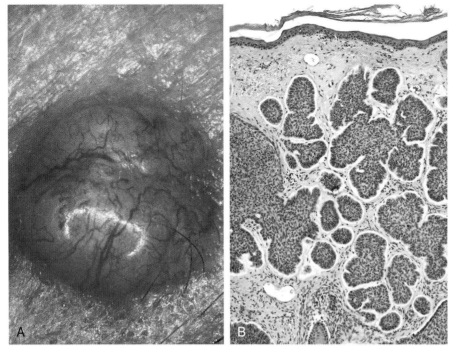

Fig. 18.20 Basal cell carcinoma. (A) A prototypical pearly, smooth-surfaced papule with telangiectatic vessels. (B) Tumor is composed of nests of basaloid cells infiltrating a fibrotic stroma.

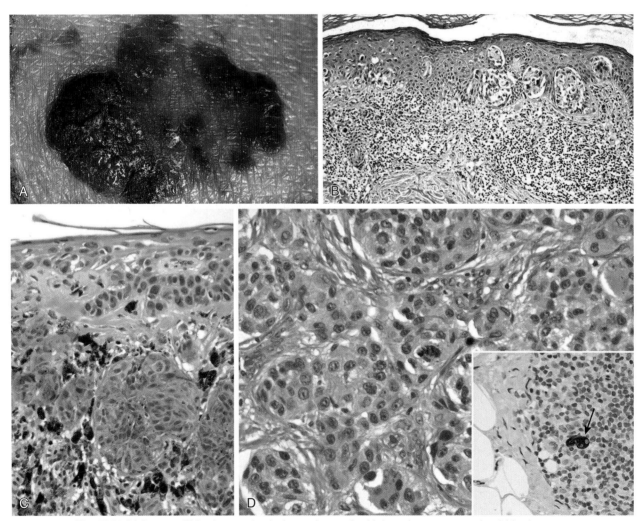

Fig. 18.21 Melanoma. (A) Lesions tend to be larger than nevi, with irregular contours and variable pigmentation. Macular areas indicate superficial (radial) growth, whereas elevated areas indicate dermal invasion (vertical growth). (B) Radial growth phase, with spread of nested and single melanoma cells within the epidermis. (C) Vertical growth phase, with nodular aggregates of infiltrating tumor cells within the dermis. (D) Melanoma cells with hyperchromatic irregular nuclei of varying size that have prominent nucleoli. An atypical mitotic figure is present in the center of the field. The *inset* shows a sentinel lymph node containing a tiny cluster of metastatic melanoma *(arrow)*, detected by staining for the melanocytic marker HMB-45.

Morphology. Unlike benign moles (nevi), melanomas often exhibit striking variations in pigmentation, including shades of black, brown, red, dark blue, and gray (Fig. 18.21A). The borders are irregular and often "notched." Microscopically, malignant cells grow as poorly formed nests or as individual cells at all levels of the epidermis (pagetoid spread) and in expansile dermal nodules (Fig. 18.21B,C). Melanoma cells usually have large nuclei, prominent "cherry red" eosinophilic nucleoli, and variable amounts of melanin granules (Fig. 18.21D).

Clinical Features. Melanoma of the skin usually is asymptomatic. The most important clinical sign is a change in the color or size of a pigmented lesion. These principles are expressed in the so-called "ABCs" of melanoma: *a*symmetry, *b*order, *c*olor, *d*iameter, and *e*volution (change of an existing mole). It is vitally important to recognize melanomas and intervene as rapidly as possible, because superficial lesions are usually cured by simple excision. The probability of metastasis is predicted by the thickness of the lesion and its mitotic rate. When metastases occur, they most often involve a sentinel lymph node, but on occasion, they may appear virtually anywhere in the body.

Once melanoma spreads, there are two main treatment strategies. Tumors with activating *BRAF* mutations often respond to BRAF inhibitors. Furthermore, melanomas are highly antigenic, due to the presence of UV light-induced passenger mutations in coding sequences of genes that create tumor neoantigens. As a result, melanomas often respond to immune checkpoint inhibitors, antibodies that release the brakes on cytotoxic T cell responses (see Chapter 5), leading to tumor killing. Current efforts are focused on building upon these successes by using combinations of different checkpoint inhibitors, as well as checkpoint inhibitors together with targeted therapies such as BRAF inhibitors.

19

Environmental Disease

OUTLINE

Metals as Environmental Pollutants, 314
    Lead, 314
    Mercury, 315
Tobacco, 315
Alcohol, 316
Injury by Therapeutic Drugs and Drugs of Abuse, 317
    Injury by Therapeutic Drugs: Adverse Drug Reactions, 317
    Injury by Drugs of Abuse, 318

Injury Produced by Ionizing Radiation, 318
    Acute and Chronic Effects of Radiation on Organ
      Systems, 319
Nutritional Diseases, 319
    Malnutrition, 319
    Vitamin Deficiencies, 321
    Obesity, 323

Many diseases are caused or influenced by factors in the environment, which can be defined broadly as the various outdoor, indoor, and occupational settings in which humans live and work. Exposure to some potentially dangerous environmental factors is largely determined by public health measures, including the existence (or absence) of governmental laws that ensure water and air quality and provide protections from physical dangers and toxins in the workplace and elsewhere in the community. Other environmental exposures are a matter of personal choice, including tobacco use, alcohol ingestion, "recreational" drug consumption, diet, exercise, and the like. Such threats are likely to become more pronounced over the coming decades as climate change alters weather patterns, sea levels, food production, and the distribution of infectious diseases. In this chapter, we will focus on some of the environmental factors that currently have the greatest impact on human health.

METALS AS ENVIRONMENTAL POLLUTANTS

Lead, mercury, arsenic, and cadmium are heavy metals commonly associated with harmful effects in human populations. Of these, lead exposure is preeminent as a cause of human disease and mercury exposure is an important consideration for pregnant women.

Lead

Lead has multiple effects that cause hematologic, skeletal, neurologic, gastrointestinal, and renal toxicities.

With recognition of its dangers, lead has been largely eliminated from paints and gasoline, but many sources persist in the environment, such as mines, foundries, and batteries. However, the highest risk is seen in children living in older houses with flaking lead paint. Ingested lead is particularly harmful to children because they absorb more than 50% of lead from food (whereas adults absorb ~15%) and have a more permeable blood–brain barrier, increasing their susceptibility to brain damage.

Pathogenesis. Most absorbed lead (80% to 85%) is taken up into bone and developing teeth, where it competes with calcium for binding to phosphates. About 5% to 10% of the absorbed lead remains in the blood, and the remainder is distributed throughout the soft tissues. The following mechanisms appear to contribute to lead toxicity:

- *Lead binds sulfhydryl groups* and interferes with the activity of several enzymes that are required for heme synthesis, leading to anemia.
- *Lead competes with calcium* for binding to proteins that participate in mitochondrial and neural functions, effects that may underlie its neurotoxicity.
- *Lead interferes with certain membrane ion transporters,* which may contribute to renal toxicity.

Morphology. The major targets of lead toxicity are the bone marrow, nervous system, and kidneys. One of the earliest signs of lead accumulation is a microcytic, hypochromic anemia associated with punctate basophilic stippling of red cells. Brain damage tends to occur in children, and in its most severe form results in brain edema, demyelination of white matter, necrosis of neurons, and astrocytic proliferation. In adults, the CNS is less often affected and neural damage usually takes the form of a peripheral demyelinating neuropathy, typically involving motor neurons, leading to wristdrop and footdrop. The kidneys may develop proximal tubular damage associated with intranuclear lead inclusions. Chronic renal damage may lead to interstitial fibrosis, gout, and eventual renal failure.

Clinical Features. The main clinical features of lead poisoning are shown in Fig. 19.1. Depending on exposure levels, the neurologic effects of lead in children range from subtle forms of cognitive dysfunction to cerebral edema, neuronal necrosis, and death. Lead-induced peripheral neuropathies in adults generally resolve with the elimination of exposure, but neurologic abnormalities in children are usually irreversible. Other effects of lead exposure include the following:

- *Abnormal remodeling* of calcified cartilage and bone trabeculae in the epiphyses in children, causing increased bone density detected as radiodense "lead lines" (Supplemental eFig. 19.1)

- *Poor healing of fractures,* due to increased chondrogenesis and delayed cartilage mineralization
- *Renal insufficiency* and *gout*

Lead poisoning may be suspected on the basis of neurologic changes or the presence of unexplained anemia. Blood tests showing elevated levels of lead in the blood and heme precursors in red cells are required for diagnosis. Treatment entails prevention of further exposure and administration of chelating agents that enhance the excretion of lead in the urine.

Mercury

Mercury damages the CNS, particularly in the developing fetus, and other organs such as the GI tract and kidneys.

The main source of exposure to mercury is from eating contaminated fish. Inorganic mercury from environmental sources or from industrial contamination is converted to organic compounds such as methyl mercury by bacteria. Methyl mercury enters the food chain and is concentrated in carnivorous fish such as swordfish, shark, and bluefish: Mercury levels may be 1 million times higher in their flesh than in the surrounding water. Ingested methyl mercury is efficiently absorbed in the GI tract and distributes widely in the body. The developing brain is extremely sensitive to methyl mercury; for this reason, the Centers for Disease Control (CDC) in the United States has recommended that pregnant women avoid the consumption of fish known to contain mercury. Ingested mercury can injure the gut and cause ulcerations and bloody diarrhea. In the kidneys, mercury can cause acute tubular necrosis and renal failure.

TOBACCO

Tobacco contains numerous carcinogens and toxins that cause several cancers and contribute to cardiovascular disease.

The main culprit is cigarette smoking, but smokeless tobacco in its various forms (snuff, chewing tobacco) is an important cause of oral cancer. In the United States alone, tobacco is responsible for more than 400,000 deaths per year, with one third of these attributable to lung cancer.

Adverse effects of smoking in various organ systems are shown in Fig. 19.2. Tobacco products are not only harmful for the user but also can cause lung cancer in nonsmokers who inhale smoke from the environment (second-hand smoke). There is also an increased risk of coronary atherosclerosis and fatal myocardial infarction in those exposed to second-hand smoke, which is estimated to cause 30,000 to 60,000 cardiac deaths annually in the United States. The frequency of respiratory illnesses and asthma in children living in a household with an adult who smokes is also increased.

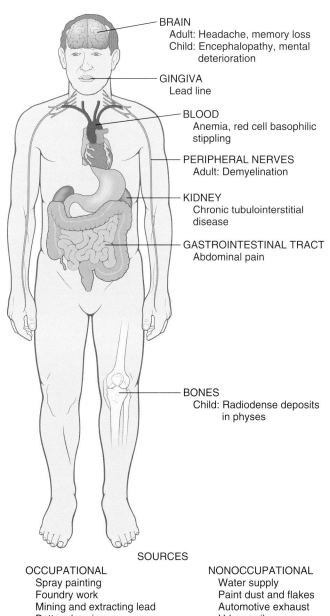

BRAIN
Adult: Headache, memory loss
Child: Encephalopathy, mental
deterioration

GINGIVA
Lead line

BLOOD
Anemia, red cell basophilic
stippling

PERIPHERAL NERVES
Adult: Demyelination

KIDNEY
Chronic tubulointerstitial
disease

GASTROINTESTINAL TRACT
Abdominal pain

BONES
Child: Radiodense deposits
in physes

SOURCES

OCCUPATIONAL	NONOCCUPATIONAL
Spray painting	Water supply
Foundry work	Paint dust and flakes
Mining and extracting lead	Automotive exhaust
Battery burning	Urban soil

Fig. 19.1 Pathologic features of lead poisoning.

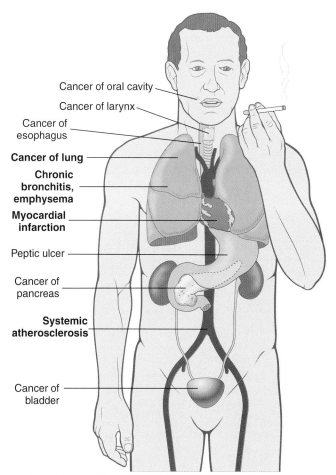

Cancer of oral cavity

Cancer of larynx

Cancer of
esophagus

Cancer of lung

**Chronic
bronchitis,
emphysema**

**Myocardial
infarction**

Peptic ulcer

Cancer of
pancreas

**Systemic
atherosclerosis**

Cancer of
bladder

Fig. 19.2 Adverse effects of smoking. The more common are in boldface.

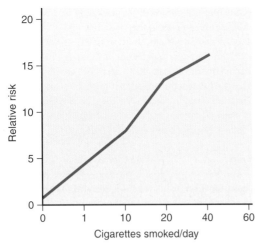

Fig. 19.3 The risk of lung cancer is determined by the number of cigarettes smoked. (Data from Stewart BW, Kleihues P, editors: World cancer report, Lyon, 2003, IARC Press.)

Pathogenesis. The addictive nature of tobacco is attributable to nicotine, which binds nicotinic receptors in the brain and peripheral tissues, producing changes in alertness, blood pressure, and heart rate. The most common diseases caused by cigarette smoking involve the lung and include emphysema, chronic bronchitis, and lung cancer (see Chapter 10), but virtually no organ is spared. The major disorders caused by tobacco smoking include the following:

- *Chronic obstructive pulmonary disease.* Agents in smoke have a direct irritant effect on the tracheobronchial mucosa, producing inflammation and increased mucus production (bronchitis). Cigarette smoke also causes the recruitment of leukocytes to the lung, increasing local elastase production and injury to lung tissue that leads to emphysema.
- *Carcinogenesis.* Components of cigarette smoke, particularly polycyclic hydrocarbons and nitrosamines, are potent carcinogens. The risk of lung cancer is related to the intensity of exposure, frequently expressed in terms of "pack years" (e.g., one pack daily for 20 years equals 20 pack years) or in cigarettes smoked per day (Fig. 19.3). This risk is multiplied by exposure to other carcinogens, such as asbestos and radiation. Tobacco smoke also has been linked to the development of cancers of the oral cavity, esophagus, pancreas, bladder, and other tissues.
- *Myocardial infarction.* Various factors in tobacco smoke increase platelet aggregation, decrease myocardial oxygen supply, and decrease the threshold for ventricular fibrillation. Almost one third of all heart attacks are associated with cigarette smoking, and smoking has a multiplicative effect on risk when combined with hypertension and hypercholesterolemia. It remains to be determined if e-cigarettes and vaping share these risks, and if so to what degree.
- *Spontaneous abortions, preterm births, and intrauterine growth retardation.* These effects stem in part from the deleterious effects of carbon monoxide in cigarette smoke on oxygen delivery to the fetus.

ALCOHOL

Excessive acute or chronic use of ethyl alcohol may cause marked physical and psychological damage.

In the United States, it is estimated that there are approximately 10 million chronic alcoholics and alcohol consumption is responsible for more than 100,000 deaths annually, about half from alcohol-related accidents, homicides, and suicides, and about 15% from cirrhosis of the liver.
Pathogenesis. After consumption, ethanol is absorbed in the stomach and small intestine and distributes throughout the body in direct proportion to the blood level. Less than 10% is excreted in the urine, sweat, and breath. Under normal circumstances, most of the remainder is metabolized to acetaldehyde in the liver by alcohol dehydrogenase. However, in chronic alcoholics, cytochrome P-450 isoenzymes are induced and may greatly enhance the rate of alcohol metabolism. Small amounts of alcohol are also metabolized by catalase. Acetaldehyde produced by these enzymes is in turn converted by acetaldehyde dehydrogenase to acetate (Fig. 19.4).

Some of alcohol's toxic effects are direct, but others stem from the consequences of its metabolism. The stomach is particularly prone to direct injury, and the deleterious effects of alcohol metabolism are particularly important in the liver, where alcohol oxidation by alcohol dehydrogenase causes a decrease in nicotinamide adenine dinucleotide (NAD+) and an increase in NADH (the reduced form of NAD+). NAD+ is required for fatty acid oxidation in the liver, and its deficiency leads to fat accumulation (fatty liver or hepatic steatosis). Other toxic effects of alcohol are not well characterized; some acute effects may be related to high levels of acetaldehyde, particularly in susceptible individuals of Asian descent with inherited defects in acetaldehyde dehydrogenase; generation of reactive oxygen species by cytochrome P-450 enzymes; and by affecting the gut mucosal barrier, release of endotoxin from the intestinal flora, possibly leading to systemic inflammation.

Clinical Features. The effects of alcohol on various organ systems can be divided into acute and chronic toxicities.

- *Acute alcoholism* exerts its effects primarily on the CNS, the stomach, and the liver. Alcohol directly depresses neural activity in the CNS, leading to impaired motor, sensory, and cognitive function and, at high doses, stupor, coma, and potentially death. Gastric damage occurs in the form of acute gastritis and ulceration. Even with a moderate intake of alcohol, multiple fat droplets accumulate in the cytoplasm of hepatocytes (fatty change or hepatic steatosis).
- *Chronic alcoholism* leads to significant morbidity and a shortened life span due to damage to the liver, GI tract, CNS, cardiovascular system, and pancreas. The liver is the main site of chronic injury, which may take the form of steatohepatitis, alcoholic hepatitis, and (ultimately) cirrhosis (described in Chapter 13). Obstruction of blood flow by cirrhosis may in turn lead to portal hypertension, and chronic injury increases the risk of hepatocellular carcinoma. In the GI tract, chronic alcoholism can cause bleeding from gastritis, gastric ulcer, or esophageal varices (associated with portal hypertension), which may be massive and prove fatal. Thiamine deficiency is common in chronic alcoholic patients; the principal lesions resulting from this deficiency are peripheral neuropathies and the Wernicke-Korsakoff syndrome, a disorder caused by damage to the thalamus and mammillary bodies that leads to cognitive and memory defects. Cerebral atrophy, cerebellar degeneration, and optic neuropathy also may occur. Injury to the myocardium may produce dilated congestive cardiomyopathy (alcoholic cardiomyopathy), and excess alcohol intake increases the risk of pancreatitis (see Chapter 13). Chronic alcohol consumption also is associated with an increased incidence of cancers of the oral cavity, esophagus, liver, and, possibly, breast in females. The mechanisms of the carcinogenic effect of alcohol are uncertain, although chronic injury and inflammation likely contribute.

Alcohol also takes a toll on the unborn; consumption of alcohol by pregnant women, particularly during the first trimester of pregnancy, may cause fetal alcohol syndrome. This consists of microcephaly, growth retardation, and facial abnormalities in the newborn, and a reduction of mental functions in older children.

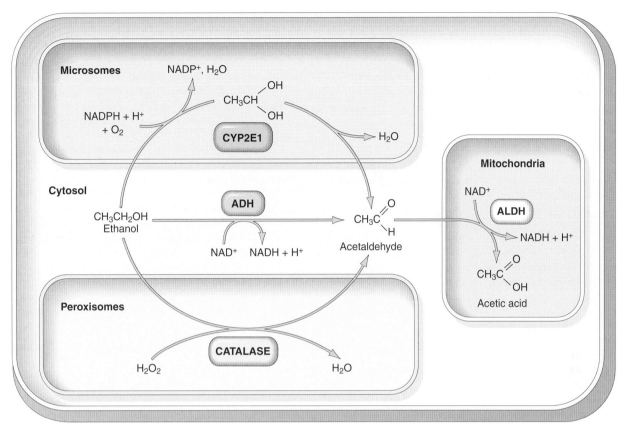

Fig. 19.4 Metabolism of ethanol: oxidation of ethanol to acetaldehyde by three different routes, and the generation of acetic acid. Note that oxidation by alcohol dehydrogenase (ADH) takes place in the cytosol, whereas the cytochrome P-450 isoform CYP2E1 is located in the ER (microsomes), and catalase is located in peroxisomes. Oxidation of acetaldehyde by aldehyde dehydrogenase (ALDH) to create acetic acid occurs in mitochondria. (Data from Parkinson A: Biotransformation of xenobiotics. In Klassen CD, editor: *Casarett and Doull's toxicology: The basic science of poisons,* ed 6, New York, 2001, McGraw-Hill, pp 133.)

INJURY BY THERAPEUTIC DRUGS AND DRUGS OF ABUSE

Injury by Therapeutic Drugs: Adverse Drug Reactions

Adverse drug reactions (ADRs) are untoward effects of drugs that are administered in conventional therapeutic settings.

These reactions are extremely common in the practice of medicine and are believed to affect 7% to 8% of patients admitted to a hospital. About 10% of such reactions prove fatal. Because they are widely used, estrogens and oral contraceptives (OCs) are discussed in detail.

Menopausal Hormone Therapy (MHT)

The most common type of MHT consists of the administration of estrogens together with a progestogen. They are used primarily to counteract "hot flashes" and other symptoms of menopause. The current risk-to-benefit consensus can be summarized as follows:

- Combination estrogen-progestin increases the risk of breast cancer after a median time of 5 to 6 years.
- MHT may have a protective effect on the development of atherosclerosis and coronary artery disease in women younger than 60 years of age, but there is no protection in women who started MHT at an older age.
- MHT increases the risk of stroke and venous thromboembolism, including deep vein thrombosis and pulmonary embolism. The increase in venous thromboembolism is more pronounced in women who have other risk factors such as immobilization and hypercoagulable states (see Chapter 3).

Assessment of the risks and benefits of MHT in women is complex. The current view is that these agents have a role in the management of menopausal symptoms in early menopause but should not be used over the long term for prevention of cardiovascular disease.

Oral Contraceptives (OCs)

Although OCs have been used since the 1960s, uncertainty persists about their safety and adverse effects. They usually contain a synthetic estradiol and a variable amount of a progestin, but a few preparations contain only progestins. There is reasonable evidence to support the following conclusions:

- *Breast carcinoma:* The prevailing opinion is that OCs are associated with a small (~1.2-fold) increased risk of breast cancer. Because breast cancer is rare in young women, the overall number of excess cancers that may be attributable to OCs is small.
- *Endometrial cancer and ovarian cancers:* OCs have a protective effect against these tumors.
- *Cervical cancer:* OCs may be associated with an increased risk of cervical carcinomas in women infected with human papillomavirus, but this may reflect an association with sexual activity and consequent risk of human papillomavirus infection rather than the effects of OCs per se.
- *Thromboembolism:* Most studies indicate that OCs are associated with a three- to six-fold increased risk of venous thrombosis and pulmonary thromboembolism resulting from increased hepatic synthesis of coagulation factors.

- *Cardiovascular disease:* There is uncertainty about the risk of atherosclerosis and myocardial infarction in users of OCs. OCs do not increase the risk of coronary artery disease in women younger than 30 years or in older women who are nonsmokers, but the risk is approximately double in women older than 35 years who smoke.
- *Hepatic adenoma:* There is a well-defined association between the use of OCs and this rare benign hepatic tumor, especially in older women who have used OCs for prolonged periods.

Injury by Drugs of Abuse

Drug abuse generally involves the use of mind-altering substances beyond therapeutic or social norms. Drug addiction and overdose are serious public health problems. Considered here are opioids, which are now the most widely abused drugs in the United States, as well as two other commonly used drugs, cocaine and marijuana.

Opioids

The past several years has seen an epidemic of opioid use in the United States, fostered by the ready availability of cheap heroin, an addictive opiate derived from the poppy plant; extremely potent synthetic opioids such as fentanyl and carfentanil; and an increased use of prescription opioids for pain relief. It was estimated that 10.3 million people in the United States used opioids in 2018, with the vast majority (>90%) misusing prescription pain killers. The results have been disastrous: Opioid overdoses are now the leading cause of death in the United States in adults under the age of 50 years.

Opioids have a wide range of adverse physical effects that can be categorized according to (1) the pharmacologic action of the agent, (2) reactions to the cutting agents or contaminants, (3) hypersensitivity reactions to the drug or its adulterants, and (4) diseases contracted through the sharing of needles. Some of the most important adverse effects of heroin and other opioids are the following:

- *Sudden death* related to overdose is an ever-present risk, particularly with synthetic opioids, which may be as much as 10,000-fold more potent than morphine or heroin. The chief mechanism of death is profound respiratory depression, an effect that can be rapidly reversed by the opioid antagonist naloxone if the victim is reached in time.
- *Pulmonary disease.* Pulmonary complications include edema, septic embolism, lung abscess, opportunistic infections, and foreign body granulomas from talc and other adulterants.
- *Infections.* Infectious complications are common in the skin and subcutaneous tissue, heart valves, liver, and lungs. One common complication is endocarditis, which often involves right-sided heart valves, particularly the tricuspid, because of injection of the drug into peripheral veins with contaminated needles. Most cases are caused by *Staphylococcus aureus,* but fungi and a multitude of other organisms have also been implicated. In the United States, sharing of needles has led to a high incidence of HIV infection in intravenous drug users.
- *Skin lesions* probably are the most frequent telltale sign of heroin addiction. Acute changes include abscesses, cellulitis, and ulcerations resulting from subcutaneous injections. Scarring at injection sites and thrombosed veins are the usual sequelae of repeated intravenous inoculations.
- *Renal disease* is a relatively common hazard in those with chronic heroin addiction. The two forms most frequently encountered are amyloidosis (generally secondary to skin infections) and focal glomerulosclerosis; both induce heavy proteinuria and the nephrotic syndrome.

Cocaine

In 2018, it was estimated that there were 5.5 million users of cocaine in the United States, and use appears to have risen since that time.

Cocaine is extracted from the leaves of the coca plant and sold as powder or as "crack", crystals of cocaine hydrochloride. It may be snorted, smoked, or injected subcutaneously or intravenously. The drug produces intense euphoria and mental alertness and profound psychologic dependence, making it highly addictive.

The following are the important manifestations of cocaine toxicity:

- *Cardiovascular effects.* The most dangerous acute physical effect of cocaine is on the cardiovascular system. Cocaine is a sympathomimetic agent, both in the CNS, where it blocks the reuptake of dopamine, and at adrenergic nerve endings, where it blocks the reuptake of epinephrine and norepinephrine while stimulating the presynaptic release of norepinephrine. These neurotransmitters accumulate in synapses and the hyperstimulation results in tachycardia, hypertension, and peripheral vasoconstriction. Cocaine also causes coronary artery vasoconstriction and promotes thrombus formation by facilitating platelet aggregation. The net effect of these actions (increased cardiac demand in the face of decreased cardiac blood flow) may result in myocardial ischemia or infarction. Cocaine may induce fatal cardiac arrhythmias by causing myocardial ischemia and through independent effects on cardiac ion transporters. These toxicities are only loosely dose-related, and fatal arrhythmias may occur in first-time users taking a typical dose.
- *CNS effects.* The most common neurologic findings are hyperpyrexia (due to effects on pathways that control body temperature) and seizures (due to hyperstimulation).
- *Effects on the fetus.* In pregnant women, cocaine may decrease blood flow to the placenta, resulting in fetal hypoxia and spontaneous abortion. Neurologic development may be impaired in the fetuses of pregnant women who are chronic drug users.
- *Chronic effects.* Chronic use may cause (1) perforation of the nasal septum in snorters, (2) decreased lung diffusing capacity in users who inhale the smoke, and (3) dilated cardiomyopathy.

Marijuana

Marijuana is the most widely used illegal drug, and its recent legalization in multiple states and the District of Columbia may increase its use further. A survey conducted in 2018 estimated that 43.5 million people (15.9% of the population) used marijuana during the previous year in the United States. Marijuana, which contains the psychoactive substance Δ9-tetrahydrocannabinol (THC), is made from the leaves of *Cannabis sativa, Cannabis indica,* or hybrids of the two species. When marijuana is smoked, about 5% to 10% of the THC content is absorbed. Whether marijuana use causes persistent adverse physical and functional effects remains unresolved; some beneficial effects, including its capacity to decrease intraocular pressure in glaucoma and to combat intractable nausea secondary to cancer chemotherapy, have been noted. The acute and chronic effects of marijuana use can be summarized as follows:

- *CNS.* Marijuana distorts sensory perception (time, speed, distance) and impairs motor coordination, effects that generally clear in 4 to 5 hours.
- *Cardiovascular.* Marijuana increases the heart rate and sometimes blood pressure, effects that may lead to angina in people with coronary artery disease.
- *Pulmonary.* Chronic marijuana smoking may be associated with laryngitis, pharyngitis, bronchitis, cough, asthma-like symptoms, and mild airway obstruction. Associations with the more severe complications of tobacco smoking (chronic obstructive pulmonary disease, lung cancer) have not been established.

INJURY PRODUCED BY IONIZING RADIATION

Ionizing radiation has sufficient energy to remove tightly bound electrons from molecules with which it interacts.

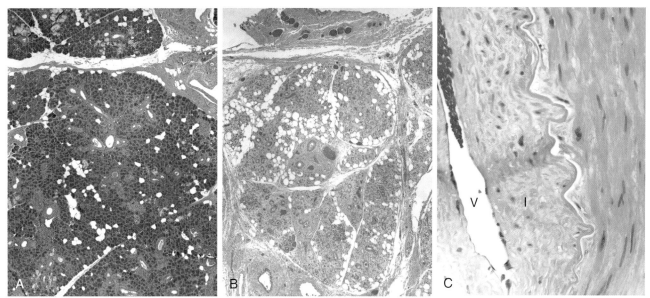

Fig. 19.5 Vascular changes and fibrosis of salivary glands produced by radiation therapy of the neck region. (A) Normal salivary gland; (B) fibrosis caused by radiation; (C) fibrosis and vascular changes consisting of fibrointimal thickening and arteriolar sclerosis. V, Vessel lumen; I, thickened intima. (**A** to **C,** Courtesy Dr. Melissa Upton, Department of Pathology, University of Washington, Seattle.)

Collision of these free electrons with other atoms releases additional electrons, a reaction cascade referred to as ionization. The main sources of ionizing radiation are (1) x-rays and gamma rays, electromagnetic waves of very high frequencies, and (2) high-energy neutrons, alpha particles (composed of two protons and two neutrons), and beta particles. At equivalent amounts of energy, alpha particles induce greater damage in a restricted area, whereas x-rays and gamma rays dissipate energy over a longer course and produce considerably less damage per unit of tissue.

About 50% of the total dose of ionizing radiation received by the U.S. population is iatrogenic, mostly from medical devices such as CT scanners. Ionizing radiation is used to treat some cancers; therapeutic ionizing radiation is a double-edged sword, however, as it is mutagenic, carcinogenic, and teratogenic. The most important cellular target of ionizing radiation is DNA. The effects of radiation include DNA breakage and cross-linking of DNA with proteins, which interfere with gene expression and cellular proliferation. To a point, DNA damage can be repaired by cellular repair enzymes. DNA damage that is not repaired leads to mutations, which may manifest years later as cancer. Another common consequence of cancer radiotherapy is the development of fibrosis in the irradiated field, perhaps as a result of vascular injury and ischemic damage to tissues.

Morphology. Cells surviving radiant energy damage have a wide range of *structural changes in chromosomes,* including deletions, breaks, translocations, and fragmentation. This damage may manifest as abnormal nuclear morphology that persists for years, including giant cells with pleomorphic nuclei or more than one nucleus that can mimic malignancy. Fibrosis may develop in the irradiated field, weeks or months after irradiation, as dead parenchymal cells are replaced by connective tissue (Fig. 19.5). Ionizing radiation may damage endothelial cells, leading to sclerosis of vessels due to deposition of compact collagen (hyalinization) and thickening of the media. Vascular insufficiency in turn contributes to fibrosis, scarring, and contractions.

Acute and Chronic Effects of Radiation on Organ Systems

The effects of radiation on organ systems are summarized in Fig. 19.6. Acute effects are most striking in organs and tissues composed of rapidly

dividing cells: the gonads, the hematopoietic and lymphoid systems, and the lining of the GI tract. Radiation directly destroys lymphocytes, both in the blood and in tissues. Hematopoietic precursors in the bone marrow are also quite sensitive, producing a dose-dependent marrow aplasia. Because neutrophils and platelets are short-lived, the destruction of precursors in the marrow results in neutropenia and thrombocytopenia within 1 to 2 weeks, whereas anemia appears after a longer time period. Very high doses of radiation kill marrow stem cells and induce permanent aplasia (aplastic anemia); such doses are often used in patients undergoing hematopoietic stem cell transplantation. Damage to the gut may result in bloody diarrhea, and the oropharynx may develop ulceration, leading to the development of infections exacerbated by neutropenia and lymphopenia. Damage to oocytes and spermatogonia may lead to sterility.

Chronic effects of radiation are related to vascular damage, fibrosis, and carcinogenesis. For example, radiation to the chest may lead to myocardial fibrosis, coronary artery disease, pulmonary fibrosis, and an increased risk of neoplasms such as carcinoma of the breast. The risk of cancer also depends on the site of exposure and the type and dose of radiation received. Among the most common neoplasms related to radiation exposure are certain leukemias and carcinomas of the lung (e.g., in uranium miners who inhaled radioactive dust), thyroid carcinoma in those exposed to radioactive iodine, and breast carcinoma, melanoma, and sarcomas within the radiation fields used to treat other cancers. Notably, the greatest risk appears to be to children, in whom as few as two CT scans may be sufficient to impart a small but significantly increased risk of leukemia and certain brain tumors.

NUTRITIONAL DISEASES

Both malnutrition and overnutrition are major sources of human disease across the globe.

Malnutrition

A healthy diet provides sufficient calories for the body's daily metabolic needs, essential amino acids and fatty acids, and critical vitamins and minerals. Malnutrition occurs when one or more of these components are missing from the diet, or when they are present in inadequate amounts because of malabsorption, impaired use

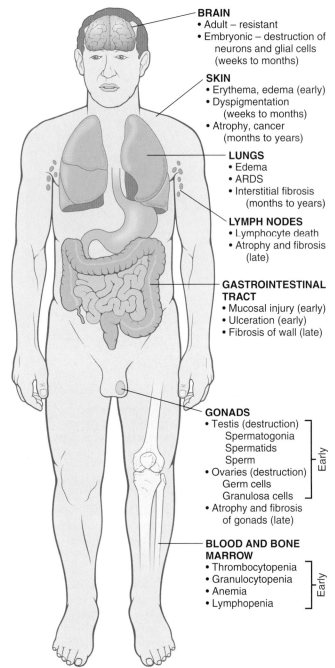

BRAIN
- Adult – resistant
- Embryonic – destruction of neurons and glial cells (weeks to months)

SKIN
- Erythema, edema (early)
- Dyspigmentation (weeks to months)
- Atrophy, cancer (months to years)

LUNGS
- Edema
- ARDS
- Interstitial fibrosis (months to years)

LYMPH NODES
- Lymphocyte death
- Atrophy and fibrosis (late)

GASTROINTESTINAL TRACT
- Mucosal injury (early)
- Ulceration (early)
- Fibrosis of wall (late)

GONADS
- Testis (destruction)
  Spermatogonia
  Spermatids   ⎤
  Sperm   ⎥ Early
- Ovaries (destruction)
  Germ cells   ⎥
  Granulosa cells   ⎦
- Atrophy and fibrosis of gonads (late)

BLOOD AND BONE MARROW
- Thrombocytopenia   ⎤
- Granulocytopenia   ⎥ Early
- Anemia   ⎥
- Lymphopenia   ⎦

Fig. 19.6 Overview of the major morphologic consequences of radiation injury. Early changes occur in hours to weeks; late changes occur in months to years. ARDS, Acute respiratory distress syndrome.

or storage, excess losses, or increased requirements. In addition to resulting from the poor or inadequate diet prevalent in underdeveloped countries, malnutrition occurs in a number of other settings, as follows:

- *Infants, adolescents,* and *pregnant women* have increased nutritional needs that may go unrecognized; ignorance about the nutritional content of various foods also contributes to malnutrition.
- *Chronic alcoholics* are prone to deficiency of several vitamins, especially thiamine, pyridoxine, folate, and vitamin A, as a result of dietary deficiency, defective GI absorption, abnormal nutrient utilization and storage, increased metabolic needs, and increased rate of loss.
- *Acute and chronic illnesses* raise the basal metabolic rate, resulting in increased daily requirements for all nutrients.

- *Self-imposed dietary restriction* in the form of eating disorders such as anorexia nervosa and bulimia may lead to malnourishment.
- *Other causes* include GI diseases, acquired and inherited malabsorption syndromes, drug therapies that block the uptake or use of particular nutrients, and total parenteral nutrition without supplemental vitamins.

The remainder of this section focuses on protein energy malnutrition, deficiencies of vitamins and trace minerals, and obesity.

Severe Acute Malnutrition

Severe acute malnutrition (previously called protein energy malnutrition) is a serious, often lethal disease that stems from an inadequate intake of protein and calories.

It is common in poor countries and in war-torn areas of the world, where it contributes to high death rates among the very young. A lack of protein and calories in the diet causes a range of clinical manifestations that have at their two extremes syndromes known as marasmus and kwashiorkor. To understand the distinction between these conditions, it is important to note that the body's proteins are largely compartmentalized in skeletal muscles (the somatic compartment) and the liver (the visceral compartment). The somatic compartment is affected more severely in marasmus, and the visceral compartment is depleted more severely in kwashiorkor.

Marasmus develops when the diet is severely lacking in calories leading to loss of protein from the somatic compartment. A marasmic child suffers growth retardation and loss of muscle mass (Fig. 19.7A). By contrast, the visceral protein compartment is initially largely unaffected, so serum albumin levels are normal or only slightly reduced. In addition to muscle proteins, subcutaneous fat is also mobilized and used as fuel. Due to losses of muscle and subcutaneous fat, the extremities are emaciated and the head appears too large for the body. Anemia and manifestations of multivitamin deficiencies are present, and there is evidence of immune deficiency, particularly of T cell–mediated immunity, often leading to concurrent infections.

Kwashiorkor occurs when protein deprivation is relatively greater than the reduction in total calories and is marked by loss of protein from the visceral compartment. This results in hypoalbuminemia and gives rise to generalized or dependent edema (Fig. 19.7B), which masks the true extent of weight loss. There is relative sparing of the muscle mass as well as the subcutaneous fat. Children with kwashiorkor have characteristic skin lesions with alternating zones of hyperpigmentation, desquamation, and hypopigmentation. Hair changes include loss of color or alternating bands of pale and darker color, straightening, fine texture, and loss of firm attachment to the scalp. Other features that distinguish kwashiorkor from marasmus include its association with fatty liver and apathy, listlessness, and loss of appetite. As in marasmus, vitamin deficiencies, defects in immunity, and secondary infections are frequently present. Recovery of malnourished children upon return to an adequate diet may be hampered by changes in the gut microbiome that impair nutrient absorption, and studies are now underway to determine if restoration of the microbiome can help starving children rebuild their health.

So-called secondary malnutrition often develops in chronically ill, older, and bedridden patients in the United States. It is common in nursing home residents and in cancer patients, in whom a particularly severe form of secondary malnutrition called cachexia often develops. The underlying mechanisms are complex, but appear to involve "cachectins" secreted by tumor cells, and cytokines, particularly tumor necrosis factor (TNF), which are released as part of the host response to advanced tumors. Both types of factors directly stimulate the degradation of skeletal muscle proteins, and cytokines such as TNF, which causes loss of appetite and also stimulates fat mobilization from lipid stores.

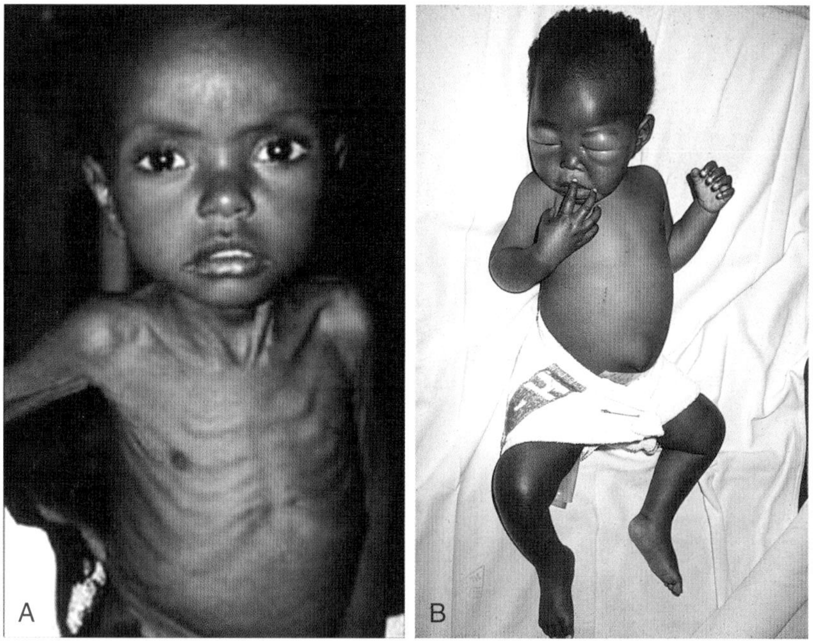

Fig. 19.7 Childhood malnutrition. (A) Marasmus. Note the loss of muscle mass and subcutaneous fat; the head appears to be too large for the emaciated body. (B) Kwashiorkor. The infant shows generalized edema, seen as ascites and puffiness of the face, hands, and legs. (A, From Clinic Barak, Reisebericht, Kenya.)

Vitamin Deficiencies

Before discussing the functions of individual vitamins and the consequence of their deficiency, some general comments are in order.

- *Thirteen vitamins are necessary for health; four (A, D, E, and K) are fat soluble and the remainder are water soluble.* Fat-soluble vitamins are more readily stored in the body, but also may be poorly absorbed in GI disorders characterized by fat malabsorption.
- *Certain vitamins can be synthesized endogenously*, vitamin D from precursor steroids, vitamin K and biotin by the intestinal microflora, and niacin from tryptophan, an essential amino acid.

In the following sections, vitamins A, D, and C are presented in some detail because of their wide-ranging functions and the morphologic changes of deficient states.

Vitamin A

Vitamin A is a generic name for a group of related fat-soluble compounds that include retinol, retinal, and retinoic acid, each with similar biologic activities. Retinol is the chemical name for vitamin A. Animal-derived foods such as liver, fish, eggs, milk, and butter are important dietary sources of preformed vitamin A. Yellow and leafy green vegetables such as carrots, squash, and spinach supply large amounts of carotenoids that are metabolized to active vitamin A in the body.

Absorption of vitamin A requires bile, pancreatic enzymes, and some level of antioxidant activity in the food. In healthy persons with a normal diet, hepatic reserves are sufficient to support the body's needs for at least 6 months.

Important normal functions of vitamin A include the following:

- *Vision* involves four forms of vitamin A–containing pigments; rhodopsin, located in rods, is involved in perception of light, and 3 forms of iodopsins, located in cones, are involved in perception of colors. Exposure to light triggers changes in the conformation of these pigments, known as rhodopsin or iodopsins, setting in motion events that produce a nerve impulse in the retina that is transmitted to the vision centers in the brain.
- *Regulation of cell growth and differentiation.* Vitamin A and related compounds (retinoids) regulate the differentiation of mucous-secreting epithelium by binding to retinoic acid receptors and regulating gene expression. Retinoid deficiency disrupts normal gene expression and causes *squamous metaplasia.*
- *Regulation of lipid metabolism.* Some retinoic acid receptors form complexes with other nuclear receptors, such as peroxisome proliferator-activated receptors (PPARs), key regulators of fatty acid metabolism, and other aspects of adipogenesis.
- *Host resistance to infections,* probably due in part to its ability to stimulate the immune system through unclear mechanisms.

Vitamin A deficiency leads to vision loss and susceptibility to infection.

Vitamin A deficiency occurs worldwide as a consequence of poor nutrition or fat malabsorption. Bariatric surgery and the continuous use of mineral oil laxatives also may lead to deficiency.

The effects of vitamin A deficiency (summarized in Fig. 19.8) are as follows:

- *Visual effects.* One of the earliest manifestations of vitamin A deficiency is impaired vision, particularly in reduced light (night blindness).
- *Epithelial changes.* Persistent deficiency gives rise to epithelial metaplasia and keratization. In the eyes, this leads to buildup of keratin debris, erosion of the roughened corneal surface, and eventual softening and destruction of the cornea *(keratomalacia),* producing blindness. Squamous metaplasia of the upper respiratory passages and the urinary tract predisposes affected patients to pulmonary infections and renal and bladder stones, respectively, while plugging of the ducts of the adnexal glands leads to skin changes, as well.
- *Immune deficiency* is a serious consequence of vitamin A deficiency, which has been linked to higher mortality rates from measles, pneumonia, and infectious diarrhea.

Vitamin D

Vitamin D is required to maintain adequate plasma levels of calcium and phosphorus and to support metabolic functions, bone mineralization,

VITAMIN A DEFICIENCY

EYE CHANGES

CELL DIFFERENTIATION

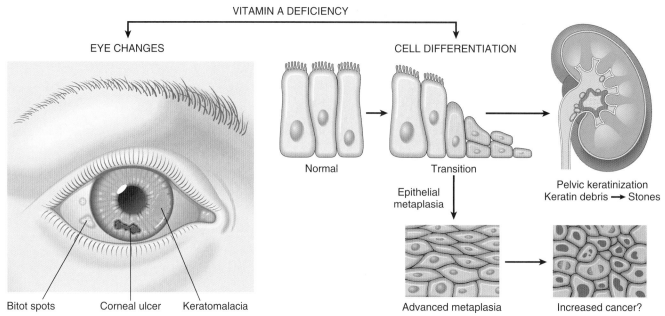

Normal

Transition

Epithelial
metaplasia

Pelvic keratinization
Keratin debris ➝ Stones

Bitot spots   Corneal ulcer   Keratomalacia

Advanced metaplasia   Increased cancer?

Fig. 19.8 Vitamin A deficiency: major consequences in the eye and in the production of keratinizing meta-plasia of specialized epithelial surfaces, and its possible role in epithelial metaplasia. Not depicted are night blindness and immune deficiency.

and neuromuscular transmission. The major source of vitamin D for humans is its endogenous synthesis, a process that requires UV light from the sun or artificial sources. Production is less efficient in individuals with darker skin because of melanin pigmentation. The remainder of vitamin D comes from dietary sources, such as fish, plants, and grains.

Synthesis of the active form of vitamin D occurs through sequential reactions that are carried out in the liver and the kidney (Fig. 19.9). The last step, renal production of dihydroxy vitamin D, is regulated by three mechanisms:

- *Hypocalcemia* stimulates secretion of parathyroid hormone (PTH), which increases the production of dihydroxy vitamin D by activating α1-hydroxylase.
- *Hypophosphatemia* directly activates α1-hydroxylase, increasing dihyroxy vitamin D synthesis.
- *High levels of dihydroxy vitamin D* suppresses its synthesis by inhibiting the action of α1-hydroxylase.

Like retinoids, dihydroxy vitamin D acts by binding to nuclear receptors, which increase the transcription of specific genes. Vitamin D maintains normal plasma levels of calcium and phosphorus by stimulating intestinal absorption of calcium and resorption of calcium in the kidney, and also has effects on osteoclasts and osteoblasts that influence bone resorption and calcification (Fig. 19.9).

Pathogenesis. **Vitamin D deficiency causes hypocalcemia and a failure of bone mineralization, leading to rickets in growing children and osteomalacia in adults.**

These skeletal diseases are mainly caused by dietary deficiencies of calcium and vitamin D in concert with limited exposure to sunlight. Less common causes include renal disorders that decrease the synthesis of dihydroxy vitamin D and malabsorption disorders. Mild forms of vitamin D deficiency leading to bone loss and hip fractures are common among elderly persons.

Vitamin D deficiency causes hypocalcemia and stimulates PTH production, leading to release of calcium from bone, decreased renal calcium excretion, and increased renal excretion of phosphate. This restores serum calcium levels to near normal, but hypophosphatemia persists, leading to impaired bone mineralization. Inadequate mineralization of

bone in rickets is exacerbated by decreased calcification of epiphyseal cartilage. This leads to overgrowth of epiphyseal cartilage, which enlarges and expands osteochondral junctions (Fig. 19.10B). The weakened bone is prone to fractures and deformations induced by mechanical stress. In infants, there is frontal bossing of the skull and a squared appearance to the head. Overgrowth of the costochondral junction deforms the chest, the "*rachitic rosary.*" Rickets in an ambulating child produces deformities of the spine and long bones, causing lumbar lordosis and bowing of the legs (Fig. 19.9C). In adults with vitamin D deficiency, inadequate mineralization produces bone that is weak and vulnerable to fractures, which are most likely in the vertebrae and femoral neck.

Vitamin C (Ascorbic Acid)

Vitamin C deficiency leads to the development of scurvy, characterized principally by bone disease in growing children and by hemorrhages and healing defects in both children and adults.

Unlike vitamin D, ascorbic acid is not synthesized endogenously in humans, who therefore are entirely dependent on the diet for this nutrient. Vitamin C is present in milk and some animal products (liver, fish) and is abundant in a variety of fresh fruits and vegetables.

The most clearly established function of vitamin C as a cofactor for prolyl and lysyl hydroxylases, which are required for hydroxylation of procollagen. Inadequate hydroxylation due to vitamin C deficiency destabilizes procollagen and prevents it from forming covalent cross-links. This decreases collagen secretion from fibroblasts and lowers its tensile strength while also increasing its solubility, making it more vulnerable to enzymatic degradation.

Vitamin C deficiency and acquired abnormalities in collagen lead to bleeding in the skin and gums, joint and muscle pain, and impaired wound healing. Fortunately, because of the abundance of ascorbic acid in foods, scurvy has largely disappeared. It is sometimes encountered as a secondary deficiency, particularly among elderly persons, people who live alone, and chronic alcoholics, groups often characterized by erratic and inadequate eating patterns.

Other vitamins and some essential minerals are listed and briefly described in Tables 19.1 and 19.2. Folic acid and vitamin B$_{12}$ are discussed in Chapter 9.

NORMAL VITAMIN D METABOLISM

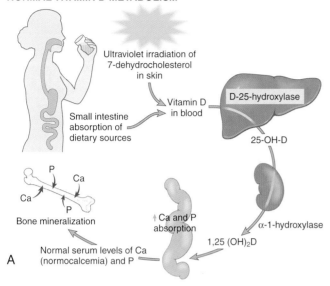

A

VITAMIN D DEFICIENCY

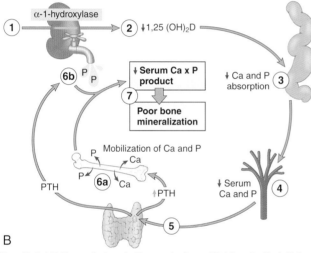

B

Fig. 19.9 (A) Normal vitamin D metabolism. (B) Vitamin D deficiency. There is inadequate substrate for the renal hydroxylase *(1)*, yielding a deficiency of 1,25-(OH)2D (dihyroxy vitamin D) *(2)*, and deficient absorption of calcium and phosphorus from the gut *(3)*, with consequent depressed serum levels of both *(4)*. The hypocalcemia activates the parathyroid glands *(5)*, causing mobilization of calcium and phosphorus from bone *(6a)*. Simultaneously, parathyroid hormone (PTH) induces wasting of phosphate in the urine *(6b)* and calcium retention. Consequently, the serum levels of calcium are normal or nearly normal, but the phosphate is low; hence, mineralization is impaired *(7)*.

Obesity

Excess adiposity (obesity) and body weight are associated with an increased incidence of several of the most important diseases of humans, including diabetes, cardiovascular disease, and cancer.

In the United States, obesity has reached epidemic proportions, and globally the World Health Organization (WHO) estimated that in 2015, 700 million adults were obese. If current trends continue, it is projected that by the year 2030, approximately half of American adults will be obese and that 25% of the population will have severe obesity.

Obesity is a state of increased body weight caused by adipose tissue accumulation that is sufficient to produce adverse health effects. Fat accumulation is assessed by measuring the body mass index (BMI),

defined as (weight in kilograms)/(height in meters)^2 or kg/m^2. BMIs in the range 18.5 to 25 kg/m^2 are considered normal, whereas BMIs between 25 and 30 kg/m^2 identify the overweight, and BMIs greater than 30 kg/m^2, the obese. For simplicity's sake, we apply the term *obesity* to both the overweight and the truly obese.

Pathogenesis. The etiology of obesity involves genetic, environmental, and psychological factors. It is a disorder of energy balance, which is regulated by neural and hormonal mechanisms that normally maintain body weight within a narrow range for many years. These neurohumoral mechanisms may be divided into three components (Fig. 19.11):

- *The peripheral or afferent system* generates signals in the form of hormones. These include leptin and adiponectin produced by fat cells, insulin from the pancreas, ghrelin from the stomach, and peptide YY from the ileum and colon. Leptin reduces food intake and is discussed in further detail below. Ghrelin stimulates appetite. Peptide YY is released postprandially and is a satiety signal.
- *The arcuate nucleus in the hypothalamus,* which integrates the peripheral hormonal signals and generates neural signals that are transmitted by (1) POMC (pro-opiomelanocortin) and CART (cocaine- and amphetamine-regulated transcript) neurons; and (2) NPY (neuropeptide Y) and AgRP (agouti-related peptide) neurons.
- *The efferent system,* hypothalamic neurons that control food intake and energy expenditure. Input from POMC/CART neurons reduces food intake and activates neurons that enhance energy expenditure and weight loss, whereas input from NPY/AgRP neurons activates neurons that promote food intake and weight gain.

Several components of the afferent system that regulate appetite and satiety deserve a brief discussion.

- *Leptin* is secreted by fat cells. When adipose tissue is abundant, leptin secretion is stimulated. The hormone reduces food intake by stimulating POMC/CART neurons and inhibiting NPY/AgRP neurons. Leptin also increases energy expenditure by stimulating physical activity and thermogenesis. In obese individuals, the cellular response to leptin is blunted, despite high circulating levels.
- *Gut hormones* are initiators and terminators of volitional eating. Ghrelin increases food intake, most likely by stimulating the NPY/AgRP neurons in the hypothalamus. Ghrelin levels rise before meals and fall 1 to 2 hours afterward, but the drop is attenuated in obese persons. *PYY* is secreted from endocrine cells in the ileum and colon in response to food consumption. It decreases appetite and augments satiety by stimulating POMC/CART neurons in the hypothalamus. PYY also reduces the rate of gastric emptying and intestinal motility, further contributing to satiety.
- *Adiponectin* is produced in the adipose tissue. It increases oxidation of fatty acids by muscle and decreases the liver uptake of fatty acids and liver gluconeogenesis. Together, this increases insulin sensitivity and protects against the metabolic syndrome. Its serum levels are lower in obese than in lean individuals, which may contribute to obesity-associated insulin resistance, type 2 diabetes, and nonalcoholic fatty liver disease (NAFLD) (see Chapter 13).
- *Adipose tissue.* In addition to leptin, adipose tissue produces other mediators that link lipid metabolism, nutrition, and inflammatory responses. The total number of adipocytes is established by adolescence and is higher in people who were obese as children. Although in adults approximately 10% of adipocytes turn over annually, the number of adipocytes remains constant. Diets fail in part because the loss of fat from adipocytes causes leptin levels to fall, stimulating the appetite and diminishing energy expenditure.

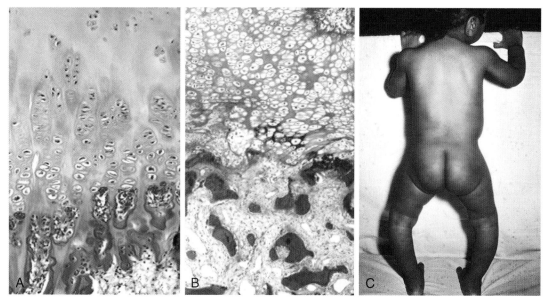

Fig. 19.10 Rickets. (A) Normal costochondral junction of a young child. Note cartilage palisade formation and orderly transition from cartilage to new bone. (B) Rachitic costochondral junction in which the palisade of cartilage is absent. Darker trabeculae are well-formed bone; paler trabeculae consist of uncalcified osteoid. (C) Note bowing of legs as a consequence of the formation of poorly mineralized bone in a child with rickets. (B, Courtesy Dr. Andrew E. Rosenberg, Massachusetts General Hospital, Boston.)

Table 19.1 Vitamins: Major Functions and Deficiency Syndromes

Vitamin	Functions	Deficiency Syndromes
Fat-Soluble		
Vitamin A	A component of visual pigment	Night blindness, xerophthalmia, blindness
	Maintenance of specialized epithelia	Squamous metaplasia
	Immune function	Vulnerability to infection
Vitamin D	Intestinal absorption of calcium and phosphorus and mineralization of bone	Rickets in children
Osteomalacia in adults
Vitamin E	Antioxidant; scavenges free radicals	Spinocerebellar degeneration, hemolysis
Vitamin K	Synthesis of procoagulants—factors II (prothrombin), VII, IX, and X; and protein C and protein S	Bleeding diathesis
Water-Soluble		
Vitamin B_1 (thiamine)	Coenzyme in decarboxylation reactions	Dry and wet beriberi, Wernicke syndrome, Korsakoff syndrome
Vitamin B_2 (riboflavin) 4	Cofactors for many enzymes in intermediary metabolism	Cheilosis, stomatitis, glossitis, dermatitis, corneal vascularization
Niacin	Incorporated into nicotinamide adenine dinucleotide (NAD) and NAD phosphate; involved in a variety of oxidation-reduction (redox) reactions	Pellagra—"three Ds": dementia, dermatitis, diarrhea
Vitamin B_6 (pyridoxine)	Coenzymes in many intermediary reactions	Cheilosis, glossitis, dermatitis, peripheral neuropathy
Vitamin B_{12}	Folate metabolism and DNA synthesis
Maintenance of myelinization of spinal cord tracts	Combined system disease (megaloblastic anemia and degeneration of posterolateral spinal cord tracts)
Vitamin C	Redox reactions and hydroxylation of collagen	Scurvy
Folate	Transfer and use of one-carbon units in DNA synthesis	Megaloblastic anemia, neural tube defects
Pantothenic acid	Incorporated in coenzyme A	No nonexperimental syndrome recognized
Biotin	Cofactor in carboxylation reactions	No clearly defined clinical syndrome

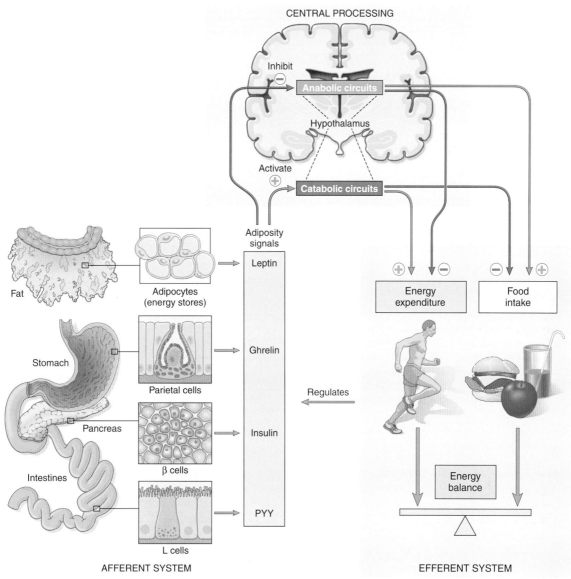

Fig. 19.11 Energy balance regulatory circuitry. When sufficient energy is stored in adipose tissue and the individual is well fed, afferent adiposity signals (insulin, leptin, ghrelin, peptide YY) are delivered to the central neuronal processing units, in the hypothalamus. Here the adiposity signals inhibit anabolic circuits and activate catabolic circuits. The effector arms of these central circuits then influence energy balance by inhibiting food intake and promoting energy expenditure. This in turn reduces the energy stores, and proadiposity signals are blunted. Conversely, when energy stores are low, the available anabolic circuits take over, at the expense of catabolic circuits, to stimulate food intake and generate energy stores in the form of adipose tissue.

Table 19.2 Ten Selected Trace Elements and Deficiency Syndromes

Element	Function	Basis of Deficiency	Clinical Features
Zinc	Component of enzymes, principally oxidases	Inadequate supplementation in artificial diets; interference in absorption by other dietary constituents; inborn error of metabolism	Rash around eyes, mouth, nose, and anus called acrodermatitis enteropathica Anorexia and diarrhea Depressed mental function Depressed wound healing and immune response Infertility
Iron	Essential component of hemoglobin and iron-containing metallo-enzymes	Inadequate diet Chronic blood loss	Hypochromic, microcytic anemia
Iodine	Component of thyroid hormone	Inadequate supply in food and water	Goiter, hypothyroidism causing cretinsm (congenital) and myxedema in adults
Copper	Component of cytochrome c oxidase, dopamine β-hydroxylase, tyrosinase, and lysyl oxidase	Inadequate supplementation in artificial diet	Muscle weakness
Fluoride	Mechanism unknown	Inadequate supply in soil and water Inadequate supplementation	Dental caries
Selenium	Component of GSH peroxidase Antioxidant with vitamin E	Inadequate amounts in soil and water	Myopathy Cardiomyopathy (Keshan disease)

As already mentioned, obesity, and particularly central obesity, is associated with type 2 diabetes, cardiovascular disorders such as atherosclerosis and hypertension, and a wide variety of cancers. In part, these risks are related to a constellation of findings often found in obese individuals that are referred to as *metabolic syndrome,* characterized by glucose intolerance, hyperlipidemia, hypertension, and a systemic proinflammatory state. The initiating events for metabolic syndrome may be obesity-associated insulin resistance and hyperinsulinemia, which set the stage for pathogenic changes in lipid metabolism and blood pressure. Included among its complications is nonalcoholic fatty liver disease, which is commonly associated with obesity and type 2 diabetes and may progress to fibrosis and cirrhosis (see Chapter 13), and cholelithiasis (gallstones), which is six times more common in obese than in lean subjects (see Chapter 13). Several other disorders are also associated with obesity:

- *Hypoventilation syndrome* stems from respiratory compromise in very obese persons. Hypersomnolence is characteristic and is often associated with sleep apnea, polycythemia, and eventual right-sided heart failure (cor pulmonale).
- *Degenerative joint disease (osteoarthritis)*
- *Cancer*

Obesity is associated with a modest but measureable increase in cancers of the esophagus, thyroid, colon, and kidney in men and cancers of the esophagus, endometrium, gallbladder, and kidney in women. The underlying mechanisms are unknown and are likely to be multiple, and include trophic effects of insulin, increased peripheral production of estrogen, reduced secretion from adipose tissue of adiponectin, and the proinflammatory state associated with obesity.

INDEX

A

"ABCs" of melanoma, 313
Abnormal immune function, trisomy 21 and, 100
Abnormal mitotic activity, 67
Abnormal remodeling, in lead exposure, 314, 314.e1f
Abnormal uterine bleeding, 254, 254t
Abscess, inflammation and, 23
Acantholysis, 309
Acetaminophen toxicity, 230f
Achondroplasia, 296
Acquired genetic aberrations, in carcinoma of prostate, 244
Acquired immunodeficiency syndrome (AIDS), 58–59, 58b
  clinical course, 59, 60f
  pathogenesis of, 59, 59b, 60f
  structure and life cycle in, 58–59, 58f, 58b
Activated RAS, 75
Active tuberculosis, 177
Acute adrenal insufficiency, 277–278
Acute alcoholism, 316
Acute appendicitis, 215–216
Acute cellular rejection, 53, 54f
Acute cholecystitis, 235
Acute diabetic ketoacidosis, 276
Acute eczematous dermatitis, 307–308, 308f
Acute endocarditis, 130
Acute humoral (or vascular) rejection, 53, 55f
Acute hypertensive encephalopathy, 283
Acute inflammation, 15, 15b, 16t
  clinicopathologic features of, 23–25, 23t, 23b
    morphologic features, 23
    systemic manifestations, 23–25, 23b, 25t
  cytokines in, 22t
  mechanisms of, 16–26, 16b
  outcomes of, 25–26
  resolution of, 20
Acute inflammatory dermatoses, 307–308
Acute kidney injury (AKI), 187, 197
Acute leukemias, 148–150, 148f–149f
  clinical features of, 149–150
  pathogenesis of, 148–149
  pathology of, 149
Acute liver failure, 222
Acute myeloid leukemia (AML), 148, 148t
Acute pancreatitis, 236–237, 236f
Acute-phase proteins, plasma levels of, 25
Acute plaque change, 110
Acute poststreptococcal glomerulonephritis, 186t, 192–193, 194f
Acute pyelonephritis, 195–196, 196f–197f
Acute pyogenic osteomyelitis, 298–299, 299f
Acute rejection, 53
Acute renal failure, 186
Acute respiratory distress syndrome, 163, 164f
Acute self-limited colitis, 211
Acute tubular injury (ATI), 195, 197–198, 199f
Acute tubular necrosis, 187
Acute viral hepatitis, 226–227
AD. See Alzheimer disease

Adaptations, of cells, 1
Adaptive immunity, 41
Addison disease, 277–278
Adenocarcinomas, 207, 207.e1f
  of colon, 217–219
    clinical features of, 218–219
    morphology of, 218, 219f
    pathogenesis of, 217b
  gastric, 209–210, 210f
  of lung, 182, 183f
  pancreatic, 237–238, 239f
Adenomas, 216–217, 217f
  gastric, 209, 209.e1f
  thyroid, 270, 270f
Adenomatous polyposis coli, 77
Adenomatous polyposis coli (APC) gene, 209
Adenomatous polyps, 216
Adhesion, of intestine, 219
Adiponectin, 323
Adipose tissue, 323
Adrenal glands, 276–279
  Addison disease, 277–278
  adrenal medulla tumors, 278–279, 278f
  adrenogenital syndromes, 276–277
  Cushing syndrome, 276, 276f–277f
  hyperaldosteronism, 276
  multiple endocrine neoplasia (MEN) syndromes, 279
Adrenal medulla tumors, 278–279, 278f
Adrenogenital syndromes, 276–277
Adrenoleukodystrophy, 288
ADRs. See Adverse drug reactions
"Adult" form, of coarctation, 120–121, 121f
Adult T-cell leukemia/lymphoma, 152t, 156
Advanced glycation end-products (AGEs), 274
Adverse drug reactions (ADRs), 317–318
Age
  atherosclerosis and, 108
  in carcinogenic mutations, 71
AGEs. See Advanced glycation end-products
Aging, osteoporosis and, 297
Agranulocytosis, 146
AIDS. See Acquired immunodeficiency syndrome
AIDS-associated (epidemic) KS, 115
Air embolism, 37
AIRE, 277
AKI. See Acute kidney injury
Alcohol, 316, 317f
  dilated cardiomyopathy and, 131
Alcoholic liver disease, 228, 229f
ALK (anaplastic lymphoma kinase) gene, 279
Allergic contact dermatitis, 307
Allergies, 14, 42
Allografts, 52–53
Alport syndrome, 194
Altered cellular metabolism, 77–79, 77b
Alternative pathway, 44
Alveolar macrophages, 16
Alzheimer disease (AD), 289, 289f, 289f–290f
Alzheimer's disease, 100
AML. See Acute myeloid leukemia

Amniotic fluid embolism, 37, 38.e1f
Amyloid, 13, 13.e3f
Amyloidosis, 13.e3f, 59–61, 59b, 133, 133.e1f
  clinical features of, 61
  morphology of, 61, 62f
  pathogenesis of, 61f
Amyotrophic lateral sclerosis, 291, 291.e1f
Anaphylactic shock, 38
Anaplasia, 66
Anaplastic astrocytomas, 292–293
Anaplastic carcinomas, 270
Anasarca, 30
Ancylostoma duodenale, 213
Androgens, 276–277
Anencephaly, 280t
Aneuploid, 97
Aneuploidy, 69–70
Aneurysm formation, 124, 125f
  of atheromas, 109
Aneurysms, 110–112
  aortic, 110–111, 111f
Angelman syndrome, 102, 103f
Angina pectoris, 109, 121
Angina, unstable, 121
Angiogenesis, 28, 29f
  sustained, 80, 80b
Angiosarcomas, 116, 117f
Angiotensin, active form of, 106
Anitschkow cells, 129
Ankylosing spondylitis (AS), 303–304
Antibody-mediated (type II) hypersensitivity, 42, 44–47
  activation and functions of complement, 44, 46f
  clinical features of, 45–47, 46t
  pathogenesis of, 44
Anticipation, 101
Anti-GBM antibody, deposition of, 187
Antigen-receptor gene rearrangements, 87
Antineutrophil cytoplasmic antibody (ANCA)-associated vasculitides, 114
Antiphospholipid antibody syndrome, 36
α1-Antitrypsin deficiency, 231, 231.e1f
Anuria, 186
Aortic coarctation, 120–121, 121f
Aphthous ulcers, 220, 220.e1f
Aplastic anemia, 146, 146.e1f
Apoptosis, 2–6, 2f, 2b
  causes of, 4
  features of, 3t
  genes regulate, 69
  intrinsic pathway of, 79, 80f
  killing stressed cells through, 77
  mechanisms of, 5–6, 5b, 6f
  pathologic, 5, 5t
  physiologic, 4–5, 5t
Apoptotic cells, morphologic appearance of, 6, 7f
Apoptotic fragments, clearance of, 6
Appendicitis, 215–216
Arachnodactyly, 90
Arboviruses (arthropod-borne viruses), 286
Architectural disarray, 67, 67f

Page numbers followed by 'f' indicate figures, 'b' indicate boxes, and 't' indicate tables.

Arnold-Chiari malformation, 280t
Arrhythmia, 123, 125–126
Arteriovenous fistulas, 105
Arthritis, 301–305, 302t
    forms of, 303–304
Articular cartilage, degeneration of, 302
AS. See Ankylosing spondylitis
Asbestosis, 170, 170f, 170.e1f
Ascaris lumbricoides, 212
Ascending cholangitis, 234
Ascending infections, placental, 258
Aschoff bodies, 129
Ascorbic acid. See Vitamin C
Aseptic (viral) meningitis, 285, 285t
Aspiration pneumonias, 174
Asthma, 166
    clinical features of, 166
    morphology of, 166, 166.e1f
    pathogenesis of, 166, 167f
Astrocytoma, 292, 292f–293f, 293f
Asystole, 125–126
Ataxia-telangiectasia, 83
Atheromas, 107
Atheromatous plaques, 107, 109f
Atherosclerosis, 107–110
    clinical features of, 109–110
    morphology of, 109, 109f, 109.e1f
    pathogenesis of, 107–109, 108f
Atherosclerotic stenosis, 109
ATI. See Acute tubular injury
Atopic asthma, 166
Atopic dermatitis, 307
Atopy, 42
Atresia, 118
Atrial fibrillation, 135
Atrial natriuretic hormone, 106
Atrial septal defects, 119
Atrophy, 11
Atypical cytotoxic T lymphocytes, 147
Atypical mitoses, 66, 67f
Atypical (or complement-mediated) HUS, 201
Auer rods, 148
Autoantibodies, 160
Autoimmune diseases, 14, 41, 49–52, 50t
    environmental factors of, 50
    genetic susceptibility of, 50
    systemic lupus erythematosus as, 50
    systemic sclerosis (scleroderma) as, 51, 51b
Autoimmune gastritis, 209, 209.e1f
Autoimmune hepatitis, 229, 229.e1f
Autoimmune pancreatitis, 237
Autoimmune thyroid disease, 268
Autoimmunity, 41, 49
    mechanisms of, 49–50, 49b
Autophagy, 6–7, 78
Autosomal dominant disorders, 88
Autosomal dominant polycystic kidney disease, 198, 200f
Autosomal recessive disorders, 83
Autosomal recessive inheritance, 88–89
Autosomal recessive polycystic kidney disease, 198
Avascular necrosis, of bone, 298, 299f
Azoospermia, cystic fibrosis and, 92
Azotemia, 186

B
B cell dysfunction, type 2 diabetes and, 273
Bacillus Calmette-Guérin (BCG), 246

Backward failure, 135
Bacterial (acute pyogenic) meningitis, 285, 285t, 286f
Bacterial cystitis, 245
Balanced reciprocal translocation, 97–98
Balanitis, 240
Balanoposthitis, 240
B-ALL. See B-cell acute lymphoblastic leukemia
Barrett esophagus, 206, 206f
Basal cell carcinoma, 311, 312f
B-cell acute lymphoblastic leukemia (B-ALL), 148, 148t
BCG. See Bacillus Calmette-Guérin
BCL2, overexpression of, 79
BCL2 protein expression, 79
Becker muscular dystrophy, 305–306
Beckwith-Wiedemann syndrome, 203
Benign epithelial lesions, breast, 260, 260.e1f
Benign neoplasms, 63–64, 63b
    characteristics of, 66–69, 66f, 66b
Benign nephrosclerosis, 199
Benign prostatic hyperplasia, 243, 243f
Benign teratomas, ovarian, 258, 258f, 258.e1f
Berry aneurysms, 105
Beta-amyloid (Aβ), 289, 289f
Bicuspid aortic valve, 127
Biliary atresia, 235
Biliary cirrhosis, 233
Biliary system, disorders of, 233–236
    cholangitis, 234
    cholelithiasis, 235
    primary biliary cholangitis, 234–235
    tumors of, 236
Bilirubin-rich gallstones, 137
Bladder cancer, 245, 245f–246f
Blastomyces dermatitidis, 179, 179f
Blastomycosis, 178–179, 179f
Blistering (bullous) disorders, 309–310, 309f
Blood flow, abnormal, 35
Blood vessels, 186
    diseases of, 105–117, 199–202
        aneurysms, 110–112
        atherosclerosis, 107–110
        dissections, 110–112
        hypertension, 106, 106f–107f
        vasculitis, 112–114
    in SLE, 51
    tumors of, and lymphatics, 115–116
        angiosarcomas, 116
        hemangiomas, 115
        Kaposi sarcoma, 115–116, 117f
Bloom syndrome, 83
Bone remodeling, 296
Bones, 296–301
    avascular necrosis of, 298, 299f
    congenital disorders of, 296–297
    metabolic diseases of, 297–298
    metastatic tumors of, 301
    Paget disease of, 298, 298f, 298.e1f
    tumors, 299–301, 300t
Borrelia burgdorferi, 133–134
Bovine spongiform encephalopathy, 287
Bowen disease. See Squamous cell carcinoma in situ
Bradycardia, 125–126
Brain abscess, 285, 285t, 286f
Brain damage, lead poisoning and, 314
Brain infarction, 281–282, 281f–282f

Branching vessel, obstruction of, abdominal aortic aneurysms and, 110
Breast
    female, 260–263
        benign epithelial lesions, 260, 260.e1f
        carcinoma, 261–263, 261t
        inflammatory processes, 260
        origin of disorders, 260f
        stromal neoplasms, 260, 261f
    fibroadenoma of, 68f
    invasive ductal carcinoma of, 68f
Breast carcinoma, 317
Bronchiectasis, 168, 168f
"Brown tumors", 297–298
Budd-Chiari syndrome, 231, 231.e1f
Bullous pemphigoid, 310, 310f
Burkholderia cepacia, 93
Burkitt lymphoma, 152t, 155, 155f

C
C3 glomerulonephritis, 186t, 191, 193f
Cachexia, 320
CAH. See Congenital adrenal hyperplasia
Calcific aortic degeneration, 127–128, 128f
Calcifications, in degenerative valve disease, 127, 128f
Calcium, 13
Calcium pyrophosphate crystal deposition disease, 305, 305.e1f
Calor, 22, 23t
Campylobacter jejuni, 211
Campylobacter spp., 211, 212t
Cancer, 326
    chronic inflammatory disorders and, 72t
    diagnosis, 85, 85b
    epigenetic alterations in, 70
    genes, 74, 74t
    grading and staging of, 84–85
    hallmarks of, 73–83, 73f, 73b
    inherited predisposition to, 72t
    molecular profiling of, 87
    morphologic methods for, 86–87
        cytogenetic markers as, 86, 87t
        nucleic acid markers as, 86–87, 87t
        protein markers as, 86
    role of infectious agents in, 72–73, 72b, 73t
Cancer genes, 69–70, 69b
Candida
    in vaginitis, 251
    in vulvitis, 250
Candida albicans, 180
Candida infection, 220
Candidiasis, of upper respiratory tract, 180–181, 182f
Capillary hemangiomas, 115, 116f
Capillary walls, fluid movement, 31f
Capsule, 68, 68f
Caput medusa, 115
Carcinogenesis, 70–71, 70b, 71f, 316, 316f
Carcinogenic mutations, 71–72, 71b
Carcinoid tumors, 210, 210.e1f
    of lungs, 184, 184f
Carcinoma, 64
    breast, 261–263, 261t
        clinical features of, 263
        epidemiology of, 261–262
        morphology of, 262, 262f–263f
        pathogenesis of, 262

Carcinoma (Continued)
    prostate, 243–244, 244f
    thyroid, 270–271, 271f, 271.e1f
    vulva, 250, 251.e1f
Carcinosarcomas, 64
Cardiac cirrhosis, 136
Cardiac failure, 30
Cardiogenic shock, 38, 39t, 123
Cardiomegaly, 135
Cardiomyopathies, 131–135, 131f, 132t
    dilated, 131–132, 132f
    hypertrophic, 132–133, 133f
    restrictive, 133
Cardiotoxic drugs, 134
Cardiovascular disease, 318
Cardiovascular system
    cocaine in, effects of, 318
    marijuana in, effects of, 318
    in SLE, 51
Caseous necrosis, 3, 5f
Caspases, 5
Catecholamines, 134–135
Cavernous hemangiomas, 115, 116f
CD4+ T cells, 53
Celiac disease, 215, 215f
Cell cycle, 75–76, 76f
    arrest, 77, 78f
Cell death, 1–13.e3, 1–6
    causes of, 1, 1b
    evasion of, 79, 79b
    mechanisms of, 7–11, 7b
    overview of, 1
    pathways of, 6–7
Cell-derived mediators, 20, 21t
Cell injury, 1–13.e3
    mechanisms of, 7b
    toxin-mediated, 9
Cell lineage, 77
Cell-mediated immunity, 41
    in tuberculosis infection, 175
Cell stress, sensors and effectors of, 79
Cell surface receptors, 264
Cells
    pathologic accumulations in, 12–13
    stress and, 1, 1b
Cellular aging, 9–11, 9b, 11f
Cellular dysfunction, 44
Cellular membranes, 7, 8f
Cellular proliferation, in carcinogenic mutations, 71, 71t–72t
Cellular reactions, 17–20, 17b
Cellular senescence, 77
Central nervous system
    effects of cocaine in, 318
    effects of marijuana in, 318
Central tolerance, 49
Centric fusion type translocation, 97–98
Centrilobular necrosis, 30, 136
Cerebral amyloid angiopathy, 283
Cerebral artery thrombosis, 281–282, 281f–282f
Cerebral edema, 280–281, 281.e2f
Cerebral palsy, 284
Cerebrovascular diseases, 281–283
    acute hypertensive encephalopathy, 283
    cerebral amyloid angiopathy, 283
    cerebral artery thrombosis, embolism, and brain infarction, 281–282, 281f–282f

Cerebrovascular diseases (Continued)
    intracranial hemorrhage, 282, 282t, 283f–284f
    with sustained hypertension, 283
Cervical cancer, 317
Cervicitis, 251
Cervix, 251–252
    cervicitis, 251
    invasive carcinoma of, 252
    neoplasia of, 251, 252f
    squamous intraepithelial lesions (SILs), 251–252, 253f
CF. See Cystic fibrosis
CF transmembrane conductance regulator (CFTR) gene, 91
Chagas disease, 133–134
Chagas myocarditis, 134, 134f
Chemical carcinogens, in carcinogenic mutations, 71, 71t
Chemical esophagitis, 206
Chest movement, diseases affecting, 126
Childhood acute leukemia, 100
Chimeric nucleic acid sequences, 86–87
Chlamydia trachomatis
    in cervicitis, 251
    in endometritis, 253
Cholangiocarcinomas, 233, 236, 236.e1f
Cholangitis, 234
Cholecystitis, 235–236
Cholelithiasis, 235
Cholera, 211, 212t
Cholestasis, 233
Cholesterol, 12
Cholesterol esters, 12, 13.e1f
Cholesterol stones, 235, 235.e1f
Cholesterolosis, 13.e1f
Chondrosarcoma, 300, 300.e1f
Choriocarcinoma, 242, 242f, 257t
Chromosomal instability pathway, 217, 218f
Chromosome rearrangements, 69, 70f
Chronic adrenal insufficiency, 277–278
Chronic alcoholism, 316
Chronic cholecystitis, 235–236, 235.e1f
Chronic diarrhea, 211
Chronic inflammation, 15, 15b, 16t, 26–27, 26b
    anemia of, 143, 144f
    cellular reactions of, 26, 26f, 26b
    clinicopathologic features of, 27, 27b
        morphologic features, 27
        systemic manifestations, 27
    cytokines in, 22t
Chronic inflammatory dermatoses, 308
Chronic inflammatory disorders, 72t
Chronic ischemic heart disease, 109
Chronic kidney disease, 187
Chronic liver failure, 223
Chronic lymphocytic (Hashimoto) thyroiditis, 268, 268f
Chronic lymphocytic leukemia, 152–153, 152t, 153f
Chronic lymphoid leukemias, 151–156, 152t
Chronic meningitis, 285, 285t, 286f
Chronic myeloid leukemia (CML), 148t, 150–151, 150f
Chronic obstructive pulmonary disease (COPD), 165–166, 316
    clinical features of, 165–166
    morphology of, 165, 165f–166f
    pathogenesis of, 165

Chronic pancreatitis, 237, 237f
Chronic pyelonephritis, 196, 197f
Chronic rejection, 53, 55f
Chronic thromboembolic pulmonary hypertension, 172
Chronic traumatic encephalopathy, 284
Chronic viral hepatitis, 227
Cigarette smoking, 315
    adverse effects of, 315, 315f
Ciliopathy, 198
CIMP. See CpG island methylator phenotype
Circulating tumor markers, 86, 87t
Circulatory disorders, of liver, 231, 231f
Cirrhosis, 228
CJD. See Creutzfeldt-Jakob disease
Classic KS, 115
Classical pathway, 44
Claudication, intermittent, 109
Clear cell carcinoma, 202
Clonal hematopoiesis, 109
Clostridium difficile, 211, 211.e1f
CML. See Chronic myeloid leukemia
Coagulation cascade, 33–34, 34f
Coagulation control, 34–35, 34f
Coagulation disorders, of hematopoietic system, 160–162
Coagulative necrosis, 3, 4f
Coagulopathy, in liver disease, 222–223
Coarctation
    of aorta, 120–121, 121f
    postductal, without patent ductus, 121
    preductal, with patent ductus, 121
Cobalamin deficiency anemia, 145–146
Cocaine, 318
Coccidioides immitis, 179, 179f
Coccidioidomycosis, 178–179, 179f
Colloid, 267
Comminuted fractures, 298
Common variable immunodeficiency, 56
Community-acquired bacterial pneumonias, 173–174, 173f–174f
Community-acquired viral pneumonias, 173t, 177–179, 178.e1f
Compensated heart failure, 135
Complement activation, 21
Complement-mediated HUS, 201t
Complement system, 21
Compound fractures, 298
Concussion, 284
Condyloma acuminatum, 250, 251f
Condylomata acuminata, 249, 249.e1f
    of penis, 249.e1f
Condylomata lata, 247
Congenital adrenal hyperplasia (CAH), 276–277
Congenital anomalies, heart and, 118
Congenital disorders, causing jaundice, 235
Congenital early onset diabetes, 273–274
Congenital heart disease, 100, 118–121, 119t
    malformations associated with left-to-right shunts, 119–120, 119f
    malformations associated with right-to-left shunts, 120, 120f
    malformations leading to obstruction, 120–121
Congenital hypothyroidism, 267–268
Congenital immunodeficiency, 56
Congenital malformations, of CNS, 280, 280t
Congenital syphilis, 247

Congenital vascular anomalies, 105
Congestion
    clinical features of, 31
    morphology of, 30–31
    pathogenesis of, 30b
Congestive heart failure, 135–136
Congestive hepatomegaly, 136
Congestive splenomegaly, 136
Conjugated bilirubin, 233
Consumptive coagulopathy, 161
Contractile dysfunction, 123
Contrecoup injury, 283–284
Contusions, 283–284
COPD. *See* Chronic obstructive pulmonary
    disease
Cor pulmonale, 126, 136
Corticotroph adenoma, 265t, 266
Coup injury, 283–284
CpG island methylator phenotype (CIMP), 218
Craniopharyngioma, 267, 267.e1f
Crescendo angina, 121
Crescentic GN, 193
Creutzfeldt-Jakob disease (CJD), 287, 287f
Crigler-Najjar syndrome, 235
Critical stenosis, 109
Crohn disease, 213–214, 213f–214f, 213t
Cryptococcosis, 181, 182f
Cryptococcus gattii, 181
Cryptococcus neoformans, 181
Cryptorchidism, 240, 240.e1f
Curling ulcers, 208
Cushing disease, 276
Cushing syndrome, 84, 276, 276f–277f
Cushing ulcers, 208
Cyanosis, 118
Cystic diseases, 198–199
Cystic fibrosis (CF), 91–93, 92f–93f
Cystic medial degeneration, 111, 111.e1f
Cystic medionecrosis, 90
Cystic tumors, of pancreas, 237
Cysticercosis, 286
Cystine stones, 201–202
Cytogenetic disorders, 97–101
    involving autosomes, 98–100, 99f
    involving sex chromosomes, 100–101
    numerical abnormalities in, 97
    structural abnormalities in, 97–98, 98f
Cytogenetic markers, 86, 87t
Cytokines, 21, 17b, 43
    of acute and chronic inflammation, 22t
Cytologic (Papanicolaou) preparations, for cancer,
    86, 86f
Cytomegalovirus (CMV) infection, 180, 180f

D
Dandy-Walker malformation, 280t
DDD. *See* Dense deposit disease
Death receptor (extrinsic) pathway, of apoptosis,
    5–6
Decompensated heart failure, 135
Deep venous thromboses (DVTs), 36
Deficiency of galactocerebroside β–galactosidase,
    287
Degenerative joint disease (osteoarthritis), 326
Degenerative valve disease, 127
Delayed-type hypersensitivity, 47–48
Deletion 22 syndrome, 100
Deletion, of chromosomes, 98

Demyelinating diseases, 287–288, 287f–288f
Dendritic cells, 16
Dense deposit disease (DDD), 186t, 191, 193f
Denys-Drash syndrome, 203
Dermatitis herpetiformis, 310, 310.e1f
Dermatomyositis, 305.e1f, 306
DHT. *See* Dihydrotestosterone
Diabetes mellitus, 272–276
    clinicopathologic features of, 274–276, 274f
    insulin physiology, 272–273, 272f
    other forms of, 273–274
    overview of, 272
    pathogenesis of, 273
    type 1, 273
    type 2, 273, 273f
Diabetic nephropathy, 186t, 191–192, 275, 275f
Diabetic neuropathy, 276, 295
Diabetic retinopathy, 275–276
Diacylglycerol, 274
Diarrheal diseases, 211
Diastolic failure, 135
DIC. *See* Disseminated intravascular coagulation
Diffuse alveolar hemorrhage syndromes, 172
Diffuse astrocytomas, 292
Diffuse axonal injury, 284
Diffuse large B cell lymphoma (DLCBL), 152t,
    154, 155f
Diffuse lupus nephritis, 193
DiGeorge syndrome (thymic hypoplasia), 57, 100
Dihydrotestosterone (DHT), 243
Dilated cardiomyopathy, 131–132
    clinical features of, 132
    morphology of, 132, 132f
    pathogenesis of, 131
Direct bilirubin, 233
Direct implantation, of microbes, 284
Dissections, 110–112
    aortic, 111–112, 111f
Disseminated intravascular coagulation (DIC),
    161–162, 161f, 162t
Diverticulitis, 215
Diverticulosis, 215
DLCBL. *See* Diffuse large B cell lymphoma
DNA damage, 9, 9b
DNA rearrangement, 71
Dolor, 22, 23t
Dominant negative protein, 88
Double-barreled aorta, 111
Double-hit lymphoma, 155
Down syndrome, 98–100
"Driver" mutations, 69–70, 69b, 71b
Drug-induced hepatitis, 229–230
Drug-induced tubulointerstitial nephritis, 197,
    198f
Drug-related eczematous dermatitis, 307
Drugs of abuse, injury by, 318
Dry gangrene, 3
Dubin-Johnson syndrome, 235
Duchenne muscular dystrophy, 305–306, 305f
Duret hemorrhages, 281, 281.e2f
DVTs. *See* Deep venous thromboses
Dwarfism, 296
Dysfunctional uterine bleeding, 254
Dysgerminoma, 257t
Dysostoses, 296
Dysplasia, 67, 67f, 67b, 296
Dyspnea, 135, 165–166
Dystrophic calcification, 13

Dystrophic neurites, 289
Dystrophin, 305–306
Dystrophin gene, 305–306
Dystrophinopathies, 305

E
Early-phase reaction, of asthma, 166
Ecchymoses, 32
Echinococcal infections, 228
Eclampsia, 259–260
Ectopia lentis, 90
Ectopic pregnancy, 258
Eczema, 307
Edema
    clinical features of, 31
    morphology of, 30–31
    pathogenesis of, 30b, 31t
EDSs. *See* Ehlers-Danlos syndromes
Effusion, 30, 31t
Ehlers-Danlos syndromes (EDSs), 90
Eisenmenger syndrome, 118
Elementary body, 249
Elephantiasis, 240
Embolism, 30, 36b, 281–282, 281f–282f
    abdominal aortic aneurysms and, 110
    of atheromas, 109
    paradoxical, 119
    types of, 37
Embryonal carcinoma, 241, 242f
Encephalitis, 284, 285t
Encephalocele, 280t
Endemic African KS, 115
Endemic goiter, 269
Endocardial infarcts, 122
Endocrine pancreas, 236, 272–276
Endocrine system, 264–279
    adrenal glands, 276–279
        Addison disease, 277–278
        adrenal medulla tumors, 278–279, 278f
        adrenogenital syndromes, 276–277
        Cushing syndrome, 276, 276f–277f
        hyperaldosteronism, 276
        multiple endocrine neoplasia (MEN)
            syndromes, 279
    endocrine pancreas, 272–276
    overview of, 264
    parathyroid glands, 272
    pituitary glands, 264–267
        craniopharyngioma, 267, 267.e1f
        hyperpituitarism, 265–266, 265t
        hypopituitarism, 266
        posterior pituitary syndromes, 267
    thyroid, 267–271
        adenoma, 270, 270f
        autoimmune thyroid disease, 268
        carcinoma, 270–271, 271f, 271.e1f
        chronic lymphocytic (Hashimoto) thyroiditis,
            268, 268f
        goiter, 269, 269f, 269.e1f
        Graves disease, 268
        hyperthyroidism, 267, 267.e1f
        hypothyroidism, 267–268
        Riedel thyroiditis, 269
        subacute granulomatous (de Quervain)
            thyroiditis, 269, 269.e1f
        subacute lymphocytic thyroiditis, 269
        tumors of, 269
Endometrial cancer, 317

Endometrial carcinoma, 254, 255f
Endometrial hyperplasia, 254, 254.e1f
Endometrial intraepithelial neoplasia, 254
Endometrioid carcinoma, 254
Endometriosis, 253–254, 253f, 253.e1f
Endometritis, 253
Endometrium, proliferative lesions of, 254
Endomyocardial fibrosis, 133
Endoplasmic reticulum (ER)
    stress, 9, 9b, 10f
    swelling of, 1
Endothelial activation, 18f, 19
    in septic shock, 39
Endothelial injury, atherosclerosis and, 107
End-stage renal disease, 187
Entamoeba histolytica, 213, 228
Enteric (typhoid) fever, 212t
Enteroaggregative E. coli, 212t
Enterohemorrhagic E. coli, 211, 212t
Enteroinvasive E. coli, 211, 212t
Enteropathogenic E. coli, 212t
Enteropathy-associated T-cell lymphoma, 215
Enterotoxigenic E. coli, 212t
Envelope glycoproteins, 224
Environmental antigens, reactions against, 42
Environmental disease, 314–326
Eosinophilic esophagitis, 206, 206f
Eosinophils, 16
Ependymomas, 293, 293.e1f
Epidermal edema (spongiosis), 307
Epididymis, 240–242
Epidural hematomas, 282
Epithelioid cells, 27
Epstein-Barr virus (EBV)-associated diffuse large
    B-cell lymphoma, 154
ER. See Endoplasmic reticulum
Erythema multiforme, 308
Erythroplakia, 220, 220.e2f
Escherichia coli, 195, 211, 212t
Esophageal lacerations, 206
Esophageal obstruction, 205
Esophageal tumors, 207, 207.e1f
Esophageal varices, 115, 205, 205.e1f
Esophagitis, 180, 205–207, 206f
    chemical, 206
    eosinophilic, 206, 206f
    infectious, 206, 206.e1f
    reflux, 206, 206.e1f
    viral, 206.e1f
Esophagus, disorders of, 205–207
Essential hypertension, 106
Ethanol, 316
Eunuchoid body habitus, in Klinefelter syndrome,
    100
Euploid, 97
Ewing sarcoma, 300, 302f
Excess free fatty acids, 228
Exogenous estrogens, 317
Exophthalmos, 268
Exostosis, 299
Extracellular destruction, 20
Extracellular matrix
    alterations in, degenerative valve disease and,
        127
    invasion of, 80–81
Extrahepatic obstruction, of liver, 231
Extranodal marginal zone lymphoma, 152t,
    153–154

Extravascular hemolysis, 137
Extrinsic pathway, 33
Exudative diarrhea, 211

F
Factor V Leiden, 35
Fallopian tubes, 256, 256f
Familial adenomatous polyposis, 217, 218f
Familial hypercholesterolemia, 90–91, 91f
Familial juvenile nephronophthisis, 198–199
Fanconi anemia, 83
Fasting, 273
Fat embolism, 37, 38.e1f
Fatty liver, 13.e1f, 228, 229f
Fecalith, 215–216
Fetus, effects of cocaine in, 318
Fever
    in acute inflammation, 25
    in chronic inflammation, 27
Fibrillin, 90
Fibrinoid necrosis, 3, 5f, 199
Fibrinous inflammation, 23, 24f
Fibroadenoma, of breast, 68f
Fibrocystin, 198
Fibromuscular dysplasia, 105
Fibrosing disease, 168–169, 169f, 169.e1f
Fibrous scar, 28
Fine-needle aspiration (FNA), for cancer, 86
FISH. See Fluorescence in situ hybridization
Floppy valve syndrome, 90
Flow cytometry, 86
Fluorescence in situ hybridization (FISH), 102,
    104f
FNA. See Fine-needle aspiration
FNH. See Focal nodular hyperplasia
Focal nodular hyperplasia (FNH), 232, 232f
Focal segmental glomerulosclerosis (FSGS), 186t,
    189–191, 191f
Folate deficiency anemia, 145
Follicular carcinoma, 270, 271f
Follicular lymphoma, 152t, 153, 154f
Forebrain malformations, 280t
Foreign bodies, inflammation and, 14
Forward failure, 135
Fractures, 298
    poor healing of, in lead exposure, 315
Fragile X syndrome, 101–102
Frank-Starling mechanism, 135
Frataxin, 291
Free fatty acids, 228
Frontotemporal lobar degeneration, 289–290, 290.
    e1f
FSGS. See Focal segmental glomerulosclerosis
Fulminant liver failure, 222
Fungal encephalitis, 285t
Fungal infections, of upper respiratory tract,
    179–180

G
Gallbladder
    adenocarcinoma, 236.e1f
    carcinoma of, 236
Gangliosides, 94
Gangrenous cholecystitis, 235
Gangrenous necrosis, 3
Gastric adenocarcinomas, 209–210, 210f
Gastric adenoma, 209, 209.e1f
Gastric lymphomas, 210, 210.e1f

Gastric polyps, 209, 209.e1f
Gastritis, 207–208, 207f
    Helicobacter pylori, 208, 208f
    stress-related, 208
Gastroesophageal reflux disease (GERD), 206,
    206.e1f
Gastrointestinal stromal tumors (GISTs), 210–211,
    210.e1f
Gastrointestinal system, 205–221.e1
    congenital anomalies of, 205, 205.e1f
    esophagus, disorders of, 205–207
    oral cavity and salivary glands, disorders of,
        220–221
    small and large intestines, disorders of,
        211–220, 212t
    stomach, disorders of, 207–211
Gastropathy, 207
Gaucher cells, 95, 96f
Gaucher disease, 95, 96f
Gender, atherosclerosis and, 109
Gene amplifications, 69, 70f
Generalized osteitis fibrosa cystica, 297–298
Genes, modifier, 88
Genetic analysis, indications for, 104
Genetic diseases, 88–104
    complex multigenic disorders, 96–97
    cytogenetic disorders, 97–101
        involving autosomes, 98–100, 99f
        involving sex chromosomes, 100–101
        numerical abnormalities in, 97
        structural abnormalities in, 97–98, 98f
    diagnosis of, 102–104
    Mendelian disorders, 88–96
        biochemical basis and inheritance patterns
            of, 89t
        prevalence of, 89t
    single-gene disorders, 88–96
        with atypical patterns of inheritance, 101–102
        Ehlers-Danlos syndromes, 90
        mutations in genes encoding enzyme
            proteins, 93–96
        mutations in genes encoding receptor
            proteins or channels, 90–93
        mutations in genes encoding structural
            protein, 90
        transmission patterns of, 88–90
    testing modalities for, 103t
Genetic factors, in osteoarthritis, 302
Genetic heterogeneity, 70–71
Genetic test, modalities and applications of,
    102–104, 104f
Genetics
    atherosclerosis and, 108
    type 2 diabetes and, 273
Genital herpes simplex, 249
Genital tract, female, 250–263
    cervix, 251–252
        cervicitis, 251
        invasive carcinoma of, 252
        neoplasia of, 251, 252f
        squamous intraepithelial lesions (SILs),
            251–252, 253f
    fallopian tubes, 256, 256f
    ovaries, 256–258
        surface epithelial tumors, 256, 256f–257f
        tumors of, 256, 257t
    pregnancy diseases, 258–260
        ectopic pregnancy, 258

Genital tract, female (Continued)
 gestational choriocarcinoma, 259, 259f, 259.e1f
 gestational trophoblastic disease, 258
 hydatidiform mole, 258–259, 259f, 259.e1f
 placental inflammations and infections, 258
 preeclampsia and eclampsia, 259–260
 uterus, 253–256
  abnormal uterine bleeding, 254, 254t
  endometrial carcinoma, 254, 255f
  endometrial hyperplasia, 254, 254.e1f
  endometriosis, 253–254, 253f, 253.e1f
  endometritis, 253
  leiomyoma, 254–256, 255f
  leiomyosarcoma, 256, 256.e1f
  proliferative lesions of the endometrium and myometrium, 254
 vagina, 250–251
 vulva, 250
Genomic instability, 83
GERD. See Gastroesophageal reflux disease
Germ cell neoplasia in situ, 241
Germ cell origin tumors, 257t
Gestational choriocarcinoma, 259, 259f, 259.e1f
Gestational trophoblastic disease, 258
Giant cell myocarditis, 134, 134f
Giant cell (temporal) arteritis, 112, 112f
Giant cell tumor, 299, 299.e1f
Giardia lamblia, 213
Gilbert syndrome, 235
GISTs. See Gastrointestinal stromal tumors
Gleason system, 244
Glioblastoma (grade IV tumor), 293, 293f
Glomerular diseases, 186t, 187–194
Glomerular injury, mechanisms of, 187, 189f
Glomeruli, 186
Glucagon, 273
Glucocerebrosidase, 95
Glucose, 272
 intracellular concentrations of, 274
Glucose-6-phosphate dehydrogenase deficiency (GPD), 142, 142.e1f
Gluten enteropathy, 215
Glycogen, 13
Glycogen storage diseases, 96, 97t
Glycogenoses, 96
 hepatic type, 96, 97f, 97t
 myopathic type, 96, 97t
 Pompe disease (type II glycogenosis), 96, 97t, 97.e1f
 subgroups of, 97t
G_{M2} Gangliosidosis, 94
Goiter, 269, 269f, 269.e1f
Gonadotroph adenomas, 265t, 266
Gonorrhea, 248–249, 248.e1f
Goodpasture syndrome, 172, 193
Gout, 304–305, 304f
 lead exposure and, 315
Gradual remodeling, of fracture, 298
Graft rejection, treatment of, 53–54
Graft-versus-host disease (GVHD), 54–56
Granulomas, 27, 27f
Granulomatosis, 172
Granulomatous disease, of upper respiratory tract, 170–171
Granulomatous inflammation, in tuberculosis infection, 175
Granulosa-theca cell, 257t

Graves disease, 268
Great arteries, transposition of, 120, 120f, 120.e1f
Greenstick fractures, 298
Growth factor receptors, 74–75
Growth-inhibitory signals, insensitivity to, 75–77, 75b
Guillain-Barre syndrome, 295
Gumma, formation of, 247, 247.e1f
Gut hormones, 323
Gut microbiome, 228
GVHD. See Graft-versus-host disease

H

Haemophilus influenzae, 173
Hairy cell leukemia, 152t, 155
Hamartomatous polyps, 216
Hand-Schüller-Christian triad, 158
Hashimoto thyroiditis, 268, 268f
HAV. See Hepatitis A virus
HbH disease, 140
HBV. See Hepatitis B virus
HBx protein, 224
HCC. See Hepatocellular carcinoma
HCV. See Hepatitis C virus
HDV. See Hepatitis D virus
Heart, 118–136.e1, 118
 arrhythmia, 123, 125–126
 cardiac tumors of, 136
 cardiomyopathies, 131–135, 131f, 132t
  dilated, 131–132, 132f
  hypertrophic, 132–133, 133f
  restrictive, 133
 congenital heart disease, 118–121, 119t
  malformations associated with left-to-right shunts, 119–120, 119f
  malformations associated with right-to-left shunts, 120, 120f
  malformations leading to obstruction, 120–121
 congestive heart failure, 135–136
 hypertensive heart disease, 126, 127f
 ischemic heart disease, 121–125
  angina pectoris, 121
  chronic, 125
  myocardial infarction, 121–125
 myocarditis, 131–135, 134f
 valvular heart disease, 126–131, 127t
  calcific aortic degeneration, 127–128, 128f
  degenerative valve disease, 127
  infective endocarditis, 130–131, 130f
  myxomatous mitral valve disease, 128, 128f
  nonbacterial thrombotic endocarditis, 131, 131.e1f
  rheumatic valvular disease, 128–130
Heart disease, pulmonary hypertension from, 172
Heart failure cells, 30
Heberden nodes, 302
Helicobacter pylori gastritis, 208, 208f
Hemangiomas, 115
Hematogenous spread, of infection, 284
Hematoma, 31, 32f
Hematopoiesis, ineffective, 145
Hematopoietic stem cell transplantation, 54–56, 288
Hematopoietic system, 137–162
 anemias of, 137–146, 138t
  hemolytic, 137–139
  hereditary spherocytosis, 139, 139f

Hematopoietic system (Continued)
  megaloblastic, 145–146, 145f
  sickle cell, 139–143, 139f–140f
  underproduction, 143–145
 bleeding disorders of, 158–162, 159t
  coagulation disorders, 160–162
  heparin-induced thrombocytopenia, 160
  immune thrombocytopenic purpura, 159–160
  thrombocytopenia, 159, 159t
  thrombotic microangiopathies, 160
 splenomegaly of, 162, 162t
 thymus of, disorders of, 162
 white cell disorders of, 146–158
  neoplastic proliferations, 147–158, 148t
  nonneoplastic, 146–147
Hemizygosity, 89
Hemochromatosis, 230–231
Hemodynamic disorders, 30–40
Hemodynamic factors, atherosclerosis and, 108
Hemoglobinemia, 137
Hemoglobinuria, 137
Hemolytic anemia, 137–139
Hemolytic-uremic syndrome (HUS), 199
Hemophilia A, 161
Hemophilia B-factor IX deficiency, 161
Hemorrhage, 31–32, 31b, 32f
 of atheromas, 109
Hemorrhagic cystitis, 245
Hemorrhoids, 115
Hemosiderin, 13, 13.e2f, 135
Hemosiderinuria, 139
Hemostasis, 32b, 33f
Heparin-induced thrombocytopenia, 160
Heparin-induced thrombocytopenia (HIT) syndrome, 35–36
Hepatic adenoma, 232, 232.e1f, 318
Hepatic encephalopathy, 222
Hepatic necrosis, 222
Hepatic vein thrombosis, 231
Hepatitis
 drug- and toxin-induced, 229–230
 other forms of, 229
Hepatitis A virus (HAV), 223, 224t
Hepatitis B virus (HBV), 223–225, 224f–225f, 224t, 227f
Hepatitis C virus (HCV), 224t, 225, 226f–227f
Hepatitis D virus (HDV), 224t, 225
Hepatitis E virus (HEV), 224t, 225–226, 226f
Hepatocellular carcinoma (HCC), 228, 232–233, 233f
Hepatomegaly, 151
Hepatorenal syndrome, 223
Hepatosplenomegaly, 94
Hereditary Fe [iron] (HFE), 230
Hereditary hemochromatosis, 230, 231f
Hereditary nephritis, 186t, 194
Hereditary nonpolyposis colon cancer syndrome, 83
Hereditary nonpolyposis colorectal cancer syndrome, 217–218
Hereditary spherocytosis (HS), 139, 139f
Herniation, 280–281, 281f
 of intestine, 219
Herpes simplex virus (HSV), 285
 infection, 220
 in vulvitis, 250
HEV. See Hepatitis E virus

HFE. *See* Hereditary Fe [iron]
High-grade serous tumors, 256, 256.e1f
High-grade SIL, 251
Hirschsprung disease, 219
Histamine, 20, 43
Histiocytic neoplasms, of hematopoietic system, 158
Histoplasma capsulatum, 179, 179f
Histoplasmosis, 178–179, 179f
HIV. *See* Human immunodeficiency virus
Hodgkin lymphoma, 156–157, 156f
Homeostasis, 1
Honeycomb fibrosis, 169
"Honeycomb" lung, 168
Hormone production, 84
Hormone-receptor complex, 267
Hormones, decreased levels of, osteoporosis and, 297
Host cells, genes regulate, 69
HPV. *See* Human papillomavirus
HPV-negative squamous carcinoma, 250
HS. *See* Hereditary spherocytosis
HSV. *See* Herpes simplex virus
HSV-2, in cervicitis, 251
Human herpesvirus type 8 (HHV8), 154–155
Human immunodeficiency virus (HIV), 286
    clinical course, 59, 60f
    pathogenesis of, 59, 59b, 60f
    structure and life cycle in, 58–59, 58f, 58b
Human papillomavirus (HPV)
    infection, 249
    in neoplasia of cervix, 251
    in vulvitis, 250
Humoral immunity, 41
Hunter syndrome, 96
Huntington disease, 291, 291f
Hurler syndrome, 96
HUS. *See* Hemolytic-uremic syndrome
Hutchinson triad, 247
Hyaline arteriolosclerosis, 106, 108f, 199
Hyaline membranes, of alveoli, 163
Hydatidiform mole, 258–259, 259f, 259.e1f
Hydrocephalus, 280–281, 281.e1f
Hydronephrosis, 202, 202f
Hyperacute rejection, 53, 54f
Hyperaldosteronism, 276
Hyperbilirubinemia, 137
Hypercalcemia, 84, 272
Hypercholesterolemia, 107–108
Hypercoagulability, 35, 35t, 84
Hypercortisolism, 276, 276f–277f
Hyperemia
    clinical features of, 31
    morphology of, 30–31
    pathogenesis of, 30b
Hypermethylation, of CpG island, 218
Hyperparathyroidism, 272, 297–298, 297.e1f
Hyperpituitarism, 265–266, 265t
Hyperplasia, 11
Hyperplastic arteriolosclerosis, 106, 108f
Hyperplastic arteriosclerosis, 199
Hyperplastic polyps, 216
Hypersensitivity disorders, 41–48, 41b
Hypersensitivity myocarditis, 134, 134f
Hypersensitivity, occurrence of, 14
Hypersensitivity pneumonitis, 171, 171t, 171.e1f
Hypersensitivity reactions, 41, 42t, 42b
Hypertension, 198

Hypertensive heart disease, 126, 127f
Hyperthyroidism, 267, 267.e1f
Hypertrophic cardiomyopathy, 132–133, 133f
Hypertrophy, 11, 12f
Hypocalcemia, 322
Hypogonadism, in Klinefelter syndrome, 100
Hypoparathyroidism, 272
Hypophosphatemia, 322
Hypopituitarism, 266
Hypospadias, 240
Hypotension, 106
Hypothyroidism, 267–268
Hypoventilation syndrome, 326
Hypovolemic shock, 38, 39t
Hypoxia, 8–9, 8f–9f, 8b
    pulmonary hypertension from, 172
Hypoxic encephalopathy, 135–136

I

IBD. *See* Inflammatory bowel disease
Icterus, 222
Idiopathic pulmonary fibrosis, 168–169, 169f, 169.e1f
Idiosyncratic reactions, drug-and toxin-induced hepatitis and, 230
IgA nephropathy, 186t, 194, 194.e1f
IgG4-related disease, 245
Immediate (type I) hypersensitivity, 42–44, 42b, 43f
    clinical features of, 43–44, 44t
    morphology of, 43
    pathogenesis of, 42–43, 44f
Immune complex deposition, 187
Immune complex-mediated (type III) hypersensitivity, 47, 42, 47
    clinical features of, 47, 47t
    morphology of, 47
    pathogenesis of, 47, 47f
Immune deficiency, 321
Immune escape, 82–83, 82f
Immune hydrops, 142
Immune-mediated demyelination, 287
Immune reactions, 14
Immune surveillance, evasion of, 81–83, 81b
Immune system, diseases of, 41–62
Immune thrombocytopenic purpura, 159–160
Immunocyte-associated amyloidosis, 158
Immunodeficiency disorders, 56–57, 56b
Immunohemolytic anemia, 142, 142t
Immunohistochemistry, 86
Impingement, abdominal aortic aneurysms and, 110
Inclusion body myositis, 306
Indirect bilirubin, 233
"Infantile" form, of coarctation, 120
Infarction, 3, 37–38, 37b
    morphology of, 38, 38f
Infection
    in CNS, 284–287, 285f–286f, 285t, 286.e1f
    dilated cardiomyopathy and, 131
    of epididymis, 241
    Helicobacter pylori causing, 208
    opiates and, 318
    placental, 258
Infectious diarrhea, 211–213
Infectious esophagitis, 206, 206.e1f
Infectious mononucleosis, 147
Infectious vasculitis, 114

Infective endocarditis, 130–131, 130f
Infertility
    cystic fibrosis and, 92
    Klinefelter syndrome and, 100
Inflammation, 30, 44, 228
    acute and chronic, 15, 15b, 16t
    cells of, 15–16, 15b
    chronic, low-level of, osteoarthritis and, 302
    in COPD, 165
    definition of, 14b
    features of, 22
    major causes of, 14, 14b
    mediators of, 20–23, 20b, 21t, 23t
    placental, 258
    and repair, 14–29.e1, 27–29, 27b, 28f
    substances that triggered, 19, 19f
Inflammatory bowel disease (IBD), 213–215, 213f
Inflammatory diseases, 215–216
Inflammatory/infectious lesions, in penis, 240
Inflammatory lesions, of penis, 240
Inflammatory processes, in breast, 260
Inflammatory responses
    in septic shock, 39
    sequential steps in, 14, 14b, 15f
Influenza, 178–179
Inherited defects, 235
Inherited gene defects, dilated cardiomyopathy and, 131
Inherited metabolic disease, of liver, 230–231
Inherited syndromes, associated with CNS tumors, 294
Inhibitory receptors, 50
Innate immunity, 41
Insufficiency, in valvular heart disease, 126
Insulin resistance, 228
Integrin activation, 18f, 19
Intermittent gross hematuria, 198
Interstitium, 186
Intestinal obstruction, 219, 220f
Intracellular concentrations, of glucose, 274
Intracellular destruction, 19f, 20
Intracellular receptors, 264
Intracranial hemorrhage, 282, 282t, 283f–284f
Intrahepatic obstruction, of liver, 231
Intrauterine growth retardation, 316
Intravascular hemolysis, 137
Intrinsic pathway, 33
Intussusception, 219
Invasion
    of cancer cells, 80–81, 80b
    of extracellular matrix, 80–81
Invasive candidiasis, 180
Invasive carcinoma, of cervix, 252
Invasive ductal carcinoma, of breast, 68f
Inversions, of chromosomes, 98
Ionizing radiation, injury produced by, 318–319, 319f
Iron deficiency anemia, 143–145, 145f
Iron overload, dilated cardiomyopathy and, 131
Ischemia, 8–9, 8f–9f, 8b
Ischemia-reperfusion injury, 8–9, 8b
Ischemic bowel disease, 220, 220.e1f
Ischemic heart disease, 121–125
    angina pectoris, 121
    chronic, 125
    myocardial infarction, 121–125
Ischemic necrosis of the legs (gangrene), diabetes and, 275

Ischemic necrosis of the pituitary (Sheehan syndrome), 266
Islets of Langerhans, 272
Isochromosomes, 98

J

Jaundice, 137, 222
    congenital disorders causing, 235
    major causes of, 233t
JIA. *See* Juvenile idiopathic arthritis
"Joint mice", 302
Joints, 301–305
    in SLE, 51
Juvenile hemangiomas, 115
Juvenile idiopathic arthritis (JIA), 303

K

Kaposi sarcoma herpesvirus (KSHV), 154–155
Kaposi sarcoma (KS), 115–116, 117f
Karyolysis, 3
Karyorrhexis, 3
Kawasaki disease, 114
Kayser-Fleischer rings, 231
Keratoconjunctivitis sicca, 52
Keratomalacia, 321
Kidney, 186–204
    blood vessels, diseases of, 199–202
    diseases, 186–187
    glomerular diseases, 186t, 187–194
    in SLE, 51
    structural components of, 186
    tubules and interstitium, disease of, 195–199
    tumors of, 202–204
Klatskin tumors, 236
Klebsiella pneumoniae, 173
Klinefelter syndrome, 100
Krabbe disease, 287, 287.e1f
KS. *See* Kaposi sarcoma
KSHV. *See* Kaposi sarcoma herpesvirus
Kupffer cells, 16
Kwashiorkor, 320

L

Lactase (disaccharidase) deficiency, 211
Lactotroph adenoma, 265–266, 265t
Lacunar infarcts, 281
Lambert-Eaton syndrome, 295
Langerhans cell histiocytoses, 158
Large cell carcinomas, of lung, 183
Large deletions, 69
Large intestine, disorders of, 211–220, 212t
Larynx, carcinoma of, 185
Late-phase reaction, of asthma, 166
Lead poisoning, 314–315, 314f–315f
Lectin pathway, 44
Left-sided cardiac failure, 30
Left-sided heart failure, 135–136
Left-sided (systemic) hypertensive heart disease, 126, 127f
Left-to-right shunts, 118
    malformations associated with, 119–120, 119f
Legionella pneumophila, 173
Legionnaire disease, 173
Leiomyoma, 254–256, 255f
Leiomyosarcoma, 256, 256.e1f
Leptin, 323
Letterer-Siwe disease, 158
Leukemias, 64

Leukemoid reactions, in reactive leukocytosis, 146–147
Leukocyte margination, 17, 18f, 18t
Leukocyte rolling, 18f, 19
Leukocyte transmigration, 19
Leukocytosis, 25
    reactive, 146–147, 147f, 147t
Leukodystrophies, 287–288
Leukoerythroblastosis, 146, 151
Leukopenia, 146
Leukoplakia, 220, 220.e2f
Leukotrienes, 20
Limitless replicative potential (immortality), 79–80, 79b
Lines of Zahn, 36
Lipid mediators, 43
Lipofuscin, 13, 13.e2f
Lipoproteins, accumulation of, atherosclerosis and, 107
Lipoxins, 16–21
Liquefactive necrosis, 3, 4f
Liquid biopsy, 102
Liver, disorders of, 160, 222–233
    alcoholic liver disease, 228
    circulatory, 231, 231f
    clinical consequences of, 222–223
    drug- and toxin-induced hepatitis, 229–230
    infections of, 228
    inherited metabolic disease, 230–231
    laboratory evaluation of, 223t
    nodules and tumors, 231–233
    nonalcoholic fatty liver disease, 228–229
    other forms of hepatitis, 229
    other infections of, 228
    viral hepatitis, 223–226
Liver fluke infection, 228
Liver involvement, cystic fibrosis and, 92
Local extension, of infection, 284
Loeffler endomyocarditis, 133
Long QT syndrome, 126
Low-grade SIL (LSIL), 251
Lung abscess, 174–175, 174.e1f
Lung carcinoma, 181–184, 183f–184f
    clinical features of, 183–184
    morphology of, 182–183, 183f–184f
    pathogenesis of, 181–182
Lung disease, pulmonary hypertension from, 172
Lupus nephritis, 186t, 193, 195f
Lyme arthritis, 304
Lyme disease, 133–134
Lymphadenitis, reactive, 147
Lymphocytes, 16
Lymphocytic lymphoma, small, 152–153, 152t, 153f
Lymphoid leukemias, chronic, 151–156, 152t
Lymphomas, 64
Lymphomas, gastric, 210, 210.e1f
Lymphoplasmacytic lymphoma, 158
Lyonization, 89–90
Lysosomal enzymes, 20
Lysosomal storage diseases, 93–94, 94f, 95t
Lysosomes, 93–94
Lysyl hydroxylase, deficiency of, 90

M

Macroovalocytes (MCV), in megaloblastic anemia, 145
Macrophages, 7
    entry of mycobacteria in, 175

Malabsorptive diarrhea, 211
Malakoplakia, 245, 245.e1f
Malaria, 142–143, 143f, 286
Malformations, of penis, 240
Malignant hypertension, 106, 199, 201f
Malignant mesothelioma, 184–185, 185f
Malignant neoplasms, 63–64, 63b
    characteristics of, 66–69, 66f, 66b
    spread by, 69
Malignant teratomas, ovarian, 258, 258.e1f
Malnutrition, 319–320
Mammosomatotroph adenomas, 265t
Mantle cell lymphoma, 152t, 153
Marasmus, 320
Marfan syndrome, 90
Marginal zone lymphoma, extranodal, 152t, 153–154
Marijuana, 318
Marrow infiltration, anemia from, 146
Mast cells, 16
Maturity-onset diabetes of the young (MODY), 273–274
McArdle disease (type V glycogenosis), 96, 97t
MCV. *See* Macroovalocytes
MDS. *See* Myelodysplastic syndromes
Mechanical trauma, to red cells, 142, 143f
Meconium ileus, 92
Mediastinal large B-cell lymphoma, 155
Medullary carcinoma, 270–271, 271.e1f
Medulloblastoma, 293, 294f
Megaloblastic anemia, 145–146, 145f
Melanoma, 311–313, 312f
Membranoproliferative glomerulonephritis (MPGN), 191, 192f
    type I, 186t
Membranous nephropathy, 186f–190f, 186t, 187–189
MEN-1, 279
MEN-2, 279
Mendelian disorders, 88–96
    biochemical basis and inheritance patterns of, 89t
    prevalence of, 89t
Meningiomas, 293, 294f
Meningitis, 284, 285t
Menorrhagia, 254
Mental impairment, in Klinefelter syndrome, 100
Mercury, as environmental pollutants, 315
Metabolic abnormalities, 40
Metabolic diseases, of bone, 297–298
Metabolic reprogramming, 78, 79f
Metabolic syndrome, central obesity associated with, 326
Metachromatic leukodystrophy, 288
Metals, as environmental pollutants, 314–315
    lead, 314–315, 314f–315f
    mercury, 315
Metaplasia, 11–12, 13f
Metastasis
    of cancer cells, 80–81, 80b, 81f
    to ovary, 257t
Metastatic calcification, 13
Metastatic cascade, 80, 81f
Metastatic tumors, of bones, 301
Metrorrhagia, 254
MGUS. *See* Monoclonal gammopathy of undetermined significance
MHT. *See* Menopausal hormone therapy

Microangiopathic hemolytic anemia, 142
Microangiopathy. *See* Small-vessel disease
Microbes, excessive reactions against, 42
Microbial infection, in COPD, 165
Microcephaly, 280t
Microglia, 16
Micronodular cirrhosis, 228
Microsatellite instability (MSI), 217–218
Microsatellites, 217–218
Miliary tuberculosis, 176, 176.e1f
Minimal change disease, 186t, 187–194, 190f
Misfolded proteins, 9, 10t
Mismatch repair pathway, 217–218, 219f
Mitochondria, 7, 8f
  swelling of, 1
Mitochondrial genes, mutations in, 102
Mitochondrial (intrinsic) pathway, of apoptosis, 5, 6f
Mitral valve prolapse, 128
Mixed-cellularity Hodgkin lymphoma, 156
Mixed tumor, 64, 65f
MODY. *See* Maturity-onset diabetes of the young
Molecular profiling of cancers, 87
Monoclonal gammopathy of undetermined significance (MGUS), 157
Moraxella catarrhalis, 173
Mosaicism, 97
MPGN. *See* Membranoproliferative glomerulonephritis
MPS. *See* Mucopolysaccharides
MPS type I, 96
MPS type II, 96
MSI. *See* Microsatellite instability
Mucinous cystadenomas, 237
Mucocele, 220
Mucoepidermoid carcinoma, 221, 221.e1f
Mucopolysaccharidoses (MPS), 95–96
Mucormycosis, 181
Multifocal unisystem disease, 158
Multiple endocrine neoplasia (MEN) syndromes, 270–271, 279
Multiple myeloma, 157, 158f
Multiple sclerosis, 287, 287f–288f
Multisystem disease (Letterer-Siwe disease), 158
Mumps infection, 241
Mural thrombus, 36, 36f, 124, 125f
Murmurs, 126
Muscle tumors, 306–307, 307t
Muscular dystrophies, 305–306
Musculoskeletal system, 296–313
Mutagenesis, 71
Myasthenia gravis, 295
Mycobacterial infection, 212t
Mycobacterium tuberculosis, 175
Mycoplasma pneumoniae, 173
Mycosis fungoides, 156
Mycotic aneurysms, 130
Myelin figures, 2
Myelodysplastic syndromes (MDS), 148t, 150
Myeloma nephrosis, in multiple myeloma, 157
Myelomeningocele, 280t
Myeloproliferative neoplasms (MPNs), 150
Myocardial infarction, 121–125, 316
  clinical features of, 122–125, 124f
  complications of, 123, 125f
  diabetes and, 275
  morphology of, 122, 123f–124f
  pathogenesis of, 121–122, 122f–123f

Myocardial rupture, 123, 125f
Myocardial structural changes, 135
Myocarditis, 129, 131–135, 134f
  causes of, 134–135
Myometrium, proliferative lesions of, 254
Myositis, 306, 306f
Myxedema, 267–268
Myxoma, 136, 136.e1f
Myxomatous mitral valve disease, 128, 128f

N

NAFLD. *See* Nonalcoholic fatty liver disease
Nasopharyngeal carcinoma, 185
NBTE. *See* Nonbacterial thrombotic endocarditis
NEC. *See* Necrotizing enterocolitis
Necator americanus, 213
Necroptosis, 6
Necrosis, 2b–3b, 2f, 3, 14
  caseous, 3, 5f
  coagulative, 3, 4f
  features of, 3t
  fibrinoid, 3, 5f
  gangrenous, 3
  hallmarks of, 3
  liquefactive, 3, 4f
  pathologic patterns of, 4f
Necrotizing enterocolitis (NEC), 216, 216f
Neisseria gonorrhoeae
  in cervicitis, 251
  in endometritis, 253
  in vulvitis, 250
"Neoantigens", 303
Neonatal hepatitis, 235
Neonatal herpes infection, 249
Neoplasia, 63–87, 63b, 64f
  benign and malignant, 63–64, 63b
    characteristics of, 66–69, 66f, 66b
  of cervix, 251, 252f
  clinical aspects of, 83–87
  definition of, 63, 63b
  differentiation of, 66–67, 66b
  local invasion of, 68, 68f, 68b
  metastasis of, 68–69, 68b, 69f
  molecular basis of, 69–73
  nomenclature of, 64, 65t
    benign tumors, 64, 65t
    malignant tumors, 64, 65t
Neoplasms, in penis, 240
Neoplastic proliferations, of white cell disorders, 147–158, 148t
Nephritic syndrome, 187
Nephritis, 187
Nephrosclerosis, 199, 200f
Nephrotic syndrome, 187
Nervous system disorders, 280–295.e1
  cerebral edema, herniation, and hydrocephalus, 280–281, 281f, 281.e1f, 281.e2f
  cerebrovascular diseases, 281–283
    acute hypertensive encephalopathy, 283
    cerebral amyloid angiopathy, 283
    cerebral artery thrombosis, embolism, and brain infarction, 281–282, 281f–282f
    intracranial hemorrhage, 282, 282t, 283f–284f
    with sustained hypertension, 283
  congenital malformations of CNS, 280, 280t
  demyelinating diseases, 287–288, 287f–288f
  infections, 284–287, 285f–286f, 285t, 286.e1f
  neurodegenerative diseases, 288–291, 288t

Nervous system disorders (*Continued*)
  Alzheimer disease (AD), 289, 289f, 289f–290f
  amyotrophic lateral sclerosis, 291, 291.e1f
  frontotemporal lobar degeneration, 289–290, 290.e1f
  Huntington disease, 291, 291f
  Parkinson disease, 290–291, 290f
  spinocerebellar ataxias, 291
  peripheral nerve disorders, 295
    neuromuscular junction diseases, 295
    peripheral neuropathy, 295
    tumors, 295, 295.e1f
  trauma, 283–284
  tumors, 292–294
    astrocytoma, 292, 292f–293f, 293f
    inherited syndromes associated with, 294
    retinoblastoma, 294, 294.e1f
Neural tube defects, 280, 280t
Neuroblastoma, 279
Neurodegenerative diseases, 288–291, 288t
  Alzheimer disease (AD), 289, 289f, 289f–290f
  amyotrophic lateral sclerosis, 291, 291.e1f
  frontotemporal lobar degeneration, 289–290, 290.e1f
  Huntington disease, 291, 291f
  Parkinson disease, 290–291, 290f
  spinocerebellar ataxias, 291
Neuroendocrine tumors, 210, 210.e1f
Neurofibromatosis type 1 (NF1), 295, 295.e1f
Neurofibromatosis type 2 (NF2), 295
Neurogenic shock, 38
Neurohumoral feedback loops, activation of, 135
Neuromuscular junction diseases, 295
Neuronal injury, patterns of, 281.e1f
Neuronal migration or differentiation, defects in, 280t
Neurosyphilis, 247
Neutropenia, 146
Neutrophils, 7
  hypersegmented, in megaloblastic anemia, 145
  killing mechanisms of, 20
NF1. *See* Neurofibromatosis type 1
NF2. *See* Neurofibromatosis type 2
Niemann-Pick disease, 95.e1f
  type C, 94–95
  types A and B, 94
Nitric oxide (NO), 7, 20
NO. *See* Nitric oxide
Nodular sclerosis Hodgkin lymphoma, 156
Nodules/tumors, of liver, 231–233
Nonalcoholic fatty liver disease (NAFLD), 228–229, 230f
Nonatopic asthma, 166
Nonbacterial thrombotic endocarditis (NBTE), 131, 131.e1f
Non-Hodgkin lymphomas, 151–156, 152t
Noninvasive low-grade papillary urothelial carcinoma, 245f
Nonneoplastic disorders, of white cells, 146–147
Nonreactive tuberculosis, 175
Nonsteroidal antiinflammatory drugs (NSAIDs), 207–208
Nontreponemal antibody tests, for syphilis, 248
Norovirus infection, 212
Nosocomial bacterial pneumonias, 174
Noxious particles, inhalation of, in COPD, 165
NSAIDs. *See* Nonsteroidal antiinflammatory drugs
Nuclear abnormalities, 66

Nuclear-cytoplasmic asynchrony, 145
Nuclei, 7, 8f
Nucleic acid markers, 86–87, 87t
Nucleic acids, 50
Nucleocapsid "core" protein, 224
Nutmeg liver, 30, 32f, 136
Nutritional diseases, 319–326

O

Obesity, 323–326, 325f
 type 2 diabetes and, 273
Obstructive diseases, 219–220
OCs. See Oral contraceptives
Oligodendrogliomas, 293, 293.e1f
Oliguria, 186
Oncogenes, 69
Oncology, 63
Oncometabolism, 78
Open (surgical) biopsy, for cancer, 86
Opiates, 318
Opportunistic infections, of upper respiratory
 tract, 180–181
Opportunistic molds, in upper respiratory tract,
 169–170, 182f
Oral cavity
 disorders of, 220–221
 inflammatory, 220
 tumors and tumor-like lesions of, 220, 221f
Oral contraceptives (OCs), 317–318
Organ allografts, immune responses to, 53, 53b
Organ dysfunction, in septic shock, 40
Organ systems, acute and chronic effects of
 radiation on, 319, 320f
Organization, of acute inflammation, 25
Organizing stage, of acute respiratory distress
 syndrome, 163
Orthopnea, 135
Osmotic demyelination syndrome, 287
Osmotic diarrhea, 211
Osteoarthritis, 301–302, 302f. See also
 Degenerative joint disease
 comparative features of, 302t
Osteochondroma, 299, 299.e1f
Osteogenesis imperfecta, 296, 296f–297f
Osteogenic sarcoma, 299
Osteoid, 296
Osteomalacia, 297
Osteomyelitis, 298–299
Osteonecrosis, 298
Osteopenia, 297
Osteopetrosis, 296–297
Osteoporosis, 297, 297f, 297.e1f
Osteosarcoma, 299–300, 301f
Ovarian cancers, 317
Ovaries, 256–258
 surface epithelial tumors, 256, 256f–257f
 tumors of, 256, 257t
Oxidative stress, 7–8

P

p53-mediated cell cycle arrest, 77, 78f
Paget disease, of bone, 298, 298f, 298.e1f
PAH. See Phenylalanine hydroxylase
Palpitations, 126
Pancreas, disorders of, 236–238
 adenocarcinoma, 237–238, 239f
 pancreatitis, 236–237
 tumors of, 237–238, 238f

Pancreatic abnormalities, cystic fibrosis and, 92
Pancreatic cancer, model for development of, 239f
Pancreatic intraepithelial neoplasia (PanIN), 237
Pancreatitis, 236–237
PanIN. See Pancreatic intraepithelial neoplasia
Pannus, 303
Papillary carcinoma, 270, 271f
Papillary muscle dysfunction, 123
Papillary necrosis, 195, 196.e1f
Papilloma, 64
Paradoxical embolus, 281
Paraneoplastic syndromes, 84, 85t, 184
Parasitic infections, 212–213
 in CNS, 285t
Parenchymal brain injury, 283–284
Parenchymal hemorrhages, 282
Parenteral transmission, of AIDS, 58
Parkinson disease, 290–291, 290f
Paroxysmal nocturnal dyspnea, 135
Partial thromboplastin time (PTT), 158
Passenger mutations, 73
Passive congestion, of liver, 231
Patent ductus arteriosus, 119–120
Patent foramen ovale, 119
Pathologic adaptations, to stress, 11
Pathologic apoptosis, 5, 5t
Pathologic fractures, 298
Pauci-immune crescentic GN, 193
PBC. See Primary biliary cholangitis
PCV. See Polycythemia vera
Pemphigus (vulgaris and foliaceus), 309, 309f–310f
Penis, 240
 carcinoma of, 240.e1f
Pentraxins, 22
Peptic ulcer disease, 207–209
Pericarditis, 123–124, 125f, 129
 in SLE, 51
Perinatal brain injury, 284
Peripartum cardiomyopathy, 131
Peripheral nerve disorders, 295
 neuromuscular junction diseases, 295
 peripheral neuropathy, 295
 tumors, 295, 295.e1f
Peripheral neuropathy, 295
Peripheral T-cell lymphoma, 152t, 156
Pernicious anemia, 146
Petechiae, 31, 32f
Peutz-Jeghers syndrome, 216, 216.e1f
Phagocytes, 16, 17t
Phagocytosis, 19–20, 19f, 44
Phenylalanine hydroxylase (PAH), 93
Phenylketonuria (PKU), 93
Pheochromocytoma, 278–279, 278f
Phimosis, 240
Photoeczematous dermatitis, 307
Physical activity, reduced, osteoporosis and, 297
Physiologic adaptations, to stress, 11
Physiologic apoptosis, 4–5, 5t
Pigment stones, 235, 235.e1f
Pigments, 13
Pili, 248
Pilocytic astrocytomas, 293, 293.e1f
Pituitary adenomas, 265, 265t, 266f
Pituitary glands, 264–267
 craniopharyngioma, 267, 267.e1f
 hyperpituitarism, 265–266, 265t
 hypopituitarism, 266
 posterior pituitary syndromes, 267

PKU. See Phenylketonuria
Plaque formation, in malignant mesotheliomas,
 185
Plasma cell neoplasms, of hematopoietic system,
 157–158
Plasma protein-derived mediators, 21–23, 21t
Platelet count, 158
Platelet function, test of, 158
Platelets, 32–33, 32b
 activation, 32
 adhesion, 32, 33f
 aggregation, 32
Pleiotropy, 88
Pleomorphic adenoma, 221, 221.e1f
Pleomorphism, 66–67, 66f
PML. See Progressive multifocal
 leukoencephalopathy
Pneumoconioses, 169–170, 169t
Pneumocystis infection, 180, 181f
Pneumocystis jiroveci, 180
Pneumonia, community-acquired
 bacterial, 173–174
 clinical features of, 174
 morphology of, 173–174, 173f–174f
 viral, 173t, 177–179
 clinical features of, 178
 morphology of, 178, 178.e1f
 pathogenesis of, 177
Polarity, loss of, 66–67
Poliovirus, 285
Polyangiitis, 172
Polyarteritis nodosa, 113–114, 113f
Polycythemia vera (PCV), 148t, 151
Polydipsia, 267
Polymerase (Pol), 224
Polymyositis, 306
Polyps, 64, 65f, 216
 gastric, 209, 209.e1f
Polyuria, 267
Portal hypertension, 136, 223
Portal vein obstruction, of liver, 231
Posterior fossa abnormalities, 280t
Posterior pituitary syndromes, 267
Prader-Willi syndrome, 102, 103f
Predictable reactions, drug-and toxin-induced
 hepatitis and, 229–230
Preeclampsia, 259–260
Pregnancy diseases, 258–260
 ectopic pregnancy, 258
 gestational choriocarcinoma, 259, 259f, 259.e1f
 gestational trophoblastic disease, 258
 hydatidiform mole, 258–259, 259f, 259.e1f
 placental inflammations and infections, 258
 preeclampsia and eclampsia, 259–260
Preterm births, 316
Primary amyloidosis, 59, 158
Primary biliary cholangitis (PBC), 233f–234f,
 234–235, 234t
Primary biliary cirrhosis, 234
Primary chancre, 247
Primary (congenital) immunodeficiencies, 56–57,
 56b, 57t
Primary hemochromatosis, 230
Primary hemostasis, 32
Primary hyperaldosteronism, 276
Primary hyperparathyroidism, 272, 272.e1f,
 297–298
Primary irritant dermatitis, 307

Primary myelofibrosis, 148t, 151, 151f
Primary pulmonary tuberculosis, 175, 176f
Primary sclerosing cholangitis, 234, 234t, 234.e1f
Primary syphilis, 247
Prinzmetal angina, 121
Prion diseases, 286–287, 287f
Procoagulant state, induction of, 39–40
Progression, to chronic inflammation, 25–26
Progressive multifocal leukoencephalopathy
    (PML), 286
Progressive pulmonary tuberculosis, 176
Proliferative endarteritis, 247
Prostaglandins, 20
Prostate, 242–244, 243f
    benign prostatic hyperplasia, 243
    carcinoma of, 243–244, 244f
Prostate-specific antigen (PSA) level, 244
Proteases, in COPD, 165
Protein droplets, 13, 13.e1f
Protein markers, 86
Proteins, 13
Proteus vulgaris, 201–202
Prothrombin time (PT), 158
Protooncogenes, 69
Pseudocyst, 237
    pancreatic, 238f
Pseudogout, 305
Pseudomembranous colitis, 211, 212t
Pseudomonas aeruginosa, 93
Psoriasis, 308, 308f
PT. See Prothrombin time
PTT. See Partial thromboplastin time
Pulmonary arterial hypertension, 172
Pulmonary disease
    cystic fibrosis and, 92
    opiates and, 318
Pulmonary embolism, 171–172, 171f
Pulmonary hemorrhage, 171–172
Pulmonary hypertension, 172, 172.e1f
Pulmonary infarction, 171–172, 171.e1f
Pulmonary parenchyma, diseases of, 126
Pulmonary (right-sided) hypertensive heart
    disease, 126, 127f
Pulmonary system, effects of marijuana in, 318
Pulmonary thromboembolism, 37, 37f–38f
Pulmonary vascular constriction, diseases causing,
    126
Pulmonary vessels, diseases of, 126
Purpura, 32
Purulent (suppurative) inflammation, 23, 24f
Pyelonephritis, 195
    acute, 195–196, 196f–197f
    chronic, 196, 197f
Pyknosis, 3
Pyogenic granuloma, 116f, 220, 220.e1f
Pyroptosis, 6

R
Rabies, 285, 285.e1f
"Rachitic rosary", 322
Rapidly progressive glomerulonephritis (RPGN),
    186t, 193–194, 196f
RAS genes, 75
RB. See Retinoblastoma
Reactivation tuberculosis, 175
Reactive arthritis, 249, 304
Reactive oxygen species (ROS), 20, 228
Reactive secondary amyloidosis, 59

Red neurons, 281
Reduction-oxidation (redox) reactions, 7
Regeneration, 27
Regulatory T cells, 49
Rejection, 52–53
    mechanisms of, 53–54, 53b
    treatment of, 53–54
Renal cell carcinoma, 202, 202f–203f
Renal colic, 202
Renal disease, opiates and, 318
Renal failure, 186
Renal insufficiency, lead exposure and, 315
Renal stones, 201–202
Renin, 106
Renovascular hypertension, 105
Replication, of mycobacteria, 175
Resolution, of acute inflammation, 25
Respiratory tract, upper, 163–185.e1
    acute respiratory distress syndrome of, 163, 164f
    diseases of vascular origin in, 171–172
        diffuse alveolar hemorrhage syndromes, 172
        hemorrhage, 171–172
        infarction, 171–172, 171.e1f
        pulmonary embolism, 171–172, 171f
        pulmonary hypertension, 172, 172.e1f
    infections of, 172–181, 173t
        aspiration pneumonias, 174
        community-acquired bacterial pneumonias,
            173–174, 173f–174f
        community-acquired viral pneumonias, 173t,
            177–179, 178.e1f
        fungal, 179–180
        lung abscess, 174–175, 174.e1f
        nosocomial bacterial pneumonias, 174
        opportunistic, 180–181
        tuberculosis, 175–177, 176f, 176f–178f
    obstructive lung diseases of, 164–168, 165t
        asthma, 166, 166f–167f
        bronchiectasis, 168, 168f
        chronic obstructive pulmonary disease,
            165–166, 165f–166f
    restrictive lung diseases of, 168–171, 168t
        fibrosing disease, 168–169, 169f, 169.e1f
        granulomatous disease, 170–171
        pneumoconioses, 169–170, 169t
    tumors of, 181–185
        carcinoid, 184, 184f
        carcinoma of larynx, 185
        lung carcinoma, 181–184, 183f–184f
        malignant mesothelioma, 184–185, 185f
        nasopharyngeal carcinoma, 185
Restrictive cardiomyopathy, 133
Reticulate body, 249
Reticulocytes, definition of, 137
Retinoblastoma (RB), 13.e2f, 75–76, 77f, 294, 294.
    e1f
Retinol, 321
Retrograde spread, of infection, 284
Retroperitoneal fibrosis, 245
Reversible cell injury, 1
    sequence of events in, 1b, 2f
Rheumatic valvular disease, 128–130
    clinical features of, 129–130
    morphology of, 129, 129f
    pathogenesis of, 128–129
Rheumatoid arthritis, 301, 303, 303f, 303.e1f
    comparative features of, 302t
Rheumatoid factor, serum, 303

Rickets, 297
Riedel thyroiditis, 269
Right-sided cardiac failure, 30
Right-sided heart failure, 136
Right-sided (pulmonary) hypertensive heart
    disease, 126, 127f
Right-to-left shunts, 118
    malformations associated with, 120, 120f
Ring abscess, 130
Ring chromosome, 98
Ring sideroblasts, 150
Robertsonian translocation, 97–98
ROS. See Reactive oxygen species
Rotavirus, 212
RPGN. See Rapidly progressive
    glomerulonephritis
Rubor, 22, 23t
Rupture
    abdominal aortic aneurysms and, 110
    of atheromas, 109, 110f

S
Salivary glands
    disorders of, 220–221
    tumors of, 221
Salmonella, 211
Salmonella paratyphi, 211
Salmonella typhi, 211
Salmonellosis, 212t
Salpingitis, 256
Sarcoidosis, 170–171, 170.e1f
Sarcomas, 64
Schistocytes, 201
Schistosomiasis, 228
Schwannoma, 295, 295.e1f
SCID. See Severe combined immunodeficiency
Scleroderma. See Systemic sclerosis
Scrotum, 240–242
Second messengers, 264
Secondary hemochromatosis, 230
Secondary hemostasis, 32
Secondary hyperaldosteronism, 276
Secondary malnutrition, 320
Secondary syphilis, 247
Secondary tuberculosis, 175
Second-hand smoke, 315
Secretory diarrhea, 211
Self-sufficiency, in growth signals, 74–75,
    74b, 75f
Self-tolerance, defined, 49
Seminoma, 241
Senile osteoporosis, 297
"Sentinel" lymph node, 69
Sepsis
    acute inflammation in, 25
Septic (infectious) arthritis, 304
Septic shock, 38–40, 39t, 40f
Sequestrum, 299
Serous carcinomas, 256, 256.e1f
Serous cystadenomas, 237
Serous endometrial carcinoma, 254
Serous inflammation, 23, 23f
Sertoli-Leydig cell, 257t
Serum sickness, 47
Severe acute malnutrition, 320, 321f
Severe combined immunodeficiency (SCID), 56
Sex cord tumors, 257t
Sexual transmission, of AIDS, 58

Sexually transmitted diseases, 246–249, 246t
  cervicitis, 249
    genital herpes simplex, 249
    gonorrhea, 248–249, 248.e1f
    human papillomavirus infection, 249
    nongonococcal urethritis, 249
    syphilis, 246–248
    trichomoniasis, 249
Sézary syndrome, 156
Sheehan syndrome, 266. See also Ischemic necrosis
    of the pituitary
Shiga toxin-associated HUS, 201, 201t
Shigella, 211
Shigellosis, 212t
Shock, 30–40, 38b
    clinical features of, 39
    morphology of, 39
    pathogenesis of, 38–39
    septic, 39–40, 40f
    types of, 39t
Short telomeres, 80
Shunt, 118
SIADH. See Syndrome of inappropriate ADH
    secretion
Sialadenitis, 220
Sickle cell anemia, 139–143, 139f–140f
Sigmoid diverticulitis, 215, 215.e1f
Silicosis, 169–170, 170f
SILs. See Squamous intraepithelial lesions
Simple cysts, 198
Simple fractures, 298
Single-gene disorders, 88–96
    with atypical patterns of inheritance, 101–102
    Ehlers-Danlos syndromes, 90
    mutations in genes encoding enzyme proteins,
        93–96
    mutations in genes encoding receptor proteins
        or channels, 90–93
    mutations in genes encoding structural
        protein, 90
    transmission patterns of, 88–90
Single-nucleotide substitutions, 69
Single-nucleotide variants, 87
Sinoatrial node, 125–126
SIRS. See Systemic inflammatory response
    syndrome
Sjögren syndrome, 51–52, 51b
    clinical features of, 52
    morphology of, 52, 53f
    pathogenesis of, 52
Skeletal muscle, 305–307
Skin, 296–313
    in SLE, 51
    tumors of, 310–313
Skin infection, 180
Skin lesions, opiates and, 318
SLE. See Systemic lupus erythematosus
Small cell lung carcinomas, 183, 184f
Small intestine, disorders of, 211–220, 212t
Small-intestinal adenocarcinoma, 215
Small-vessel disease (microangiopathy), 275
Small-vessel vasculitides, 114
    immune-complex, 114
Soap-bubble lesions, 181
Soft callus, 298
Soft tissue tumors, 306–307, 307t
Soles, increase in length between pubic bone and,
    Klinefelter syndrome and, 100

Solid-organ allografts, mechanisms of rejection of,
    53–54, 53b
Somatotroph adenoma, 265t, 266
Specialized teratomas, ovarian, 258
Spent phase, 151
Spermatocytic tumor, 242
Sphingomyelinase, 94
Spina bifida, 280t
Spinocerebellar ataxias, 291
Splenomegaly, 162, 162t
Spontaneous abortions, 316
Sporadic goiter, 269
Squamous cell carcinoma, 207, 207.e1f, 220,
    310–311, 311f
    of lung, 182, 183f
Squamous cell carcinoma in situ (Bowen disease),
    240, 240.e1f
Squamous intraepithelial lesions (SILs), 251–252,
    253f
Stable adhesion of leukocytes, 18f, 19
Stable angina, 121
Staphylococcus aureus, 130, 173
    in inflammatory breast diseases, 260
Stasis, 17, 35
Status asthmaticus, 166
Steatohepatitis, 228
Steatosis, 12, 13.e1f
Stenosis, 126
Sterility, in Klinefelter syndrome, 100
Stomach, tumors of, 209–211
Strawberry hemangiomas, 115
Streak ovaries, 100–101
Streptococcus pneumoniae (pneumococcal)
    pneumonia, 173
Streptococcus viridans, 130
Stress
    cells and, 1, 1b
    cellular adaptations to, 11–12
    endoplasmic reticulum (ER), 9, 9b, 10f
Stress fractures, 298
Stress-related gastritis, 208
Stromal neoplasms, breast, 260, 261f
Strongyloides stercoralis, 212–213
Subacute endocarditis, 130
Subacute granulomatous (de Quervain)
    thyroiditis, 269, 269.e1f
Subacute lymphocytic thyroiditis, 269
Subarachnoid hemorrhage, 282
Subcapsular infarcts, in splenomegaly, 151
Subcutaneous edema, 31
Subdural hematomas, 282
Subfalcine (cingulate) herniation, 281
Subluxation, of lens, 90
Sudden death, opiates and, 318
Surface epithelial tumors, in ovaries, 256,
    256f–257f
Sustained hypertension, cerebrovascular diseases
    with, 283
Sydenham chorea, 129–130
Syncope, 126
Syndrome of inappropriate ADH secretion
    (SIADH), 267
Syphilis, 246–248, 247f
Syphilitic aortitis, 247
Syphilitic chancre, of scrotum, 248f
Systemic amyloidosis, 303
Systemic inflammatory response syndrome (SIRS),
    197–198

Systemic (left-sided) hypertensive heart disease,
    126, 127f
Systemic lupus erythematosus (SLE), 50, 50b, 193
    clinical features of, 51
    morphology of, 51
    pathogenesis of, 50
Systemic sclerosis (scleroderma), 51, 51b
    clinical features of, 51
    morphology of, 51, 52f
    pathogenesis of, 51
Systemic thromboembolism, 37
Systolic failure, 135

T
T cell-mediated macrophage activation, in
    tuberculosis infection, 175
T cell-mediated (type IV) hypersensitivity, 47, 42,
    47–48
    clinical and pathologic features of, 48, 48f, 49t
    pathogenesis of, 48, 48f
Tachycardia, 125–126
Takayasu arteritis, 113, 113f
T-ALL. See T-cell acute lymphoblastic leukemia
Tangles, 289
Tau, in Alzheimer disease, 289
Tay-Sachs disease, 94, 95f
T-cell acute lymphoblastic leukemia (T-ALL), 148,
    148t
Telomerase, 80
Teratoma, 64, 64.e1f, 242, 242.e1f
Tertiary syphilis, 247
Testicular atrophy, in Klinefelter syndrome, 100
Testicular germ cell tumors, 241, 241f, 241t
Testicular neoplasms, 241–242
Testis, 240–242
Tetralogy of Fallot, 120
α-Thalassemia, 140
    trait, 140
β-Thalassemia, 140
    intermedia, 140
    major, 140
    trait, 140
Thalassemias, 140, 141f, 141t
Thanatophoric dysplasia, 296
Thecoma-fibroma, 257t
Therapeutic drugs, injury by, 317–318
Thiamine deficiency, in chronic alcoholic patients,
    316
Thin basement membrane disease, 194
Thrills, 126
Thrombocytopenia, 159, 159t
Thromboembolic phenomena, 51
Thromboembolism, 30–40, 317
Thrombophlebitis, 115
Thrombosis, 30, 35b
    clinical features of, 36
    morphology of, 36, 36f, 36.e1f
    pathogenesis of, 35–36
    Virchow triad in, 35, 35f
Thrombotic microangiopathies (TMAs), 160,
    199–201, 201t
Thrombotic thrombocytopenia purpura (TTP),
    199, 201, 201t
Thrush, 180
Thymic follicular hyperplasia, 162
Thymic hyperplasia, 295
Thymic hypoplasia. See DiGeorge syndrome
Thymoma, 162, 295

Thyroid gland, 267–271
  adenoma, 270, 270f
  autoimmune thyroid disease, 268
  carcinoma, 270–271, 271f, 271.e1f
  chronic lymphocytic (Hashimoto) thyroiditis,
        268, 268f
  goiter, 269, 269f, 269.e1f
  Graves disease, 268
  hyperthyroidism, 267, 267.e1f
  hypothyroidism, 267–268
  Riedel thyroiditis, 269
  subacute granulomatous (de Quervain)
        thyroiditis, 269, 269.e1f
  subacute lymphocytic thyroiditis, 269
  tumors of, 269
Thyroid-stimulating hormone (TSH), 267
Thyrotoxicosis, 267
Thyrotroph (TSH-producing) adenomas,
        265t, 266
Thyrotropin, 267
Thyroxine (T₄), 267
Tissue damage, in tuberculosis infection, 175
Tissue injury, 50
Tissue repair, 27–29, 27b, 28f
  angiogenesis, 28, 29f
  clinicopathologic features of, 17f, 28–29,
        28b–29b
Tissue-resident macrophages, 16
TMAs. See Thrombotic microangiopathies
Tobacco, 315–316, 315f–316f
Tolerance, defined, 49
Tonsillar herniation, 281
Tophi, 304–305
Toxic multinodular goiter, 269
Toxin-induced hepatitis, 229–230
Toxin-mediated cell injury, 9
Toxoplasmosis, 286, 286.e1f
TP53 mutation, 79
TP53 tumor suppressor gene, 76–77
Translocation, 97–98
Transmural infarcts, 122
Transplantation-associated KS, 115
Transplants, rejection of, 52–56
Transtentorial (uncinate) herniation, 281
Trauma, in nervous system, 283–284
Traumatic hemolysis, 142
"Traveler's diarrhea", 211
Treponema pallidum, 247.e1f
  in vulvitis, 250
Treponemal antibody tests, for syphilis, 248
Trichomonas vaginalis, 249
  in cervicitis, 251
  in vaginitis, 251
Trichomoniasis, 249
Triiodothyronine (T₃), 267
Triplet repeat mutations diseases, 101–102
Trisomy 21, 98–100, 99f
Tropheryma whipplei, 211–212
Trypanosoma cruzi, 133–134
TSH. See Thyroid-stimulating hormone
TTP. See Thrombotic thrombocytopenia
        purpura
Tuberculosis, 175–177, 241
  etiology of, 175, 176f
  morphology of, 175–176, 176f–177f
  pathogenesis of, 175, 176f
Tuberculous osteomyelitis, 299
Tuberculous salpingitis, 256

Tuberous sclerosis, 294
Tubules, 186
Tubulointerstitial nephritis, 195
Tumor antigens, 82
Tumor cachexia, 84
Tumor cells
  genes regulate, 69
  homing of, 81, 81b
  vascular dissemination of, 81, 81b
Tumor destruction, immune mechanisms
        of, 82
Tumor-promoting inflammation, 83, 84f
Tumor suppressor genes, 69
Tumors, 22, 23t
  of biliary system, 236
  clinical effects of, 84
  CNS, 292–294
        astrocytoma, 292, 292f–293f, 293f
        inherited syndromes associated with, 294
        retinoblastoma, 294, 294.e1f
  esophageal, 207, 207.e1f
  of intestine, 219
  of kidney, 202–204
  of oral cavity, 220, 221f
  of ovaries, 256, 257t
  of pancreas, 237–238
  of peripheral nerve, 295, 295.e1f
  of salivary glands, 221
  of stomach, 209–211
  of thyroid, 269
  of vulva, 250, 251f
Turbulent blood flow, 35
Turner syndrome, 100–101, 101f
Type I glycogenosis. See Von Gierke disease
Type III collagen, deficient synthesis of, 90
Type V collagen, deficient synthesis of, 90
Typhoid, 211

U
Ulcer, inflammation and, 23, 24f
Ulceration, of atheromas, 109, 110f
Ulcerative colitis, 213–215, 213f, 213t, 215f
Unconjugated bilirubin, 233
Underproduction anemia, 143–145
Unfolded protein response (UPR), 9, 10f
Unifocal unisystem disease, 158
Unstable angina, 121
UPR. See Unfolded protein response
Ureaplasma urealyticum, in cervicitis, 251
Uremia, 186
        Helicobacter pylori causing, 208
Ureter, 245
  urinary bladder, 245–246
Ureteropelvic junction obstruction, 245
Urinary bladder, 245–246
Urinary infection, 198
Urolithiasis, 201–202
Urushiol, 307
Uterus, 253–256
  abnormal uterine bleeding, 254, 254t
  endometrial carcinoma, 254, 255f
  endometrial hyperplasia, 254, 254.e1f
  endometriosis, 253–254, 253f, 253.e1f
  endometritis, 253
  leiomyoma, 254–256, 255f
  leiomyosarcoma, 256, 256.e1f
  proliferative lesions of the endometrium and
        myometrium, 254

V
Vagina, 250–251
Vaginitis, 180, 251
Valve dysfunction, 135
Valvular heart disease, 126–131, 127t
  calcific aortic degeneration, 127–128, 128f
  degenerative valve disease, 127
  infective endocarditis, 130–131, 130f
  myxomatous mitral valve disease, 128, 128f
  nonbacterial thrombotic endocarditis, 131, 131.
        e1f
  rheumatic valvular disease, 128–130
Valvulitis, 129
Variable expressivity, 88
Variant angina, 121
Varicella zoster, 285
Varicose veins, 114–115
Vascular congestion, 17
Vascular diseases, 220, 220.e1f
  mechanisms of, 105
Vascular lesions, in diabetes mellitus, 275
Vascular permeability, increase in, 16–17
Vascular reactions, 16–17
Vasculitis, 112–114
  giant cell (temporal) arteritis and, 112, 112f
  infectious, 114
  Kawasaki disease and, 114
  polyarteritis nodosa and, 113–114, 113f
  small-vessel, 114
  Takayasu arteritis and, 113, 113f
Vasoactive amines, 43
Vasodilation, 16
Vegetations, 36
Veins, disorders of, 114–115
Velocardiofacial syndrome, 100
Venereal warts. See Condylomata acuminata
Venoocclusive disease, 231
Ventricular dilation, 124, 125f
Ventricular fibrillation, 125–126
Ventricular septal defects, 119, 119.e1f
Vessel wall, abnormalities of, 35
Vessel wall inflammation, atherosclerosis and, 107
Vibrio cholerae, 211
Viral encephalitis, 285–286, 285t
Viral esophagitis, 206.e1f
Viral hepatitis, 223–226, 224t
Viral myocarditis, 134, 134f
Virchow node, 183
Vitamin A, 321, 322f
  deficiency, 321
Vitamin B₁₂ deficiency anemia, 145–146
Vitamin C (ascorbic acid), 322
  deficiency, 322
Vitamin D, 321–322, 323f–324f
  deficiency, 322
Vitamin deficiencies, 321–322, 324t–325t
Vitamin K deficiency, 160
Volvulus, 219
Von Gierke disease (type I glycogenosis), 96, 97t
von Hippel-Lindau disease, 115, 202, 294
Von Willebrand disease, 160–161, 160f
Vulva, 250
Vulvitis, 250

W
WAGR syndrome, 203
Waldenström macroglobulinemia, 158
Warburg effect, 77

Warthin tumor, 221, 221.e1f

Waterhouse-Friderichsen syndrome, 277–278

Watershed infarcts, 281

Wegener granulomatosis, 172

Well-differentiated squamous cell carcinoma, 67, 67f

Wet gangrene, 3

Whipple disease, 211–212, 211.e1f, 212t

Wilms tumor, 203–204, 203f

Wilson disease, 231

WNT signaling pathway, 77

X

Xanthomas, 91

Xeroderma pigmentosum, 83, 311

Xerostomia, 52, 220

X-inactivation, 89–90

X-linked agammaglobulinemia, 56

X-linked disorders, 89–90

X-linked hyper-IgM syndrome, 56

Y

Yersinia spp., 211, 212t

Yolk sac tumor, 241–242, 242f

Z

Zollinger-Ellison syndrome, 210